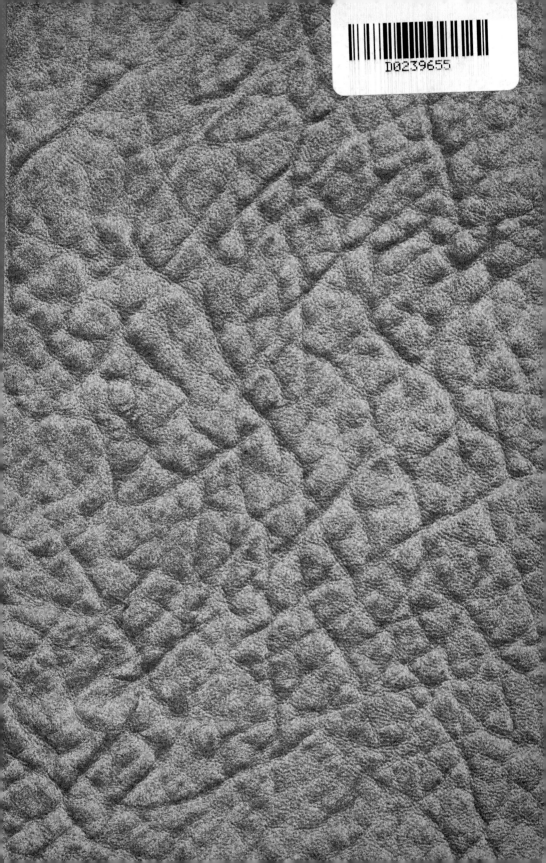

THE COMPLETE FAMILY DOCTOR

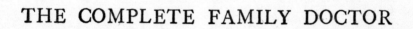

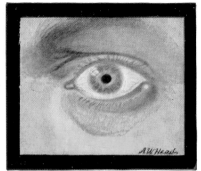

Fig 1. Sty.

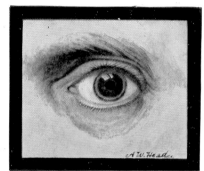

Fig. 2. Arcus Senilis.

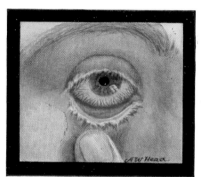

Fig. 3. Catarrhal Conjunctivitis.

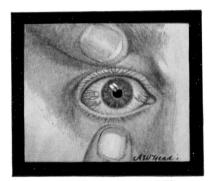

Fig. 4. Phlyctenular Conjunctivitis.

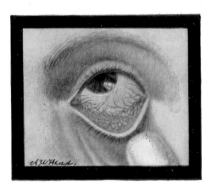

Fig. 5. Follicular Conjunctivitis.

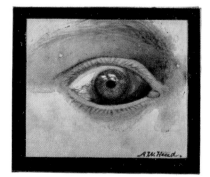

Fig. 6. Subconjunctival Ecchymosis.

PLATE I. AFFECTIONS OF THE EYE.

THE COMPLETE
FAMILY DOCTOR

Edited by
A LONDON PHYSICIAN

WITH FOUR COLOUR AND TEN
BLACK AND WHITE PLATES AND
ILLUSTRATIONS IN THE TEXT

ODHAMS PRESS LIMITED
LONG ACRE - - LONDON, W.C.2

Printed in Great Britain

EDITOR'S PREFACE

Now that physiology and hygiene are taught in so many schools, and an active health and first-aid propaganda is being carried out by a great variety of public organizations, some interest in Medicine is pretty widely felt. In those who have had some education in the laws of health a curiosity as to the processes of disease is but natural, and it is well that works free from sensationalism and informed by sound medical knowledge should be published to meet the need that thus arises.

Such works fulfil a useful purpose also because they enable the reader to avoid certain illnesses by revealing the causes of them. Moreover, they tend to interest him in those preventive measures which the health authorities of the land are busily engaged in carrying out. If these measures are to reach the highest level of effectiveness they must have the enlightened sympathy and co-operation of the public. It is all to the good, therefore, that people generally should be encouraged to take an instructed interest in all that pertains to their health.

The present work aims, *inter alia*, at imparting an intelligent conception of the common diseases to which we are liable—the causes to which they are due, the symptoms by which they may manifest themselves, and the treatment they require. There are emergencies, such as accidents and cases of poisoning, in which first aid has to be given. Such emergencies are provided for in these pages, and since the arrangement is alphabetical, the reader will find it to be a book of ready reference, as by its title it claims to be. There are also many simple ailments which every mother feels she ought to be able to treat. How to recognize such ailments and how to treat them are here described. Even in the more serious diseases it is well that the mother and other members of the household who may undertake nursing duties should not only have instruction in nursing, but should be able to appreciate the significance of symptoms as they arise, the course the illness may be expected to run, and the reasons for the treatment that is administered. All such information as this is given in these pages. At the same time the necessity for promptly summoning medical aid in all but trivial complaints is insisted upon ; again and again the reader is cautioned to call in the doctor without delay in cases of real illness. If the common saying that at forty a man is either a fool or a physician means that at that age he ought to be capable of acting as his own doctor, no sanction for such a notion will be found in this volume.

Readers of the work will find that it is well up to date. Those who wish to be informed concerning diseases of recent development such as so-called " sleepy sickness " will not seek such information in vain. Nor will those be disappointed who are curious about new methods of diagnosis such as that associated with the name of Schick in connexion with diphtheria. If, again, an appraisal of methods of treatment that have recently come into vogue, such as artificial sunlight and diathermy, is desired, it will here be found. And if the reader would learn something about those ductless glands upon which much fruitful research work has been and is being done, he will be helped by the articles in which that subject is dealt with.

It should be pointed out, further, that THE COMPLETE FAMILY DOCTOR is a book of Health as well as of Medicine. It contains brief statements of the elements of anatomy and physiology, has much to say about food and dietetics, stresses the importance of vitamins, and discusses the feeding and hygiene of infants and children. It shows how the hair and the teeth may be cared for, gives sound advice about baths and bathing, enunciates the principles of ventilation, and outlines the activities of Preventive Medicine. Finally, it misses no opportunity of inculcating healthy modes of life, and of urging how much better it is that disease should be avoided than that it should be cured.

THE EDITOR.

LIST OF PLATES

THE COMPLETE FAMILY DOCTOR

ABSCESS.—An abscess, or " gathering," is an accumulation of pus, popularly styled " matter," as the result of inflammation. When an abscess begins to form, the patient first notices a sensation of tension, gradually increasing to a heavy, throbbing pain, greater when the part hangs down and less when it is raised. The part is hot, red, swollen, and hard ; presently the centre turns blue, the skin here becomes shiny and thin and more prominent, and beneath it the white or yellowish pus can be seen ; this is the stage known as " pointing." Finally the skin gives way, and through the minute opening the pus escapes. As soon as the abscess has broken the redness disappears, and the pain and swelling gradually subside. An abscess allowed to take its own course, and break, may not heal quickly, and may leave an unsightly scar, and it is usually better that it should be opened as soon as, in the judgment of the medical attendant, it has reached the right stage.

Treatment.—Apart from operation, the treatment of abscess consists for the most part in the application of moist heat. Poultices should not be used for this purpose if the abscess is to be opened, for they cannot be rendered absolutely free from germs. It is better to soak the part in hot water, or to apply warm boric-acid lotion on lint covered with oil-silk. An aperient should be administered. When the abscess has been opened or has ruptured, it should be protected from contamination by covering it with lint wetted in boric-acid lotion, and should be occasionally washed with the warm lotion. The wound must not be allowed to close up until the discharge has quite ceased, otherwise there may be a fresh accumulation of matter. While the abscess is pursuing its course the patient should have a nourishing diet and the general health should be attended to.

So far we have been considering acute abscess. In *chronic* abscess there is usually no redness, and while the affected part may be tender when pressed, there is frequently little or no pain. Treatment should be directed to the general health, or to the particular cause of the condition—such as tuberculosis—if there is one.

ACETIC ACID POISONING.— In these cases the mouth is burnt, and the breath has an odour of vinegar. The treatment is to give soap, chalk, or whitewash off wall or ceiling, in water and freely. Lime water, or saturated solution of lime in teaspoonful doses, may be frequently repeated, and may be followed by an ounce of castor oil. Milk, oil and thick gruel are suitable. No emetic must be given.

ACNE ROSACEA.—Rosacea, as this affection is often called, begins in a flushing of the face, due to such causes as menstruation or the cessation thereof, pregnancy, the secretion of milk, defective circulation, chlorosis, dyspepsia, and alcoholic intemperance. As the condition becomes chronic, the skin in the middle of the face becomes permanently red. The sebaceous glands may now be stimulated to over-activity by the extra supply of blood, and the secretion may block the ducts, which become the seat of

2

1

pimples. The case has now become one of " grog blossoms," a poetical but misleading designation, for drink is but one of the many causes of the condition. If the last step of the affection is reached, the skin of the nose becomes greatly thickened and is formed into lobes ; this is known as *rhinophyma*, and is mostly (though not exclusively) seen in habitual spirit-drinkers who are much exposed to the weather. Rosacea is an affection of middle and advanced life, and is less frequent in men than in women.

Treatment.—Everything in the form of food or drink that causes flushing should be avoided. The bowels must be carefully regulated, and the digestive organs maintained in good working order. One of the best drugs for this affection is ichthyol, of which a 2½-grain tablet may be taken on an empty stomach night and morning, the dose being gradually increased under medical direction. The external treatment should follow the same lines as that advised for ordinary acne (*see* the next article). In the more advanced stages of the affection good results have been yielded by various mechanical forms of treatment—the cautery, electrolysis, X-rays and radium. In cases due to the absorption of intestinal poisons, vaccines have been found beneficial.

ACNE VULGARIS.—This, the ordinary form of acne, arises from obstruction of the sebaceous glands of the skin, and is possibly due to the action of microbes. The glands themselves, or the mouths of the ducts which bring their oily secretion to the surface, become blocked, so that the secretion is unable to escape. Thus tiny red pimples are formed, which may become inflamed, and may contain " matter " (pus). Many of the pimples become comedones, popularly called " blackheads ; " these blackheads are simply particles of dirt which have been deposited on the blocked-in secretion. The pimples either fade away or break, but the tendency is for fresh crops to come out to take their place. If much pus forms, they leave behind them scars. Their favourite situations are the face, especially the cheeks, nose, forehead and chin, the back of the neck, the back between the shoulders, and the chest ; but they may appear wherever there are sebaceous glands. Acne vulgaris is a disease of adolescence, the ages at which it is most common being those between twelve and twenty-five. In the activity excited in many glands with the approach to puberty the sebaceous glands share, and in persons in whom these glands are naturally well developed, as indicated by a coarse, greasy skin, more secretion may easily be formed than is able to escape.

Treatment.—If pus has not yet formed, the contents of the pimples should be squeezed out between the nails covered with a clean handkerchief, or by means of an instrument which the chemist will supply ; the part should then be washed frequently with soft soap and coarse flannel. An ointment consisting of 10 grains of sulphur to 1 ounce of vaselin, or of 15 grains of resorcin to the same quantity of vaselin, may then be rubbed in. When pus has formed the pustules should be pricked with a clean needle, and the part bathed with hot water to encourage bleeding. If the covered parts are affected, the undergarments should be frequently changed to avoid reinfection. In some cases vaccines are useful.

Preventive measures consist in attention to the general health, the observance of a simple dietary, the avoidance of everything likely to cause flushing of the face, and the correction of anæmia, if present, by a course of iron (*see* ANÆMIA). The affected parts should be rubbed at night with cold cream, or with the sulphur ointment mentioned above, and scrubbed next morning with soap and a flannel.

ACONITE POISONING.—Aconite is obtained from the plant known variously as monkshood, wolfsbane, and blue rocket. In cases of aconite poisoning give an emetic (*see* EMETICS), and when it has acted give alcohol, strong tea or coffee, apply hot bottles and blankets, and keep the patient lying down. Artificial respiration may be necessary.

ACROMEGALY.—In this strange affection certain of the bones of the body, and especially those of the face and head, the hands and the feet, undergo enlargement, and other tissues may also be similarly affected. The cause of the change is over-activity of the pituitary gland, which lies at the base of the brain, and forms a secretion that stimulates the growth of the body. If this change occurs early in life, the growth of the whole body is excessive (*see* GIGANTISM); if later, the over-development is more local. Neither medical nor surgical treatment can do much more than mitigate the headache, partial blindness, and other symptoms that develop. In the later stages the pituitary secretion becomes deficient in quantity; some benefit may then be derived from pituitary extract.

ACTINOMYCOSIS.—This serious disease, which affects chiefly the bones and the internal organs, but occasionally attacks the skin, is named after the fungus called the actinomyces, otherwise the ray-fungus. It is chiefly a disease of cattle and horses, and may

be conveyed to human beings by grasses and cereals on which the parasite lives. The drug which is most used is iodide of potash, in large doses. This may be supplemented by vaccine treatment. Surgical measures may be necessary to provide drainage.

ACUTE YELLOW ATROPHY OF LIVER (*see* PREGNANCY, DISORDERS OF).

ADDISON'S DISEASE.—This rare affection is named after the physician who first identified it as a distinct disease—Thomas Addison, who flourished in the first half of the nineteenth century, and was on the staff of Guy's Hospital. It is in most cases due to tuberculosis of the suprarenal capsules, small ductless glands situated above the kidneys (*see* DUCTLESS GLANDS). The symptoms of Addison's disease—anæmia, great enfeeblement of the heart's action, extreme general weakness, irritability of the stomach, and bronzing of the skin—are believed to be due to lack of the powerful stimulus which the secretion of the suprarenal glands normally furnishes. It was hoped, therefore, that by administering suprarenal extract, manufactured from these glands in animals, the disease might be successfully combated, but the results have been on the whole disappointing. The affection sometimes ends fatally in a few weeks, but under careful treatment the patient may survive for years, and cases of complete recovery have been reported.

ADENITIS.—This term simply denotes inflammation of a gland, but it is lymphadenitis—inflammation of the lymph-glands (*see* BLOOD AND LYMPH)—which will here be considered. These glands may become inflamed from a variety of causes, but the commonest cause is tuberculosis, and the glands that are most frequently attacked by the tubercle bacillus are those in the neck, the cervical glands, the affection then being styled *cervical adenitis*. At first there is nothing to attract attention except a slow enlargement of the cervical glands. Later there is, perhaps, an evening rise of temperature. Then, as " matter " forms, the patient complains of pain and tenderness, and stiffness of the head and neck. Presently the skin becomes red and discoloured, and finally the abscess bursts. The disease may spread from one group of glands to another, until both sides of the neck are involved.

Treatment.—In the early stages of adenitis, whether tuberculous or due to other causes, the pain and stiffness may be treated by hot fomentations, and the swellings smeared over with a liniment of equal parts of belladonna and glycerin, and covered with a warm compress (*see* COMPRESSES). If the tenderness is thus subdued, a small piece of iodide of lead or mercury ointment—say the size of a pea—may be rubbed in night and morning. Fresh air and sunlight are of the first importance if the case is tuberculous, and cod-liver oil should be given. If the affection is the result of disease elsewhere, such as decayed teeth, enlarged tonsils, adenoids, eczema, or ear disease, such conditions should be corrected. These various measures failing, the glands must be excised. The operation should be done before an abscess has formed, for healing will then be more rapid, no prominent scar will be left, and the disease will not recur. In some cases of cervical adenitis, tuberculin has been employed with good results.

ADENOIDS.—This very common affection in children is due to overgrowth of the pharyngeal tonsil, situated at the back of the nose. Sometimes present at birth, the condition is most frequent between the ages of three and twelve. It may persist into adult life, but as puberty approaches the overgrowth tends to atrophy, though its effects remain. In infants the blocking of the nose produces difficulty of breathing, convulsions, and vomiting. Children above the age of three affected with this disease present what is styled the " adenoid facies "—the mouth open ; the lips thick ; the teeth projecting ; the chin receding ; the nose pinched and atrophied because it is not used for breathing, the child being able to breathe only through the mouth ; the face flat, smooth, and expressionless. The child breathes noisily during the day, snores and is restless at night, and gets out of breath with the least exertion ; he may be afflicted with night terrors, bed-wetting, epilepsy, St. Vitus's dance, stammering, convulsions, and various other nervous affections, and he is very likely to be rickety. This affection, though simple in itself, is serious because of its direct and indirect effects, and it is most important that it should not be allowed to run on indefinitely. If the overgrowth is but slight, careful attention to the general health may be sufficient. In more pronounced cases the redundant tissue should be removed.

AGUE (*see* MALARIA).

ALASTRIM (*see* SMALLPOX).

ALBINISM.—This term denotes an hereditary deficiency or absence of pigment in the skin and the coloured parts of the eye. The lack of colour in the iris leads to dazzling, especially in a strong light. Glasses of a special kind, which an oculist will prescribe, should be worn to counteract this dazzling, while relief may be afforded out of doors by tinted glasses.

ALBUMINURIA (*see* URINE, NORMAL AND ABNORMAL).

ALCOHOL (*see* STIMULANTS).

ALCOHOLISM, ACUTE.—There are two main varieties of acute alcoholism, viz. drunkenness and delirium tremens. A third form is considered separately under DIPSOMANIA. The symptoms of *drunkenness* are too familiar to observation to need description. The only condition with which drunkenness is likely to be confused is apoplexy; even such experienced observers as policemen occasionally make this mistake, and the unfortunate victim of a " stroke " is detained in a police cell under the impression that he is dead drunk (*see* APOPLEXY).

Treatment.—The patient—for such he really is—may be left to sleep off his bout, nothing more being necessary than to keep him well covered. In more extreme cases, in which it is impossible to awaken him by shouting, hot and cold douches should be given, and if by this and other means he can be aroused sufficiently to swallow, an emetic should be administered. The patient must be kept warm by plenty of coverings and hot bottles (care being, of course, taken to prevent him from being burnt). This point is of importance, for the secondary effect of a large dose of alcohol is considerably to lower the body-temperature. The symptoms that follow a drinking debauch may be relieved by a purge and gentle exercise in the open air, alcohol being, of course, rigidly avoided.

Delirium tremens is the crisis of a long course of excessive drinking, a crisis which may be provoked by a variety of causes, such as an exceptionally heavy drinking bout, an accident or operation, acute disease or mental distress. The patient is subject to hallucinations and delusions; he sees repulsive insects, hears noises, may rave and become violent, and may have murderous or suicidal impulses. The medical man—for such cases are too serious for domestic treatment—will administer hypnotics and sedatives, and the patient's strength must be maintained by feeding him with soups, beef tea, milk, etc. He must also be efficiently nursed and closely watched, to see that he does neither himself nor any one else mischief. In ordinary cases the symptoms subside in the course of a few days.

ALCOHOLISM, CHRONIC.—Chronic alcoholism is the condition caused not by a drinking bout but by the habitually excessive use of alcoholic drinks. The only hope for the chronic dram-drinker is entire abstinence from alcohol. Compromise is almost inevitably doomed to failure. If, however, the health has become seriously impaired, the patient should make his attempt at total abstinence under the direction of a medical man, who by a judicious choice of drugs will help to tide the damaged organism over its time of trial. Of the special methods of curing drunkenness, the most scientific is that of hypnotism (q.v.).

ALIMENTARY CANAL (*see* DIGESTION).

ALMONDS, OIL OF, POISONING BY.—Almond flavouring, essence of peach kernels, or essential oil of almonds, is sometimes taken in mistake; the treatment is similar to that for prussic-acid poisoning (q.v.).

ALOPECIA AREATA.—Baldness is considered under its own name; here we are concerned with the loss of hair in patches, a condition mostly affecting young people, but not limited to them. In many cases it appears to be the result of nerve strain, or of debility, but some authorities believe that it is caused by the action of microbes. In most cases the hair grows again, either spontaneously or as the result of improved nutrition and tonic treatment. Among other measures, massage, electricity, and sea-bathing may be recommended; or the growth of hair may be stimulated by painting the bald spots with tincture of iodine or using a liniment of turpentine and acetic acid (glacial acetic acid 11, liniment of camphor 44½, turpentine to 100).

AMAUROSIS (see BLINDNESS).

AMBLYOPIA. — Derived from Greek words which mean "dulled sight," this name is generally used at present to denote defective vision not due to errors of refraction, and not associated with obvious lesions of the eye. The forms of amblyopia most often met with are those due to the excessive use of quinine—in malaria, for example—and to immoderate smoking. The latter condition is considered under its popular name of Tobacco Blindness (see BLINDNESS).

AMENORRHŒA.—The function known as the courses or periods, and its natural cessation, are considered under the heading of MENSTRUATION AND THE MENOPAUSE. Here we are concerned with that disorder of the function which is known as amenorrhœa, in which menstruation is suppressed—that is, fails to begin, or, having begun, fails to recur.

Causes.—A not infrequent cause of delayed menstruation is the form of anæmia known as chlorosis. Menstruation may be suppressed also by loss of blood as from a severe operation, by a profuse discharge from the genital organs in the nature of the "whites," by protracted discharge from a wound or abscess, by the exhaustion resulting from illness, or by the wasting consequent upon tuberculosis of the lungs. It may be suppressed, again, by overwork in unhealthy surroundings, by insufficient or unsuitable food, and by the subject becoming plethoric or fat, as well as by sudden changes in the mode of life. Marriage, too, in some cases has the effect of checking the periods. Other conditions unfavourable to menstruation are exposure to cold and wet during the period, and mental shock. One group of cases is attributable to malformation or maldevelopment. For example, the ovaries may be absent, and as menstruation is dependent upon the functioning of these organs, it cannot, of course, take place. Other parts of the sexual apparatus may also be undeveloped; or the suppression may be due to obstruction, as when the orifice of the vagina may be entirely closed up by the fold of membrane forming the hymen—imperforate hymen; in this case menstruation actually occurs, but the discharge is unable to find its way through the genital passage. At the time when menstruation should begin the girl feels pains in the back, and other marks of commencing activity in the womb, but there is no loss of blood. The symptoms recur at monthly intervals and grow more severe, and at last the accumulated blood so distends the vagina and womb that a swelling is felt in the lower part of the abdomen. The vagina may also be obstructed by inflammation of its walls, which causes them to adhere together.

The results of long-continued absence of menstruation, especially if the condition should arise after the function has been well established, are in many cases injurious ; the digestion is disturbed, the patient grows thin, suffers from throbbings, headaches, and mental confusion, and is liable to bleeding from the nose, stomach or lungs. It is important on another ground that the condition should be inquired into and treated, for cessation of the periods is one of the earliest and most characteristic signs of pregnancy, and many girls have thus fallen under wholly undeserved suspicion.

Treatment.—The treatment of anæmia is described in the article on that subject. In all cases the general state of the health must receive careful attention. If the patient is living under unhealthy conditions, these must be changed. In many cases a nourishing diet and tonics are required. Any digestive disturbances must be corrected, and the bowels kept in regular action. For nervous girls a " rest-cure " combined with massage often yields good results. If the suppression is due to cold or to nervous shock the patient should take a hot hip-bath, a little mustard having been added to the water ; she should go to bed, and should take sweet spirit of nitre or solution of acetate of ammonia to promote perspiration. If she is in pain, hot poultices may be placed on the abdomen, and the doctor may direct that a few leeches be applied to the groin or to the region of the anus. In some cases hot vaginal douches (*see* DOUCHES) are useful. If there is obstruction, from imperforate hymen or other causes, it should be removed by operation with the least possible delay.

AMMONIA POISONING.—Solution of ammonia, or " spirit of harts-horn," is sometimes taken by mistake for sal-volatile or in a liniment. Give milk, olive oil, beaten-up eggs, lemon- or orange-juice in water ; weak vinegar and water may be sipped— a tablespoonful of vinegar to a tumblerful of water.

AMŒBIC DYSENTERY (*see* DYSENTERY).

ANÆMIA.—The popular expression for anæmia is " poverty of the blood." This phrase does not quite cover all the ground, for anæmic symptoms may be the result of a diminution of the *volume* of the blood, as in profuse hæmorrhage, but in most instances anæmia means a reduction either in the number of red corpuscles or in their colouring matter (hæmoglobin). In the one case there are too few red corpuscles ; in the other, the red corpuscles are not red enough. The phrase " poverty of blood " is not, therefore, very wide of the mark. Anæmia may be secondary to many other conditions, or it may be a primary disease, i.e. a disease in itself. It is anæmia in the latter of the two senses—as a distinct disease —that we shall consider first.

Primary anæmia, also termed chlorosis or " green sickness," from the yellow-green complexion which is one of its signs, occurs chiefly in girls, especially between the ages of fourteen and seventeen ; in them it is closely associated with sexual development, with irregularities of menstruation, and with hysteria. Lack of sunshine, working or living in vitiated air, an insufficiency of nourishing food, and the absorption of poisons from the intestine in cases of constipation, are believed to be promotive of anæmia. It is now much less frequent than it was a few years ago—a change which by some is thought to be due to the discontinuance of tight lacing.

Symptoms.—The complexion is not only pallid, as in secondary anæmia, but yellowish-green, and the nails, the lips, the gums, and the inner sides of the eyelids are similarly affected ; the eyes glitter, and the sclerotics— the white part—are sky-blue. The patient suffers from breathlessness, palpitation, fainting fits, indigestion, constipation, neuralgia, and dropsy and coldness of the extremities. Humming noises may be heard, spots and shadows may float before the eyes, the muscles may feel sore, and there may be backache and sideache. In some cases the appetite is very capricious ; the patient may crave for all sorts of food, and may even eat mud and filth. But although the health is in these various ways seriously affected, she may remain plump.

Treatment.—Constipation, if present, must be relieved by an aperient, such as cascara tablets. If the stomach is irritable, shown by nausea, vomiting and pain after eating, the following mixture may be taken for a few days :—

> Carbonate of bismuth ......80 grains
> Tincture of nux vomica.....80 minims
> Bicarbonate of soda .... 2 drachms
> Mucilage of gum .... ½ ounce
> Tincture of orange .... 2 drachms
> Chloroform water to 8 ounces.
> Two tablespoonfuls three timesa day, 20 minutes before meals.

These measures, however, in cases where they are called for, are merely preparatory to a course of *iron*, which is the great remedy for anæmia. One popular form is found in Blaud's pills, which represents the carbonate of iron. One of these should be taken after meals two or three times a day, and the dose gradually increased to three pills three times a day. Iron may also be taken in the form of reduced iron powders, 2 to 6 grains three times a day, immediately after or during a meal. Easton's syrup, which contains quinine and strychnine in addition to iron, is useful in some cases.

The efficacy of iron when taken in the form of natural mineral water is often remarkable, although the quantity of iron so taken is very small. There are chalybeate springs in this country at Bath, Builth Wells, Cheltenham, Harrogate, Leamington, Llandrindod Wells, Tunbridge Wells and elsewhere.

While reliance is placed chiefly on the administration of iron, *diet* and *hygienic measures* must receive their due share of attention. Milk and cream are valuable, and so also is raw or slightly cooked meat, reduced to pulp and flavoured with broth. Cod-liver oil, if it can be digested, is to be recommended. Egg-yolk, beaten up with a little boiling water and flavoured with sugar and spice, is a valuable food because it is rich in iron. As the patient gains ground, solid but not rich animal food may be taken. As to hygiene, the most important points are to avoid stuffy, ill-ventilated rooms, to spend as much of the day as possible in the open air, and to take a sufficiency of exercise, passive at first, or quite gentle, and more vigorous as sound health returns.

Secondary anæmia.—What has been said about the treatment of anæmia proper applies for the most part to anæmias that are the result of some other condition, whether it be hæmorrhage, Bright's disease, consumption, cancer, chronic poisoning by such metals as lead, mercury, arsenic, or copper, or disease of the organs which are concerned in the making of blood. There is one form of secondary anæmia, however, which must be considered separately—the form known as *pernicious anæmia*, of which the cause is involved in much obscurity. It is sometimes ushered in by gastric and intestinal troubles, or by nervous shock or worry. More often, however, it comes on insidiously, the first symptoms to attract attention being pallor, lassitude, and muscular feebleness. Breathlessness and fainting fits, with a tendency to palpitations, are next complained of. The appetite fails, the mucous membranes of the eye, mouth, etc., become pale, the skin takes on a waxy or " lemon " tint, the muscles grow flabby, the temperature is often high but not considerably so, vomiting and diarrhœa are frequently present, and there is usually dropsy in the feet and ankles. The disease is remarkable for its intermittency. Iron is useless ; the drug usually given is arsenic, in the form of Fowler's solution. Transfusion of blood is also practised, sometimes with temporary benefit. Treatment must begin with rest in bed, free exposure to fresh air and sunshine, and an abundant and nourishing diet where food can be taken without difficulty. Some benefit may be derived from the use of ultra-violet rays (artificial sunlight treatment).

ANÆSTHESIA.—The artificially induced anæsthesia under which operations are performed may be either (1) general or (2) local. In the former case the anæsthetic acts upon the central nervous system and the patient is reduced to unconsciousness ; in the latter he remains conscious, but sensation is suspended in the area of the operation. The drugs chiefly used in **general anæsthesia** are *chloroform* (usually mixed with ether, or with alcohol and ether), *ether, ethyl chloride,* and *nitrous-oxide gas,* popularly styled " laughing gas." These drugs are often employed in combination ; thus ether may be preceded by nitrous-oxide gas so that the patient may be spared the unpleasantness of the ether vapour, or by ethyl chloride. The safest of the general anæsthetics is nitrous-oxide gas, mixed with oxygen or air, but it is suitable only for short operations such as the extraction of teeth, the opening of abscesses, the removal of small tumours or sebaceous cysts. If, however, the air-passages are obstructed, this anæsthetic is not used. Ethyl chloride is suitable for short operations in which " gas " ought not to be used. The next safest general anæsthetic is ether, which, however, should be avoided in acute diseases affecting the air-passages, such as diphtheria, acute bronchitis, and active tuberculosis of the lungs. Ether, by the way, and not chloroform, was the first drug to be employed as an anæsthetic. Sir James Simpson, the discoverer of chloroform, himself repudiated as " wild and extravagant " the fiction that the latter drug was used as an anæsthetic before ether. In **local anæsthesia** the priority belongs to cocaine, but this has been virtually displaced by drugs which are less dangerous, such as novocain and alypin, supplemented by adrenalin, which reinforces the action of the anæsthetic by constricting the local blood-vessels and so preventing it from being diffused. **Spinal analgesia** is a form of local anæsthesia in which sensation can be suspended in large portions of the body without the patient being deprived of consciousness, by injecting a local anæsthetic, such as stovaine or novocain, into the sheath of the spinal cord. By this means long operations can be performed on the lower parts of the body and on the abdomen.

ANAL FISSURE AND FISTULA
(*see* FISSURE AND FISTULA, ANAL).

ANAPHYLAXIS. — Anaphylaxis
denotes a condition of hyper-sensitiveness to the action of a substance introduced into the body. The term, derived from the Greek, means *without guard*, the idea being that a person in the anaphylactic state is caught with his guard down when a substance that affects him abnormally is taken. The word is most often used in connexion with serums (*see* VACCINE AND SERUM TREATMENT); for example, there are some persons who, having received a serum injection, are rendered so sensitive to its action that the injection of a second dose after a short interval has deleterious effects. There is, however, a *natural* as well as an acquired form of anaphylaxis. Examples of this natural hyper-sensitiveness are hay-fever, in which the patient is abnormally sensitive to contact with the pollen of certain grasses, etc., and the rashes and digestive disturbance set up in some persons by the eating of strawberries or some other article of diet which most people can consume with impunity.

ANASARCA (*see* DROPSY).

ANEURYSM (*see* ARTERIES' DISEASES OF).

ANGINA PECTORIS.—This disorder, known also as " breast pang," is one of the most agonizing affections to which mankind is liable. Fortunately, in many cases the paroxysm is of short duration, and drugs are available which usually afford rapid relief. Angina pectoris is due in some instances to degeneration of the heart muscle; in others the coronary arteries—the arteries that nourish the heart itself—are diseased; in

yet others there appears to be no organic disease, but the heart is enfeebled, or is irritated by some poison. These are the primary causes of the affection. The secondary causes include anything that throws a sudden strain upon the heart—active exercise, such as walking uphill, an indigestible meal, exposure to a blast of cold air, an attack of severe pain due to some other cause. Or the secondary causes may be of an emotional kind—unexpected good news, mental excitement, or anger. Thus the great John Hunter, the anatomist, who suffered from this disease, was rudely contradicted while speaking at a meeting of the Governors of St. George's Hospital (October 16, 1793) at which feeling ran high. He stopped, left the room in silent rage, and had just time to reach an adjoining room when he fell down dead. In some cases, however, no exciting causes can be traced : the paroxysm may even come on while the patient is asleep.

Symptoms.—Intense pain is suddenly felt in the chest, accompanied by a feeling of constriction, as though the chest were compressed in a vice ; the pain may shoot through to the back and down the left arm, and sometimes also down the right. The agony is such that the patient stands motionless, apprehensive of sudden death, and fearing to breathe. Usually the face is deadly pale, but in rare cases is flushed, the hands are cold, very often the surface of the body is covered with a cold clammy sweat, the pulse is usually slow and feeble, the breathing short and hurried. As a rule the attack lasts but a few minutes or even seconds, but it may continue, with varying intensity, much longer, or may be broken up into a series of paroxysms. As it passes off there is generally a discharge of gas through the mouth, and often a copious discharge of urine.

Treatment.—The drug which is most used in angina pectoris is nitrite of amyl, of which a glass capsule containing 3 or 5 minims can be carried in the pocket and crushed in a pocket handkerchief when an attack comes on. The inhalation of this powerful drug, which must, of course, be used with caution, and under medical direction, immediately dilates the small blood-vessels throughout the body, and in most cases at once cuts short the attack. In cases in which it fails of this effect hot brandy and water may give relief ; but in bad cases it may be necessary for the doctor to inject morphia under the skin, or to give a whiff or two of chloroform. The patient should be so placed that air is freely accessible, and should be encouraged to draw a few deep breaths, which will sometimes cut short an attack. Treatment between the attacks must be directed to any condition that is known to excite the paroxysms. The diet should be simple, light and nutritious, and the bowels kept in regular action. The patient must be careful to rest for a while after a meal. At other times gentle exercise may be taken, always, however, stopping short of fatigue, or, if ordinary exercise is out of the question, it may be replaced by massage.

ANGULAR CURVATURE (*see* SPINAL CURVATURE, ANGULAR).

ANIMAL EXTRACTS, TREATMENT BY (*see* ORGANOTHERAPY).

ANKLES, WEAK.—Weakness of the ankle, so that the foot has a tendency to turn on its side in walking, may exist independently, or may be an accompaniment of flat-foot (*see* FLAT-FOOT). In either case shoes should be avoided in favour of well-made boots, of which the sides may, if necessary, be made stiffer than usual. In children who suffer from enlargement of the ankle-bones, bathing in sea-water, or with water in which sea-salt has been dissolved, is beneficial.

ANKYLOSTOMIASIS(*see*MINER'S ANÆMIA).

ANOREXIA (*see* APPETITE).

ANTE-NATAL DEATH (*see* MISCARRIAGE).

ANTHRAX.—This disease, due to a bacillus, is sometimes communicated to man by contact with the living or dead bodies or the hides of cattle or other animals infected with it. It may begin as a red pimple on the skin, which presently becomes filled with " matter " (pus), or it may start in the respiratory or the alimentary tract and there may be no external lesion. The one form is known also as *malignant pustule,* the other as *woolsorters' disease.* In malignant pustule the bacillus finds entrance through the skin, usually when this is abraded, and it is sometimes conveyed by shaving-brushes; in woolsorters' disease it is usually inhaled.

Malignant pustule is the more frequent and less dangerous form. When a case comes under early treatment there is good hope of recovery. Nothing may be required but the application of an antiseptic compress. If, however, the pustule shows no sign of spontaneous healing, it should be cauterized, and then dressed ; at the same time Sclavo's anti-anthrax serum should be injected.

Woolsorters' disease is much more serious. Sclavo's serum should be injected, and repeated whenever the symptoms become urgent.

ANTIBODIES (*see* IMMUNITY).

ANTITOXINS (*see* IMMUNITY).

ANTIMONY POISONING.—Tartarated antimony, otherwise tartar emetic, has occasionally been taken in mistake for Epsom salts. Give tepid water to encourage vomiting, plenty of strong tea or coffee, and afterwards milk, barley water, or white of egg in water. If collapse is threatened, stimulants are called for, and warmth should be applied to the extremities.

ANTISEPTICS.—The office of antiseptics is to prevent the multiplication of harmful germs. Those used in surgery, such as biniodide of mercury, corrosive sublimate, and carbolic acid, are strong poisons, but there are certain drugs and preparations which are safe for domestic use, such as boric acid, a dessert-spoonful to a pint of water, permanganate of potash, enough to give water a pale purple tint, Condy's Fluid, Sanitas, Jeyes' Fluid and friar's balsam (compound tincture of benzoin). Tincture of iodine (2½ per cent. strength) is also a serviceable lotion, especially in the treatment of chronic sores. Another is peroxide of hydrogen (of 5-volume strength), much used for cleansing suppurating cavities, such as the cavity left by a boil or carbuncle. (*See also* DISINFECTANTS AND DISINFECTION.)

ANUS, IMPERFORATE (*see* IMPERFORATE ANUS).

APERIENTS (*see* CONSTIPATION).

APHASIA.—This is an affection of the brain—due to such causes as tumours, bloodclot, hæmorrhage, inflammation—in which the patient loses his command over words. It manifests itself in many different forms, but chiefly thus : the patient

either cannot read, or cannot write, or cannot speak, or cannot understand what is said to him. The lost power may be to some extent regained by a system of re-education, which includes teaching the patient the lip-reading method.

APHONIA (*see* VOICE, LOSS OF).

APOPLEXY.—The popular term for this symptom is a " stroke," which exactly corresponds in meaning with the Greek verb from which the word apoplexy is derived. The condition of which apoplexy is ordinarily one of the manifestations is hæmorrhage on or into the brain from the rupture of one of the arteries supplying that organ, but in some cases the trouble is set up in other ways, such as arterial obstruction, so that the supply of blood to a part of the brain is cut off. An artery ruptures because it has degenerated as the result, say, of chronic alcoholism, syphilis, or prolonged muscular strain as in athletic competitions, or because of old age, or because of abnormally high blood-pressure, etc. (*see* ARTERIES, DISEASES OF).

Symptoms.—An apoplectic seizure does not always begin in the same way. Sometimes the patient falls down suddenly, deprived of sense and motion, and lies like one in a deep sleep, the face flushed, the breathing laboured, the pulse full, and usually less rapid than normal. There may be convulsions, or contractions of the muscles of the limbs, often confined to one side. In other cases the attack begins with a sharp pain in the head, the patient becomes pale and faint, and usually vomits ; he may fall down insensible, with a cold and bloodless skin and feeble pulse, or may remain standing, the pain being attended only by slight and transient confusion ; he may soon recover from these symptoms and be quite sensible and able to walk about, but the headache continues, and after an interval varying from a few minutes to several hours he becomes heavy and incoherent, and sinks into a state of insensibility. In yet other cases the seizure begins with an abrupt attack of paralysis of one side of the body, often with loss of speech ; after a while unconsciousness may come on, or there may be no further urgent symptoms, or the paralysis may pass off and the patient recover. If there is no loss of consciousness it is because the hæmorrhage on or into the brain is but slight ; if unconsciousness is deferred for some time the explanation is that, although the hæmorrhage is considerable, the blood escapes from the vessel slowly.

The attack gradually passes off, the patient being apparently none the worse for the " stroke ; " or terminates in incomplete recovery, the mind being impaired and some parts of the body paralysed ; or issues in death. In any particular case it is very difficult to say what the result will be ; but the degree of danger may be roughly estimated by the depth of the insensibility, the degree of prostration, and the difficulty in swallowing. The common notion that a person suffers from three successive attacks of apoplexy, the first being mild, the second ending in paralysis, and the third terminating fatally, is rather wide of the mark, but has in it this amount of truth—that the danger increases with every successive attack. In fatal cases death rarely occurs immediately upon the " stroke ; " there is almost always an interval of some hours, so that there is time to send for relatives or friends. In favourable cases, even when partial recovery has taken place, there is still a fear, especially during the first fortnight, that there may be a recurrence of the bleeding, or that the clot which forms at the site of the bleeding may set up inflammation. If the symptoms gradually diminish there is, in the first place, a recovery of mental power. For a time this may be imperfect, the patient being more or less childish, with impaired memory, and difficulty in expressing his wants. This, however, soon passes off, and simultaneously there is an improvement in the paralysed limbs.

Treatment.—The first thing to do is to send for the doctor. Next, unfasten the neckwear, open the windows so as to admit plenty of fresh air, put the patient in an easy chair and let him remain in a half-recumbent position, or lay him on the bed or on the floor, being careful that the head is well supported, but not so as to throw the chin down on the chest, for then breathing would be obstructed by the tongue. The less he is moved about the better, for the thing to aim at in this stage is to prevent, if possible, the further outpouring of blood from the ruptured artery. Sponge the head with the coldest water that can be got, and as soon as ice is available put it in a bag and apply it to the head, cutting short the hair if it is long. At the same time hot bottles may be applied to the feet, with due care that they are not hot enough to burn the patient. On no account should any attempt be made to feed the patient, for this would probably result in his being choked ; if necessary, the medical man will order a nutrient injection into the rectum.

When the patient has recovered consciousness the greatest care must be taken to avoid a recurrence of the hæmorrhage. He must be kept still and quiet, the cold applications to the head must be continued, and free action of the bowels kept up, and a mustard leaf may be applied to the nape of the neck. The diet should consist of nothing more stimulating than milk, milk puddings, and the like. In due time the patient will have sufficiently recovered to undergo treatment for the hemiplegia, as the one-sided paralysis which follows apoplexy is termed ; this treatment is described in the article PARALYSIS.

Preventive treatment, in the case of persons who have had a " stroke," or are predisposed to one, consists in living an easy, placid, regular life, free from excitement and from vigorous exertion, either bodily or mental. The diet should be limited to cereals, vegetables, and ripe fruits, with a little chicken or white fish occasionally, and strict moderation in everything must be observed. Gentle aperients must, if necessary, be taken to keep the bowels regular and the motions fluid ; the action of the skin may be assisted by warm baths, and gentle and regular exercise in the open air should be taken.

APPENDICITIS.—The appendix, a small blind tube, which projects from the cæcum, the beginning of the large intestine (*see* Fig. 15, p. 109), is apt to become inflamed, and when this occurs the case is one of appendicitis. In the great majority of instances bacilli, and particularly the colon bacillus, play a leading part in the affection. Formerly it was thought that appendicitis was usually set up by the presence of fruit-seeds or other " foreign bodies " in the appendix, but this is found to occur so rarely that it is now regarded as a curiosity. There can be no doubt, however, that the accumulation of hard fæces in the intestine is a not

infrequent contributory cause of appendicitis. The chief symptom is severe pain all over the abdomen, which later becomes localized to the right and lower part of it. This is followed by vomiting and rise of temperature, with a rapid pulse. The abdomen soon becomes rigid and tender and is usually distended, and soon a swelling appears low down on the right side, where the appendix is situated. In many cases the symptoms disappear spontaneously after a few days. In others an abscess forms which, if left untreated, breaks either on the surface or internally ; in the latter event it may set up the serious condition known as peritonitis.

Treatment.—Absolute rest in bed must be ordered. The medical attendant will have to determine whether the case is one for operation. If he decides against operation, hot fomentations, freely sprinkled with belladonna liniment, may be applied to the abdomen to relieve the pain, and aspirin given by the mouth. No aperient medicine should be used ; if the bowels are loaded, an enema of soap and water may be employed. Opium should only be given in cases in which it is absolutely necessary to relieve the patient's suffering. Food at first must be entirely fluid—slops, milk and soda, or meat broths.

In many cases in which the appendix has not been removed by operation the attack is followed, after a longer or shorter interval, by another, and this by others. In these cases the best thing to do is to remove the appendix. These are what are called " interval cases." There are also cases of chronic appendicitis, and here again removal of the appendix should be advised.

APPETITE.—When the body is in good working order, the desire for food is Nature's reminder that the fire, so to speak, needs a fresh supply of fuel. It is well, however, to keep a firm control over even a healthy appetite. It is easy for those who are not engaged in physical work and who take little exercise to eat more food than the body requires to hold the balance even between income and expenditure ; and for all normal persons it is a wholesome rule to leave off eating before the appetite is quite satisfied. **Excessive appetite** may be the result of disease, as in convalescence from acute fevers, when the great waste the body has undergone creates an abnormal craving for food, or in diabetes, in which there is an enormous loss of sugar from the body, or in chronic diarrhœa ; and it is sometimes present in pregnancy (*see* Pregnancy, Disorders of). Appetite, without being excessive, may recur too frequently, from imperfect digestion and assimilation of the food. The remedy in cases of this group is not to be always eating, but to have the digestive organs toned up so that they may do their work efficiently. In children undue craving for food is often a symptom of worms, and will disappear as soon as the parasites have been expelled. Excess of appetite, from whatever cause, is not so common as **defective appetite**, known medically as *anorexia*. This is usually an indication that something is wrong with the stomach, the organ of digestion. It is to be treated by restoring the stomach to its normal condition (*see* Indigestion).

ARCUS SENILIS.—In some persons a grey line, beginning as a crescent, appears near the edge of the coloured part of the eye, but always separated from it by a narrow margin. This is the arcus senilis (**senile bow**),

so called because it occurs mostly in old people, though occasionally it is met with in the young and middle-aged. It is a fatty degeneration of the cornea (*see* Eye), but although it may grow into a complete circle, as shown in Fig. 2 of the frontispiece, it never spreads over the centre, and does not interfere with the sight. No treatment, therefore, is required.

ARSENIC POISONING.—In *acute* poisoning by arsenic, the symptoms include burning pain in the stomach, retching and vomiting, diarrhœa, and a metallic taste in the mouth, followed by exhaustion, fainting and coma. Give an emetic at once, if no medical man is at hand to wash out the stomach, and repeat it after milk, or beaten-up eggs, or olive oil and strong tea have been taken. The pain may be relieved by poultices applied over the pit of the stomach, the thirst by barley water. In *chronic* arsenic poisoning the symptoms come on gradually. The appetite fails, the gums are tender, the tongue is white and slimy, the throat dry and sore, the eyes are red and watery and sensitive to light, nausea, vomiting and looseness of the bowels follow, and the nervous system is seriously affected. In some cases there is an itching eruption. Treatment consists in removing the source of the poison, and improving the digestion and the general health by tonics and fresh air.

ARTERIAL HÆMORRHAGE (*see* Hæmorrhage).

ARTERIES (*see* Blood, Circulation of).

ARTERIES, DISEASES OF.—The arteries are the tubes which convey the blood from the heart to all the various parts of the body. They are very strong and elastic, their walls being made up of three distinct coats. The innermost of these coats, the *tunica intima*, is thin, and has a smooth surface over which the blood is able to flow without friction ; the middle coat, the *tunica media*, is composed mainly of muscle, by which the channel can be contracted ; the outer coat, the *tunica adventitia*, possesses great elasticity. The important rôle the arteries play in the human economy is suggested by the saying, " A man is as old as his arteries." Unfortunately they are very liable to inflammation, and in this way arises the condition of **arterio-sclerosis,** in which the artery is thickened and hardened but at the same time weakened. If the inflammation becomes chronic the inner coat of the artery is affected, and then the condition is styled **atheroma ;** this term, however, is sometimes used in a wider sense as synonymous with arterio-sclerosis. An inflamed artery may undergo fatty degeneration, or lime may be deposited in its walls until it loses its elasticity, when it is said to be calcified. Further, it may be so thickened that the channel is too small for the proper conveyance of the blood, so that some part of the body, deprived of its due blood supply, degenerates, as in the affection popularly known as " softening of the brain." Or the channel may be blocked altogether, and then " mortification " (gangrene) is produced. Or the weakened wall may at one point undergo such great stretching that it is abnormally expanded, a swelling, which may be of considerable size, being formed (*see* ANEURYSM, below). Or the wall may give way altogether and permit the blood to escape ; the cerebral arteries, owing to the thinness of their walls and to their receiving little support from the soft tissues of the brain through which they run, are especially liable to this accident, and thus many cases of apoplexy arise (*see* APOPLEXY). Or the artery becomes calcified, its inner coat loses its smoothness, and the blood, as it passes over the roughened surface, forms clots, and so **thrombosis** (from *thrombos*—a clot) occurs. The clots may be carried along by the blood-stream until at some point one is arrested and the vessel is plugged ; the patient is then said to be suffering from **embolism.** The travelling clot is sometimes brought to a stop in an artery of the brain, and in this way, again, apoplexy may be produced.

There can be little doubt that in many cases there is an hereditary predisposition to arterial disease. In other cases the arteries become inflamed or degenerate in old age as the result of wear and tear. In the comparatively young they may become diseased from immoderate indulgence in athletics or excessive and long-continued physical work. Many cases are due to poisons circulating in the blood as the result of syphilis, gout, rheumatism, malarial and other fevers, or alcoholism, or the poison may be derived from lead, etc.

Treatment.—When the arteries have once degenerated no cure is possible, but by careful treatment the mischief may be prevented from going further, and some improvement may be hoped for. If the degeneration is due to the diseases enumerated, they must be dealt with as far as possible. Violent exertion must be avoided, but a moderate amount of gentle open-air exercise should be taken. The diet should be light and easily digested ; excess, both in eating and drinking, is positively dangerous ; tobacco and stimulating drink, whether alcoholic or in the form of strong tea or strong coffee, should be proscribed.

One of the most serious sequels of arterial degeneration is the formation of an **aneurysm,** by a process which has been briefly explained above. When the aneurysm is external, as in one of the limbs, it may be the result of an injury ; but the cause of most aneurysms, especially aneurysm of the aorta, the largest of the arteries, into which the blood is pumped by the heart to begin its course through the body, is syphilis. Arteries of the limbs may be dealt with surgically, but this is not practicable in the case of aneurysm of the aorta. Occasionally Nature effects a cure of this aneurysm by forming a blood-clot. The physician's aim is to follow Nature's lead and endeavour to bring about the formation of a clot by slowing the blood-stream and making the blood more coagulable.

ARTERIO-SCLEROSIS (*see* AR-TERIES, DISEASES OF).

ARTHRITIS DEFORMANS.—A large group of inflammations of the joints was formerly styled *rheumatic gout.* But there is none but the most superficial resemblance between these affections on the one hand and rheumatism or gout on the other hand, and essentially they are neither rheumatic nor gouty. The name is therefore being discarded in favour of *arthritis deformans*—an inflammation of a joint or joints which causes deformity. The group is divisible into cases of *rheumatoid arthritis* and cases of *osteo-arthritis.* In rheumatoid arthritis the soft parts of a joint become thickened, the cartilages, tendons and muscles waste away, and the bone is thinned. In osteo-arthritis the cartilages and bones of a joint become enlarged, the bones become grooved, and outgrowths (osteophytes) are formed. The causes of these affections have not yet been clearly established, but in many cases there is ground for believing that the inflammation is set up by poisons produced by germs. Exposure to cold and damp, prolonged worry, privation and overwork, appear also to be factors.

Acute arthritis deformans affects many joints at the same time, and is accompanied by some amount of fever. In the chronic type of the disease the hands are usually attacked first, then the knees and feet, and lastly, in very bad cases, nearly all the other joints of the body ; but in most cases sooner or later the course of the disease is arrested, and although the joints remain deformed and crippled, the pain ceases and the general health is fairly good. In children arthritis deformans is sometimes called Still's disease, after the physician who first described it.

Treatment.—In acute cases the inflamed joints must have complete rest, and it is well to wrap them in cotton-wool. The pain may be relieved by hot fomentations sprinkled with laudanum, while aspirin may be taken internally. It is important that as soon as the joints cease to be painful, movements should begin to be practised, and these must be continued perseveringly when the disease has passed into the chronic stage, so as to prevent or lessen deformity. To this end light massage of the joints and neighbouring muscles is of great importance, and benefit may also be derived from hot-air baths. In bad cases of deformity, in which the joint is contracted and fixed, an extension apparatus, consisting of weights and a pulley, should be employed. Various internal remedies are used ; these of course would only be taken under medical direction. In many cases warm mineral baths are beneficial. The diet must be generous, and should include as much animal food and fat as can be digested. Cod-liver oil should be taken regularly, either alone or with syrup of iodide of iron. In feverish cases quinine should be administered. Iodide of iron, instead of being taken with cod-liver oil, may be combined with arsenic. Warm clothing should be worn, and cold and damp carefully avoided.

ARTIFICIAL RESPIRATION (*see* RESPIRATION, ARTIFICIAL).

ARTIFICIAL SUNLIGHT (*see* SUNLIGHT TREATMENT).

ASCITES (*see* DROPSY).

ASPHYXIA.—This word means, literally, pulselessness. In practice it denotes the symptoms produced by any cause which prevents air from entering the lungs and so supplying the blood with oxygen. The chief causes of asphyxia are enumerated and the appropriate treatment is described in the article RESPIRATION, ARTIFICIAL.

ASTHMA.—Directly or indirectly, this affection, so frequently met with, so distressing to witness, and so obdurate to treatment, is probably a nervous disorder, which causes a spasmodic contraction of the muscles in the walls of the bronchial tubes. The trouble is not necessarily in the respiratory mucous membrane ; in some cases it is due to irritability of the nerve-centre which governs respiration. There can be no doubt that asthma is sometimes hereditary. It is also liable, apart from heredity, to run in families. It occurs at all ages, but usually begins in childhood and, when it begins thus early, is often outgrown by the time maturity is reached. In other cases it persists throughout life. In some patients an attack of asthma is excited by fatigue and physical exhaustion. In others it may be induced by irritation of the bronchial mucous membrane, as by common dust, by the pollen of grasses and plants, or by certain odours such as those of ipecacuanha, new-mown hay, pitch, phosphorus fumes, or even the smell of such animals as cats, dogs and horses. These cases are examples of what is called *anaphylaxis* — hyper-sensitiveness (*see* ANAPHYLAXIS). Just as some persons cannot eat strawberries without suffering digestive disturbance and breaking out into a rash, so these persons cannot eat certain foods without having to endure an attack of asthma. Some patients are prejudicially affected by heat, others by cold, some by a damp atmosphere, others by an unusually dry atmosphere. The slightest change of locality may bring on an attack or may cut one short. But of all the causes of asthma, bronchitis is probably the commonest.

Symptoms.—An attack often comes on in the early morning, between 3 and 6 o'clock, after the patient has had a part of his night's rest. It is sometimes preceded by warning symptoms which may take the form of flatulent dyspepsia, of languor, headache, depression and sleepiness, of unusually high spirits, or of slight cough. After a shorter or longer sleep the patient's breathing becomes distressed, and the characteristic wheezing begins ; he half wakes up and changes his position, and then dozes off, but the difficulty of breathing returns and becomes worse, and at last he sits up in bed and gasps for breath, placing himself in what seems to him the most favourable position for breathing. His respiration is noisy and whistling, and is accompanied with a low humming sound, and at every breath his head is thrown back ; his expression is anxious and depressed, the eyes are wide open, the face is pallid and perhaps slightly blue ; beads of sweat stand on his forehead, or run in drops down his face. The heat of the body falls and the extremities become cold, blue and shrunken ; during a severe attack the pulse may be so feeble as to be hardly perceptible. The attack may last a few minutes only, or be spread over several days. Happily it seldom remains long at its maximum intensity ; after an hour or two the severity of the paroxysm abates, and a sense of relief is experienced. There may, however, be a succession of aggravations and abatements, especially if the patient should take food. When the spasm finally subsides, mucus is expectorated, first as semi-transparent masses like little balls of jelly, and afterwards as ordinary phlegm.

Treatment.—During an attack the patient should place himself in the position which he finds to be most comfortable and most conducive to breathing. If in bed, he should get up, bolster himself up in an arm-chair in front of a table of convenient height, with a pillow on it, on which he can rest his elbows and throw himself forward. In many cases this position is not only comfortable, but disposes the spasm to yield. If the difficulty of breathing renders the sitting posture impossible, the same arrangement should be adapted to the standing position.

A good mixture for rendering the sputum less viscid is the following :

Iodide of potash .... 20 grains
Citric acid ....160 grains
Syrup .... 16 drachms
Chloroform water to 8 ounces.
Two tablespoonfuls thrice a day.

The drugs which are used to relieve the spasm are known as antispasmodics. The following mixture may be recommended :

Ethereal tincture of lobelia ......2 drachms
Spirit of ether ....2½ drachms
Compound tincture of chloroform.40 minims
Camphor water to 8 ounces.
Two tablespoonfuls every two or three hours during an attack.

Another drug used for asthma is that obtained from the Californian plant *Grindelia robusta*. It may be combined with lobelia and other drugs in the following mixture :

Fluid extract of grindelia
   robusta..................15 minims
Tincture of lobelia ....40 minims
Tincture of belladonna ..... ½ drachm
Iodide of ammonia .... 1 drachm
Syrup of Virginia prune .... 1 ounce
Water to 8 ounces.
Two tablespoonfuls every three or four hours.

Drugs may be applied directly to the mucous membrane in the form of smokes, sprays, or clouds. A very useful smoke, which is cheap and easily made at home, is nitre paper, prepared by dipping a piece of fairly thick ordinary blotting-paper into water in which nitre (nitrate of potash) has been dissolved, and drying it. There is no difficulty in making the solution : it requires as much nitre as the water will dissolve. These papers are sometimes made stronger by adding some chlorate of potash to the solution; they are soaked in boiling water to which has been added equal parts of nitre and chlorate of potash in as large quantities as the water will dissolve, much thicker blotting-paper being used than for nitre alone. The papers will keep for any length of time without losing their virtue. The best time to use these " touch papers " is when going to bed. The paper should be folded across the middle and stood up on a metal plate, the cover of a tin box, or the fender, and lighted at the upper corners. The milder papers gradually smoulder, the stronger burn more quickly, and give off, in doing so, thick fumes of smoke, which cause a feeling of drowsiness.

In using smoke for asthma the smoke should be inhaled well into the lungs, and not simply drawn into the mouth and puffed out again.

Among favourite asthma cigarettes are Cigares de Joy, cubeb cigarettes, and arsenical cigarettes. In some cases tobacco is found to ward off attacks ; it can be used in a pipe, cigar, or cigarette, but for preference a pipe. For women and children, a few whiffs of a mild cigarette may suffice.

Stramonium, or thorn apple, may also be smoked in a pipe. But if while using it the throat becomes very dry or the pupils are dilated, the remedy should be discontinued for a time.

It should be added that most of the preparations that are inhaled as smoke act better if they are taken early in an attack as a preventive, rather than when the asthma has become well established.

Coffee is useful in many cases, and should certainly be tried. It should be taken hot, strong, and in small quantity, and on an empty stomach.

Chloroform is an excellent remedy, but when it is inhaled from a handkerchief great caution must be exercised, and another person should always be present. A case is on record of a patient who, administering chloroform to himself in this mode, when partly under its influence placed his handkerchief on the table and buried his mouth in it. Soon he was too far gone to raise his head, but he went on breathing the chloroform and never recovered consciousness. Glass capsules encased in cotton-wool and silk may be bought, containing 10,

20, or 30 drops of chloroform in each ; the capsule is broken in the handkerchief and the vapour inhaled without danger of an overdose. Glass capsules containing 5 drops of ethyl iodide with 10 drops of chloroform may be employed in the same way. Alcohol should be used, if at all, very cautiously.

In asthma, *prevention* is of great importance. The general health must be maintained by good habits, by healthy exercise, fresh air, cold bathing, freedom from worry, and careful avoidance of all the risks likely to lead to an attack of bronchitis, which, as we have said, is perhaps the commonest cause of asthma. In the dietetic group of cases the individual patient must find out what he can eat and drink with impunity, and what he must avoid. The doctor may help him here by carrying out a cutaneous test. A little of any food that comes under suspicion, or a watery extract of it, is rubbed into a scratch in the skin, and if a reaction follows, it shows that that food must be avoided. Gouty asthmatics sometimes find themselves benefited by taking 2 grains of blue pill pretty regularly once or twice a week.

In **children** asthma may be met with at so early an age as two months. It is in some cases an accompaniment of bronchitis. The symptoms have a general resemblance to those of asthma in adults. One attack may be followed by others on succeeding days or after longer intervals, but the tendency is for them gradually to diminish in frequency, and there may then be a long period of immunity. In some children the asthma entirely disappears as they grow older, but more frequently it develops into chronic asthma, or into emphysema, in which the walls of some of the air-cells of the lungs give way and cavities are formed. Treatment may consist in the inhalation of the fumes of pyridine, 5 to 6 drops being poured on to cotton-wool or lint at the bottom of a tumbler, or nitre wafers may be burned in the room. During the attack iodide of potassium 1 to 3 grains, with tincture of lobelia 5 minims, may be given every three hours; in the intervals, cod-liver oil. The general health should be carefully attended to; precautions should be observed against catching cold; a course of gymnastic and breathing exercises should be taken, and if possible the child should spend some time at the seaside or in mountain air, whichever may be found the more suitable. The nose and throat should be examined, and any unhealthy conditions corrected.

ASTIGMATISM (*see* SIGHT, DE-FECTS OF).

ATHEROMA (*see* ARTERIES, DIS-EASES OF).

AURA (*see* EPILEPSY).

AURICULAR FIBRILLATION (*see* Myocarditis, *under* HEART DIS-EASE).

AURICULAR FLUTTER (*see* Myocarditis, *under* HEART DISEASE).

AUSCULTATION (*see* DIAGNOSIS)

B

BACILLARY DYSENTERY (*see* DYSENTERY).

BACILLI (*see* GERMS).

BACKACHE.—One of the commonest ills to which women are subject is pain in the back; we shall accordingly consider this affection first as it is met with in women, and afterwards more generally.

The pain due to **disease of the female generative organs** is of a dull, wearing character, and is situated low down in the back not far from the end of the spine. It is frequently due to a backward displacement of the womb, or it may be set up by inflammation and ulceration of that organ, or by disease of the ovaries. Another cause of pain in this situation is difficult menstruation; a bad attack of the " whites " (leucorrhœa) is yet another. The pain is always aggravated by exertion, especially if carried to the point of fatigue. Chronic constipation is an accompaniment of the pain, and also aggravates it; in some cases indeed, it may be the actual cause of the backache. The remedy in all these cases is to remove the cause of the symptom. What that cause is it will be for the doctor to discover from other symptoms, for the pain itself affords no clue to the precise nature of the affection.

Backache in women unrelated to any affection of the generative organs is believed to be due to **weakness of the muscles of the back**—those which are called into action when the erect posture is assumed. The pain, chiefly felt in the small of the back, is much increased by exercise, and is always more severe when the patient is fatigued or out of health; it is particularly liable to attack those who have had frequent pregnancies, or who have nursed their babies too long. Sedentary habits are a predisposing cause. The trouble is relieved by rest in the recumbent position and by massage of the painful muscles. All causes of exhaustion should be avoided, the general health should be carefully attended to, and while moderate exercise is distinctly beneficial, it should always be followed by a spell of complete recumbency.

Even when backache is due to general causes, women are often more liable to it than men. It is so in the backache of **movable kidney** (q.v.)

and also in **coccygodynia,** a word which denotes pain in the coccyx, the curved bone in which the spinal column ends. This is not strictly a pain in the back, but it may be considered here. One of the most frequent causes of this trouble is injury during labour, especially if forceps have had to be used; another is a sudden descent upon some hard object; others are diseases of the womb and of other neighbouring structures, severe constipation, and piles, while some cases are considered to be of a rheumatic or neuralgic character. However caused, the pain is usually considerable, and in some cases almost unbearable. If the trouble is caused by injury, hot fomentations and a lotion such as that of lead and opium (*see* LOTIONS) should be used; this treatment, with complete rest, will soon give relief. In long-neglected cases, and in those thought to be due to neuralgia and rheumatism, the pain is prone to persist. General treatment consists in nutritious food, tonics, change of air and, where necessary, care of the bowels; and special attention must be paid to the nervous system. If local treatment, in the form of sedative lotions and counter-irritation—say by a mustard leaf—is not successful, operation may be necessary.

Another cause of backache is **strain of the muscles of the back,** the result of violent exertion or injury. The remedy is rest in the recumbent posture, together with anti-rheumatic medicine (*see* RHEUMATISM, CHRONIC) should there be ground for thinking that the weakened or injured muscles are attacked by rheumatism, as they are very apt to be.

In some cases backache is caused by **disease in the spinal column,** or in the spinal cord or the membranes that cover it; these serious conditions are considered elsewhere. If the pain is high up in the back, between the shoulders, it may be an indication that there is something wrong with the digestion; if so, it will probably be worse after the taking of food, and there may be vomiting, and pain in the pit of the stomach (*see* INDIGESTION). Pain due to kidney trouble is felt lower down in the back, in the loins, and may spread round to the abdomen and down to the groins. If the cause is stone in or inflammation of the kidney, or cancer, pressure over the spot will cause tenderness; the bladder will be irritable, so that water has to be passed frequently; the urine also will probably show some definite change from the normal. In healthy young women an aching pain in this region is sometimes caused by their taking too little fluid, the urine in consequence being concentrated and setting up irritation in the kidneys. The remedy is to drink more water or other liquid, so that the solid substances in the urine may be kept in a state of solution.

One other form of backache may, in conclusion, be mentioned—that due to intestinal irregularity in the form of chronic constipation or of distension of the bowel with wind. In the former case the pain may be accompanied by irritation of the bowel set up by the hardened fæces. *See* CONSTIPATION.

BACTERIA (*see* GERMS).

BALDNESS.—Loss of hair (alopecia), though usually a sign of old age, may occur quite early in life, and may even be congenital. It is said to be much more frequent among men than among women, and although this statement is denied by some authorities, it appears to agree with general observation. When it occurs in old age, it is a sign of physical decay and is irremediable. **In**

younger people the chief cause is chronic scurfiness of the scalp (*see* DANDRUFF). Another factor in the case is the wearing of hard hats, which compress the arteries—the temporal arteries—that supply the scalp with blood and so nourish the papillæ, the little projections from which the hairs grow. Hats are still more injurious if besides being hard they are unventilated. After bad attacks of enteric and some other fevers the hair may fall out as the result of the enfeeblement of the body, but with the return to health the hair will grow as before. If the condition is due to dandruff, the treatment described in the article under that heading should be followed. In other cases a stimulating lotion should be well rubbed into the skin of the scalp (not the hair) night and morning with a piece of flannel or one of the small sponges sold for the purpose. The following lotion will be found useful :

Tincture of cantharides ....1 ounce
Distilled vinegar ....1½ ounces
Elderflower water..........3 ounces
Rose water to 8 ounces.

For baldness in patches, *see* ALOPECIA AREATA.

BANDAGES.—Surgical bandages are of four main types—(1) the triangular bandage, (2) the roller bandage, (3) the elastic bandage, (4) the plaster-of-Paris bandage. We shall consider them briefly in that order. How they are applied in cases of broken bones is described under FRACTURES.

1. Triangular bandages. — The triangular bandage, also called the Esmarch bandage, after Professor Esmarch, of Kiel, who introduced it into the German army, is particularly useful in first-aid work because it can be so easily improvised out of old garments, towels, scarves, etc. Thus,

a bandage of this kind can be made out of a large pocket-handkerchief by cutting it into two diagonally. It may be doubled in size by stitching the two pieces together along one of the shorter sides. Regulation bandages are cut from material measuring from 36 in. to 42 in. square ; smaller sizes are better for children. The parts are named as follows (Fig. 1, A) : The *apex* or *point*, the *sides*, the *ends* or *tails*, the *base* or lower border.

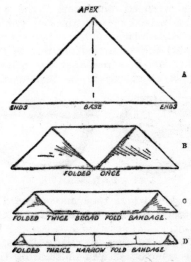

Fig. 1.—Triangular bandage, folded for application. (*See* text.)

MATERIALS.—The material most used is *cotton*, in the form of unbleached calico, or of bleached calico ; the latter is the more easy to adapt and the more pleasant to wear. Linen is quite suitable in itself, but its expensiveness is an obvious drawback.

FOLDED AND UNFOLDED BANDAGES. —When a bandage has to cover a large surface of the body it may be used unfolded. To fold a bandage, spread it out on the table, bring the point down to the middle of the lower border (Fig. 1, B) and then fold it upon itself lengthwise (Fig. 1, c). This is known as the *broad* or *broad-fold* bandage. The *narrow* or *narrow-fold* bandage is made by folding the broad bandage lengthwise (Fig. 1, D). For most purposes the narrow bandage is the more convenient of the two, for it adapts itself more easily to the part to which it is applied. It is also suitable for tying round splints to keep them in position. For this purpose it may be carried round the splint and limb two or three times and then tied, or it may be folded in two and then wrapped round, one of the ends being passed through the loop (which should be placed on the outside of the splint) and then tied securely to the other end in a reef-knot (*see* below). Knots should never be tied against

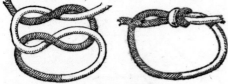

Fig. 2.—Reef-knot.

the skin, where they may cause discomfort, but on the outside of the splint.

SECURING THE BANDAGE ENDS.— The commonest way of securing the ends of the bandage is by *tying*. There are two ways of tying them— the reef-knot and the " granny " knot. The latter is the ordinary knot made in tying string, etc., and it should never be used in bandaging because of its liability to slip. The reef-knot is shown in Fig. 2 ; in the excellent " First Aid Manual " of the British Red Cross Society the following directions are given for tying it : " Pass a narrow-fold bandage round your own or another person's neck, make the first half of the knot—this is the same for either a granny- or a reef-knot. It will be observed that in the half-knot thus tied there is an

upper and a lower end to the bandage. Bring the upper end across the lower end, and with it (the upper end) complete the knot. The ends when pulled will be found lying parallel to the course of the bandage. It will be seen that in making the second half of the reef-knot the upper end is made to do the work, the lower end being kept steady. The reverse is the case in the second half of the granny-knot ; it is the lower end that is made to do the work, the upper end being passive." It is added that " tucking the ends of the bandage away out of sight after the reef-knot is completed is a necessary part of applying the bandage ; when the bandage is completed the ends should never be seen. In some diagrams the ends are visible ; this is done on purpose to show where the knot should be, and it is not intended to indicate that leaving out the ends is ever correct."

Another method of securing the ends of a bandage is by *pinning*. For this purpose safety pins should always be used. A third method, which may be used when pins are not at hand or pinning is not suitable, is to include the apex of the bandage between the halves of a knot.

By referring to the figures in Plate II the reader will find illustrations of the application of triangular bandages to the scalp and the eye (1), the shoulder (2), the foot (3) and the chest (4, 5).

2. Roller bandages.—Besides unbleached *calico*, which is most frequently used for roller bandages, various other materials may be employed, among them *bleached calico* or *sheeting material ; flannel*, most suitable for the trunk and for rheumatic joints ; *stockinette*, especially adapted for cases of dropsy and varicose veins, owing to its elasticity ;

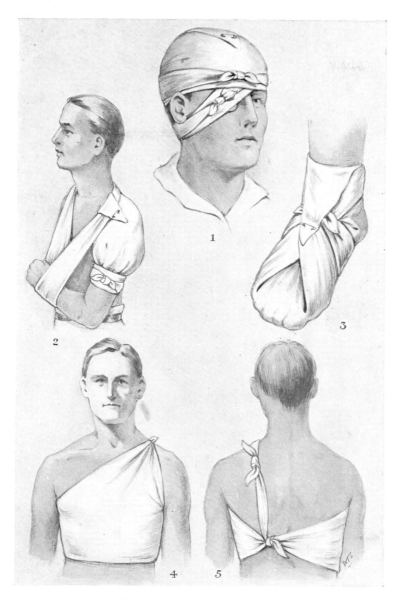

PLATE II. TRIANGULAR BANDAGES APPLIED.

1. Scalp and Eye Bandage. 2. Shoulder Bandage. 3. Foot Bandage.
4, 5. Chest Bandage, front and back.

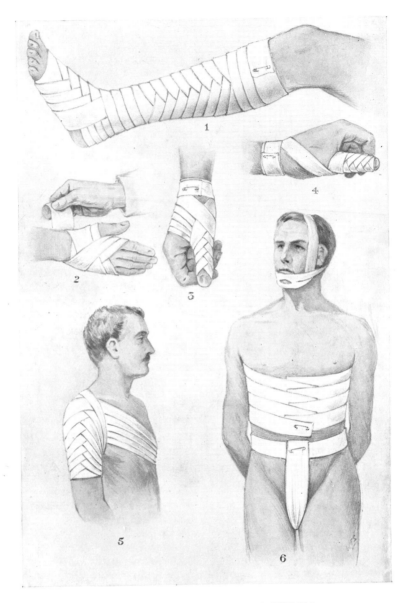

PLATE III. ROLLER BANDAGES APPLIED.

1. Figure-of-8 Bandage for Foot, Ascending Simple Spiral for lower part of Leg, Ascending Reversed Spiral for calf of Leg, and Ascending Simple Spiral just below Knee. **2.** Figure-of-8 Bandage for Hand. **3.** Thumb Spica. **4.** Reversed Spiral for Thumb. **5.** Spica for Shoulder. **6.** Four-tailed (Head), Many-tailed (Chest) and T-bandage (Crutch).

tape, for bandaging the fingers ; and *gauze* for retaining bandages.

For home use, strips of any soft material are suitable ; thus an old cotton sheet may be torn into strips of the requisite width (*see* below), and two or more of the strips may, if necessary, be stitched together ; the selvedge and loose threads must be trimmed up. When a bandage is ready for use the roll is termed the

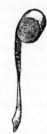

Fig. 3.—Single-headed roller bandage.

head, the loose end the *tail* or *free end*, and the surfaces the *outer surface* and the *inner surface*.

SIZES OF ROLLER BANDAGES.—For the *trunk* a roller bandage should measure 8 yd. by 6 in. ; for the *lower limb*, 6 yd. by $3\frac{1}{2}$ in. for men and 6 yd. by 3 in. for women ; for the *upper limb*, 4 yd. by $2\frac{1}{4}$ in. ; for the *finger*, $1\frac{1}{2}$ yd. by $\frac{3}{4}$ in.

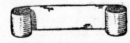

Fig. 4.—Double-headed roller bandage.

SINGLE-HEADED AND DOUBLE-HEADED BANDAGES.—The roller bandage in ordinary use is the single-headed (Fig. 3) ; the double-headed roller bandage (Fig. 4) is rolled from both ends towards the centre of the material, or it may be made by stitching together the ends of two single-headed bandages which are equal in length and width. In the case of both single-headed and double-headed

bandages, the rolling, whether by a bandage roller or by hand, must be done evenly and tightly.

RULES FOR ROLLER BANDAGING.—The chief rules to be observed are the following :—

1. Stand in front of the patient.

2. Hold the bandage securely between the finger and thumb of the right hand.

3. Apply it firmly, with equal pressure to the whole of the part. (A slack bandage is useless, an over-tight one is not only painful but also dangerous, for it will impede the circulation. Beginners, in their anxiety to avoid wrinkles, generally err in the latter direction.)

4. Begin by fixing the bandage by two or three turns one over the other, applying the outer surface of the roller to the skin.

5. Each turn of the bandage should cover two-thirds of the one preceding it.

6. Keep all the margins parallel, and the crossings and reverses in one line.

7. Make the end secure with a safety pin or a few stitches.

8. Bandage the abdomen from above downwards, the chest and limbs from below upwards.

9. In bandaging a limb, (i) stand exactly opposite to it, not on either side. (ii) Hold the bandage in the left hand when the limb is on the patient's right side, and in the right hand when the limb is on his left side. (iii) Begin by applying the bandage to the inner side of the limb ; that is, bandage from within outwards. (iv) When dressings or splints have to be retained, it is a mistake, as the authors of the " First Aid Manual " insist, to cover the tips of the fingers or toes, because these enable you to see whether the pressure is too great and is affecting the circulation. (v) For

the same reason, leave the tip of the elbow and the heel uncovered when a bandage is applied along the length of a limb—unless, of course, the elbow or the heel is wounded. (vi) Avoid taking turns round the wrist or above the ankle before carrying the bandage round the hand or the foot, so that the superficial veins may not be compressed. (vii) In approaching the elbow, be careful to bend it, so as not to impede the flow of blood in the large veins.

VARIETIES OF ROLLER BANDAGES. —A *spiral* bandage consists of a series of spiral turns, each overlapping the one below for about two-thirds of its width. This is the simplest form of roller bandage, but it can be applied only to those parts which are of uniform size, such as a finger, or which increases in girth very gradually. If it were applied to a part of which the girth varies abruptly, the lower edge would be loose. (It is illustrated in the lower part of the leg in Plate III, 1.) A *reversed spiral* (Plate III, 4) is made by turning the bandage over so as frequently to change the upper and lower edges, by which the whole width is enabled to grip the part to which the bandage is applied. This is the most frequently used of all the methods of bandaging. Chiefly employed for the limbs, it may also be used for the trunk, or for the fastening of splints. It is not, however, suitable for the neighbourhood of joints, and it has the defects of being inelastic and liable to slip. The *double-headed spiral* with reverses requires a long double-headed bandage, the two rolls or heads, however, being of unequal size, and the larger being employed to form the reverses. This bandage is not easy of application, but it has substantial advantages in that it secures great firmness, nor are the turns liable to slip, each layer of the spiral being securely fixed by the next layer of the reverse. Another very efficient bandage is that known as the *figure-of-8* (Plate III, 2, and the foot in 1). At once firm and elastic, it is capable of being applied to all parts, but is especially useful for the limbs, and it is the best method for carrying a bandage over a joint; it is also an excellent way of covering the points of the elbow, the heel and the knee-cap. The *spica* bandage (Plate III, 3, 5), so called because the crossings of the turns bear some resemblance to the position of the grains in a head or spike of barley, is a modification of the figure-of-8 bandage combined with a firm attachment to a limb in the neighbourhood of a joint. It is especially useful for applying firm pressure to a joint, for retaining dressings, and for bandaging the groin or the breast or the shoulder. It is also often employed for injuries to the joint of the thumb. The *four-tailed* bandage (*see* the head of the figure in Plate III, 6) is made from a strip of roller bandage from 2 to 6 in. wide and from 1 to 1½ yd. long, split in two from each end to within a few inches of the centre; it is useful for supporting the chin, or the breast; in the latter case the centre is placed under the breast, the two lower tails being carried one across the chest, the other across the back, and tied over the opposite shoulder, while the two upper tails cross the lower and are tied under the arms. The *many-tailed* bandage, used to retain dressings or poultices on the chest, breast or abdomen, is especially suitable when it is important to avoid movement, either of the patient or of the part; it consists of a wide piece of calico, flannel or domette (the width depending upon the part to be covered), torn into strips from each

side to within an inch or two of the centre, which is left entire; or it may be made by tearing the material into strips of 1½ yd. by 2 or 3 in., laying them parallel with and rather overlapping one another, and stitching them to another strip placed at right angles across their centres (*see* the chest of the figure in Plate III, 6). The *T-bandage* is used for retaining dressings on the perineum, as after operations in that region (*see* the lowest bandage in Plate III, 6). It can be quickly prepared by tying one piece of roller bandage round the body as a waist-band; another, fixed to it at the back and passed between the thighs, is carried forward and tied to the waist-band in front.

3. The elastic bandage.—Elastic bandages, made of indiarubber or other elastic material, are used to reduce or prevent swelling and to furnish support to varicose veins. They should be rolled up rather loosely before being used, and special care must be taken to prevent them from being too tight. They are much more simple in application than ordinary bandages, for it is sufficient merely to roll them on in a simple spiral, and no turns or reverses are required.

4. Plaster-of-Paris bandages.—These bandages, usually made of gauze upon which powdered plaster of Paris has been rubbed, although starch, gum and chalk, glue and liquid glass answer the same purpose, are used when a part has to be rendered immobile for some time, as in the case of a fractured limb. The limb should first be swathed with flannel. The plaster-of-Paris bandage, having been well soaked in salted water, is put on evenly over the part; some powdered plaster-of-Paris may then be wetted and rubbed over the surface to make the whole firm. In five or

ten minutes the plaster will have set; it should be allowed to become perfectly dry before being covered over. If the bandage, when the time comes for removal, cannot be unwound, it should be softened with dilute hydrochloric acid, rubbed along in a line on one side; the bandage can then be divided along this line with a large pair of scissors.

BANDY LEGS (*see* Bow-Legs).

BANTINGISM (*see* Obesity).

BARBER'S ITCH.—This is an infectious disease of the beard or moustache, known also as chin whelk and medically as coccogenic sycosis, which may be "caught" from the infected brush of a barber, or may be set up by a discharge from the nose, or ear, or some other part of the body. If the upper lip is the seat of the trouble, the cause is usually a chronic discharge from the nose. The organism which is the cause of the disease gains access to the hair-follicles, the little pits in which the hairs are rooted, and there sets up inflammation, with resulting pimples, some of which contain pus ("matter"). The disease is a very refractory one, which may persist for years. Even when the hairs have been removed (depilation) by the X-rays, it may recur, for some of the germs may have been left behind in the follicles, and it may be necessary to remove the hairs again and again. After depilation a mild antiseptic lotion and ointment should be employed. Vaccine treatment is sometimes useful as an adjunct.

BATHS.—The subject of bathing in mineral waters is briefly considered in the article Mineral Waters; in this place we shall deal only with ordinary and with artificially medicated baths.

27

Varieties of baths and their uses.—Baths are hot, warm, tepid, temperate, or cold, according as they conform roughly to the following temperatures :—

Hot bath	101° to 110° Fahr.
Warm bath ...	96° to 100° ,,
Tepid bath......	85° to 95° ,,
Temperate bath .	75° to 84° ,,
Cold bath.......	34° to 74° ,,

Hot baths are beneficial when one or more of the internal organs is congested—i.e. is too full of blood. It must not, however, be too prolonged, or the heart or the brain, or both, may be so deprived of blood as to be incapable of performing their functions, in which case faintness will ensue. Hot baths are unsuitable for persons with weak hearts or with high blood-pressure. *Warm* baths are useful in rheumatism and gout and to relieve muscular spasm in convulsions and colic. *Tepid* baths have a slightly stimulating effect on the body generally and a sedative influence on the nervous system. They should be followed by friction with a rough towel, so as to remove the dead scales of the upper or scarf skin, clear the glands of retained secretion, and stimulate the action of the skin. *Temperate* baths may be regarded chiefly from the " morning tub " point of view. *Cold* baths, in the sense defined by our table, should only be taken, except in very hot weather, by those in vigorous health, whose organs are all sound ; they are certainly not suitable for elderly people, whose arteries may not be able to stand the strain to which they are exposed by the rush of blood from the surface of the body. They are sometimes used in cases in which there is high fever, the patient being placed in water of about the temperature of his body,

gradually cooled down to 60° Fahr. or lower, when he is quickly dried and put back to bed. The same effect is produced by wrapping him in a sheet wrung out of cold water which is further chilled by being rubbed with ice, and continuing the process until his temperature falls to about 100° Fahr. In both instances the patient must be carefully watched to guard against collapse. These are measures which should be carried out only under medical supervision. The caution applies equally to the *wet pack* (q.v.).

In connexion with cold baths, a few words may be said about *sea-bathing*. It is even more important than in the case of ordinary cold baths that this kind of bathing should be indulged in cautiously by all who are not in robust health, for the stimulating effect of sea water is much enhanced by the presence in it of a large quantity of salt and by the fact that it is in constant motion. Sea-bathing should never be practised after a full meal, nor is before breakfast the best time, although that is the time preferred by many enthusiastic bathers. The vital powers, including the circulation, which have ebbed during the night, are not in full flow in the early morning. Nor are the water and the air so warm as they become during the forenoon. The best time, therefore, for the plunge into the sea is about midway between breakfast and the mid-day meal. Contrary to the prevalent belief, a sea bath—and the same remark applies to a cold fresh-water bath—may be taken without harm while one is heated from exercise, but should never be taken when one is cooling. The affections in which a course of sea-bathing is frequently advantageous are scrofula, enlarged glands, diseased joints, and chronic and

muscular rheumatism. Those who easily " catch cold " will often find that bathing in the sea braces up their powers of resistance and makes them less susceptible to this annoying affection. A substitute for sea-bathing is available by adding to ordinary water sea salt in the proportion of ¼ lb. to the gallon.

In the *Turkish* bath the patient is exposed to hot air, in the *Russian* bath to steam ; they both induce very free perspiration and are found useful in rheumatism, sciatica, gout and other affections, as well as by persons who want to keep down their weight and are unable or unwilling to take an ample amount of exercise. Hot air is sometimes applied locally, as to stiffened joints, the limb being placed in a metal cylinder containing air which is heated up to a temperature of 180° Fahr. or even beyond ; the immediate effect is to relax the joint. The stiffness will return, but it may not be quite so bad as it was before, and by persevering in the treatment the condition is in many cases permanently ameliorated. In *douche* baths a stream of either hot or cold water is directed upon a part from a height or from a hose. In the *shower* bath, water issues through small apertures (like those in the " rose " of a watering can) in a cistern overhead. A *needle* bath is somewhat similar to a shower bath, but the fine streams of water come through apertures in a coiled pipe, to play either upon the whole body or upon some particular region.

Medicated baths.—*Alkaline* baths may be made with carbonate of soda, ¼ ounce to a gallon of water, or with carbonate of potash, a teaspoonful to a gallon ; they are employed in skin diseases and in rheumatism and gout for steeping the painful part. *Acid* baths are oc-

casionally useful in some liver affections, but are more often applied locally, as in a footbath. The average strength is ½ ounce of dilute nitro-hydrochloric acid to a gallon of water ; a wooden or earthenware vessel must be used. *Sulphur* baths —¼ ounce of sulphuretted potash for each gallon of water—are employed in certain skin affections, as also are *mercury* baths—2 drops of hydrochloric acid and 6 grains of corrosive sublimate (a powerful poison) to a gallon of water ; these latter baths are also specially beneficial in syphilis. *Pine* baths, prepared by adding about 1 lb. of the extract of pine leaves, with a little of the essence, to a full-sized bath of hot water, are of service in hysterical, rheumatic and gouty affections. If a *mustard* bath is desired, it may be obtained by adding 1 ounce of mustard for each gallon of water. *Bran* baths, advantageous in acute eczema and other irritable conditions of the skin, in which the external application of plain water has to be avoided, are prepared by mixing with a small quantity of boiling water 2 ounces of bran for each gallon of bath water, the mixture being then well stirred into the bath. *Ozone* or *seaweed* baths are made by adding to the bath water enough chopped-up seaweed or decoction of seaweed to make it glutinous.

BEDSORES.—In the nursing of the sick, especially if the patient is very aged and infirm, or is suffering from an exhausting disease such as typhoid fever, or, still more, is affected with paralysis, it is often difficult to prevent bedsores. Patients who are compelled to use the bed-pan or the urinal, and most of all those paralysed patients whose motions and water pass involuntarily, are particularly liable to develop this trouble. In all such cases the greatest care must be taken to secure cleanliness. If the discharges from bladder and bowels are involuntary the patient should wear an india-rubber urinal, and a sponge or cotton-wool should be so placed as to catch the motions. The drawsheet must be kept free from creases and changed as often as it becomes damp or soiled; and the bedclothes and the night-dress must also be often changed. Whenever possible, the posture should be frequently altered so as to vary the pressure. Water- or air-beds and cushions should be used in all cases in which there is any danger of the occurrence of bedsores, but it will still be necessary to observe most scrupulously all the precautions we have mentioned; in addition, all the parts subject to pressure, after being washed and thoroughly dried, should be rubbed gently with a little cotton-wool soaked with some stimulant of the skin, such as eau-de-Cologne, or methylated spirit, until this has quite dried in, and should then be dusted over with a starch and oxide-of-zinc powder.

While carefully carrying out all these preventive measures, the nurse must ever be on the watch for the earliest indication of a bedsore—a pale, mottled and sodden aspect of the skin at the affected part. If the sore is quite small it may be painted over with collodion; if larger, it must be cleansed twice or thrice a day with boric-acid lotion, carefully dried, and covered with a small piece of lint smeared with zinc ointment or with carbolized vaselin. Over this, to protect the sore from pressure, should be placed a pad formed of thick felt or gamgee tissue, with a hole cut in the centre rather larger than the piece of skin to be protected; it may be kept in place with a few turns of a bandage. If the piece of skin mortifies, which will be shown by its turning black, its separation may be expedited by a compress of boric lint wetted with hot water. The raw surface left must be kept clean, and should be dressed two or three times a day with slightly stimulating applications, such as a lotion of compound tincture of benzoin or balsam of Peru and zinc or resin ointment.

BED-CRADLE (*see* NURSING, DoMESTIC).

BED-WETTING.—Juvenile incontinence of urine, as this troublesome infirmity is termed medically, occurs more frequently in boys than in girls. Usually appearing when the child is 7 or 8 years of age, it is in most cases cured before puberty is approached, but in girls it may persist to the age of eighteen, and in many cases, in both girls and boys, the affection is apt to recur after apparent cure. The involuntary passing of urine mostly takes place during sleep, but in boys it may occur during the day as well. It is met with chiefly in families prone to epilepsy or St. Vitus's dance. But there may be some physical cause for the trouble. The boy may have a long foreskin which cannot be drawn back, or the urine may be unusually acid, or there may be a stone in the bladder, or worms in the lower bowel. Occasionally the trouble has been traced to chronic hip-joint disease. Sometimes it is associated with the process of teething, and not infrequently it is the result of indigestion.

Treatment.—The first thing to do is to remove any of the local causes of irritation which have been mentioned. The child should be well fed, but no indigestible food should be allowed, meat should be given sparingly, and rhubarb, on account of its irritating acid, prohibited. A tonic —iron or nux vomica—should be administered. The child should have his last meal an hour or so before going to bed, should take no drink with it, should pass water before getting into bed, should be waked an hour later for the same purpose, and, if possible, once again during the night. He should not sleep on his back, and the bedclothes must not be heavy. This treatment failing, belladonna may be given—four drops for a child 2 years, and larger doses for older children, one dose in the afternoon and a second at bedtime if the incontinence is only nocturnal, three doses a day if it is general. If the affection persists, the doses may be gradually increased at weekly intervals for three weeks, unless complaint should be made of persistent thirst or the pupils of the eyes should be enlarged. In nervous cases, especially in girls, bromide of potash or soda is beneficial, in 15- to 20-grain doses, taken at bedtime. In many cases of bed-wetting extract of thyroid gland is useful.

BELLADONNA POISONING.—

The glistening black berries of the belladonna or deadly nightshade plant are sometimes eaten by children, but there is little danger to life if only a few of the berries are consumed; the poison in the root and leaves is much stronger. Belladonna liniment, a very powerful poison, has occasionally been swallowed by mistake for medicine. First give an emetic (*see* EMETICS), then a stimulant—strong coffee, or sal volatile, or brandy or whisky. If the patient is drowsy, flicking with a wet towel should be tried, or alternate hot and cold douches to the head. A mustard leaf or plaster should be applied to the calves of the leg, over the abdomen and heart, etc., and hot-water bottles to the feet. The antidote for this poison is pilocarpine, a half-grain tabloid.

BELL'S PALSY (*see* FACIAL PARALYSIS).

BENIGN TUMOURS (*see* TUMOURS).

BERIBERI.—This disease is a form of neuritis frequently met with in most tropical and sub-tropical climates, and also under appropriate conditions in temperate latitudes. It is favoured by a moist atmosphere. At one time it was believed to be a germ disease, but there is now ground for believing that the beriberi of the Eastern Archipelago, of China, and of Japan is mainly the result of a diet of rice that has been overmilled. The effect of the overmilling is to remove from the rice the entire pericarp, which contains a vitamin necessary to the nutrition of the nervous system (*see* Vitamins, under FOOD). The most important point in treatment is the diet. Rice, especially white rice, should be entirely avoided, and its place taken by oatmeal, wheat and flour which has not been too much milled, beans, peas and peanuts. Milk, eggs, and meat should be given freely; extracts of rice polishings, prepared in various ways, have been found to be very beneficial. The extract of yeast known as *marmite* has been used with good results; it is given in doses of $1\frac{1}{2}$ grammes daily. If the patient lives in a moist region he should be removed to a dry one. When recovery has begun, a suitable muscle tonic, such as Fowler's solution of arsenic, 5 drops three times daily in water, may be given. The atrophy of muscles and numbness of the skin should be treated by electricity and massage, and the deformities due to the wasting by surgery.

BILHARZIASIS.—In this disease the bladder or the rectum is inflamed owing to the presence in the urine or fæces of the eggs of a parasite, the *Schistosoma hæmatobium,* and the disease is now often called schistosomiasis. It is common in Egypt and in many other parts of Africa, and is also met with in the western parts of Asia. The parasites, in an immature stage of their existence, enter the body of man or of some other vertebrate either through the skin in bathing or from the drinking of polluted water, take up their abode in the liver, and attain maturity. The female lays an immense number of eggs, which are carried to various regions of the body, especially the bladder and the rectum. In cases in which the disease is active, and the patient is not suffering from disease of the heart or arteries or kidney, tartar emetic should be injected into the veins. In certain cases surgical treatment has to be employed either before or after the treatment by injections. In all case alike the diet should be nutritious, but light and unirritating.

BILIARY COLIC (*see* GALL-STONES).

" BILIOUSNESS."—The liver is often blamed unjustly for those attacks of nausea, headache, and general malaise with which most of us are much too familiar. One considerable group of these attacks is due to migraine, or megrim (*see under* HEAD-ACHE), and in many of the remaining cases it is the stomach rather than the liver that is at fault. The chief cause of this gastric irregularity is believed to be excessive indulgence in food, especially fatty and sweet foods, by those who take little exercise ; in some cases the irritation is caused by alcohol, particularly in the form of heavy malt liquors and sweet wines.

The symptoms, however, may be the result of cumulative irritation rather than of any specific dietetic indiscretion ; in these cases either a little more food, or richer food, is habitually taken than can be digested, or the diet includes some article which happens not to agree with the patient.

Symptoms and treatment.—The symptoms of these attacks are so well known that they need be only briefly described. In many cases the patient wakes up in the morning with a headache, generally a dull, heavy pain, either at the back of the head or in the forehead. He may also be giddy, and is drowsy, and mentally confused, and generally " out of sorts." He has no appetite, and even if he is wise enough to abstain entirely from food, he may vomit, without experiencing immediate relief. He has a " dirty " furred tongue ; there may be an unpleasant taste in the mouth, and a secretion of somewhat viscid saliva. Sometimes there is a scalding sensation in the palms and soles ; in some cases, too, there is a dull pain or a sense of weight in the region of the liver. These symptoms may last for days, but more frequently, if the patient abstains from food and keeps in bed in a well ventilated room, or sits or gently strolls about in the fresh air, they subside in the course of a few hours. A blue pill at night and a black draught next morning may then be taken by way of speeding the parting guest. This time-honoured form of treatment may also be adopted preventively when a " bilious " attack appears to be imminent ; or compound cascara sagrada tablets may be taken. For prevention, however, the most important things are to avoid food that is known from experience to be unsuitable, to eat at regular intervals and observe strict moderation, to take a fair amount of open-air exercise, to keep the bowels in regular action, and to avoid excitement as far as possible. Plenty of water, either hot or cold, should be drunk, between rather than with meals, for thus the stomach and intestines will be flushed.

BIRTHMARKS.—The reddish spots or patches which are variously termed birthmarks, port-wine stains, strawberry marks, cherry marks, and (medically) nævi, are caused by an overgrowth of the blood-vessels of the skin. In all cases they are present at birth, though at first they may be so small as to escape notice; they may either remain stationary, increase in area, or disappear in the course of a few months—it may be after an illness. Nothing is known of the cause of birthmarks, but the popular opinion is that they are the record, so to speak, of some fancy or longing that seized the mother's mind during pregnancy. If they are not by their size and their situation disfiguring, it is better to let them alone. In other cases they may be treated surgically.

BITES (*see* STINGS AND BITES).

BLACKHEADS (*see* ACNE VULGARIS).

BLACKWATER FEVER.—In many warm regions there occurs, sometimes in epidemics, a fever of which a striking, though not an absolutely constant symptom is the dark-brown, almost black colour of the urine. This is blackwater fever, otherwise, in medical language, *hæmoglobinuric* or *melanuric fever*, the one term signifying that hæmoglobin, the colouring matter of the blood, is present in the urine, the other having just the same meaning as the popular name. Until recently the relation between this disease and malaria, by

which it is usually preceded, was not understood; but the view now gaining acceptance is that it is not a disease in itself but rather a complication of severe forms of malaria to which Europeans who contract malaria are especially liable. When the disease declares itself the patient should at once go to bed, should be kept warm and free from draughts, and should take a dose of calomel, say 10 or 15 grains, to clear the bowels. A drug often used to counter the disease is Sternberg's mixture. In some cases quinine is beneficial. Careful nursing is important.

BLADDER, FUNCTIONS OF (*see* URINARY ORGANS).

BLADDER, INFLAMMATION OF.—Cystitis, or inflammation of the membrane lining the inner surface of the bladder, may be either acute or chronic. **Acute** cystitis may be induced by exposure to cold, as from sitting on wet grass; by the presence of a stone or some " foreign body " in the bladder; by the passage of a catheter to draw off the urine; or, in women, by pregnancy or displacement of the womb, etc. The exciting cause of the affection, however, in chronic as well as in these acute cases, is the action of germs; the influences just enumerated are only predisposing causes, which give the bacteria their opportunity. The main symptom is a frequent and very urgent desire to pass water, attended with pain and slight fever. The *treatment* is to keep the patient in bed, to put him on a milk diet, with plenty of barley-water, to see that the bowels act freely, to give him two or three hot hip-baths a day, and to apply hot fomentations to the lower part of the abdomen. The doctor may order a mixture containing boric acid, tincture of hyoscyamus, and infusion of buchu. Suppositories of morphia and belladonna will be found useful in subduing the pain.

Chronic inflammation of the bladder may follow an acute attack, or may be set up by something that interferes with the passage of the water, such as enlarged prostate, stricture of the urethra, a stone in the bladder, or a tumour. When any of these troubles is present the bladder is not entirely emptied and the water that is left behind irritates and at last inflames the mucous membrane. This residual urine, as it is called, may decompose in the bladder and be as offensive to the smell when passed as is stale urine. *Treatment* does not involve keeping the patient in bed, nor need he be debarred from a moderate amount of animal food, so long as highly spiced dishes are avoided. If the urine is offensive or characterized by acidity, the doctor will order appropriate medicine. The predisposing cause of the cystitis, whatever it may be, must of course be dealt with.

BLADDER, IRRITABLE.— Inflammation of the bladder has been considered in the preceding article; here we are concerned with cases in which the only symptom is the need to pass water more frequently than normal. It may be due to the use of some article of food or some beverage which irritates the mucous membrane of the bladder; or to nervousness, or emotional excitement, or hysteria, or to the urine being too acid, or too concentrated from insufficient fluid being taken. Little more is called for in the way of treatment than to avoid the cause of the trouble. Belladonna, 10 drops of the tincture in a glass of water three times a day, may be recommended.

BLADDER, STONE IN (*see* STONE IN THE BLADDER).

BLEAR EYE.—Some children and young people suffer from a chronic soreness and redness of the edges of the eyelids. There is discharge from the edges, and the eyelids become matted together. In neglected cases the follicles in which the eyelashes are rooted may be permanently injured, so that the hairs cease to grow; this is the condition known as blear eye. Sometimes the disfigurement is made worse by the lids being everted—that is, turned outwards. Or one or several of the hairs may turn towards the eyeball (*see* EYELASHES, INGROWING). The remedy for the inflammation which has these disagreeable sequels is to paint yellow oxide of mercury ointment (9 grains of the oxide to 1 ounce of vaselin) along the margins of the lids with a brush. The eyelashes may be cut short, and the crusts formed by the discharge as it dries should be removed night and morning. Blear eye is generally associated with delicate health; and the patient should take cod-liver oil and syrup of iodide of iron.

" BLEEDERS " (*see* HÆMOPHILIA).

BLEEDING (*see* HÆMORRHAGE).

" BLIND SPOT " (*see* EYE).

BLINDNESS.—Before the invention of the ophthalmoscope by Prof. Helmholtz, in 1851, many cases of blindness were described as *amaurosis*, a word which, signifying simply darkness, covered all forms of loss of vision in which there was no discoverable defect in the structure of the eye. It has been wittily defined as a condition of the eye " in which neither the patient nor the surgeon can see anything." Now that, by means of the ophthalmoscope, the interior of the eye can be examined, cases of blindness are grouped according to their cause, and little scope is left for a term which was formerly a convenient veil for ignorance. In many cases children lose their sight in the act of birth, from inflammation contracted from the mother (*see* OPHTHALMIA). Blindness, too, is sometimes caused in children and young people by inherited syphilis. Other poisons which may produce blindness, temporary or permanent, are lead, alcohol, tobacco, opium, and quinine, and those generated in such affections as Bright's disease and diabetes. Some cases are due to the affection of the lens which is termed cataract (*see* CATARACT), others to disease of the retina, of the optic nerve, etc., yet others to such affections as hysteria and tumours of the brain. Blindness may also follow heavy blows on the face, forehead or temple, when it is believed to be caused by concussion of the retina, or it may come on gradually months after an injury to certain nerves of the face, or as a sequel of decayed teeth. It may be produced, too, by exposure to the glare of sunlight on snow (snow blindness), or to an exceptionally vivid lightning flash.

In **tobacco blindness,** said to attack especially those who smoke cigars and short pipes, the patient gradually becomes conscious of a general dimness of sight, for both near and distant objects. If smoking is entirely renounced for a time, and the eyes are rested, and attention is paid to the general health, the trouble, as a rule, gradually disappears; but in patients who are past middle age recovery may be a tedious process.
Night blindness.—This curious form of visual defect is nearly always if not invariably associated with a disease of the conjunctiva—the membrane lining the front part of the eyeball and the inner surfaces of the lids. Just as a person with no visual defect finds it difficult to see objects on first entering a darkened room, until his sight has adapted itself to the situation, so the sufferer from night blindness fails to see objects in a dim light. An exciting cause is believed to be the dazzling produced by glaring light as in the tropics; this, and not the influence of the moon, as they believe, is the reason why the affection is often met with in sailors. The probable predisposing causes are defective nutrition and malaria. As the general health improves with good food, fresh air, and tonics, the sight gradually improves. There is a precisely opposite condition termed **day blindness,** in which objects can only be seen comfortably in a more or less dim light. It is rather a symptom of several different affections of the eye than a disease itself, and the treatment must be adapted to the morbid state of which it is a manifestation.

BLISTERS.—The treatment of *accidental* blisters is considered under BURNS AND SCALDS. Blisters in the *pathological* sense of the term are met with in various skin diseases, but they are termed by dermatologists bullæ, or blebs. It is with a third class of blister, *surgical* blisters, that we are concerned here.
The object of applying a blister to the skin is, by setting up counter-irritation, to draw blood to the surface of the body from a part in which there is congestion. A blister may take the form either of a plaster of the desired size or of a blistering fluid, which is painted on with a camel's-hair brush, the skin having first been well washed and dried. Care must

be taken to prevent the fluid from running over to other parts of the skin, for in that case they would also be blistered. A second application is frequently necessary after the first coat has dried. The application finished, the part should be protected with a layer of cotton-wool. The length of time a plaster should be allowed to remain on varies with the sensitiveness of the skin, but six or eight hours may be taken as an average. When the plaster or fluid has done its work, the bleb produced may be pricked in one or two places to give exit to the contained fluid,

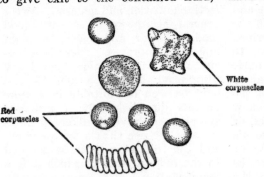

Fig. 5.—Blood-corpuscles.

which should be dabbed up with lint or cotton-wool. The loose skin should not be dragged away, but should be left as a protection for the very sensitive part beneath, and covered with cotton-wool or with lint smeared with cold cream or with an ointment.

BLOOD AND LYMPH.—Blood consists of a colourless fluid, the plasma, and a large number of small floating bodies, the corpuscles, which are suspended in it. The great majority of these floating bodies (Fig. 5) are the *red corpuscles* or cells, disc-shaped bodies which give to the blood its familiar bright-red hue. They tend to run together into rolls or rouleaux (Fig. 5), like coins placed one on

another. There are, approximately, five million red corpuscles in a space of one cubic millimetre, which is about equal to the size of a large pin's head. The remaining corpuscles are called *leucocytes*, because they are white cells (Fig. 5). They are capable of movement of a crawling kind, can penetrate the walls of blood-vessels, and have the property of seeking out and engulfing any bacteria which may find their way into the body, and perhaps killing them. There are several different kinds of white corpuscles ; some, called *lymphocytes*, have but one nucleus, others a nucleus divided into several parts, attached to each other, however, by slender strands ; these are the *polymorpho-nuclears*. The proportion of leucocytes to red corpuscles is as 1 to 500, and there are about ten thousand of them in a cubic millimetre. In addition to the red and white corpuscles, the blood also contains bodies called blood-platelets, which are smaller still ; they are believed to be in part the source of the materials which produce clotting of the blood (*see* below).

The chief source from which both red and white corpuscles are derived is the red marrow of the bones. The red corpuscles are composed of colouring matter, called hæmoglobin, and a framework of supporting substance. The importance of hæmoglobin in the living body consists in its power of taking up oxygen from the air and giving it off again to the plasma, and so, when the plasma escapes from the capillaries (*see* below), to the cells of the tissues.

CLOTTING.—The property of clotting, or coagulation, which the blood possesses is due to the presence of ferments in the plasma, its fluid part, which lead to the formation of fibrin. If freshly drawn blood is whipped with a bundle of twigs, this fibrin will be seen adhering to them as a mass of colourless threads, the corpuscles remaining behind in the serum, which in consequence is red. Serum, then, is the plasma divested of the substance concerned in blood-clotting. The importance of blood-clotting need hardly be pointed out.

When small vessels are severed, the bleeding ceases because a clot has formed and plugged the cut ends. When a large vessel is opened the blood escapes too quickly for a clot to form spontaneously, but if the flow is stopped by the application of pressure or of a ligature, then clotting takes place.

Lymph.—In its passage through the very tiny tubes called capillaries (*see* BLOOD, CIRCULATION OF) the fluid part of the blood oozes out into the tissues, giving up to them its oxygen and nutritive material, and taking from them their carbonic-acid gas. When it has left the capillaries, the fluid part of the blood, now known as lymph, passes along ducts called lymphatics and through the lymphatic glands. The small ducts form larger ones, and finally the lymph is poured into the thoracic duct and the right lymphatic duct, and is returned to the blood by way of the large vessels in the neck called the subclavian veins.

This group of ducts and glands forms the *lymphatic system.* One of the offices of the lymphatic glands is to deal with any intruders that may have found their way into the lymph, such as bacteria ; these are arrested in the glands, and are here brought into contact with their natural foes, the leucocytes. It is in the discharge of this duty that lymphatic glands often become inflamed.

BLOOD, CIRCULATION OF.— The mechanism of the circulation of the blood consists of the heart, the arteries and capillaries, and the veins. The *heart,* a hollow muscular organ, in the middle of the chest but rather more on the left side than on the right (Fig. 6), acts as a powerful double pump which drives the blood through the tubes bearing those various names. It is enclosed in a fibrous sac, the

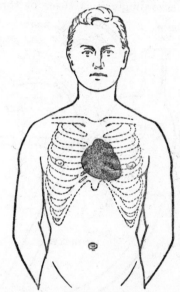

Fig. 6.—Position of the heart.

pericardium, and is lined inside by a membrane called the *endocardium ;* the muscle of which it is largely composed is the *myocardium.* It is completely divided into two parts, the right and the left, by a partition running across it from the base, the upper end, to the apex or pointed end, and each half is partially divided into two by an incomplete partition at right angles with the other partition. Thus, it has four cavities, two at the base, called the **auricles,** and two towards the apex, the **ventricles** (Fig. 7). Between the auricle and ventricle in each side of the heart are openings which are provided with valves—on the right side the tricuspid valve (Fig. 8), on the left side the mitral valve (Fig. 8). These valves are so arranged that the blood can flow only from the auricle into the ventricle, and not vice versa. The left ventricle does the chief share of the work, for it has to pump the blood to all the extremities of the body, and accordingly it is twice or thrice

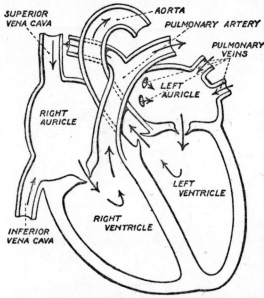

Fig. 7.—Diagram of the heart, laid open.

as thick as the right ventricle, which has to drive the blood only to the lungs. The *arteries* into which the blood is forced are strong tubes, muscular and elastic, which gradually grow smaller and thinner until they shrink into tubes so tiny that they can only be seen with the microscope. These tiny tubes are the *capillaries* (Fig. 9); they are formed of membranes so thin that the fluid part of the blood can ooze freely through; they are spread out in almost every part of the body as a network. These

minute vessels in turn merge into tiny *veins* (venules) which gradually become larger. The walls of the veins are thinner than those of the arteries, and contain less muscle and elastic tissue, and they are supplied at intervals with valves to prevent the stream from flowing backwards.

Let us now follow the blood (Plate IV) from the beginning of its course as it is pumped by the left ventricle of the heart into the chief artery, the aorta (Fig. 7). From the aorta it passes to all parts of the body except the lungs, presently entering the capillaries, and being returned by the veins, and finally, by the great trunk vein called the vena cava, to the right auricle of the heart. This is called the *general* or *systemic circulation*. The blood, it will be observed, though it has got back to the heart, has not yet reached the *left* side of the heart, whence it started. To do this it has to be pumped by the right ventricle into the pulmonary artery (Fig. 7), the only artery that contains venous blood, and so into the lungs, whence it returns by the pulmonary veins, the only veins that contain arterial blood, to the left auricle, and so into the left ventricle. This subsidiary circulation is called the *pulmonary circulation*. The blood is now ready to start another journey round the body. There is yet another subsidiary circulation, the *portal circulation*. The blood from the stomach, spleen, pancreas and intestinal canal, instead of passing from their capillaries into veins leading directly to the inferior vena cava, flows into a large vessel called the portal vein, which carries it first to the liver. Here it undergoes certain changes and then passes into

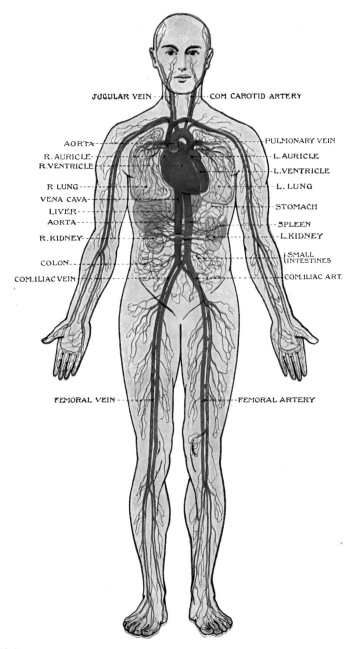

JUGULAR VEIN	COM. CAROTID ARTERY
AORTA	PULMONARY VEIN
R. AURICLE	L. AURICLE
R.VENTRICLE	L.VENTRICLE
R LUNG	L. LUNG
VENA CAVA	STOMACH
LIVER	
AORTA	SPLEEN
R. KIDNEY	L.KIDNEY
COLON	SMALL INTESTINES
COM.ILIAC VEIN	COM.ILIAC ART.
FEMORAL VEIN	FEMORAL ARTERY

PLATE IV.   COURSE OF THE CIRCULATION OF THE BLOOD.

THE BLOOD, PURIFIED BY ITS PASSAGE THROUGH THE LUNGS, IS SEEN (RED) IN THE LEFT SIDE OF THE HEART, WHENCE IT IS CARRIED BY THE ARTERIES DOWNWARDS TO THE ABDOMINAL ORGANS AND THE LEGS, AND UPWARDS TO THE ARMS AND THE HEAD.   FROM THE ARTERIES IT PASSES INTO TINY VESSELS CALLED CAPILLARIES, AND THENCE (NOW BLUE) INTO THE VEINS, AND SO UPWARDS AND DOWNWARDS TO THE RIGHT SIDE OF THE HEART, WHENCE IT IS PUMPED INTO THE LUNGS.   THEN IT RETURNS TO THE LEFT SIDE OF THE HEART TO BEGIN ITS COURSE AGAIN.

veins which conduct it to the inferior vena cava, whence it is conveyed to the right auricle.

In its course the blood undergoes important changes in composition. When it leaves the left ventricle to enter upon its systemic journey, it is bright red, but by the time it flows into the veins, after having traversed the capillaries and there parted with oxygen and taken up carbonic acid

BLOOD-POISONING—The germs which cause blood-poisoning may come from some diseased part of the body, such as an infected tonsil, but more usually they come from without the body and find entrance through a breach in the skin, which may be a mere prick with a dirty pin, but more often is a bruised and lacerated wound. The symptoms set up by the poisons they produce in the blood are high fever, violent shivering fits, headache and irritability, sweats, and rapid exhaustion. This is the condition known medically as *septicæmia ;* if, in addition, abscesses form in various

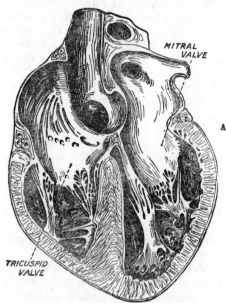

MITRAL VALVE

TRICUSPID VALVE

Fig. 8.—The heart laid open to show the tricuspid and mitral valves.

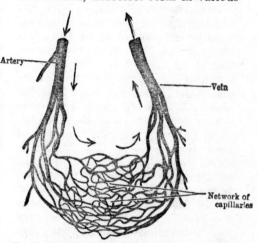

Artery

Vein

Network of capillaries

Fig. 9.—Shows how the capillaries form the connecting link between an artery and a vein.

gas, it has become dark-coloured. The bright-red blood is called arterial blood, the dark-coloured blood is called venous blood. Venous blood only becomes bright red again when it has passed through the lungs and has there been relieved of carbonic acid gas and recharged with oxygen.

BLOOD IN URINE (*see* URINE, NORMAL AND ABNORMAL).

BLOOD-CLOTTING (*see* BLOOD AND LYMPH).

parts of the body, it is called *pyæmia*. It is a very serious but fortunately a rare condition. The wound is treated with carbolic acid or some other antiseptic, a febrifuge such as quinine is administered to bring down the temperature, and strenuous efforts are made to support the patient's strength with food and stimulants. In some cases either vaccine or serum treatment is employed.

BLOOD-PRESSURE.—Stated in its simplest terms, the blood-pressure is the resultant of the force which propels the blood through the arteries and capillaries and of the resistance which those vessels offer to the flow of the current. Low blood-pressure occurs in wasting diseases such as tuberculosis ; high blood-pressure in kidney disease, in arterial disease (*see* ARTERIES, DISEASES OF), and also in a group of cases known as cases of hyperpiesis (= high pressure), in which no organic disease is discoverable. Blood-pressure is measured by an instrument called the sphygmomanometer.

BLOOD-SPITTING.—Under this heading it will be convenient to group together all cases in which there is a discharge of blood from the mouth. The blood may come from inflamed gums, or from some other part of the mouth, or it may run back from the nose into the throat. The more serious cases are those in which the blood comes either from the lungs or from the stomach. The former is styled *hæmoptysis*, which means the coughing up of blood ; the latter, *hæmatemesis*, the vomiting of blood. If the blood comes from the lungs it is usually because they are affected with tuberculosis (consumption), but that is not always so, for in a certain kind of heart disease in which the circulation of the blood through the lungs is impeded, small congested vessels in them may give way and the blood be coughed up ; in these latter cases, unless the bleeding is excessive or much prolonged it is not serious, and some patients feel all the better for it. If the blood comes from the stomach the symptom may be due to disease of that organ—congestion, ulceration, cancer ; to acute infectious fevers ; to scurvy, purpura, persistent jaundice, or certain diseases of the liver and the heart. In most cases it is not difficult to determine whether the blood comes from the lungs or from the stomach. If from the lungs, it is coughed up in mouthfuls, is bright red and frothy, is mixed with phlegm, and is not followed by the presence of blood in the motions ; and the patient has a history of cough, shortness of breath, or other chest symptoms. If from the stomach, it is vomited profusely, is not frothy and is dark-coloured, is mixed with food, is often followed by motions stained black with blood, or even consisting of blood, and the patient has a history of vomiting, loss of appetite, or other stomach symptoms. This makes the task of identifying the seat of the bleeding appear to be simple, but in reality it is not quite so easy as it might seem. For instance, a person who is spitting blood from his lungs may accidentally swallow some of it, and this may give rise to nausea and vomiting ; or on the other hand, one who is vomiting blood may in his hurry and excitement draw some into his lungs, and then it would set up coughing, and might be expelled again mixed with phlegm.

Treatment.—Bleeding from the *gums* or *mouth* or *throat* may easily be stopped by a simple astringent mouth-wash, such as a teaspoonful of alum in a tumblerful of water. How to stop bleeding from the nose is described under NOSE-BLEEDING. If the blood comes from the *lungs* in quantity a doctor should at once be sent for. Pending his arrival, put the patient to bed and keep him perfectly quiet and cool. If nothing else is at hand, give him some salt and water to sip. Send for ice and give him some to suck ; when a lump has been sucked small it may be swallowed. If the bleeding persists, crush some ice into small pieces, put them in a waterproof bag (an ordinary sponge-bag will answer the purpose), and apply this to the chest or back, next the skin ; if no bag is available, use a towel or pocket-handkerchief. Turpentine is a very good remedy ; wet a pocket-handkerchief with it and let the patient inhale the vapour. Be careful to give no stimulants, even if the patient should seem to need them, for they will only aggravate the bleeding. Fainting may be relieved by raising the foot of the bed, so that the blood may be helped to return to the brain, by sprinkling cold water on the face, by applying smelling salts to the nostrils, etc. What further treatment is necessary will be ordered by the doctor.

In cases of serious bleeding from the *stomach* there is the same need for instantly summoning medical aid, the same need, too, for absolute rest and quiet. The patient should suck ice, and an ice-bag should be placed over the upper part of the abdomen. Fainting may be relieved in the ways described above.

BLOODY FLUX (*see* DYSENTERY).

BLUE DISEASE (*see* CYANOSIS).

BLUSHING.—In many young persons blushing is an expression of self-consciousness and shyness which is the cause of great mortification. The very fear of blushing is sometimes enough to give rise to it. It cannot be called an affection, though to its victims it involves so much mental discomfort that it is by no means trivial. The only way of avoiding it is to think as little as possible of oneself by keeping the mind occupied with external things.

BODY-WEIGHT.—By comparing the weights and heights of a large number of persons it has been found possible to compile tables showing the average weight of men and of women for a given height. In consulting the following tables, reduced from those which appear in Wellcome's "Excerpta Therapeutica," it should be remembered that nothing is more variable than the weight of quite healthy men and women of the same height. No misgiving need, therefore, be felt by anyone whose variation from the average standard does not exceed 15 per cent., whether on the side of excess or of deficiency. It should be borne in mind, further, that in middle life weight tends to increase with age—about ¾ lb. should therefore be deducted for each adult under 30 and added for each year above that age. The average weight of a man's clothing is about one-twentyfourth of his body-weight ; of a woman's about one-twentieth or less.

AVERAGE WEIGHT FOR HEIGHT OF A MAN, DRESSED, AGED 30.

Height.		Weight.		Chest Circumference.
ft.	in.	st.	lb.	in.
5	0	8	0	33½
5	1	8	4	34
5	2	9	0	35
5	3	9	7	35
5	4	9	13	36
5	5	10	2	37
5	6	10	5	37½
5	7	10	8	38
5	8	11	1	38½
5	9	11	8	39
5	10	12	1	39½
5	11	12	6	40
6	0	12	10	40½
6	1	13	0	41

AVERAGE WEIGHT FOR HEIGHT OF A WOMAN, DRESSED.

Height.		Weight.	
ft.	in.	st.	lb.
4	10	7	0
4	11	7	4
5	0	7	7
5	1	7	12
5	2	8	2
5	3	8	9
5	4	9	2
5	5	9	9
5	6	9	13
5	7	10	8
5	8	11	4

BOILS AND CARBUNCLES.

Boils.—In medical language a boil is a *furuncle* and the disorder of which it is a manifestation is *furunculosis*. A boil may be described as an inflammatory swelling of the skin, originating either in one of its glands or in a hair-follicle, i.e. a depression in the skin in which the root of a hair is embedded. The exciting cause is a germ, which often finds entrance through some break in the surface of the skin; hence the frequency with which boils present themselves in spots exposed to friction, as in the neck where it is chafed by the collar. In those who are troubled by boils again and again, with intervals between which show that it is not a case of auto-infection (*see* below), there is probably some predisposing condition of a constitutional kind, such as anæmia. Boils may also occur as a sequel of one of the infectious fevers, or of such skin diseases as eczema and the itch, or in association with diabetes. One boil is very prone to be quickly followed by a series of others; in many cases this is the result of auto-infection—that is to say, a boil when it has burst discharges germs which contrive to effect an entrance elsewhere in the skin.

Symptoms.—A boil usually starts as a little red pimple, which is very tender. Soon it begins to harden and become inflamed. In some cases, those of " blind boils," little or no matter is formed, and there is no " pointing "—that is, the swelling does not become conical, but the pain is none the less acute; when it breaks it discharges a core which is usually much smaller than that of an ordinary boil. The course a boil more often takes is for the swelling to enlarge, meanwhile irritating the surrounding tissues, which look " angry." After a time the swelling points and acquires a bright-red blush on the surface. In from four to eight days from the beginning the boil bursts and lets out a little matter, disclosing a little opening leading straight down to a greenish-yellow core, which in a day or two comes away, when the pain is at once relieved.

Treatment.—The course of a boil may be cut short by painting it three or four times a day with tincture of iodine or glycerin of belladonna. If these measures fail, the pain may be to some extent relieved by a compress of carbolic acid, 1 in 80. Poultices should never be used, for they prepare the surrounding skin for infection by the germs when the boil discharges. The patient may escape a prolongation of his pain by allowing the doctor to make an incision when pus is definitely formed, an antiseptic dressing being then applied. If this course is not adopted, the " ripening " of the boil may in some cases be expedited by taking sulphide of calcium in a pill containing $\frac{1}{10}$ grain—one pill every hour; or $\frac{1}{4}$ grain three or four times a day after food. If the patient is debilitated he will need a generous diet, and should take a course of iron and quinine, or a teaspoonful of Easton's syrup, or of the compound syrup of hypophosphites, three times a day after meals. A good quinine and iron mixture is the following:

Sulphate of quinine .... 8 grains
Sulphate of iron .... 16 grains
Diluted sulphuric acid ..... 8 minims
Water to 8 ounces.
Two tablespoonfuls three times a day.

In many cases benefit has been derived from the injection of collosol manganese or the taking of stannoxyl tablets. Vaccine treatment is worth trying if there is a succession of boils.

Carbuncle.—This is a large boil affecting several neighbouring hair-follicles, and often choosing the nape of the neck for its site. Due to the same cause as boils, carbuncles are more deeply seated, and set up severer symptoms. In ten days or a fortnight the swelling becomes as large as the palm of the hand, or larger, covered by purple skin. The centre now softens and the surface is dotted with mattery points, which break, giving exit to bloodstained " matter." The carbuncle is not necessarily, however, at the end of its career; it may still go on spreading, until the core separates, which it may take from a fortnight to two months to do. The patient feels ill, and has shivering fits, fever, and aching in the back and limbs. In elderly or weakly subjects death may result from exhaustion or from blood-poisoning, especially when the face is the seat of the trouble. For small carbuncles the same treatment should be adopted as for boils. If the pain is very severe the doctor may give morphia, and under an anæsthetic will probably make incisions into the carbuncle and scrape out the diseased tissue. The patient's strength must be supported in every possible way : he must have a liberal diet and take such tonics as those mentioned above ; the bowels must be carefully regulated.

BONE, DISEASES OF.—Bone, including its covering membrane, the periosteum, is subject to various affections ; most of them require surgical treatment and may therefore be dealt with very briefly. One of the commonest of them, rickets, is considered separately (*see* RICKETS).

Acute periostitis, that is, inflammation of the membrane of the bone, is one of the most serious of children's diseases, which sometimes issues in mortification of the bone and death by blood-poisoning. It is most frequent in growing boys who are feeble and ill-nourished. The exciting cause is a germ, but there are certain predisposing causes, such as a blow or a kick, exposure to cold or wet, an attack of rheumatism, gonorrhœa, etc., or the inflammation may follow the extraction of a tooth. The first symptom may be a rise of temperature, followed by pain and swelling in the affected limb ; the skin soon becomes red and tense. Early treatment is important. It may be necessary to make incisions down to the bone and insert drainage-tubes ; or the whole bone may be removed from its sheath of periosteum ; or, in rare cases amputation may have to be performed.

Chronic periostitis.—The causes of chronic periostitis are similar to those of acute periostitis. Among the diseases by which it is set up are syphilis and tuberculosis. The symptoms are less severe, and there is no death of bone, though there may be thickening. The swelling is tender but pain may be absent, or there may be a dull aching which is worse at night. In feeble, emaciated children extensive abscesses sometimes form, and in these cases death sometimes ensues from pneumonia, diarrhœa, or exhaustion. In syphilitic cases there may be disease of the underlying bone. *Treatment.*—In cases in which there is much pain the limb should be put on a splint and raised on a pillow, and leeches and hot fomentations may be applied. In less severe cases a lotion of glycerin of belladonna may be used to relieve the pain, or the part may be painted with iodine. In some instances relief can only be obtained by opening the shaft of the bone. In syphilitic cases grey powder or iodide of potash should be resorted to. For delicate children cod-liver oil and iron should be prescribed.

Periosteo=myelitis, most frequent between the ages of twelve and seventeen, is another condition due to infective germs. Not only the bone and its periosteum are affected, but also, as the name myelitis implies, the marrow ; matter forms in the cavity containing the marrow, and elsewhere, and may spread until it reaches the surface. The symptoms begin with sudden and severe pain in one of the long bones, most frequently the bones of the thigh and leg, followed by swelling and redness of the soft parts. There is fever, the pulse is rapid, the face flushed, the tongue furred and dry, and delirium may supervene. If the case is left untreated, either the " matter " may find its way to the surface externally or the patient will die of exhaustion. Treatment, which must be promptly applied, is surgical. The patient's strength must be maintained by cod-liver oil, tonics, and a suitable diet.

Epiphysitis is an inflammation of the growing ends of bones which occurs in syphilitic infants and children, and in those affected with rickets or scurvy. Cases of a chronic character generally follow some accident—it may be a slight one—in scrofulous children. There is sudden and very acute pain with swelling in the neighbourhood of a joint, and the joint itself is often affected. The disease sometimes takes a very mild form, manifesting itself in pain in the ends of the bones and feverishness, symptoms which soon pass away ; in these cases it is sometimes known as " growing fever." In treatment, rest and care of the general health are important. Any constitutional affection from which the child is suffering must also be treated. Surgical measures are frequently necessary.

Tuberculosis of bone.—In this condition the neighbouring joint or joints are frequently affected also, and the two conditions may be considered together. The exciting cause is, of course, the tubercle bacillus, but the mischief is frequently started by an injury, which is usually trivial in itself —a slight blow or a moderate strain. Another great predisposing cause is lack of fresh air, sunlight and good food, to which addiction to drink may be added. The inflammation of bone leads to the formation of an abscess. When a joint is affected, early symptoms are loss of free movement, swelling and muscular wasting ; pain may take the form of " night starts," a sudden contraction of muscles occurring as the patient is dropping off to sleep ; later there is deformity. In the very young and in the very old the prospect of cure is not hopeful. Treatment consists largely in rest, fresh air, and a generous diet, supplemented by cod-liver oil or olive oil. Tuberculin is sometimes administered, but it is not a generally accepted remedy in these cases. Operation on the bone or the joint may be necessary.

BONES AND JOINTS. 1. Bones. —The human skeleton is made up of 200 distinct bones, divided into four groups—long (those of the limbs), short, flat and irregular.

How Bone Grows.—If a long bone from a young subject is examined, it will be seen that each extremity is separated from the shaft by a layer of cartilage (Fig. 10). It is from this layer of cartilage, called the epiphysial line, that the bone grows in length. The extremity of the bone beyond this epiphysial line is called the *epiphysis ;* the part between the two epiphysial lines is called the *diaphysis* or shaft (Fig. 10). By the time the bones have finished growing in length the epiphysial cartilage has

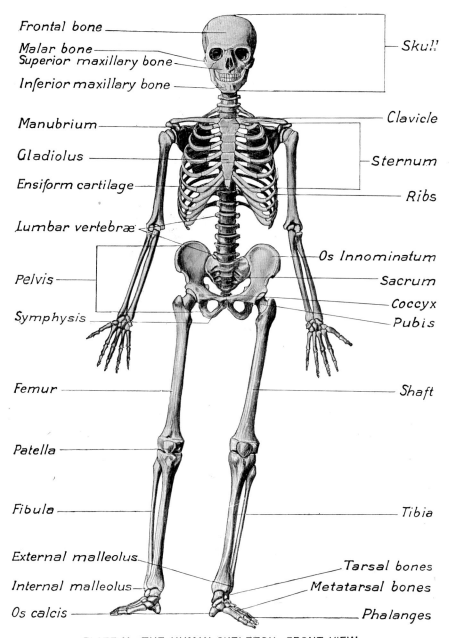

Frontal bone —
Malar bone —
Superior maxillary bone —
Inferior maxillary bone —

— Skull

Manubrium —
Gladiolus —
Ensiform cartilage —

— Clavicle

— Sternum

— Ribs

Lumbar vertebræ —

Pelvis —

Symphysis —

— Os Innominatum

— Sacrum

— Coccyx
— Pubis

Femur —

— Shaft

Patella —

Fibula —

— Tibia

External malleolus —
Internal malleolus —
Os calcis —

— Tarsal bones
— Metatarsal bones
— Phalanges

PLATE V   THE HUMAN SKELETON. FRONT VIEW.

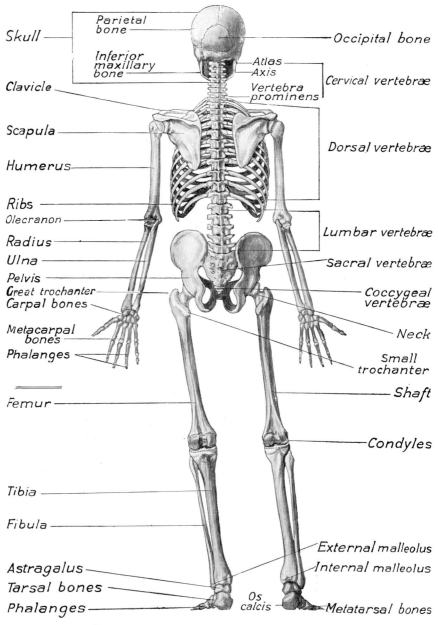

Skull — {
  Parietal bone
  Inferior maxillary bone
}

Occipital bone

Atlas
Axis
Vertebra prominens

Cervical vertebræ

Clavicle

Scapula

Dorsal vertebræ

Humerus

Ribs
Olecranon

Radius

Ulna

Lumbar vertebræ

Pelvis
Great trochanter
Carpal bones

Sacral vertebræ

Coccygeal vertebræ

Metacarpal bones

Neck

Phalanges

Small trochanter

Shaft

Femur

Condyles

Tibia

Fibula

External malleolus
Internal malleolus

Astragalus
Tarsal bones
Phalanges

Os calcis

Metatarsal bones

PLATE VI. THE HUMAN SKELETON BACK VIEW.

been converted into bone, and no trace of the epiphysial line can be seen. The growth of a bone in thickness proceeds from the *periosteum*—a dense fibrous membrane which surrounds it. The periosteum is freely supplied with blood-vessels and nerves, which pass from it into the structure of the bone.

The long bones are more or less cylindrical, with a cavity in the centre which contains the marrow, a sub-

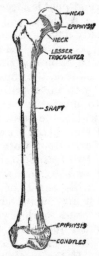

Fig. 10.—A growing thigh-bone (the femur, showing cartilage at the epiphyses before these are united to the shaft.

stance that also grows in the cancellous or less dense tissue of bones. In adult long bones the marrow consists chiefly of fat, and is yellow in colour. In the flat and short bones, and also in the long bones in young subjects, it is red, and it is in this red marrow that red corpuscles of the blood are formed, as well as some of the white corpuscles.

The names of the principal bones will be found in the illustrations of the human skeleton (Plates V, VI).

2. **Joints.**—In the human body there are 230 joints, which are bound together by strong bands or capsules

of fibrous tissue called ligaments. They are constructed on various patterns. Thus, there are ball-and-socket joints, such as those of the hip and the shoulder, capable of movement in all directions, and hinge-joints, e.g. the elbow and the ankle, in which movement is only possible in one direction. There are also two joints in which movement is rotatory ; one is the joint between the atlas and the axis at the top of the spinal column, the other is the joint between the two bones of the forearm—the radius and ulna—near the elbow. The surface of the bone that enters into the formation of a joint is covered with cartilage, and the ligaments which hold a joint together are lined with smooth membrane that secretes synovia—the glairy fluid, somewhat resembling the white of an egg, that lubricates the joint.

BONES, BROKEN (*see* Fractures).

BOTULISM (*see* Food-Poisoning).

BOWEL, FALLING OF.—In many weakly or rickety children it may happen, as the result of diarrhœa, or constipation, or threadworms, or of violent coughing, or a tight foreskin, that when there is straining in an action of the bowels, the membrane lining the rectum, the lower part of the intestine, comes down in the form of a bright-red ring. The condition is known also as *prolapse of the bowel* or *prolapsus ani*. Before undertaking its domestic treatment it is necessary to make sure that the case is not one of piles or of polypus ; this may be done by noticing the ring-like shape of the protrusion, which is not present either in piles or in polypus.

Treatment.—The bowel should be gently pressed back whenever it comes down, and if it returns often the orifice may be guarded with a pad of lint smeared with vaselin and kept in place by a bandage. If any difficulty is experienced in returning the bowel, it should be gently pressed upon with a sponge, or lightly squeezed with a piece of oiled lint or a pledget of absorbent wool dipped in cold water and wrung out. The child should be kept in bed on a nourishing diet reinforced by tonics. To prevent straining, a mild aperient should be given in the form of powdered rhubarb 3 grains, bicarbonate of soda 1 grain. Should the trouble continue, 2 to 4 ounces of infusion of quassia or decoction of oak bark may be injected into the bowel twice a day, after an action. If it should still continue, medical aid should be called in.

BOWELS, CATARRH OF.—This is a complaint from which many young children suffer, especially during the first three years of life. It most often occurs in connexion with teething, premature weaning, hot weather, or bad feeding ; but it may be due to cold, or may be a sequel of measles or of whooping-cough.

In the **acute** form several motions consisting of yellow or greenish mucus or slime mixed with undigested food are passed during the twenty-four hours, in some cases with colicky pains, and the diarrhœa may persist for a week or two, or even a month. Treatment consists in giving for two to five days, or until the diarrhœa ceases, half a teaspoonful or a teaspoonful of castor oil daily, or a daily dose of $\frac{1}{4}$ to 1 grain of calomel, either singly or divided into two or three portions, according to the child's age. If the diarrhœa becomes worse, subnitrate of bismuth may be given in doses of 5 to 20 grains daily and persevered with, while if there is much pain $\frac{3}{4}$ grain each of grey powder

and Dover's powder may be given. For diet, *see* DIARRHŒA.

Chronic catarrh of the bowels may be a sequel of an acute attack of diarrhœa occurring during the course of measles, whooping-cough, or scarlet fever, or may gradually develop as a result of chronic dyspepsia. It is most frequent in delicate children. In some cases vomiting is a more prominent symptom than the diarrhœa. If treatment is successful there may still be relapses, and the child may gradually develop rickets. Careful feeding is of most importance. For bottle-fed babies or those nursed by a sickly mother, the engagement of a healthy wet-nurse will often be sufficient to meet the case. If this is impracticable the milk should be peptonized and mixed with an equal quantity of arrowroot water, with the addition of two teaspoonfuls of cream to each 6 ounces, the whole being sweetened with sugar of milk. In some cases it may be better to substitute whey and barley-water, egg-water or meat juices for milk foods until the diarrhœa or the vomiting grows less. If the motions have an offensive odour, castor oil or small doses of calomel (*see* above) should be given, followed by a few doses of an astringent mixture such as the following :

Tannigen 60	grains
Solution of citrate of bismuth...................	$\frac{1}{2}$ ounce
Compound tincture of camphor 12	minims
Spirit of chloroform 24	minims
Dill water or cinnamon water to 1$\frac{1}{2}$ ounces	

A teaspoonful every four hours.

The child should be taken into the open air as much as possible whenever the weather is suitable.

Older children should be allowed plenty of time for out-of-door games, and a change to the seaside is very desirable. The diet must be simple, digestible, and given at regular intervals; it may include mutton broth, beef tea, eggs, white fish, broiled mutton, wholemeal bread, rice pudding, cocoa, and milk.

BOWELS, CONSUMPTION OF

(*see* CONSUMPTION OF THE BOWELS).

BOWELS, INFLAMMATION OF.

—This condition is known medically as *enteritis,* and, if the mucous membrane is chiefly affected and there is a great discharge of mucus, as *catarrhal enteritis.* If it is the colon, or large intestine, that is inflamed, the affection is termed *colitis;* if the cæcum, or first part of the colon, *typhlitis;* if the vermiform appendix, *appendicitis* (q.v.); if the rectum, or end of the bowel, *proctitis.* In popular language, enteritis is sometimes called *gastric fever,* a much-abused name that is also made to do duty for typhoid fever.

Causes.—The bowels can be inflamed by indigestible, irritating foods, and especially by food which has begun to decompose, and by unripe fruit. Other causes are wounds and injuries. Or the inflammation may arise elsewhere and extend to the bowels, or may be set up by an acute fever, such as scarlet fever or diphtheria.

Symptoms.—In severe enteritis there is a good deal of fever, and the patient is prostrated; in mild cases there is but slight fever. In an average case, besides the heightened temperature there are loss of appetite, furred tongue, bad headache, and pain and tenderness all over the abdomen, especially about the navel. When the inflammation affects chiefly the upper part of the bowel, the swelling of the mucous membrane is apt to spread up the ducts of the liver and obstruct the passage of the bile, which is taken up by the blood—producing jaundice. When the lower bowel is more affected there is severe diarrhœa, with much straining at stool, and a constant desire to pass water. In most cases of enteritis, diarrhœa is present; but in bad cases the bowel becomes paralysed, with resulting constipation. If the inflammation is chronic, the bowel will probably ulcerate.

Treatment.—The doctor will at once send the patient to bed. Food should be limited to milk, diluted with an equal quantity of soda-water or one-third of lime-water, and given very frequently. There will still be thirst, which may be assuaged by sucking ice, or by sipping barley-water or toast-water. If milk does not suit the patient, chicken or mutton broth or weak beef tea and meat essences may be substituted. Everything taken should be cold, or not more than tepid. Later, bread-and-milk, arrowroot, cornflour, tapioca, and sago may be brought into the menu, and along these lines the patient may gradually return to an ordinary diet. If the attack has been brought on by unsuitable food, a tabloid of two grains of calomel may be given as a purge, followed in three or four hours by a dose of Carlsbad salts; but if the abdomen is tender and there is much fever, an enema of soap and water should be substituted for a purge. Pain may be relieved by applying moisture and heat to the abdomen, in the form of poultices or of fomentations, and by adding 10 drops of tincture of opium to each dose of the following mixture :

Carbonate of bismuth .....80 grains
Dilute hydrocyanic acid ...24 minims
Bicarbonate of soda....... 2 drachms
Mucilage of gum........... ½ ounce
Water to 8 ounces
Two tablespoonfuls every four hours with a dessertspoonful of lemon-juice.

To guard against recurrences, which are very apt to take place, exposure to cold and all indigestible food should be avoided.

BOWELS, OBSTRUCTION OF.

—The bowels may be obstructed by various causes, which may be thrown into three groups : (1) The bowel may be pressed upon by a tumour, or it may be twisted into what is called a kink, or more learnedly a volvulus, or it may be drawn within itself (*intussusception*) as when the foot of a sock is drawn into the leg of the sock ; or in a rupture (*hernia*) it may be nipped by the surrounding parts. (2) Its walls may be diseased, as in cancer, or contracted by the formation of a scar, or it may be paralysed. (3) Its contents may be hardened and compacted as in severe constipation, or it may be blocked by collections of hair or of worms, or by large gallstones, or other foreign bodies. However it arises, intestinal obstruction is too serious a condition for domestic treatment.

In *children,* obstruction of the bowels generally takes the form of intussusception (*see* above). This arises more frequently in young children than in grown-up persons owing to greater looseness, in the former, of the attachments of the bowels. It is more likely to occur between the fourth and sixth months of life, and male children are much more prone to it than female. Unless the child is very fat the seat of the obstruction may usually be felt through the abdomen as a lump shaped something like a sausage. In the less severe cases the irregularity may correct itself and the child is gradually restored to health. Treatment consists in restoring the infolded bit of bowel to its proper place (1) by injecting water or air, (2) by mechanical means and massage, or (3) by operation. As in adults, the condition is obviously one that does not admit of domestic treatment.

BOWELS, ULCERATION OF.

—Ulcers of the duodenum, the first part of the small intestine, are considered in connexion with gastric ulcers (*see* STOMACH, ULCER OF). The forms of ulceration of the intestine met with in dysentery, typhoid fever, tuberculosis, etc., are dealt with under the diseases of which they are a symptom.

BOW - LEGS.

— This condition, termed also bandy legs, is sometimes present at birth, especially in strong babies ; in these cases it is not improbably due to compression of the legs within the womb. When it develops after birth it may be a manifestation of rickets (q.v.), but often it is the result of allowing the child, while the bones are still soft, to squat in the tailor position, and the deformity is increased by the child's weight when he walks. In many cases one leg only is affected, while the other is the subject of knock-knee ; in these instances the trouble is caused by the nurse habitually carrying the child on the same arm, one leg then becoming knock-kneed while the other grows bandy from being pressed against the bulging knee.

Treatment.—If the deformity is but slight the leg often straightens out as the child grows. Until it has done so the child must be prevented from walking. To this end a light splint, padded on both sides, should be so fixed to the inner side of the leg as to project about two inches below the heel, the foot thus being kept off the ground. The splint should be removed for about an hour night and morning while friction and massage are applied to the leg. Nutrition and the general health should be attended to as recommended in the article RICKETS. In the case of older children, whom is is not desirable to prevent from walking, a brace should be used consisting of a steel extending from the inner side of the heel to the top of the thigh, with joints at the ankle and knee. It is only in very bad cases that operation is necessary.

BRAIN (*see* NERVOUS SYSTEM).

BRAIN, COMPRESSION OF.— When a heavy blow from some blunt instrument falls upon the skull it may either fracture the bone or temporarily indent it. In the latter case the brain may be simply bruised, and the case is one of concussion (*see* the next article); on the other hand the brain may be lacerated, and when the blood has accumulated so as to press upon the brain the symptoms of compression—unconsciousness and paralysis—will appear. When the same symptoms are set up by a fracture of the skull they follow immediately upon the injury; if they are due to a slow accumulation of blood they will be delayed. The treatment is operative, the main object being to relieve the brain of the pressure to which the symptoms are due.

BRAIN, CONCUSSION OF.—The skull is not the rigid structure which it is ordinarily thought to be; when it receives a blow which is sufficient to produce unconsciousness but not sufficient to cause a fracture it bends in, and its elasticity enables it soon to recover its ordinary shape. This is what happens in cases of concussion. The immediate effect of the injury varies with the form of the blow, from complete unconsciousness to a mere passing giddiness and mental confusion, followed by some headache. In severe cases, if the patient does not

die from failure of the circulation, signs of recovery begin to appear in the course of a few minutes: he may attempt to answer when spoken to loudly, his breathing becomes perceptible, the pulse can be felt, and the pupils, though dilated, will contract in response to light. Before long, headache, giddiness, and nausea, with tremulousness and general weakness, set in, and they may be accompanied by sleeplessness. Vomiting occurs in most cases, and memory of the events just before the accident is lost. Recovery may be complete, or the patient may long suffer from headache, tenderness of the scalp, slight changes of disposition, giddiness, etc. During the stage of unconsciousness, treatment consists simply in keeping the patient well wrapped up in the recumbent position, any tight clothing being loosened. When consciousness has quite returned he should be put to bed in a darkened room and kept absolutely quiet. A purgative will be required, and no solid food should be given. If there is much headache an ice-bag may be applied to the head; if much restlessness, warm sponging should be resorted to. The patient should not attempt to get up for a week or ten days, and for at least another fortnight should avoid all exertion, especially straining at stool. If possible, he should give himself a further month's rest before resuming his ordinary activities. In certain cases there is a return of unconsciousness, with paralytic symptoms. These are cases in which the brain has been lacerated and there is an accumulation of blood which presses upon the organ; they are dealt with in the preceding article.

BRAIN, CONGESTION OF (*see* CONGESTION OF THE BRAIN).

BRAIN FEVER (*see under* MENIN-GITIS, SUPPURATIVE).

BRAIN, INFLAMMATION OF (*see* MENINGITIS, SUPPURATIVE ; MENINGITIS, TUBERCULOUS ; CEREBRO-SPINAL FEVER ; ENCEPHALITIS LETHARGICA).

BRAIN, WATER ON (*see* HYDROCEPHALUS).

BREAST, ABSCESS OF (*see* SUCKLING).

BREAST PANG (*see* ANGINA PECTORIS).

BREATH, OFFENSIVE.—Under this heading we do not propose to consider the offensive breath characteristic of such serious affections as Bright's disease, advanced phthisis, gangrene of the lung, or bronchiectasis ; here we are concerned with those ordinary cases which are due not to organic or constitutional disease, nor to bad habits such as dram-drinking or excessive smoking, but mainly to disorders which arise in the alimentary tract.

Many cases of bad breath are due to chronic indigestion and constipation. The treatment of these conditions is described in the articles INDIGESTION and CONSTIPATION ; but in the case of indigestion the breath may be benefited by taking 5 grains of powdered charcoal, or eating a charcoal biscuit half an hour after meals. Many cases of bad breath can be traced back to the beginning of the alimentary tract—the mouth. The trouble may be that the teeth are not kept clean, or that some of them are decayed. The remedy is to make a more diligent use of the tooth-brush, or to visit the dentist. Or the fault may be in the gums, which if long neglected may become spongy and produce an offensive discharge ;

or sores may have formed in the mouth. In cases such as these, formamint tablets, or tablets of chlorate of potash, cocaine and borax, are suitable. These remedies will also be found serviceable when the breath is tainted from ulcerated throat, or from long-continued inflammation of the tonsils with discharge.

Some cases of exceptionally offensive breath are caused by inflammation of the membrane that lines the antrum of Highmore, a large cavity in the upper jaw. There is a discharge from the inflamed membrane, and while part of the fluid escapes through the nose, some of it is retained in the cavity, and there decomposes and communicates an abominable odour to the breath. In these cases a slight operation is usually necessary to enlarge the opening from the antrum into the nose, so as to enable the whole of the secretion to drain away. In other cases in which the breath is overpoweringly offensive the fault may be with the nose itself, which becomes the seat of a form of chronic catarrh known as ozæna. (*See under* CATARRH, NASAL.)

BREATHING, DIFFICULTY OF. —Dyspnœa, as difficulty of breathing is termed medically, is a symptom not only of disease of the respiratory organs, but also of affections of the brain, heart, etc. It is indicated by alterations in the rate and depth of respiration, although it should be remembered that such variations are not necessarily indicative of disease ; thus, they may be due simply to vigorous exertion or to nervousness or excitement. Normally, in an adult, the act of respiration takes place from fifteen to twenty times a minute, or, roughly, once to every four beats of the pulse. It becomes more *rapid* (" shortness of breath ") in bronchitis, pneumonia, pleurisy, many affections of the heart, and fever, as well as in some forms of hysteria. When the rate is noticeably increased after some slight exertion, such as walking upstairs, anæmia, weakness, consumption, or an affection of the heart is indicated. Sometimes respiration is *deep* as well as rapid, as in diabetic coma, in which there is what is called "air-hunger," but more often it is *shallow*, as in pleurisy and peritonitis. *Slow* breathing is characteristic of compression of the brain and other affections of that organ, such as apoplexy; it also occurs in faintness. In other cerebral affections, and also in some forms of heart and lung disease and poisoning, the peculiar symptom known as *Cheyne-Stokes breathing* is encountered: respiration becomes gradually more shallow until it ceases entirely for a few seconds, and then becomes deeper and deeper until the maximum is attained, when the cycle is repeated. Other diseases of which difficult breathing is a symptom are some forms of indigestion, rickets, emphysema, asthma, croup, and diphtheria. The rough hissing or roaring noise known as *stridor*, and audible in both inspiration and expiration, indicates a block in some part of the air-passages, as in diphtheria, where the larynx is obstructed by false membrane, or in aneurysm of the aorta, where the aneurysm presses on the windpipe or on one of the bronchial tubes. Stridor may occur also when the larynx is obstructed by some object which has "gone the wrong way," or ought to have gone neither way, such as a coin. If there is an accumulation of mucus in the tubes a *rattling noise* is produced; this is the explanation of the so-called "death-rattle," the dying person being unable to expel the mucus by coughing. *Stertorous* or snoring

breathing may occur in those who are in a state of coma, as it does in ordinary sleep, from a relaxed condition of the soft palate, which vibrates with the current of air. In pneumonia there is sometimes a *grunting noise* with each expiration.

BREATHING, MECHANISM OF (*see* RESPIRATION).

BRIGHT'S DISEASE.—Inflammation of the kidneys, technically termed *nephritis*, is named after Dr. Bright, who, in 1827, first described it as a separate affection. It may be either acute or chronic.

Acute Bright's disease.—Of this form scarlet fever is one of the commonest causes; another is exposure to cold, especially after muscular exertion, which puts some strain upon the kidneys and so renders them more liable to chill. But this disease may also occur as a complication of various other diseases, or of pregnancy, or it may be set up by alcoholic excess or by the action of certain irritant drugs.

Symptoms.—The disease usually begins with shivering fits and a rise of temperature, accompanied by pain in the loins, nausea, and vomiting; other common symptoms are headache, a furred tongue and constipation. But in some cases the onset is more insidious, and is only discovered when the urine is examined. This is generally small in amount, high-coloured or "smoky," and greatly concentrated; it contains albumin, and sometimes also blood. It may be entirely suppressed, and the symptoms of uræmia—headache, drowsiness, convulsions—then begin to develop. There may or may not be dropsy. Some cases pass into the chronic form of the disease.

Treatment.—Medical attendance is, of course, necessary. The greatest care must be taken to avoid chill; the patient should therefore be clothed in flannels, and lie between blankets. The skin may be stimulated by hot-air or hot-water baths every other night, and, if no dropsy is present, plenty of water, milk and water, or barley water should be taken. The bowels may be freely opened by half a teaspoonful of compound jalap powder, followed by similar doses as required; but in mild cases it is only necessary to ensure the regular action of the bowels. The inflammation in the kidneys may be relieved at the outset by the application of leeches to the loins, and afterwards by flannels wrung out of hot water and covered with waterproof material.

At first nourishment should consist only of liquids such as those already mentioned, and even in the stage of convalescence, milk and milk puddings should still be the staple of the diet, supplemented, however, by fresh vegetables, lettuce, and ripe and cooked fruits, but not by animal food until the urine is free from albumin. In many cases a quinine and iron, or an iron and nux vomica tonic will be found beneficial.

During convalescence the patient should take only the gentlest exercise, and should be warmly clad, and he should never cease to be on his guard against chills.

Chronic Bright's disease may follow an acute attack; it may be due to habitual dram-drinking, to lead-poisoning, to gout, to the absorption of poisons from diseased bone or in exhausting illnesses, etc.; or it may be a complication of malaria. It usually comes on gradually, the early symptoms being dyspepsia and lassitude and failing appetite; in the morning the eyelids are puffy, in the evening the ankles. The urine is pale in colour and contains more or less albumin, and is sometimes mixed with blood, etc. By extreme care in avoiding strain and chill and excess of any kind the patient may survive for years, but he is no longer the man he was.

Treatment must first be directed to the cause of the disease. The more general treatment should follow the lines indicated for the convalescent stage of acute Bright's disease. Butchers' meat should be taken very sparingly; fish, chicken, poultry and game are permissible; but the diet should be ample and nourishing, so as to make up for the albumin lost in the urine. As a tonic, one teaspoonful of Easton's syrup with water may be taken three times a day before meals.

In *children* inflammation of the kidneys of the *acute* type is usually an accompaniment or sequel of scarlet fever or some other infectious disease. The symptoms resemble those of the same disease in adults (*see* above). In treatment the first thing to do is to put the child to bed in a flannel nightdress between the blankets. The body in the region of the loins should be encircled with a hot linseed poultice to which a little mustard has been added; this should be covered with oil silk and renewed as soon as it begins to get cold. The bowels should be made to act freely two or three times a day; in the case of a child of 5 years, $\frac{1}{2}$ or 1 grain of calomel may be given, followed in three or four hours by two tablespoonfuls of solution of magnesium citrate; for younger children the dose of calomel must be smaller, for older children it may be larger. In mild cases it may be sufficient to give two or three tablespoonfuls of fluid magnesia with a teaspoonful of lemon juice early in the morning, to secure regular action of the bowels. Free sweating should be encouraged by a bath of hot air, steam, or hot water. The diet must consist at first simply of milk and barley water in equal proportions given in small quantities and frequently. As the child gets better, pure milk may be given, and afterwards the doctor will allow such simple foods as arrowroot and oatmeal, with orange juice, baked apples, etc., to afford variety. Meat should only be allowed gradually, and not until some weeks after the urine is free from albumin. A simple fever mixture such as the following will be found beneficial :

Citrate of potash ....60 grains
Solution of acetate of am-
   monia .... 3 drachms
Tincture of aconite........12 minims
Glycerin .... ½ ounce
Cinnamon water to 3 ounces.
A dessertspoonful every two hours with a wineglassful of water ; for a child of 7.

During convalescence great care should be taken to prevent the child from catching cold ; warm woollen clothes should be worn, and he should only leave the house on warm dry days.

Chronic Bright's disease in children sometimes follows an acute attack which has been imperfectly cured. It may also occur from the great exhaustion caused by some antecedent disease ; this form of chronic Bright's disease is known as " waxy kidney." Treatment is on the same lines as for the acute form of the disease in children.

BROMIDROSIS (*see* SWEAT, OFFENSIVE).

BRONCHIAL TUBES (*see* RESPIRATION).

BRONCHIECTASIS.—This term means dilatation of the bronchial tubes, which is not a disease in itself, but an effect of bronchitis (*see* BRONCHITIS, CHRONIC).

BRONCHITIS, ACUTE.—Bronchial catarrh, as the affection is also styled, is one of the commonest of diseases in such climates as ours. Most prevalent in the winter months, from November to March, it finds its victims chiefly among the very young and the very old. An acute attack which takes a favourable course lasts only a few days, or at most a week or two. The chronic form of the affection, which is reserved for the next article, may persist for months and recur again and again.

In the great majority of cases the immediate cause is exposure to cold and wet, especially in those who dwell or work in warm, ill-ventilated rooms and amid unhygienic surroundings, or who are in a low state of health from some chronic disease or from being overworked or underfed.

Symptoms. — Bronchitis varies greatly in severity from a mere cold and cough to a condition in which the patient has to fight for breath. In mild cases only the large bronchial tubes are affected, but in more severe cases, known as capillary bronchitis, the inflammation at the outset attacks the small or capillary tubes also, or extends to them from the others, and even the lung tissue around may be involved, the case then becoming one of broncho-pneumonia (q.v.). The earliest symptom, as a rule, is an irritating watery flow from the nose and eyes, with frequent attacks of sneezing, sore throat, and husky voice. The patient feels hot and feverish and out of sorts, but usually the temperature is but slightly elevated ; the pulse is a little quicker than natural. Sometimes the limbs ache, and the patient seems to have a chill all over.

There is a sense of heat or rawness in the chest, particularly beneath the upper part of the breast-bone. Cough usually comes on in fits. Expectoration is at first very slight in quantity, and thin and frothy in appearance, but after a time it gets thicker and more copious, and assumes a yellow colour; it may become so thick that great difficulty is found in expelling it. Extension of the inflammation to the small tubes, which occurs more often in children than in adults, is often indicated by violent shivering fits, severe headache, and vomiting. The patient becomes short of breath; respiration is quickened and laboured; in bad cases it may be alarmingly hurried, and inspiration may be attended by distressing efforts; and there may be loud wheezing. The cough, almost continuous, is heightened into paroxysms during which the face becomes swollen, red, or purple, the arteries throb, and the veins swell. In these capillary cases the temperature may rise to 103° Fahr., or higher.

Treatment.—The patient, even in mild attacks, should keep his bed, but in any case he should not venture out of doors, but should remain in a warm but not unventilated room; the bedroom should also be warmed, transition from a warm to a distinctly colder atmosphere being dangerous. A hot bath may be taken immediately before going to bed, or the feet bathed in hot mustard and water; the bed may be warmed with a hot bottle, and a basin of hot gruel taken before settling down to sleep. If the chest is sore a hot linseed, or linseed and mustard, poultice may be applied to it, or it may be rubbed with camphorated oil until it is red. Should the patient be little or no better in the morning he must not think of getting up, and the bedroom should be kept

at a temperature of 60° to 65° Fahr. The air of the room may be moistened with a bronchitis kettle; the addition of a little eucalyptus oil or friar's balsam to the water will assist the vapour in loosening the phlegm. Throughout the illness it is important that the bowels be kept in regular action.

When the expectoration becomes thick and profuse the doctor may order a stimulating mixture such as :

Tincture of squills ....80 minims
Carbonate of ammonia .... ½ drachm
Tincture of senega .... 5 drachms
Syrup of tolu............. ½ ounce
Spirit of chloroform ...... 2 drachms
Water to 8 ounces.
Two tablespoonfuls every four hours.

The diet should be virtually limited to fluids, especially if there is much fever; the most suitable fluid foods are milk, nourishing soups and broths, and gruels; to the broths, if the tongue is not furred, a little powdered meat or chicken may be added. Milk puddings and beaten-up eggs are also suitable. In quite mild cases, fish and chicken may be allowed from the beginning; in other cases, as convalescence begins, they may be regarded as stepping-stones to an ordinary diet.

In some cases, especially in the aged and the debilitated, stimulants may be necessary to relieve the strain thrown upon the heart; from four to six tablespoonfuls of good brandy, mixed with milk or with seltzer water, may be given in the twenty-four hours.

Convalescence will be aided by tonics, such as Easton's syrup, or quinine and iron. The tendency to recurrence which is characteristic of bronchitis must be carefully guarded against. Every possible precaution must be taken against catching cold —by wearing warm clothes, by breathing through the nose, and—

except in the aged—by toning up the skin by a daily cold sponge bath, not, however, beginning with cold water.

In *children* bronchitis, both acute and chronic, is of frequent occurrence. It often develops from a cold in the head, the voice gradually becoming hoarse and the child beginning to cough, the breath at the same time being quickened and wheezy. The inflammation may spread into the finer bronchial tubes—capillary bronchitis; the cough becomes more troublesome and painful, the breathing and the pulse-rate are much quickened, and the temperature rises, it may be, to 103° or 104° Fahr. The lips turn bluish; the cheeks are flushed; the nostrils dilate with every breath; the pit of the stomach sinks in. The result in these serious cases depends upon the age of the child, the height of the fever, the extent of the disease, and the state of the general health. If the bronchitis is associated with whooping-cough, with fevers, or with constitutional diseases, the outlook is not hopeful. Instead, however, of developing into capillary bronchitis the catarrh may take a chronic course, the child suffering from an obstinate cough and having some difficulty in breathing for weeks or months. Or the catarrh may develop into asthma, or the bronchial tubes may be permanently enlarged and may undergo ulceration.

Treatment should, of course, be directed by a medical man. The child should be confined to his bed in a room of which the temperature is kept at about 65° Fahr., and should be sheltered from draughts by screens. Hot fomentations, prepared by wringing out spongiopiline in hot water and covering with jaconet, should be applied to the chest in young children. If necessary, the phlegm may be loosened by giving an emetic of powdered ipecacuanha in a teaspoonful of syrup of orange; the dose for a child under two is 5 grains, repeated if necessary in ten minutes. If the cough is irritable and a sedative is required, bromide of ammonium 15 grains, and tincture of henbane 1 drachm, may be made up into a linctus with 1 ounce of syrup of tolu; for infants the dose is one teaspoonful given occasionally. For older children codeine jelly may be recommended, or $\frac{1}{8}$ grain of codeine in a teaspoonful of syrup of cherry-bark. In chronic bronchitis in rickety children cod-liver oil is very serviceable. During an attack of bronchitis the child should be put upon a liquid diet consisting of milk, beef tea, broth, etc. A recurrence of the affection may be guarded against by the use of cold sponging, the avoidance of over-heated rooms, and by fresh air, cleanliness, and an abundance of nourishing food.

BRONCHITIS, CHRONIC.—The causes of chronic bronchitis are much the same as those of acute, with this addition, that the chronic form of the disease is often a sequel of the acute. A great many persons suffer from a mild form of chronic bronchitis without knowing it. They begin the winter with a cough and keep it until the return of spring, and this may happen regularly year after year. They speak of not being able to get rid of " this dreadful cough," but really they are victims of chronic bronchitis, and it might be some comfort to them to know it. The symptoms are like those of a mild case of acute bronchitis as described above. In certain cases, styled " dry " bronchitis, although there is violent coughing the expectoration is scanty, and is only expelled with difficulty, as small pearly masses; this is believed by some to be a gouty form of the complaint. In other cases the expectoration is abundant; this form is termed *bronchorrhœa*. Often there is shortness of breath. The bronchial tubes may in time come to be dilated—*bronchiectasis*; or, as the result of the violent coughing, frequently repeated, air-sacs of the lungs may not only be distended but rupture—*emphysema* (q.v.). The preventive and tonic measures advised for acute bronchitis should be adopted, and with them as generous a diet as the patient can tolerate. Of medicines, one of the most effective is iodide of potash—3 grains thrice a day in tablets dissolved in water, or combined with the bark and ammonia mixture (p. 289). In " dry " bronchitis a mixture consisting of bicarbonate of soda 1 drachm, chloride of soda ½ drachm, carbonate of ammonia ½ drachm, and spirit of chloroform 2 drachms, with water to 8 ounces (two tablespoonfuls, with the same quantity of hot water, every six hours), may be taken. Where, on the other hand, expectoration is profuse, turpentine is suitable, 20 or 30 drops of spirit of turpentine being added from time to time to the water in a bronchitis kettle for inhalation. The cough may be eased and expectoration, where abundant, lessened by the use of a stimulating liniment —say compound camphor, rubbed thoroughly into the back and chest every night and morning and persevered with for two or three weeks at a time. All that has been said in the preceding article about taking care to avoid cold applies with double force to persons who have long suffered from chronic bronchitis.

BRONCHO-PNEUMONIA.—This serious affection almost always begins as bronchitis, the inflammation of the small bronchial tubes extending to the surrounding lung tissue, and so setting up pneumonia, or inflammation of the lung. It is also known as *catarrhal pneumonia,* because of the exudation from the inflamed mucous membrane of the tubes, and as *lobular pneumonia,* to distinguish it from ordinary or lobar pneumonia. The significance of the terms " lobar " and " lobular " will be seen when it is remembered that each lung is divided into *lobes*—two in the case of the left lung and three in the case of the right, and that each lobe is composed of a multitude of tiny and quite separate divisions or *lobules.* In lobular pneumonia scattered groups of these lobules are attacked, not the lobe as a mass, but as the disease progresses the inflammation may spread from group to group until the condition resembles lobar pneumonia. The causes of broncho-pneumonia are virtually the same as those of bronchitis.

Symptoms.—Breathing becomes more rapid and more difficult, the pulse quicker and weaker, the cough more violent and more persistent, the expectoration thicker and more tenacious, and streaked with blood. There is usually vomiting, often accompanied by diarrhœa, and in bad cases the tongue is brown and dry and there is distressing thirst. The fever often undergoes daily fluctuation, and the temperature may attain 104° or 105° Fahr. The disease runs no definite course. If it terminates favourably, recovery is very gradual, and is apt to be incomplete, the patient being left with a tendency to some form of lung disease, or to rickets, etc.

Treatment should follow the general lines laid down for the treatment of acute bronchitis (*see under* BRONCHITIS, ACUTE). The bedroom must be kept quite warm, the temperature being steadily maintained at about 64° Fahr., and while ventilation should not be neglected, the greatest care must be taken to exclude draughts. The steam kettle may be constantly kept going; a little carbolic acid (1 in 60) may be added to the water. Liniments of compound camphor, mustard, or turpentine should be rubbed into the chest and back, and a quilted cotton-wool jacket worn. To deal with the fever, sponging with tepid or cold water is usually sufficient. In many cases, if the difficulty of breathing becomes greater and the pulse feeble, alcohol is necessary, and a mixture containing strychnine or digitalis may be prescribed. If suffocation threatens, oxygen may be inhaled, or an emetic given to get rid of the accumulated phlegm. Emetics should, however, be avoided if possible. The food must be light and nourishing—diluted milk for babes, broths, beef tea, whipped eggs and milk, whey, etc., for older patients. During convalescence the diet should include solid food and be supplemented by as much cod-liver oil as can be digested. An iron and quinine, or iron, quinine and strychnine tonic may be given with advantage. The greatest care must be taken to avoid chill.

BRONCHORRHŒA (*see* BRONCHITIS, CHRONIC).

BRUISES.—The colour of a contusion or bruise is due to bleeding from torn blood-vessels beneath the surface. The nearer they are to the surface, the sooner the bruise appears. The application of cold and pressure will do something to prevent or mitigate bruises by tightening up the bleeding vessels. Ice, cold fomentations, vinegar and water, or a metal object may be used for the purpose. There is no special virtue in the popular expedient for preventing a black eye —the application of a beefsteak : such effect as it has is due simply to its being cool. Cold-water bathing, or firm pressure of a handkerchief wrung out of cold water, is more effectual. The final disappearance of a bruise may be hastened by hot fomentations.

BUBONIC PLAGUE(*see* PLAGUE).

BUG-BITES (*see* STINGS AND BITES).

BULBAR PARALYSIS.—The medulla or bulb is that part of the brain in which are situated the nervous centres that govern respiration, the action of the heart, the processes of digestion, the blood supply, the movements of the tongue, larynx, etc. If, therefore, its functions are interfered with, the results are very serious ; instant death may ensue, while in less severe disturbances the patient may find it difficult or impossible to masticate or swallow. Little can be done in the way of treatment.

BUNIONS.—The swelling which bears this name usually occurs at the base of the big or of the little toe, as the result of ill-fitting or improperly shaped boots or shoes. The bone, covered with a water pad or bursa, as in the condition termed " housemaid's knee," projects and is subject to pressure from the boot. The bursa may become inflamed and cause acute pain, and "matter" may form and escape. The trouble may in this way be cured, or on the other hand a running sore may be left which is very disinclined to heal.

Treatment.—The bunion should be relieved from pressure in the same way as a corn, by means of a circular pad with a hole left in the centre. It may be reduced in size by an occasional painting with liniment of iodine. The pain will be mitigated by a boric-acid poultice at night ; a loose soft boot with a wide sole and square toe should be worn in the day. If the bunion becomes inflamed, a warm compress should be applied and the foot rested. If matter forms in it an incision with a surgeon's knife will be necessary. In bad cases the projecting bone, or even the joint itself, may have to be removed.

BURNS AND SCALDS.—The injuries caused by dry heat (burns) and by moist heat (scalds) are so essentially similar that they may be considered together. There is also great similarity between them and the injuries produced by corrosive liquids, such as caustic potash and nitric acid, and in legal terminology the term " burns " covers injuries of the latter group.

Degrees of burns.—Burns are classified in six degrees, according to their depth. In the *first* degree there is simply a scorching and redness of the skin, which becomes normal after some hours, or after a day or two. In the *second* degree the scarf skin is raised from the true skin in the form of blisters, containing a clear yellowish fluid ; healing takes place rapidly, and no scars are left. In the *third* degree the scarf skin and the upper part of the true skin are destroyed. The pain, considerable at first, soon passes off, to return, however, a few days later, when the burnt tissues separate. A dull scar is left after healing, but there is little contraction or deformity. In the *fourth* degree the whole thickness of the skin is destroyed, as well as some of the tissues lying immediately beneath. As the nerve-endings also are destroyed, pain is felt chiefly in surrounding parts that have been burnt

less deeply. In these burns " matter " almost always forms, and a good deal of scarring is left, which by contraction may cause serious deformity. In the *fifth* degree the destruction goes still deeper, so as to include more or less muscle, while in the *sixth* degree all the burnt part is completely charred.

Symptoms.—The first effect of a serious burn is *shock*, manifested by a rapid and feeble pulse, a lowered temperature, extreme thirst, and cold sweat. In from twenty-four to forty-eight hours the stage of *inflammation* begins, with a rise of temperature, and lasts until the tissues which have been destroyed separate—from one to two weeks. Then begins the stage of *suppuration*, or matter-formation, which only ends with the healing of the wound, and may endure for months.

Treatment.—In severe cases the first thing to do is to counteract shock. This is the business of the medical man, who will apply warmth, give brandy, and if necessary adopt further measures. The next thing is to remove the clothing from the injured part. This must be done with the greatest possible gentleness, so that the blisters may not be broken or the loosened skin dragged away. Boots should not be pulled off, but, the laces having been undone, the back of the boot should be slit open with a knife or scissors ; the stockings also should be slit up. If clothing adheres to the burnt skin the surrounding parts should be cut away and the adherent parts soaked with olive oil until they are loosened. Having been freed of clothing, the burn should be protected from the air by a sprinkling of flour, starch, arrowroot or powdered chalk, covered with a thick layer of cotton-wool which may be kept in place by an easy bandage. The doctor may snip **away** the blisters in order to apply anti-septics to the wound ; if not, the blisters should be simply pricked to give exit to the fluid, and the loose skin left to protect the tender surface from the air. In washing burns a little bicarbonate of soda or common salt should be added to the water, with a few drops of some mild anti-septic, such as Condy's fluid, to neutralize the smell. When destroyed tissues have come away in the form of what are called sloughs, ulcers will be left which will need to be dressed with boric or zinc or other ointment.

Scalds in the mouth and throat, caused by swallowing hot fluids, need to be carefully watched, even when not serious in themselves, because of the danger of suffocation from swelling. The doctor may find it necessary to open the windpipe (tracheotomy), or he may place a tube in the throat (intubation), to enable breathing to proceed. Pending his arrival a sponge or flannel wrung out of hot water should be applied to the front of the neck, the patient meanwhile sucking ice or sipping cold water or olive oil.

Electrical burns are similar to those inflicted by the more ordinary forms of heat, and require the same kind of treatment. If the patient is in contact with a live rail, and no thick rubber gloves are available, a mackintosh may be folded several times and placed on the ground, and, standing on this, the helper may push him off the rail as quickly as possible with a dry stick, held in something dry—a rubber tobacco pouch if pos-sible, or, failing this, in the folds of another mackintosh. If no mackin-toshes are at hand, it is less dangerous for one wearing rubber- or crepe-soled boots to push the patient away from the rail than for one who is wearing leather-soled boots. It should be remembered that a wet object is a better conductor of the electric current than a dry one.

BURSÆ.—A bursa may be roughly described as a water cushion which serves the purpose of diminishing friction and facilitates gliding move-ments where, as in the case of the knee-cap, one structure has to move over another. There are many of these bursæ in various parts of the body, and as the result of repeated pressure they may become enlarged and inflamed. Thus arise such con-ditions as " housemaid's knee " and " miner's elbow," caused in the one case by kneeling on the floor or ground, in the other by working while resting on the elbow. Another part in which the trouble may occur is just above the heel, where it may be caused by ill-fitting boots or by over-exertion. If the inflammation is acute, the affection is very painful, an abscess forms, and there is danger of the inflammation spreading to the joint. If it is chronic, the skin over the swelling undergoes some thickening, and may be formed into ridges. The *treatment* is to rest the limb and apply poultices or fomentations to the swelling. In chronic " housemaid's knee " nothing may be necessary beyond applying Scott's ointment on lint and covering with strapping ; this will promote absorption. In cases where the skin is much thickened it may be necessary to remove the bursa by operation. To prevent the forma-tion of bursæ, a soft object such as a cushion should be interposed between the knee, or whatever part is in question, and the hard surface which receives the pressure.

C

CACHETS (*see* MEDICINES, AND HOW THEY ARE MEASURED).

CAISSON DISEASE (*see* DIVER'S PALSY).

CALCULUS (*see* STONE IN THE BLADDER; STONE IN THE KIDNEY; GALLSTONES).

CALLUS (*see* FRACTURES).

CAMPHOR POISONING.—Sometimes camphor liniment is drunk in mistake, or an overdose of spirit of camphor, Rubini's essence, or camphorated oil may be taken. The treatment is to give an emetic, to apply warmth to the extremities, and to douche the head and chest with hot and cold water. Smelling salts may be used, but alcoholic stimulants must be avoided.

CANCER.—Tumours, as is explained in the article on that subject, may be either benign or malignant, and of the two great groups of malignant tumours, cancer (or carcinoma) and sarcoma (q.v.), the former is much the more common. Formerly every malignant tumour was termed a cancer, and the term is still sometimes used in that wide sense; the distinction between the two forms turns upon the character of the cells of which they are composed. Cancer, to use the word in its stricter sense, prevails much more among civilized than among barbarous races. It is more common in middle and later than in advanced life. It scarcely ever occurs in persons under the age of 20; between 20 and 40 there is a gradual rise in susceptibility, but the next fifteen years are pre-eminently those in which cancer flourishes, while after the age of 55 it begins to become less frequent. It attacks women more often than men, because of the great liability of the uterus and the female breast; but for this, cancer would be less common in women than in men, who are much more prone than women to cancer of the stomach. Cancer may attack almost every part of the body, but it is the three organs that have been mentioned, the uterus, the female breast, and the stomach, that are most often the seat of its ravages.

Cause.—The statistics that have been quoted to prove that cancer is infectious, and that certain dwellings, which have been styled "cancer houses," are centres of infection, have not borne the test of scrutiny. Nor has the theory that cancer is hereditary found acceptance; at most, nothing but a susceptibility to the disease can be transmitted, and even that is by no means certain.

Until recently there was little to show for all the researches that have been made throughout the civilized world into the cause of cancer. But in 1925 Dr. W. E. Gye and Mr. J. E. Barnard (the latter a skilful amateur microscopist), working together under the auspices of the Medical Research Council, announced that they had discovered both in cancer and in sarcoma a living organism which they believed to be one factor in the production of these growths. Their theory is that the organism, which Mr. Barnard succeeded in photographing by a special method, although it is invisible by the microscopic methods generally used in bacteriology, is harmless in itself but, when brought into contact with a chemical substance produced by living cells as the result, for example, of chronic irritation, it is capable of giving rise to a malignant tumour. The organism, then, if this theory is correct, is the essential factor and the chemical substance the accessory factor in malignant disease. If this discovery should come to be generally accepted, we may hope that before long the means for averting cancer and sarcoma by some form of inoculation will be devised.

It has long been known that chronic irritation of a part is sometimes followed by cancer. Thus cancer of the tongue often arises when this organ has long been irritated by an ill-fitting dental plate, or by a jagged tooth, or by overmuch smoking; workers with substances such as soot, tar and paraffin are especially liable to cancer of the skin; and prolonged action of the X-rays, in the days when the danger of setting up serious inflammation of the skin by this means was not understood, has not infrequently been followed by cancer.

Symptoms and course.—The symptoms of cancer vary with the organ attacked. Though usually accompanied by a good deal of pain of a stinging, shooting kind, it is not always, especially in the earlier stages, a painful disease. A swelling is always present, though in an internal organ it may not be perceptible until the disease has reached a late stage. Cancer almost always tends to increase, and sooner or later it is infected with microbes from other parts of the body, or from without, and there is ulceration with an offensive discharge. In the great majority of cases the general health suffers; the patient becomes thin and feeble, and his complexion acquires a sallow, earthy tint which is one of the marks of the disease; he is, in fact, poisoning himself. Further, particles of the growth are carried by the lymph or the blood to other parts of the body, and there they take root, so to speak, and grow. This is one of the distinguishing features of malignant as compared with innocent tumours; this, too, is in many cases the explanation of the recurrence that is some-

times reported after operations for cancer: the disease may have been entirely removed from the organ in which it originated, but if it had begun to disseminate, sooner or later it will reappear elsewhere. It is of the first importance, therefore, that anyone who has reasonable ground for suspecting cancer should without delay undergo medical examination. Far better consult a doctor early about a growth, even though it may seem unimportant, than continue to watch one slowly increase, afraid to know the truth. There is usually so much pain with cancer of the stomach that the patient is sure to take advice early, but in the uterus there may be nothing more than discomfort until the disease has advanced too far for effective operation. Every woman should therefore know that any escape of blood from the vagina, except during the monthly periods, any excessive loss in the monthly periods, and any coloured or other discharge after " the change of life," are suspicious symptoms, which should lead her to seek medical advice. In cancer of the breast the first sign of the disease in many cases is the presence of a lump, and there may be no pain, or other symptom, for a long time. Such a lump is not necessarily cancer, but it may be, and it should never, therefore, be disregarded, as in too many cases it is until too late.

The course the disease will run, if left untreated, or treated too late, is quite indefinite; the end may come in a few months, as when some organ like the stomach, whose functions are necessary for the maintenance of life, is affected, or it may be postponed for years, as in cancer of the female breast, or of the skin. In the old, it progresses much more slowly than in the young. It should be added that in rare cases cancer undergoes spontaneous cure.

Treatment.—The only effective treatment for cancer is early operation. If the disease is entirely extirpated before it has begun to disseminate, there is good hope that the patient is cured, but if operation is too long delayed cure is out of the question. All the many " cancer cures " that are vaunted from time to time, violet leaves and the rest, may be dismissed as not worth consideration ; when put to the test by competent experimenters, as all of them have been, they have proved to be worthless. The only non-operative measures that should be excepted from this condemnation are the X-rays and radium, and injections of specially prepared lead. In some cases of superficial cancer radium has removed all traces of the disease. But it is as adjuncts to operation, or as palliatives in cases in which operation is impossible or has failed, that radium and X-rays are chiefly valuable in cancer. They may be used to prepare the way for operation, or to follow operation and destroy any cancer-cells that have escaped removal, while in cases in which they can only be used as palliatives they are of inestimable service in retarding the progress of the disease, in assuaging pain, and in diminishing ulceration and offensive odour. There are good reports of the treatment by injections of lead, used in cases in which operation is inadmissible ; it is still in the experimental stage.

CANCRUM ORIS.—Canker, or gangrene, of the mouth is a very serious but fortunately rare affection occurring between the ages of two and nine, usually as a sequel or a complication of measles, typhoid fever, or some other exhausting disease in delicate and ill-nourished children. The gangrenous parts of the cheek come away, both inside and outside, leaving a hole which exposes the jaw. The poison from the diseased tissues infects the blood, and death may result either from exhaustion or from pneumonia. If the patient does not recover before the cheek is perforated, the disease leaves behind it deformity, which may, however, be greatly modified by operation. Treatment consists mainly in cutting out the diseased tissues, or destroying them by cauterization.

CANITIES (*see* Grey Hair).

CAPILLARY HÆMORRHAGE (*see* Hæmorrhage).

CAPSULES (*see* Medicines and how they are Measured).

CARBOHYDRATES (*see* Food).

CARBOLIC-ACID POISONING.—Carbolic-acid lotion may be given in mistake for medicine, or carbolic oil for castor oil. The lips will be found white and burnt, and the breath will smell of carbolic. If a doctor is at hand he will wash out the stomach with diluted saccharated lime-water or fresh lime-water. Milk and white of egg may be administered in abundance, with olive oil and water—$\frac{1}{4}$ pint of oil to a pint of water; but the doctor will remove the olive oil from the stomach so that the carbolic may not be absorbed by it on reaching the intestines. Epsom salts may be given in sips—a tablespoonful to a tumblerful of warm water. Shock should be counteracted by brandy, with warmth and friction to the extremities.

CARBONIC-ACID SNOW, TREATMENT BY.—The application to the surface of the human body of extreme degrees of cold produces results similar to those produced by the application of great heat. When liquefied carbonic acid gas is allowed to escape from the steel cylinders in which it is subjected to great pressure, the sudden expansion it undergoes causes a great lowering of temperature and it freezes in the form of snow. This is pressed into solid pencils or sticks, which are used to destroy warts, moles, small patches of eczema and psoriasis, the lesions of lupus vulgaris, rodent ulcer, etc. The treatment is almost painless, but for the first hour or so there may be a sense of smarting which is uncomfortable rather than painful. There is little or no scarring if proper antiseptic precautions are taken. This method of treatment is sometimes called *freezing* or *refrigeration*.

CARBUNCLES (*see* BOILS AND CARBUNCLES).

CARCINOMA (*see* CANCER).

CARIES, DENTAL (*see* TEETH, DECAY OF).

"CARRIERS."—Infections are often disseminated by persons who, though in their ordinary state of health, harbour the germs of disease, it may be in the throat, or the intestine, or the gall-bladder, or the urinary tract. In some cases these " carriers," as they are called, have had the disease in question and have not got rid of the germs ; in others, they are in the incubation stage ; in yet others, they have never had the disease, and do not subsequently develop it ; but in all cases alike they are a source of danger to those around them. Their infectivity may last for a few weeks only, or may persist for many years. The diseases most frequently spread in this way are typhoid fever, cholera, dysentery, diphtheria, and cerebro-spinal fever. Obviously, carriers of germs that haunt the urinary tract or the intestine, such as those of typhoid, cholera, or dysentery, ought not to engage in employments that involve the handling of food, and should thoroughly cleanse the hands

after unloading the bowels or the bladder. Carriers of germs which, like that of cerebro-spinal fever, have their habitat in the throat, should avoid kissing.

CARTILAGE (*see* BONES AND JOINTS).

CATALEPSY.—This condition is one of the symptoms of dementia præcox (*see under* INSANITY), and is often a manifestation of that strangest of all disorders, hysteria. It may or may not be preceded by headache, giddiness, or hiccough. The patient suddenly loses consciousness or becomes dazed, the limbs remaining in the position in which they happened to be at the moment of seizure. At first they offer firm resistance to movement, but after a time they can be moved, but will remain in the position in which they are left. The attack may last for a few minutes only or for several hours ; in some cases it never recurs. Treatment consists chiefly in applying stimulation, in the form of cold douches, ammonia to the nostrils, electricity, etc. Emetics may also be given, for if the patient can be made to vomit the attack may be cut short. Between the attacks tonic treatment is required.

CATAPHORESIS (*see* ELECTRICAL TREATMENT).

CATARACT.—Cataract is a not uncommon disease of the lens of the eye, the transparent convex structure which lies behind the iris (*see* EYE). Usually as a degeneration of old age, but sometimes from inflammation originating in other parts of the eye, or from injury, or from diabetes, while some cases are congenital, the lens loses its transparency and becomes milky in appearance, and although no pain is felt, blindness is gradually produced. The only treatment consists in removing the lens of the eye and wearing suitable convex glasses. In many cases it is necessary to wait until the cataract has reached maturity.

CATARRH, NASAL.—Literally, a catarrh is "a flowing down," and as used medically the word denotes an excessive flow of mucus from a mucous membrane as the result of inflammation. The mucous membrane of any organ may be attacked in this way—for instance, the lining membrane of the stomach as in gastritis, that of the intestine as in enteritis and colitis, that of the bronchial tubes as in bronchitis. But it is catarrh of the nasal mucous membrane with which we are most familiar, and when the term catarrh is used alone it is this affection which is signified.

Formerly cold, and especially damp cold, was regarded as sufficiently accounting for an attack of *acute nasal catarrh*, or *coryza*, as the affection is also called. Investigation has, however, shown that the action of cold or damp does not cover all the ground. For example, workers in the Ben Nevis observatory are able to live in an atmosphere of clouds, fog and rain without taking cold, and members of the arctic and antarctic expeditions of recent years have enjoyed a similar immunity. We must, therefore, look to some other source for the essential cause of nasal catarrh. That the affection is really one of the many germ diseases might have been suspected from the fact the colds are frequently infectious. Thus it is a matter of common observation that a cold will "run through" a house or a school. It has been observed, too, that the inhabitants of sequestered islands sometimes contract colds when visited by a ship containing infected persons, as polar explorers may when they return to warmer climates. There can be no doubt, therefore, that acute nasal catarrh is a microbic affection, and bacteriological investigations tend to show that it may be due to several different germs. The germs may be caught from the breath of an infected person who generously distributes them broadcast in sneezing and coughing, or they may be comfortably residing in the inner parts of the nose waiting until the nasal mucous membrane becomes irritated or temporarily enfeebled, when they fasten upon it and work their wicked will.

While, however, damp and cold are not the exciting cause of an acute cold, they undoubtedly form the chief predisposing causes, acting, no doubt, by temporarily diminishing the natural defensive powers of the nasal mucous membrane. Other predisposing influences are the hot, impure atmosphere of crowded rooms, railway carriages, etc.; living in insanitary dwellings; fatigue, hunger, anxiety and mental depression, and the excessive use of alcohol or tobacco. Some persons, even when not in a low state of health, are peculiarly liable to catch cold; in certain cases this is because of some structural defect in the nose, or it may be because of enlarged tonsils or the presence of polypi or adenoids.

Symptoms.—The incubation period of a cold varies from a few hours to two or three days. Most often the inflammation starts in the nose, whence it may spread along the Eustachian tube to the middle ear, causing slight deafness or earache; or into the mouth, making the tongue sore and the gums tender; or backwards to the throat, larynx, windpipe, and bronchial tubes, and even the lungs themselves; or upwards into the cavities of the frontal bone, where it gives rise to a sense of heaviness and headache; or along the tear-ducts to the eyes, making them red and watery. Sometimes, however, it may begin behind the nose, whence it spreads forwards to the nose and downwards to the throat. In a few cases it originates in the larynx; when it does so it is less likely to spread to the nose than to the bronchial tubes. One of the first symptoms is frequently-repeated sneezing; the nasal membrane fills with blood and is swollen, feels stopped up and uncomfortable, and secretes a thin, saltish fluid which is irritating to the skin.

Treatment.—The best remedy for a cold is to spend twenty-four hours in bed. A preliminary measure, in order to encourage perspiration, is to take a hot bath, or soak the feet in hot water and mustard, winding up with a basin of hot gruel or a glass of hot water flavoured according to choice. If the patient cannot or will not spend twenty-four hours in bed, this preliminary measure may be sufficient in itself to cure the cold if it is in a quite early stage. Dover's powder, which contains opium, is sometimes prescribed by way of increasing the perspiration and relieving the aching and feverish feelings, but this drug is better avoided, for it may give rise to headache in the morning. It is better to rely upon such a drug as aspirin or phenacetin to relieve feverishness and other uncomfortable feelings. An aperient may be taken at night, followed by a dose of mineral water in the morning. The patient should take a reasonable quantity of nourishing food, and a tonic such as the bark and ammonia or quinine and iron mixture (see pp. 89 and 42).

In some cases, though not perhaps in many, it is possible to stop a cold in its initial stages by means of drugs. One drug used for this purpose is ammoniated tincture of quinine, two or three doses of a teaspoonful in half a wineglassful of water; another is spirit of camphor, 10 drops in water or on a lump of sugar every half hour for three doses.

Among local applications, one of the most popular, by reason of its soothing effects, consists in inhalations of eucalyptus oil, a few drops of which are placed in a jugful of hot water and the steam breathed in and out of the nose for a few minutes. Another application consists of a mixture of carbolic acid (1 drachm), strong solution of ammonia (1 drachm), distilled water (2 drachms) and rectified spirit (3 drachms); a few drops are sprinkled on a pocket-handkerchief and inhaled every two or three hours. The feeling of stuffiness may also be relieved by bathing the nose and forehead in hot water. Substances applied directly to the mucous membrane are ordinary ammonia, smelling salts, and menthol snuff.

In acute nasal catarrh, prevention is much more important than treatment. Unfortunately, one attack, instead of conferring immunity, as is the case in many infectious diseases, leaves behind it greater liability to another. Care should therefore be taken to avoid exposure to damp and cold; the living room should not be overheated, the bedroom should be well ventilated, clothing should be sufficient but not excessive. The action of the skin should be maintained by friction, an abundance of open-air exercise should be taken, and a wide berth given to infected persons. Those who are exceptionally liable to colds may be advised to take a short course of vaccine treatment early in the winter—say in October or November.

Chronic nasal catarrh is sometimes a sequel of one or more acute attacks; it may be a legacy from measles, scarlatina, or some other infectious fever; it may be caused by inflamed adenoids (*see* ADENOIDS) or by some other form of nasal obstruction; or it may be set up by the inhalation of dust in occupations such as those of stonemasons, millers, and furriers. The predisposing causes are virtually the same as those of acute nasal catarrh. The affection is much more frequently met with in men than in women, in children than in adults; it seldom occurs in old age.

Symptoms.—The discharge from the nasal mucous membrane may be not much beyond the normal, or there may be a good deal of thick, tenacious phlegm. The nasal obstruction may not be constant; it is often worse after meals, and also at night, when the patient may be obliged to breathe through the mouth.

Treatment.—Hot and dust-laden atmospheres should be avoided, and attention must be paid to the general health, which should be brought up to the normal standard by exercise in fresh air, by nutritious food, cod-liver oil, quinine and iron tonic, etc. The patient should be careful not to blow the nose violently, nor to indulge in sniffing, or " hawking," for such actions only increase the congestion which is the cause of the discomfort. A lotion may be employed to free the nasal passages of stagnant mucus, such as the following: Bicarbonate of soda 5 grains, biborate of soda 5 grains, chloride of soda 5 grains, white sugar 5 grains; dissolve in 6 ounces of water. Nose lotions may be given by means of the nasal douche, one form of which consists of a tube with a nozzle which is inserted in the nostril, while the other end is placed in the vessel containing the lotion; by squeezing the bulb in the tube the liquid is made to flow into the nostril. (Fig. 11.) In using a nasal douche the patient should bend the head slightly forward, and open and breathe entirely through the mouth; the soft palate will then close up the back of the nostrils like a curtain, and the lotion, instead of passing down into the throat, will run back through the other nostril.

The douche may be followed by the

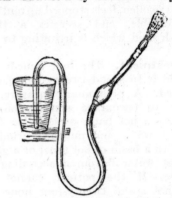

Fig. 11.—Syphon nasal douche.

application of an ointment such as the following:

Ichthyol	1 drachm
Coumarin	2 grains
Paraffin ointment	5 drachms

A short camel-hair pencil is twisted round in this ointment and then inserted in the affected nostril, which is pressed from the outside as the pencil is withdrawn.

Ozæna.—This is a special form of chronic nasal catarrh. The name is derived from a Greek word meaning stench, the characteristic symptom being that the thick secretion in the nose stagnates, putrefies, and dries into evil-smelling crusts. The odour is so offensive that the affection is sometimes styled " stink-nose." This very disagreeable affection usually begins in youth, and is much more common in women than in men. Of the cause, little is known. Treatment, which must be carried out by a medical man, consists in removing the crusts, cleansing the nose often enough to prevent the formation of further deposits, and packing it with strips of medicated ribbon gauze.

"CATHETER LIFE" (*see* PROSTATE GLAND, ENLARGED).

CAUSTIC-POTASH AND CAUSTIC - SODA POISONING.—The symptoms and treatment of poisoning by caustic potash or by caustic soda (soap lees) are the same as in poisoning by the other alkalis (*see* AMMONIA POISONING).

CAUSTICS.—These substances are used to destroy diseased tissues, or poisons that have been introduced into the body through a breach in the skin (as in snake-bite). Among the drugs used in this way are several acids, such as carbolic, nitric, hydrochloric, sulphuric, chromic, and glacial acetic acids, silver nitrate, acid nitrate, red oxide, perchloride of mercury, chloride of zinc, chloride of antimony, and arsenic. Morbid tissues may also be destroyed by the application of physical heat—*cauterization*. The galvano-cautery may be employed, or Paquelin's cautery, a hollow, platinum point heated by a current of benzene vapour, or the "actual" cautery, a white-hot iron. Another means of securing the same result is by the application of extreme degrees of cold (*see* CARBONIC-ACID SNOW, TREATMENT BY).

CELLULITIS.—Sometimes a wound of the skin—it may be a mere prick or slight abrasion—is followed by erysipelas (q.v.), which is an inflammation of the skin itself; in other cases it is followed by cellulitis—i.e. inflammation of the tissue beneath the skin, as well as of the skin itself. In cellulitis, as in erysipelas, the affection is caused by a germ. In severe cases of cellulitis there may be a high temperature, and both the skin and the underlying tissue may be destroyed. The patient must take to his bed, hot boric-acid fomentations should be used to allay the pain, and in severe cases the doctor will make incisions, and apply suitable after-treatment. Vaccines are sometimes beneficial.

CEREBELLUM (*see* NERVOUS SYSTEM).

CEREBRO-SPINAL FEVER.—This disease is known medically as epidemic cerebro-spinal meningitis—since it consists in inflammation of the meninges or covering membranes of the brain and spinal cord—and popularly as "spotted fever," from the blood spots which in some cases appear on the skin. It is caused by the germ known as the *Diplococcus intracellularis meningitidis*, and is predisposed to by physical exhaustion and mental depression. It may appear either in isolated cases or in epidemics. Prone to attack children and young adults, especially young soldiers and recruits, it is only contagious in a rather low degree, and cannot be transmitted, as can scarlet fever, by a second person to a third. It is believed to be conveyed by the secretions of the mouth, nose, and conjunctiva—the lining membrane of the eye and eyelids—where the germ ordinarily dwells.

Symptoms.—Cerebro-spinal fever is very variable in its manifestations. In the *ordinary* form it begins suddenly with shivering fits, severe aching in the back of the head, and vomiting. The muscles of the neck stiffen to a painful degree, until the head may be drawn back between the shoulder-blades ; there are severe pains in the back and limbs, tremors and spasms in various muscles, and often acute tenderness along the spine. As the headache grows worse the eyes become very sensitive to light and the ears to noise. The temperature rises to 101° or 102° Fahr. ; delirium is an early symptom, but gradually subsides into stupor. It is in the *malignant* form of the disease that the spots are more usually met with. The symptoms in this form are of the same character as in the ordinary type, but more pronounced, and death may occur in the course of a few hours. In some cases the disease assumes a *chronic* character and may last for six months or even longer. The symptoms in certain cases are so vague that they would escape recognition except during the course of an epidemic. The disease is sometimes complicated by inflammation of the lungs, of the pleura, of the heart, of the salivary glands, etc., and it may have such serious sequels as inflammation of the eye or the ear, or of nerves, producing blindness, or deafness, or facial paralysis or squint.

Treatment.—Some favourable reports have been made of Flexner and Jobling's serum, which is injected into the spinal canal ; and the withdrawal of cerebro-spinal fluid by puncturing the sheath in the region of the loins appears in some cases to have had good results. But apart from these measures, little can be done except to endeavour to combat the symptoms —the headache and spinal tenderness by ice-caps and ice-bags, etc., the fever and restlessness and pain by hot baths. The patient must lie in a cool, quiet, darkened and well-ventilated room, and be fed with milk, milk foods, and strong broths, small

doses of brandy or whisky being administered to counteract depression and exhaustion. During the frequently long convalescent period tonics such as quinine and iron, and plenty of nourishment, should be given, and, for the headache with which the patient still may be troubled, phenacetin and caffeine.

CEREBRO-SPINAL FLUID (*see* Nervous System).

CEREBRUM (*see* Nervous System).

CERVICAL GLANDS, INFLAMMATION OF (*see* Adenitis).

CHAFING.—Intertrigo, as this condition is technically termed, may occur where two surfaces of skin come into frequent contact, but it especially affects opposing surfaces which are moistened by perspiration or discharges. Its most frequent sites are the thighs, genital organs, armpits and necks of babies and of fat persons. The parts become red, shiny and sore, and unless a remedy is applied the irritation may run into eczema. To avoid chafing, soft water should be used for washing, and unirritating soap. The skin should be dried by dabbing rather than rubbing, and powdered over with good fuller's earth or equal parts of oxide of zinc and starch. To cure the condition when it has arisen the parts should be frequently washed with boric-acid lotion—a teaspoonful of the acid to a tumblerful of warm water, or with oatmeal water, then dried by dabbing with a soft towel, and dusted as recommended above.

CHANCRE, HARD (*see* Syphilis).

CHANCRE, SOFT (*see* Soft Sore).

CHAPPED HANDS AND LIPS.— As the result of exposure to cold, aggravated, it may be, by the imperfect drying of the hands after washing, the skin of the hand may become cracked and painful. The hands should be thoroughly dried after washing, and kept as warm as possible. A good plan is to moisten them with glycerin, mixed with eau-de-Cologne or with rose-water in equal proportions, to stimulate the healing of the chaps. If the lips should become cracked, as they are especially apt to do during the prevalence of easterly winds, they may be treated in the same way.

"CHELSEA PENSIONER" (*see* GOUT).

CHERRY MARKS (*see* BIRTH-MARKS).

CHEYNE-STOKES BREATH-ING (*see* BREATHING, DIFFICULTY OF).

CHICKEN - POX.—Varicella, or chicken-pox, one of the commonest of the affections of infancy and child-hood, was only distinguished from smallpox in the nineteenth century. Until then, cases of this disease were regarded as cases of mild smallpox. The name is believed to be derived from *chick-pea*, from a supposed re-semblance between the fruits of this plant and the eruption. Chicken-pox occurs in epidemics, and as there is frequently a coincident outbreak of smallpox, the two diseases are apt in the early stages to be confused with each other. Infection is active from the beginning, is given off by contact with or probably by the breath of a patient, and may also be transmitted by contaminated clothes. After an attack the patient should be kept isolated until all the scabs have disappeared. The quaran-tine after exposure to infection is twenty-one days. The same person rarely contracts the disease twice.

Incubation stage and symptoms. —From ten to sixteen days after the disease has been "caught" a rash is observed. There may be more or less fever, but in some cases there is none; when present, it usually lasts but a few hours; in some cases, however, it continues until the rash has ceased to renew itself; but the temperature is generally much less every morning and gets higher towards evening. The rash consists of little blisters surrounded by a small, rose-coloured ring. They quickly enlarge to about the size of a split pea, and become glistening and opalescent. In some cases, where there is no red ring round the spots, the patient looks as if he were sprinkled with drops of scalding water. The spots may appear on every part of the body, including the mucous membranes of the mouth and throat, but are gener-ally thickest on the back and shoulders; they are almost always seen first on the trunk, then on the face and scalp, and last of all on the limbs, where they are usually scanty. They come out in two or three crops on succeeding days, but in some cases there are four, or even five crops. About four days later they begin to dry up and then form scabs, which after a few days fall off, leaving faint red marks. In some of the worst cases this is not so, but sores form which may take weeks to heal, and which leave scars not unlike those following smallpox. The illness is usually over in a little more than a week, but not quite so soon if there are four or five crops. The number of spots is very variable. As a rule, the patient never feels really ill, but the tongue may be coated with a moist fur, and the appetite may not be so good as usual, or may be lost entirely. In some cases the eye becomes in-flamed; sometimes, too, the ear.

Treatment.—The patient should keep his room, but need not remain in bed unless the temperature is high, or there are many spots. A boric-acid bath, 1 ounce of the crystals to the gallon, may be given morning and evening, to avert or allay irritation of the skin and lessen the provocation to scratching. The food should be light, such as beef tea or broth, milk, custard, and milky farinaceous puddings, arrowroot made with milk, blancmange, simple jellies, etc. A lightly boiled egg and a little thin bread and butter may be allowed if the patient can eat them, and older children who are in the habit of taking tea need not be deprived of it. Thirst may be relieved by an abundance of water or of thin barley water. The patient will feel more comfortable if he takes a medicine which promotes perspiration, such as half a teaspoonful, or a whole teaspoonful, of solution of acetate of ammonia, sometimes called spirit of Mindererus, in a wineglassful of water, every three or four hours, the larger dose being for children of six years and over. To hasten the falling off of the remainder of the scabs, the child, at the end of a week or ten days, should be gently sponged with warm water and a little good soap. If he does not make a good recovery, he should have a change of air. It is especially important that health should be thoroughly re-established if there is any tendency to tuberculosis, otherwise the patient's enfeebled defensive resources may enable the tubercle bacillus to effect a lodgment.

CHILBLAIN.—Even so simple and ordinary an affection as chilblain has its technical name—*pernio*. More common in childhood and old age than in adult life, it especially attacks persons of feeble circulation. The blains most frequently appear on the hands and feet, but they may occur in any part distant from the heart which is especially exposed to the influence of cold, such as the ears, nose and cheeks. There is usually a good deal of itching. If the inflammation subsides the skin often peels, but in many cases it breaks, when troublesome ulcers may form.

Treatment.—To broken chilblains boric-acid ointment should be applied; unbroken ones may be rubbed with camphorated spirit or friar's balsam and painted with tincture of iodine. If ulcers form they may be dressed with salicylic acid 2 parts, menthol 3 parts, soft white paraffin 100 parts. In those who are subject to this affection the health should be maintained by an abundance of nutritious food and active exercise. The parts likely to be affected should be carefully dried after washing and should not be held before the fire. A useful dusting powder, to be used after the parts have been thoroughly dried, is composed of boric acid 15 per cent., zinc oxide 15 per cent., and finely powdered talc 70 per cent.

CHILDBED FEVER (*see* PUERPERAL FEVER).

CHILDBIRTH.—For a description of the stages of this process and its complications, the reader must be referred to Chavasse's " Advice to a Wife " (Cassell & Co. Ltd.).

CHILD-CROWING.—Laryngismus stridulus, to give this affection its technical name, is a spasm of the vocal cords, limited, as a rule, to young children between the ages of three months and two years. It is often associated with rickets, but is also met with in otherwise healthy children while they are cutting their teeth or are in the early stage of an attack of measles or some other fever. The cause is obscure. In some cases the spasm seems to be set up by adenoids, dyspepsia, or teething; in others it appears to be due to an irritant poison in the blood created in the stomach and intestines by improper food, digestive disorders, or constipation.

Symptoms.—The attacks most frequently occur during the day. The spasm begins with a long-drawn, hoarsely-sounding breath, which is suddenly interrupted, the interruption being popularly known as "a catch in the breath," and a crowing noise is made every time the little sufferer attempts to draw in his breath. After a longer or shorter period respiration temporarily ceases, but suddenly a long, deep breath is taken and the attack is at an end. In some cases the crowing continues for days together and may not even cease during sleep, though usually it does. In bad attacks, which are fortunately rare, the aspect of the child is distressing. When the breathing suddenly stops he remains with mouth open and nostrils dilated, the muscles of the face rigid and motionless, the eyeballs glistening and staring, the countenance dusky and then blue and livid, the arms twitching. In about ten seconds, or more, either spontaneously or as the result of the measures described later, a long-drawn inspiration is taken and colour and consciousness return. In other cases the attack is brought to an end by convulsions. However the attack may end, the child often falls asleep, and after a short time wakes up in his normal state. One attack may soon be followed by others, and occasionally, in spite of all attempts at treatment, the child succumbs to one of them. Recurrence is most frequent in cases which are associated with rickets; those which are due to bad

feeding or to teething improve rapidly with the removal of the cause.

Treatment.—During severe attacks the skin must be stimulated by rubbing or slapping, or by dashing cold water on the face, or by energetic fanning, and if these measures are unsuccessful the child should be put into a hot bath and the application of cold water to the face repeated. A dose of castor oil may be given. When this has operated, a nerve sedative is required, such as bromide of potash 5 grains and hydrate of chloral $2\frac{1}{2}$ grains, in a teaspoonful of sweetened water, every six hours in the case of an infant of six months. Attention must be paid to the general health. The nerve sedative may be followed by a tonic, such as arsenic, which may be used in the form of Fowler's solution, 1 to 2 drops in water after meals.

CHILDREN, FEEDING OF (*see* INFANTS AND YOUNG CHILDREN, FEEDING OF).

CHILDREN, HYGIENE OF.—Under the heading of INFANTS, HYGIENE OF, some hints are given as to the management of babies during the first year or two of life. In this place we may very briefly consider the management of children of a larger growth—from the end of the second to the beginning of the eighth year of life. The question of food is considered in the article on INFANTS AND YOUNG CHILDREN, FEEDING OF, while the cutting of the milk teeth and of the permanent teeth is dealt with in TEETHING AND ITS TROUBLES.

The child should be carefully trained in habits of *cleanliness*. A warm bath in the evening (100° Fahr.) is necessary to cleanse the body after the exercise of the day. In the morning the child should stand in a basin of warm water and be rapidly sponged down with cold water—though in wintry weather the water need not be absolutely cold. This is followed by friction—not too vigorous, of course—with a roughish towel. By the fourth or fifth year the sponge-down in the morning may be replaced by a jump in and out of a cold or nearly cold bath, followed, again, by friction with a rough towel. Having dressed, the child should be encouraged to run or skip about the garden, when the weather permits, with uncovered head.

In the early years *exercise* should consist for the most part in outdoor games. Breathing exercises and skipping are useful for developing the lungs, and tip-toe exercises to prevent flatfoot, a condition to which some children are prone.

As a rule, children should take as much *sleep* as they are capable of. Until the end of the fourth year rest for an hour in the middle of the day, in a darkened room in summer, is desirable. Even beyond this age the child should go to bed with unbroken regularity quite early in the evening, and fourteen hours of sleep in a well-ventilated room is none too long. The windows of the bedroom should be kept open both day and night except in very rough weather, but the child should be sheltered from direct draughts by a screen.

The *clothing* should consist of a woven combination stretching from neck to knee, stockings, warm woollen knickers and bodice, and an over-dress or tunic. In cold weather coats should reach below the knees, but normal children, who can keep themselves warm by trundling a hoop or running about or skipping, need very little extra clothing out of doors.

CHIN-WHELK (*see* BARBER'S ITCH).

CHLORAL POISONING.—An overdose of chloral may be taken as a sleeping draught. An emetic should be given (*see* EMETICS) and persevering efforts made to arouse the patient by flapping the face with a wet towel, and if necessary applying an electric battery. He should be covered with hot blankets, hot bottles should be put to the feet, the limbs well rubbed, and brandy and strong coffee given him to drink if conscious, or administered as an enema if he is unconscious. If the breathing appears to be failing, artificial respiration must be adopted, and the doctor may give inhalations of oxygen.

CHLORODYNE POISONING (*see* OPIUM POISONING).

CHLOROFORM POISONING.—Occasionally chloroform is drunk in mistake for some other medicine. An emetic (*see* EMETICS) must be given, and carbonate of soda, dissolved in plenty of water, and the patient must be prevented from going to sleep by the means mentioned under CHLORAL POISONING.

CHLOROSIS (*see* ANÆMIA).

CHOKING (*see* Foreign Bodies in the Larynx and Windpipe, *under* FOREIGN BODIES).

CHOLERA.—This disease has probably been endemic from time immemorial in Lower Bengal, whence from time to time it has spread as an epidemic in India generally. It has not been epidemic in Britain since 1866 ; it knocked at our door in 1884, and again in 1892, but did not succeed in gaining entrance. It is due to a germ which, from its curved shape, is styled the comma bacillus, first discovered by Koch, in 1883. In the vast majority of cases the disease is water-borne : the germ, having been swallowed in drinking-water, multiplies in the alimentary canal, and, being contained in the patient's discharges, finds its way again to water and there continues to multiply.

Symptoms.—There may be a premonitory attack of ordinary diarrhœa, which, in the course of a day or two, assumes the form of cholera ; or the disease may break out quite suddenly with the occurrence of profuse watery motions, not different in character from ordinary looseness of the bowels, but soon looking like thin rice-water, of which many pints may be passed. Before long vomiting sets in, the matter brought up being of the same rice-water appearance as the motions. The extremities and the abdomen are now seized with agonizing cramps. The surface of the body is cold and exudes a clammy sweat. The urine is suppressed, the breathing is rapid and shallow, the pulse becomes feeble, the voice sinks to a whisper. The state of collapse into which the patient passes may end in death, or on the other hand he may outlast the exhaustion and make a rapid recovery. More often, however, he emerges from the collapse to enter what is known as the stage of reaction, in which, after making distinct progress, he becomes feverish, and in fact is in very much the condition of a typhoid patient. Serious complications may arise during this stage ; if not, he finally enters the stage of convalescence.

We have described typical cases of cholera, but the disease varies greatly in severity ; thus there is the very mild type called *cholerine*, there is also the *ambulatory* type, so called because the patient is able to get about during the attack, and there is the very fatal type called *cholera sicca*, or dry cholera.

Treatment.—The first thing the doctor aims at is to stop the premonitory diarrhœa, if the attack is so ushered in. If the diarrhœa cannot be checked and the motions assume the rice-water appearance, little can be done except to keep the patient warm with hot-water bottles, etc., to relieve the thirst and exhaustion by sips of iced champagne and soda-water or iced weak brandy-and-water, and the cramps by friction with dry, powdered ginger. If the heart fails and stimulants cannot be given by the mouth, ether or brandy may have to be injected under the skin. This not sufficing, injections of saline solution into the veins or beneath the skin should be tried. During convalescence the diet must for a time be limited to thin broths, diluted milk, barley-water and the like ; the return to ordinary food should be very gradual and careful.

In India and elsewhere Haffkine's system of vaccination against cholera is now in extensive use ; although not an absolute preventive, it appears to lessen liability to the disease and to diminish its virulence if acquired.

CHOLERA, ENGLISH, and **CHOLERA, INFANTILE** (*see* EPIDEMIC DIARRHŒA).

CHOREA (*see* ST. VITUS'S DANCE)

CIRCULATION OF BLOOD (*see* BLOOD, CIRCULATION OF).

CIRCUMCISION (*see* PHIMOSIS).

CIRRHOSIS OF THE LIVER.— This is one of the medical designations of a chronic inflammation of the liver in which the organ, if cut into, is seen to be of a reddish-yellow colour. The disease is also known popularly as " hob-nailed liver "—because in many cases, in a late stage, the liver shrinks and presents a hard and irregular surface—and as " gin-drinker's liver," from the belief that it is caused by alcoholic intemperance. This theory of the origin of liver cirrhosis has now, however, been modified. There are a few cases in which there is no antecedent intemperance, the affection being a legacy, so to speak, from scarlet fever or some other infectious disease, or a manifestation of malaria or of syphilis. On the other hand, it is notorious that many who drink ardent spirits to excess do not suffer from degeneration of the liver. The probability is that excessive consumption of alcohol, especially in the form of spirits, irritates the liver and exposes it to the action of poisons to which otherwise it would be immune. It is believed that over-stimulating foods and certain metallic poisons act in the same way. The nature of the poisons is not definitely known : possibly they are manufactured by bacteria. Practically, the earlier theory was not very misleading, for the fact remains that the great majority of the patients would have escaped the disease had they not indulged too freely in strong drink. In other words, although alcohol may never be the exciting cause, it is nearly always a potent, and may even be the sole, predisposing cause. In an ordinary case the liver becomes congested with blood, first increases in size and then begins to shrink and harden, so that the organ becomes incapable of performing its functions. In some cases, however, it remains permanently enlarged, and, instead of hardening and becoming reddish-yellow in colour, presents much the appearance of a liver that has undergone fatty degeneration, being smooth and yellowish-white. This form, much more common in America than in England, is met with in beer-drinkers rather than in spirit-drinkers.

Symptoms.—A dull pain is often felt in the right side, and there are various indications that something is seriously wrong with the digestive apparatus. The patient sleeps badly, is thin and sallow, and perhaps slightly yellow from jaundice. Presently his face becomes bluish from blood which is not circulating properly ; the eyes are puffy, the legs heavy and swollen, and the abdomen enlarged—all manifestations of dropsy ; on the surface of the abdomen and lower part of the chest distended veins may be seen. The urine is scanty and turbid. There may be bleeding from the stomach, the blood being vomited, or from the bowels as a result of piles. These various symptoms go from bad to worse, and to them may be added delirium, stupor deepening into unconsciousness, or convulsions. Then, perhaps in about a year from the time when the disease became well established, comes the end. There is little hope for anyone affected with cirrhosis of the liver unless at a quite early stage he at once and entirely avoids the indulgence or habit in which the trouble originated.

Treatment.—Animal food should for a time be taboo, except in such forms as boiled chicken and boiled sole or whiting, and milk should be made the chief article of diet, mixed, if desired, with thin oatmeal gruel (equal parts), or boiled and thickened with arrowroot and isinglass. For the sake of variety, milk soup may be taken occasionally, made by adding fresh, well-cooked vegetables to hot milk and flavouring with celery salt or Spanish onion. Very little fat or sugar food should be taken. The bowels must be kept in free and regular action by saline medicines, such as Carlsbad or Epsom salts, taken in the morning, with a pill of podophyllin ($\frac{1}{8}$ grain), extract of aloes (1 grain), soap (1 grain), and a little oil of peppermint, occasionally at night. The patient should take plenty of riding or walking exercise in the open air. The dropsy will require treatment on the lines laid down in the article on that subject. For the treatment of piles and vomiting of blood, if present, *see* PILES and BLOOD-SPITTING.

CLAVUS HYSTERICUS (*see* HEADACHE).

CLEFT PALATE.—Like hare-lip, with which it is often associated, cleft palate is an error of development, the two halves of the roof of the mouth failing to unite properly, so that a gap is left. The defect exists in various degrees, and the severer deformities are sometimes accompanied by mental weakness. Besides being unsightly, cleft palate interferes with sucking, while fluid which has been introduced into the mouth may be returned, and escape through the nose. Death may be caused during the first few months of life by lack of nutrition. The child is also liable to inflammation of the mucous membranes of the mouth and nose from the lodgment and decomposition of particles of food, etc. In some cases the gap is too wide to be closed by operation, and a specially prepared dental plate must then be worn. In most cases, fortunately, operative treatment is possible. If the child is exceptionally healthy and robust, the operation may be performed during the first three months of life ; in the majority, it is better deferred until later.

CLERGYMAN'S SORE THROAT (*see* SORE THROAT).

CLINICAL THERMOMETER(*see* TEMPERATURE, BODY).

CLOTTING OF BLOOD (*see* BLOOD AND LYMPH).

CLUB - FOOT.—This deformity which is known medically as *talipes*, may either be present at birth or may come on subsequently. It may take several different forms : the foot may be twisted outwards (*talipes valgus*), so that it rests on the inner side and inner ankle ; or it may be twisted inwards (*talipes varus*), so that it rests on the outer edge ; or the heel may be drawn up so that the foot rests on the toes (*talipes equinus*) ; or the toes may be raised so that the foot rests on the back of the heel (*talipes calcaneus*). Yet another form is that known as " hollow foot " (*pes cavus*), in which the arch of the foot is too high, owing to depression of the heel or of the toes, or of both. Club-foot rarely occurs in either of these forms alone ; usually there is a combination of two or more, and the most common variety is that in which the heel is drawn up while the foot is twisted inwards (*talipes equino-varus*).

Causes.—Most cases of club-foot are congenital, and may arise from faulty position of the child, or from abnormal mechanical pressure, in the womb. In some cases, however, some of the bones of the foot or leg may be absent. When it arises subsequently to birth it is due to infantile paralysis, spasmodic contraction of muscles, or rupture of a tendon or muscle.

Treatment.—If an ordinary case of club-foot is taken in hand within a few days of birth, while the tissues are soft and pliable, it can be cured by manipulations and the use of a small splint. Neither of these measures is sufficient in itself, but if combined and applied early they will prove to be effective. The manipulation, which must, of course, be carried out under medical supervision, should be practised for at least ten minutes every night and morning. The splint has to be used both day and night except for an hour in the morning and evening when the manipulations are performed. The use of a plaster-of-Paris case to keep the apparatus in position is very undesirable, for the effect in many cases has been to deprive the growing limb of part of its blood supply, so that it ceases to develop, or actually wastes. In cases where operation is necessary it usually consists in dividing certain ligaments and tendons and then putting the limb into splints. As soon as the child begins to walk he may be fitted with an apparatus. If the deformity has not been corrected by the time the child is five years old, operations of a more extensive kind are necessary.

CLUB-HAND.—This deformity of the wrist is much less common than club-foot. Always congenital, it may sometimes be due to a cramped position in the womb with overstretching of muscles, but in most cases there is either a congenital deficiency or complete absence of one of the bones of the forearm. In the first group of cases the defect may be cured by manipulations and the use of a simple apparatus. If, however, there is deficiency or absence of bone it is necessary that tendons should be cut and an apparatus worn. Even then the deformity is not entirely cured.

COCAINE (*see* ANÆSTHESIA ; NARCOTICS AND HYPNOTICS).

COCCYGODYNIA (*see* BACKACHE).

COLD, A (*see* CATARRH, NASAL).

COLD PACK (*see* WET PACK).

COLIC.—Popular synonyms for this affection are " the gripes," " belly-ache," and, more elegantly but less accurately, " stomach-ache." Strictly speaking, colic means severe pain in the large intestine ; but as ordinarily used, it denotes such pain in the abdomen generally, whether in the large intestine, the small intestine, the stomach, the gall-bladder and bile-ducts, or the kidneys and ureters —the tubes which conduct the urine from the kidneys to the bladder. The colic most frequently met with is that due to violent spasms of the muscular tissue of the intestines, and is properly described as intestinal colic ; it is with this that the present article deals. Biliary colic, caused by the passage of gall-stones, is considered under GALL-STONES, and renal colic, due to the passage of a urinary stone, under STONE IN THE KIDNEY.

Causes.—Intestinal colic is sometimes due to poisoning by lead ; the form of the disease which attacks painters is known as painter's colic. Another cause of colic is cold, which may take the form of chill to the abdomen, or may be the result of getting the feet wet. Colic may also be a manifestation of nervous disturbance, such as is caused by fright, anger, intense anxiety, or mental fatigue resulting from overwork. But the most frequent of all causes of colic is irritation of the bowels by unsuitable or undigested food.

Symptoms.—When the stomach is the seat of the disorder, pain is felt in the upper part of the abdomen ; when the colic is intestinal the pain is usually felt first in the region of the navel, but gradually spreads over the abdomen, or may wander about from part to part. The pain may be of almost intolerable severity. In bad cases the patient is a pitiable object—the features pinched, the face pale and expressive of great anxiety, the skin bathed in a cold sweat ; he may be found wandering about with his body doubled up and his hands pressing on the abdomen, or lying down with the legs drawn up. In most cases there is great distension of the abdomen from wind. Gradually the pain passes off, but as a rule returns in all its intensity. Besides flatulence, constipation is nearly always present, either as a cause of pain or as the result of spasm. As soon as the wind has been got rid of or the bowels have been cleared the attack passes off. It may last from a few minutes to several days ; as a rule, the more violent the attack the shorter its duration. Treatment should be applied without delay, not only to shorten the duration of the patient's sufferings but also to prevent the setting up of inflammation of the bowels (enteritis), or of the peritoneum (peritonitis), or other serious troubles. It is necessary also to distinguish as early as possible between colic and more serious affections which are attended with abdominal pain. It may usually be differentiated from these other affections by absence of fever and quickened pulse, and excessive vomiting, and by the fact that the pain is relieved by pressure, whereas in obstruction or inflammation of the bowels and in peritonitis it is made worse. If there are indications that something more than colic is the cause of the patient's sufferings, the doctor must at once be called in.

Treatment.—The patient should go to bed with hot-water bottles to his feet, and the abdomen should be gently rubbed with some sedative liniment, such as belladonna. Warmth may also be applied to the abdomen, in the form either of a hot linseed poultice or of a fomentation. The large bowel may be unloaded by means of a copious soap-and-water enema, or the intestines may be cleared of offending matters by taking a tablespoonful of castor oil with 20 drops of laudanum. A glass of hot brandy-and-water, or 30 drops of sal-volatile, or some essence of peppermint or ginger with hot water will disperse the wind and get rid of the pain.

In *children* colic is a frequent trouble, generally caused by unsuitable food or improper feeding. In the case of infants the pain may be relieved by laying the child across the knee on his stomach and gently rubbing the back. Half a teaspoonful of dill water with 2 teaspoonfuls of hot water, or a dessertspoonful of equal quantities of lime water and cinnamon water, may be given, while the bowels should be cleared by an enema of warm water or by a 1-grain powder of mercury and chalk. Hot fomentations may be applied to the abdomen. The next meal may be postponed for a time, or the amount of food temporarily reduced, the feed of milk being replaced by a little sweetened barley-water or some whey. If the child is bottle-fed, more lime-water or barley-water should be added to the milk.

COLITIS (*see* Bowels, Inflammation of).

COLLAPSE (*see* Shock).

COLLES'S FRACTURE (*see* Fractures).

COLOUR-BLINDNESS. — This defect of sight may either be present at birth or may come on later. The acquired form is usually a sequel of disease of the optic nerve. In both alike the colours most frequently confused with each other are red and green, although cases are occasionally met with in which the colour sense is entirely absent. The condition is incurable. Except in the æsthetic loss to the patient, it is, speaking generally, of practical importance chiefly in the case of railwaymen and sailors.

COMA.—Partial loss of consciousness is styled *stupor ;* complete loss, *coma.* But even of coma there are different degrees, which are described by the terms *comatose condition, coma,* and *profound coma.* Coma occurs in connexion with apoplexy, sunstroke, poisoning, exposure to extreme cold, etc. Deep coma which persists for twenty-four hours usually ends **in** death.

COMPRESSES.—A compress is a device for the continuous application of moisture to an inflamed part, such as the throat. The material employed, lint, spongiopiline, or folded-up linen, is wetted with water—cold, warm, or hot—covered with oil-silk, and kept in place by a bandage or folded handkerchief. The boric-acid compress, made by dipping a doubled piece of boric-acid lint in hot water and wringing it out, or by wringing a plain piece of lint out of boric acid lotion, and applied hot, has now, in the case of wounds, taken the place of the familiar linseed poultice, which often contains a plentiful admixture of dirt and germs, and should never be applied either to broken skin or to skin which is liable to be broken.

CONCUSSION OF THE BRAIN (*see* BRAIN, CONCUSSION OF).

CONGENITAL DISEASE (*see* DISEASE, CLASSIFICATION OF).

CONGENITAL MALFORMATIONS (*see* MALFORMATIONS, CONGENITAL).

CONGENITAL SYPHILIS (*see* SYPHILIS).

CONGESTION OF THE BRAIN.—The brain may be gorged with blood as the result of habitually immoderate indulgence in alcohol, or of mental anxiety and overwork, or the congestion may occur in connexion with other diseases, especially diseases of the circulatory system, or as a sequel of blows on the head. The symptoms include giddiness, headache, sleeplessness, irritability and mental excitement or, on the other hand, dullness and drowsiness ; and to them, in more severe cases, may be added delirium, convulsions, and unconsciousness. Treatment consists in rest, quiet, abstinence from work, worry and alcohol ; the application of cold to the head, and of warmth and blisters, etc., to the surface of the body, the use of aperient medicines, and, if necessary, blood-letting. The patient's head should be raised, so that the flow of blood to the head may be hindered and the return flow assisted. During convalescence a change of air and scene is desirable.

CONGESTION OF THE LIVER.—A liver affected with congestion is enlarged from over-distension with blood, the result in some cases of indulgence in rich foods and spirituous liquors, while in other cases it may be due to chill, and in yet others to affections of the circulation, etc., which prevent the free return of blood from the liver. The symptoms more or less resemble those described in the article BILIOUSNESS, but when the condition is due to heart or lung affections symptoms of these affections will also be present. In many cases of congested liver the patient suffers from piles, and by the bleeding from these the liver symptoms are often relieved. In treatment the original affection, if there is one, must, of course, receive attention. If the congestion is the result of chill or of dietary indiscretion the patient should go to bed and have a hot poultice applied over the liver, while the bowels should be cleared by means of a grain of calomel at night and a dose of aperient mineral water the next morning. Alcohol must be avoided, and the diet should be light, simple, and chiefly fluid.

CONGESTION OF THE LUNGS.

—Sometimes "congestion of the lungs" is used as though it were synonymous with bronchitis (inflammation of the bronchial tubes), or with pneumonia, inflammation of the lung substance itself. This use of the expression is misleading; the name should be reserved for cases in which, owing to the presence of some serious heart affection or to exhaustion, there is an accumulation of blood in the vessels of the lung. It will be convenient to deal with these two varieties separately.

1. **Lung congestion due to heart disease.**—The failure of the heart to do its work properly leads to engorgement and distension of the vessels of the lungs. The symptoms include cough, difficulty of breathing, especially after exertion, rapid pulse, bluish lips, and palpitation of the heart, with a sensation of tightness over the heart region. *Treatment* must be directed to the heart affection; all that can be done besides is to avoid exertion, exposure to cold, and every other harmful or trying influence.

2. **Lung congestion due to exhaustion.**—The exhaustion may be the result of an infectious fever, or of a surgical operation, or it may be the debility of extreme old age, in which the weakened heart has lost the power to do its work properly. The lower and most dependent parts of the lungs are chiefly affected, and it is on this account that a doctor is always reluctant to order an aged

patient to remain in bed for any length of time, for when the patient remains long in one position the blood is liable to stagnate in the dependent parts. This form of congestion may easily develop into pneumonia. The lips, face, hands and feet are blue, the breath is quick, short and shallow, the general condition one of prostration. *Treatment* must aim at supporting the patient's strength and stimulating the circulation. Alcohol should be allowed in small quantities at frequent intervals, and as much nutritious food as the patient can take. The doctor may give inhalations of oxygen, and such stimulating drugs as sal-volatile, ether, strychnine, and caffeine. The patient must not be allowed to lie for many hours at a time in one position, but should be turned from one side to the other; if not too enfeebled, he should sit up in bed for a few minutes at a time, and as soon as possible he should be got out of bed every day for a short time, the sitting-out intervals being gradually extended.

CONJUNCTIVITIS.—The conjunctiva, the mucous membrane that lines the front part of the eyeball and the inner surface of the eyelid, is a delicate structure, and when it becomes inflamed, from a cold, from irritation by a foreign body or excessive glare, from eyestrain, or from germ-infection, there is an extreme degree of discomfort, which many would speak of as pain.

Forms of conjunctivitis.—*Catarrhal* conjunctivitis (Frontispiece, Fig. 3) may be caused by contact with certain liquids and gases, glare from snow and electric light, etc. *Phlyctenular* conjunctivitis (Frontispiece, Fig. 4) is found almost exclusively in badly nourished children with a tuberculous tendency, who are living under unhealthy conditions. In a typical case one or more small yellowish-white swellings appear on the margin of the cornea, where the white and the coloured part of the eye meet, and the blood-vessels around them are dilated. In *angular* conjunctivitis the inflammation appears at the inner and outer corners of the eye (hence the name), and to a certain extent along the edge of the lids. *Follicular* conjunctivitis (Frontispiece, Fig. 5) is so called because numbers of enlarged follicles appear on the membrane. In the form of conjunctivitis called *trachoma*, which flourishes where people are crowded together in unhealthy surroundings, the whole of the conjunctiva is covered with numerous sago-like granulations. *Purulent* conjunctivitis is usually due to the germ of gonorrhœa; the discharge becomes profuse, and the mucous membrane is swollen; this form is described more fully under the designation Purulent Ophthalmia in the article OPHTHALMIA.

General symptoms.—The eyes water profusely, and are bloodshot; there is a gummy discharge, which during the night sticks the eyelids together; the lids itch, and are irritable. The sight, however, is not affected. If some of the small vessels of the membrane burst, as they are apt to do, unsightly red blotches will be seen, but these, though they may alarm the patient, have no serious import and will clear up.

Treatment of ordinary conjunctivitis. — Even the simple forms of conjunctivitis ought to be taken seriously and medical aid obtained. If the inflammation is due to the presence of a foreign body, this must first be removed. The eye—as a rule only one eye is attacked, though the inflammation may spread to the other—should be washed out with lotion consisting of a teaspoonful of boric acid to a pint of warm water; cold tea, or 3 grains of alum to an ounce of water, may be used in the same way. To wash out the eye, the lids should be held apart and liquid poured into them from an undine (Fig. 12) or similar receptacle held a few inches above the eye, or it may be injected from a syringe. The eye should not be poulticed or bound up, but simply rested and protected from light, dust, and cold currents of air. If in a few

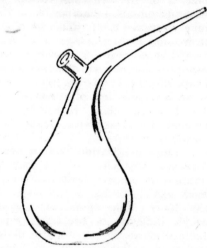

Fig. 12.—Undine.

days the inflammation does not subside under this treatment, two or three drops of a 5-per-cent. solution of argyrol should be placed on the turned-back lower lid with a little camel-hair brush two or three times a day. The eyelids may be prevented from sticking together at night by spreading a little vaselin or boric-acid ointment along the edges at bed-time. The general health should be improved, an aperient taken to clear the bowels, and the digestion toned up. As most forms of conjunctivitis are contagious, the patient's towels, handkerchiefs, etc., should be kept separate from others, and those who attend to his eyes should carefully wash their hands afterwards.

CONSTIPATION. — For most persons perfect health is not compatible with a less frequent movement of the bowels than once in the twenty-four hours. This may be taken as a rule to which there are many exceptions. Thus there are many persons who have a motion only every other day, or once in three days, or even at longer intervals, and yet complain of no discomfort and are apparently healthy. The only rule of universal applicability is that if the dejections are hard and dry and small in quantity the bowels move too infrequently ; if they are of the ordinary consistency and volume and the symptoms of constipation, presently to be described, are absent, no concern need be felt at the infrequency of the evacuations.

Causes.—The most common cause of constipation is to be found in diet. In these days bread and other kinds of food are carefully divested of those coarser elements which cannot be assimilated, and the result is that the bowels, deprived of the stimulation which such unassimilated substances would supply, become sluggish and inactive. In some cases, too, especially among women, the diet contains too little liquid, which tends to produce constipation in two different ways : the amount of fluid is insufficient to keep the contents of the intestinal canal soft, and the secretions formed from the blood by the intestinal glands will be diminished in quantity. The same deficiency may arise from excessive exercise in persons who perspire freely. On the other hand, constipation may be due to lack of exercise. Yet another cause is inattention to the calls of Nature. Some people never think of attending to the admonition unless it is urgent, and even when they do, insufficient time is allowed for the lower part of the bowel to be properly emptied. Nature is apt to show her resentment of this treatment by discontinuing her mild admonitions. On the other hand she evidently disapproves of the application of force in the form of strong purgatives, the frequent use of which leads to the cessation of her gentle stirrings, so that the bowels remain inactive unless subjected to violent stimulation. There are many cases of constipation, however, in which no neglect or injudicious behaviour can be alleged against the sufferers. They may suffer from anæmia, or hysteria, or some other affection which deprives the bowels of their tone ; or there may be an insufficient secretion of bile ; while there are also many persons in whom the bowels are naturally inactive, so that it is only by constant attention to diet and exercise and the use of medicines that they can be made to move. Possibly it may presently be discovered that the first cause of the trouble in these latter cases is deficient secretion of one or other of the ductless glands (q.v.).

Symptoms. — These include a coated tongue, a bad taste in the mouth, disordered digestion, flatulence, palpitation, and difficulty of breathing. Dark patches form under the eyes, spots appear before them, the face may be flushed, there may be a good deal of headache and giddiness. The sufferer becomes irritable, and is restless, or drowsy and heavy ; he may either have deep but unrefreshing sleep, or suffer from the opposite condition of sleeplessness ; and there is often great depression of spirits. More serious symptoms of constipation are piles, dropsy of the feet, irritation of the sexual organs from pressure on the veins, neuralgic pains in the legs from pressure on the nerves, and a high temperature set up by the absorbed poisons. The pain in the head becomes worse, and the depression of spirits may pass into melancholia, or the sufferer may become a hypochondriac and be able to think of nothing but the state of his health.

Treatment.—Before resorting to drugs the sufferer from constipation should carefully inquire whether there is anything in his diet or general habits which needs correction. If he has been using white bread he should replace it by brown or wholemeal bread ; if he can digest oatmeal porridge—it is not everyone who can —he should have it for breakfast, flavoured with treacle or golden syrup, which will not only render it palatable but will increase its effect upon the bowels. Gingerbread and oatmeal biscuits are other suitable foods. Plenty of well-cooked green vegetables should be eaten, and fruit also should form an element in the dietary, especially figs, prunes and apples. Marmalade, jams and honey are useful if sweets can be taken. Salads, dressed with oil as well as vinegar, are to be recommended, and as much fat should be taken as can comfortably be digested. In many cases, and especially where the fæces are hard and dry, liquid paraffin is a valuable aid. Water and other fluids should amount to about three pints per day, and extra fluid may be taken in the form of a tumblerful of hot water on going to bed and another on getting up. If no other exercise is taken the sufferer, unless incapacitated by age or infirmity, should make a point of having a good brisk walk for at least half an hour—an hour would be better—every day. In

cases in which the trouble is due to weakness of the intestinal muscles, massage is useful. A cold bath, or a cold douche after a hot bath, should be taken on rising. Every morning, soon after breakfast, the closet should be visited, even if no reminder is received. The visit must not be hurried, and it should be kept up regularly. Those who smoke may find that a pipe of tobacco or a cigarette will encourage Nature to do her duty.

Only when such measures as are here recommended have failed should drugs be resorted to. One of the most popular aperients is cascara sagrada ; if the liver is sluggish, it may be taken in the form of compound cascara tabloid. Castor oil is not a suitable drug in every case of constipation, because after it has acted it may increase the tendency which it is used to correct. Other time-honoured remedies for constipation are sulphur, which may be taken in lozenges, and senna tea. Senna may, if preferred, be employed in the form of an infusion of senna pods (senna tea being an infusion of the leaves) ; seven or eight of the pods, less or more according to the strength required for the individual case, are placed in half a tumblerful of cold water in the morning, and the infusion, which is devoid of taste, drunk at bedtime. It may be taken daily for a time, and then every other day, and discontinued when no longer necessary. Both senna and sulphur are present in the familiar compound liquorice powder, of which about a teaspoonful, stirred up in a little water, may be taken at night or in the morning.

Of late years the old remedy of a blue pill and black draught has lost some of its popularity, but this means of securing a brisk action of the bowels has much to recommend it. It should not, however, be used frequently, but only when there is need to effect a thorough clearance. Other forms of mercury are calomel, $\frac{1}{2}$ grain to 2 grains, and grey powder, 1 grain to 5 grains; these also should be used with care and but seldom.

In many cases natural mineral waters are very serviceable. Among

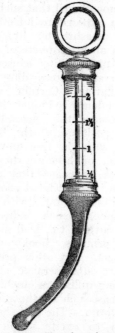

Fig. 13.—Glycerin syringe.

the most effective of them are the Hunyadi Janos, Friedrichshall, and Carlsbad waters; the one chosen should be sipped, mixed with as much or twice or thrice as much of quite hot water, on rising in the morning. In some cases, as when there is vomiting, it may be desirable to clear the lower bowel by giving an enema instead of administering aperients by the mouth. A suitable enema is from $\frac{3}{4}$ pint to a pint of soap and water, to which an ounce of castor

oil may be added, though this is not usually necessary. Instead of a copious enema a teaspoonful of glycerin may be injected into the lower bowel with a special syringe (Fig. 13), or a glycerin suppository may be introduced into the orifice. By such means as these an action can be produced in a few minutes.

Constipation in children may be due to a constitutional weakness such as rickets, or may be the result of taking too little exercise, of too close an application to lessons, of eating too much animal food, or of neglecting to go to the water-closet daily. Some cases, however, are associated with hysteria or some other manifestation of the nervous temperament. In the case of breast-fed infants, the mother should eat plenty of green vegetables and fruit, and drink Vichy water. The food of bottle-fed babies should be prepared with oatmeal-water instead of barley-water, or a small piece of manna or a pinch of phosphate of soda may be added to each bottle. The abdomen may be gently massaged. Suppositories of soap or cacao-butter or glycerin jelly may be introduced into the lower bowel, or the object may be gained by gently inserting into the orifice the little finger dipped in glycerin. Instead of suppositories, cold injections of plain water, of glycerin and water, or of olive oil may be given. Liquid paraffin should be taken in sufficient doses to prevent the stools from becoming hard; from $\frac{1}{4}$ to 1 drachm may be taken twice or thrice a day, either alone or in an emulsion, or combined with malt. Should these measures fail, a gentle laxative must be used for a few days, such as infusion of senna pods ($\frac{1}{2}$ to 2 pods may be infused for a dose), or a small dose of calomel, $\frac{1}{4}$ to $\frac{1}{2}$ grain.

In older children, reliance should be placed upon dietary and hygienic habits, as described above. If medicine is necessary, sugar-coated tabloids of compound cascara may be tried, or a small dose of one of the natural aperient waters.

CONSUMPTION.—The word " consumption," when used without qualification, denotes tuberculosis of the lungs, known also as pulmonary tuberculosis and as phthisis. Besides the lungs, tuberculosis may attack many other organs and structures (*see* TUBERCULOSIS). In all alike the mischief is due to the activities of a minute germ, the *Bacillus tuberculosis*, less formally the tubercle bacillus, which was discovered by the late Dr. Koch, the bacteriologist, in 1882. In the tissues of the lungs the bacillus brings about the formation of small, greyish-white lumps called tubercles, which grow larger and soften, and so the lung substance is destroyed and is discharged as expectoration,leaving behind it smaller or larger cavities.

Causes.—The tubercle bacillus is communicated chiefly by inhalation, or by being swallowed, as in milk or meat from tuberculous cows. Inhalation appears to be much the more common of the two processes. The germ may be inhaled either dry, as when sputum (phlegm) from a patient is discharged into the road, dries, and is blown about in the dust, or moist, as when a patient coughs or shouts and so scatters the germs broadcast for the benefit of those around him. All of us, therefore, frequently inhale the germ (*see* TUBERCULOSIS). Whether phthisis is hereditary is a question not yet finally settled, but at present most of the authorities are of opinion that what a consumptive patient may transmit to the child is, not the disease

itself, but merely a predisposition to it, in the form either of a narrow, contracted, or weak chest, or of constitutional weakness. To contract the disease, the child of such a parent must be exposed to it after birth. It is true that some consumptive parents have consumptive children, but the proportion is not greater than can be accounted for by supposing the inheritance of a predisposition, if it is also remembered that such children are often exposed to infection in an unusual measure by living, so to speak, in an atmosphere of phthisis.

Other predisposing causes of consumption are overcrowding and lack of ventilation. Certain industries have a tendency to induce the disease, either because they necessitate constrained positions of the body that interfere with the free movement of the lungs, or because they involve night work, or because they are carried on in hot, ill-ventilated rooms, or in an atmosphere charged with irritating dust ; among such industries are those of cutlers, tin, lead and copper miners, printers, bookbinders and hairdressers. Yet other predisposing causes are intemperance and other debilitating influences, including previous disease such as whooping-cough.

Symptoms.—The first sign of consumption to excite suspicion is a hacking, persistent cough. Presently a little watery or frothy mucus is coughed up, and about the same time the general health begins to decline : the patient looks pale, loses flesh, and is easily fatigued. By this time tubercles have formed in the lungs, and as they grow and multiply the expectoration becomes freer and thicker. If the evening temperature is now taken, it is found to be raised ; the pulse is quick, the patient is troubled with profuse night-sweats, which may occur several times a night, and he becomes more and more emaciated. The evening rise of temperature—it may be to about 100° Fahr., or as high as 103° or 104° —with subsidence to normal or below normal in the morning, is one of the most characteristic signs of consumption, and as the disease progresses, the difference between the two temperatures may grow. As a rule, the patient complains little of pain, beyond a dull aching under the collarbone. Blood-spitting if persistent and profuse, and accompanied by cough, wasting, or evening rise of temperature, points distinctly to consumption. As the disease progresses, the discharge from the tubercles is expectorated in large quantities; but even now, in spite of extreme emaciation, and although prostrate from weakness, the patient may still cherish sanguine hopes of recovery, for it is one of the characteristics of consumption that as a rule the patient confidently expects to get well.

Diagnosis.—Whether or not in any given case consumption can be checked depends upon the stage at which the diagnosis is made. It is therefore of the greatest importance that all suspected cases should be submitted to diagnosis with the least possible delay.

Treatment.—If a case of consumption is taken in hand at an early stage there is every reason to hope that the disease will be permanently arrested. In these days the *open-air method* of treatment is regarded as of most importance. The success of sanatorium treatment, however, is not explained merely by the open-air life, though this is its chief factor. When a patient enters a sanatorium he comes under the observation of experts who exercise a constant supervision over every detail of his life; and the treatment also includes an abundance

of nutritious food, and entire freedom from the ordinary anxieties of life. Advanced and hopeless cases are, of course, unsuitable for this treatment; such patients should be sent to a sick asylum, where they will cease to be centres of infection to the community.

The question of *food* has already been touched upon. Whether in a sanatorium or not, the patient, as a rule to which there are some exceptions, should be somewhat overfed. The special feeding must, however, be supervised with care, for at the beginning of treatment the patient's digestion is easily upset. Abundance of milk should be taken, and as much fat in the form of milk, cream, butter, fat bacon, suet, etc., as can be digested. Meat should be well cooked and combined with a moderate quantity of vegetables. The diet should include bread and other starchy foods, and sweets as far as they can be digested. Stimulants are seldom necessary, but their occasional use with food is justifiable when the patient feels weak and low-spirited and the appetite flags. If the digestion is feeble it may be necessary to fall back upon predigested foods, and upon meat essences, raw meat pounded to a pulp, beaten-up eggs, etc. The patient's weight must be regularly taken. If it increases he is gaining ground; if it grows less he must, if possible, be plied with more food.

We come now to the *drug treatment* of consumption. Cod-liver oil is prescribed somewhat less than it used to be, but it is still of the greatest value in the cases of poor and ill-fed patients, in whom to some extent it takes the place of food. It is not suitable in cases in which there is much fever or the digestion is enfeebled. The dose should at first be small, and gradually increased. The nauseous taste may be concealed with orange wine, coffee, or sherry, but the flavour is one to which most patients soon get accustomed.

Many drugs are used, especially in the form of inhalations, with a view to destroying the bacillus in the lungs, and although they do not succeed in this object, in many cases they lessen cough and expectoration. Among the inhalations which have been recommended are equal parts of creosote and spirit of chloroform, equal parts of carbolic acid and spirit of chloroform, ½ ounce each of spirit of chloroform and creosote with 10 grains of menthol. One of the best of these inhalations consists of creosote 2 parts, carbolic acid 2, tincture of (mild) iodine 1, spirit of ether 1, spirit of chloroform 2 ; 6 to 8 drops per hour are put on the sponge of a Burney Yeo respirator.

For the treatment of consumption by *tuberculin*, *see* the article TUBERCULOSIS. *Serums* have also been tried in the treatment of consumption, but the evidence of their utility has failed to secure wide acceptance.

We must now consider the treatment of the chief symptoms of phthisis, as distinct from the disease itself. If there is much *fever* a phenacetin and hydrobromide of quinine pill, 2 grains of each, may be taken three times a day. Benefit will be derived from sponging the body every night, especially over the chest and between the shoulders, with cold or tepid water containing a little vinegar or eau-de-Cologne. This will help to check the *night-sweats*. Patients troubled with this symptom should wear light woollen or flannel night-clothes, and at bedtime should take a pill containing 3 grains of oxide of zinc and ⅓ grain of extract of belladonna. The *cough* with which the patient is often troubled in the morning is usually Nature's endeavour to expel the mucus which has accumulated in the air-passages during the night, an endeavour which should be aided rather than suppressed. It may be assisted by a dose or two of a mixture containing 10 grains of bicarbonate of soda, 3 grains of common salt, and 20 minims of spirit of chloroform in each dose ; this may be taken with a little hot milk and water. The cough which sometimes occurs in the small hours may possibly be relieved by a cup of milk that has been kept hot in a thermos flask. By painting the upper part of the affected side of the chest with a liniment of iodine, not only the cough but also the pain in the chest may be relieved. When *bleeding from the lungs* occurs it is imperative that the patient should be put to bed in a cool and airy room, and should neither speak nor move. Stimulants should, as a rule, be withheld, only cold milk should at first be taken, the patient should suck ice, and ice, or rags soaked in iced water, should be placed on the upper part of the chest on the affected side. (*See also* BLOOD-SPITTING.) Constipation, diarrhœa and flatulence may be treated as recommended in the articles on those subjects.

Prevention.—Persons with a tendency to consumption should, if possible, avoid indoor occupations, especially those which are carried on in crowded and heated rooms or in which irritating dust has to be breathed. Open-air gymnastics should be practised with the view of developing the body generally, but especially the chest, which in such persons is usually flat and narrow, and a course of breathing exercises should be taken. Exposure to damp should be avoided, food should be abundant and nutritious, the digestive organs should be kept in good working order, warm but light clothing should be worn, and if a cold is caught it must be carefully nursed until it has disappeared, or, if it is long in departing, medical advice should be obtained.

Consumption in children.—The

disease may attack children in either of three forms. One, styled *acute miliary tuberculosis*, begins with weakness and rapid wasting, quick breathing, irregular rise in temperature, and in some cases slight cough. In another form, popularly known as *galloping consumption*, there are irregular rises of temperature, quick breathing and pulse, an irritable cough, excessive sweating, and great loss of strength; the child takes less and less nourishment, and in a few weeks from the beginning of the illness death ensues from exhaustion. In the third form, *chronic consumption*, the first symptom to attract attention is rapid wasting. The skin becomes harsh and dry; there is usually a rise of temperature some time during the day; in many cases there is loss of appetite, with diarrhœa, and a troublesome cough. Both in this form and in galloping consumption the tuberculosis may attack the membranes of the brain (meningitis), or the bowels, or the peritoneum, and so the end may be hastened. All three forms, indeed, are extremely serious.

Treatment of consumption in children.—In miliary tuberculosis

and galloping consumption the fever should be treated by means of cold sponging and wet packs, and the use of quinine. If there is much sweating, the skin may be dusted with a powder composed of salicylic acid 3 parts, starch 10 parts, and talc 87 parts. A good mixture for the cough is one consisting of oxymel of squills 1 drachm, compound tincture of camphor ½ drachm, spirit of nitrous

ether ½ drachm, water to 1½ ounces; a teaspoonful for a child one year old. In chronic consumption, children old enough to swallow pills should take one composed of creosote 1 minim and iodoform ½ grain, three times daily, or a palatinoid of beechwood creosote ½ minim, also three times daily. Younger children may be induced to take creosoted wine, which can be got from the chemist. The chest—the breast-bone and below the collar-bone—may be painted every night with strong tincture of iodine, diluted with twice as much glycerin and water in equal parts, and covered, after application, with wool. If this makes the skin sore it may be discontinued and resumed later on. Cod-liver oil, if it can be digested, should be given, but must be stopped if appetite should fail, or the tongue become furred. With it may be combined syrup of the hypophosphites.

Children of consumptive parents should, if possible, be removed from the home and brought up where they will not be constantly exposed to infection. It is especially important that a consumptive mother should not suckle her child. A mildly bracing regime should almost from the beginning be adopted; thus, after the morning bath, the child's body should be rapidly sponged over with cold sea-water, or water containing sea-salt, a little vinegar or eau-de-Cologne having first been added. The child's health should be most carefully watched, especially when such affections as measles or whooping-cough, or a common cold, are contracted. He should live much in the open air, and the bedroom should be thoroughly ventilated; plenty of exercise, not, however, carried to the point of fatigue, should be taken; and when the time comes for him to go to school, he must be preserved from too close an application to lessons.

CONSUMPTION OF THE BOWELS.—The intestine, like any other organ, may be attacked by tuberculosis, but when people speak of "consumption of the bowels" they more often mean tuberculosis of the glands of the mesentery—the fold of peritoneum which attaches the intestine to the back wall of the abdomen. When the bowel itself is deeply involved in tuberculosis, the result is almost always unfavourable ; when the mesenteric glands are attacked, the disease, though serious, leaves ground for hope. The symptoms in the two conditions are very similar, and it will be sufficient if we confine our attention to consumption of the glands—*tabes mesenterica*, as it is technically termed. When this disease occurs in adults it is usually preceded by consumpton of the lungs, or of the intestine, but in children— and it is much more a disease of children than of adults—it may occur independently of tuberculosis elsewhere. In these latter cases it is believed to be caused by drinking milk from tuberculous cows.

Symptoms.—There is usually a good deal of digestive trouble, accompanied either by diarrhœa or by constipation. The abdomen is swollen with gas, and the patient complains of colicky pains ; the temperature rises at night ; the patient becomes anæmic and feeble and emaciated. Cases vary much in severity, but even when the symptoms are severe the glands may presently be converted into chalky masses and the patient may recover.

Treatment.—Abundance of fresh air is required, as in other forms of tuberculosis. The food must be nutritious, and the child should be encouraged to eat as much as possible. The best diet is one made up of minced, underdone meat with red gravy from the joint, as much fat as the child can be induced to take, and eggs beaten up in milk. When diarrhœa is not excessive, cod-liver oil emulsion with maltine, or hypophosphites with maltine, may be given. If there is much diarrhœa, a grain of grey powder with two grains of Dover's powder should be given at night as an astringent.

CONTAGIOUS DISEASE (*see* DISEASE, CLASSIFICATION OF).

CONTRACTED FINGERS (*see* FINGERS, CONTRACTED).

CONTUSIONS (*see* BRUISES).

CONVULSIONS.—This manifestation of nervous disorder occurs chiefly in infants and quite young children. In those of older growth it more frequently takes the form of epileptic fits, which are considered under the heading EPILEPSY. In the first few years of life convulsions naturally cause a good deal of alarm, but, fortunately, it is exceedingly rare for them to have fatal results, nor does the symptom leave behind it any untoward effects.

Causes.—There is a sense in which convulsions are in some cases hereditary, for they are not seldom met with in children whose parents suffer from such nervous disorders as hysteria and epilepsy. One of the commonest causes of convulsions is the strain on the nervous system inseparable from teething. Another frequent cause is the irritation set up by unsuitable food, flatulence, constipation, or worms. In some cases fits are brought on by fright. Children affected with rickets are very apt to suffer from convulsions, which are also a common sequel of inflammation of the membranes of the brain, acute disease of the kidneys, and anæmia, while often they are an early symptom of one of the infectious fevers.

Treatment.—The first thing to be done is to remove tight binders and clothing, to lay the child down and give plenty of fresh air ; meanwhile a bath, of which the temperature is not over 97° Fahr., should be got ready. Into this the child is put for a few minutes until the skin is quite red ; he is then carefully wrapped up and put to bed in a darkened room, being kept perfectly quiet, and encouraged to sleep. A drug most useful in warding off or checking fits is bromide of potash—for an infant, 5 grains in syrup and water, or a 5-grain tabloid, every hour for two or three or four doses, and then in smaller doses as the fits cease ; for children 2 years old, a 10-grain dose may be given ; for children 5 years old, 15 grains. In addition to these measures steps must, of course, be taken to deal with the condition to which the convulsions are due. If teething is the cause of the trouble, relief may be given by rubbing the tender gums with a bromide-of-potash and syrup mixture. If the lower bowel seems to be loaded it may be relieved by a soap-and-water injection ; if the stomach is at fault a teaspoonful of ipecacuanha wine may be given as an emetic, or a grain or two of calomel as a purge ; and the diet must receive attention. If the child is affected with worms or with rickets the treatment described in the articles on those subjects must be instituted.

COOKERY, INVALID.—For those who are sick, or who are recovering from sickness, we give a number of recipes for invalid foods and drinks.

1. Soups, broths, etc.—Meat soups and broths are of very different nutritive value according as they do or do not contain fragments of the meat, as distinct from its extracts. The latter are powerful stimulants to digestion, and are also valuable because of their appetizing character, but their nutritive properties are inconsiderable.

Beef tea.—Freshly-killed, lean, juicy beef is required for making beef tea. Shin of beef is often chosen, but it contains more gelatin than gravy. Fine steak, or the roll of the blade-bone of beef, are perhaps the best portions that can be chosen for the purpose. Take away every morsel of fat, skin, gristle, etc., and leave nothing but the lean fibre ; cut this into very small pieces, put it in a jar, and pour cold water over it, allowing as a rule, a pint of water for a pound of meat. Let it soak for an hour, when the water should be red and the meat white ; then cover it closely, and set the jar in a deep saucepan with boiling water to come half way up its height. Simmer by the side of the fire for two or three hours. Pour out, skim from the surface with a spoon any particles of fat that may be seen, and take away the remainder with a sheet of clean paper. Season agreeably, and the beef tea is ready.

Beef tea (peptonized).—Mix one pound of finely minced lean beef with a pint of water, add 10 grains of bicarbonate of soda, simmer for an hour and a half in a covered saucepan, then pour off the beef tea into a covered jug. Beat up the meat into a pulp with a spoon, and put it also into the jug ; when the beef tea has cooled, add a teaspoonful of liquor pancreaticus, and stir well ; put in a warm place for two hours, stirring occasionally. Boil for two or three minutes, strain, and add salt.

Beef tea (quickly made).—Mince half a pound of the lean fibre of beef and put it into a saucepan with half a pint of water. Let it come slowly to the boiling-point, simmer for a few minutes (as long as can be allowed), season, strain, clear from fat, and serve.

Beef tea (flavoured).—Beef tea may be pleasantly flavoured by boiling in it a pinch of mixed herbs, or a bay leaf, or a little onion, carrot, turnip, or celery, with a few peppercorns. The roots should either be chopped small or be scraped to pulp before being put in.

Celery soup.—Wash a single head of celery and boil it in as much salted water or chicken broth as will cover it. When it is tender rub it through a sieve. Mix a dessert-spoonful of flour to a smooth paste with a little cold water, and pour on it three-quarters of a pint of hot milk. Season with pepper and salt, add the celery pulp and a quarter of a pint of cream. Boil up once and serve.

Chicken broth.—A fowl should be used for this broth, for it will make a more nourishing soup than a chicken. Pluck the fowl, draw it carefully, and remove everything that is not quite dainty—all fat, for example, and skin, if the bird is fully grown. Remove the head and feet also, wash the bird well, and cut the flesh into neat pieces; put these into a stewpan with rather less than two quarts of water. The liver and gizzard, after being carefully cleansed, may be cut into slices and put with the rest. Simmer gently for two or three hours. Take out the pieces of fowl, and leave the broth until the next day. Skim off the fat, and serve. Pepper and salt should be added by the nurse or the invalid. If flavoured broth is desired, three or four sticks of celery, a blade of mace, and a sliced onion may be stewed with the meat.

Chicken broth made from giblets.—For the sake of economy, chicken broth is frequently made from giblets of the bird—that is, from the feet, throat, gizzard and liver. When this is done the fowl can be cooked to make a separate dish, and excellent results can thus be obtained. Cleanse the giblets thoroughly, and be particularly careful to skin the feet, first pouring boiling water over them, and letting them lie in it for about a minute to loosen the skin. Put the cleansed giblets into a small saucepan with a pint of cold water, adding, if approved, a sprig of parsley, a small onion, a slice of carrot, and a little celery. Simmer very gently for two hours, then strain for use. This broth may be flavoured with a tablespoonful of sherry and a squeeze of lemon juice, or it may have a teaspoonful of sago, rice, or tapioca boiled in it to give it consistency.

Chicken cream.—Take a quarter of a pound of raw chicken or veal, three-quarters of an ounce of butter, one egg, one white of egg whipped and half a gill of cream. Pound the chicken in a mortar, add the egg and some seasoning. Rub through a sieve, stir in half the whipped white of egg and the cream whipped. Place in small buttered moulds; steam gently for about fifteen minutes. Serve with a nice white sauce. Pheasant or game may be cooked in this way if wished.

Chicken milk.—Clean a fowl carefully. cut it into small pieces and break the bones. Put it into an enamelled saucepan with two or three peppercorns and a little salt, and the white part of a head of celery, barely cover it with cold water, bring it slowly to the boil, and simmer gently for four hours or more. Strain the broth into a bowl and leave it till cold, when it should form a stiff clear jelly. Carefully remove the fat from the top by wiping the jelly with a napkin dipped in hot water and squeezed dry. Take equal quantities of the jelly and milk, put them into an enamelled pan, boil, skim and serve.

Clear soup.—Take 2lb. of fleshy beef, without fat or skin, from the silverside or buttock, and tie it round to make it compact. Put it into an enamelled saucepan or an earthenware pipkin, and let it brown over the fire for ten minutes. Turn it once during the time, and move it to keep it from burning, sticking a large fork into it to let the gravy escape. A few bones, free from marrow and fat, may be put under the meat. Pour on three pints of cold water and a small tablespoonful of salt, let the liquor come very slowly to the boil, and carefully remove the scum as it rises. Throw in a teacupful of cold water, bring to the point of boiling and skim again. Repeat this process three times. When no more scum rises, put in two carrots, a turnip, two onions, one leek, a bunch of parsley, four bay leaves, and four cloves; draw the pan to the side of the stove and simmer gently for four hours.

Meat juice.—Take freshly killed meat full of gravy, remove the skin, fat and gristle, and cut the lean part into thin strips. Put it into a bottle or jar, cover closely, set it in a saucepan of cold water, and heat gradually for an hour. At no time should the heat rise above 160° Fahr. Press the meat, strain out the juice and gravy, add a little salt, and serve. The liquid should be red and clear, not brown. Half a pound of fine beef should yield about four table-spoonfuls of gravy. Beef that is slightly broiled before being cut up yields more gravy than can be obtained from raw beef. The meat when done should be pink through-out, not brown, and the heat should have penetrated to the centre. When cut it may be squeezed in a lemon squeezer.

Meat purées.—The meat is cut very fine, and simmered in a saucepan until it is pulpy and sufficiently soft to pass through a hair sieve or tamis cloth. Sometimes it is necessary to pound the meat with a pestle and mortar before it can be got to pass through the sieve. Place the sieve upside down on a dish, put the meat on the sieve, and then proceed to rub it through the sieve by means of a spoon or a stick with a rounded end. It may be necessary to add a little water, milk, or other liquid in order to get the purée to pass the easier. The meat in a purée is in the finest possible state of division, and is consequently in a very digestible condition. A spoonful of purée meat is a welcome and valuable addition to beef tea or broth of any kind, or it may be added with advantage to farinaceous slops.

Mutton broth.—Take a pound of the scrag end of neck of mutton, two pints of water, pepper and salt, half a pound of potatoes or some pearl barley. Put the mutton into a stewpan, pour water over it, and add pepper and salt. When it boils, skim carefully, cover the pan, and let it simmer gently for an hour. Strain, let it get cold, and then remove the fat. When required for use, add some pearl barley or potatoes, first boiling the potatoes, mashing them very smoothly, so that no lumps remain, and putting them into a pan. The mutton broth is poured upon them, the whole is stirred until it is well mixed and smooth and allowed to simmer for five minutes. Serve with fried bread.

Rice-cream soup.—Wash two tablespoonfuls of Carolina rice, and boil it gently in a pint of stock for about two hours, or until quite soft. A short time before it is done, put a slice of onion and a stick of celery into a pint of milk, and simmer. When the milk is pleasantly flavoured, pour it over the rice, press the whole through a sieve, and add pepper and salt. Make the soup hot, stir a gill of scalded cream into it, and serve.

Veal broth.—Take a pound of veal free from fat and bone, cut it into small pieces the size of dice, place in a covered jar with a pint and a half of water or barley water, cold ; place in an oven not too hot, and bake for three or four hours, or leave in the oven all night. Strain, and remove fat.

Vegetable soup.—Take some cauliflower, asparagus, peas, or any vegetable that may be preferred, and cook it in the ordinary way. Drain it, put it in a saucepan and cover it well with milk. Let it simmer for a quarter of an hour, rub it through a sieve, season with salt and pepper, and serve.

2. **Milk puddings, etc.**—In combination with starchy and other foods milk is one of the sheet anchors of invalid cookery.

Arrowroot.—This may be made with either milk or water ; if made with water, however, it contains very little nourishment. A small

dessertspoonful of arrowroot will thicken about half a pint of milk. The arrowroot should be placed first in a teacup or small basin, and should be thoroughly mixed with a small quantity of cold water till quite smooth. Then add by degrees the boiling milk, and continually stir the mixture. It may be flavoured with sugar and a little nutmeg or other kind of spice, or some lemon peel may be added.

Cornflour.—Work a tablespoonful of cornflour into a paste with a little water. Take a quarter of a pint of milk and the same quantity of water, and heat them in a saucepan, without boiling. Stir in the cornflour paste, and continue the stirring for three or four minutes after the mixture has thickened

Custard.—Beat up the yolks of four eggs with an ounce of castor sugar and three-quarters of a pint of milk ; pour into a jug and heat in a saucepan of water, stirring all the time, so that the custard thickens without boiling. Serve cold in wineglasses with nutmeg grated over the surface, or flavoured with a little orange-flower water.

Gruel (peptonized).—Gruel of any kind, whether oatmeal, flour, arrowroot, sago, barley, pea, or lentil, may be peptonized by boiling it well and making it thick and strong, pouring it into a covered jug to stand until lukewarm, adding a dessertspoonful of liquor pancreaticus for each pint of gruel, putting it aside in a warm place or under a cosy for two hours, and finally boiling and straining.

Milk (peptonized).—Add to a pint of milk a quarter pint of water. Boil half of the whole, and then add the other half, which will bring it to the required temperature, 140° Fahr. Add two tablespoonfuls of liquor pancreaticus and ten grains of bicarbonate of soda. Pour into a covered jug, stand in a warm place near the fire, or under a cosy, and at the end of an hour and a half, boil for a minute or two. The second boiling is designed to prevent the digestive process from going too far and imparting to the milk an unpleasant flavour ; when it has gone far enough, a slight bitterness will be just perceptible.

Milky rice pudding.—This pudding must be slowly baked ; that is, it must be put into an oven so gentle that the grains will not simply become soft, but will swell as they soften. So long as the rice cooks at all, the more slowly it is cooked the better. The rice should be washed in two or three waters before it is cooked ; it should have a tiny piece of butter put into the dish with it, and it should not be stirred after it is put in the oven. If these precautions are observed it will not be likely to burn, even though it should be long in cooking. Two tablespoonfuls of rice are sufficient for a quart of milk. A little sugar and a pinch of salt should be mixed with the milk in the first instance, and an inch of stick cinnamon and a little lemon-rind may be allowed for flavouring. Rice that is very slowly cooked is usually done when it is covered with a brown skin. If the oven is over-hot, the pudding-dish may be placed in a dripping-tin containing boiling water, the supply of water being maintained. This will moderate the heat.

3. **Jellies.**—The popular notion that the gelatin and isinglass used in the making of jellies are nutritious is mistaken. Such nutritive properties as jellies possess they owe to the other substances they contain, not to the isinglass or gelatin, which is used simply to give them consistency.

Beef jelly.—Prepare beef tea or beef juice in the usual way, and either boil with it a pound of knuckle of veal or add a teaspoonful of soaked gelatin to each quarter of a pint of tea. The gelatin should be boiled until dissolved, and stirred into the beef tea, which may then be left till firm.

Chicken jelly.—This is made of chicken broth, with gelatin added.

Citric-acid jelly.—Soak half an ounce of gelatin in a gill of water for an hour. Boil three ounces of loaf sugar in half a pint of water, and remove the scum as it rises. Put in the soaked gelatin, and boil for five minutes, again removing the scum. Pour the liquid into a basin, stir in it until dissolved an eighth of an ounce of lump citric acid, skim again, add a glass of sherry, and mould it when it is quite cold and beginning to set.

Lemon jelly.—Take half a pint of lemon juice, a pint and a half of water, six ounces of loaf sugar, one inch of cinnamon, four cloves, two and a half ounces of sheet gelatin, the rind of four lemons thinly cut, and two whites of egg with the shells. Put all these ingredients into a saucepan together; whisk until it boils. Let it stand for five minutes. Strain through a clean cloth scalded; set in a mould when clear. When it is firm, turn out. If wine is desired, one gill of sherry may be put in, and that quantity of water omitted.

4. **Fish.**—For invalids the white-fleshed fish, and especially whiting, sole, and halibut, are the easiest to digest. They are most easy of digestion when boiled, and after this the modes of cookery to be preferred are broiling and grilling.

Halibut, boiled.—Take the quantity of fish that is required, wash it quickly, and divide it into pieces convenient for serving. Put it into a wire vegetable-basket, or lay it on a strainer, then lower it into a saucepan of boiling salted water, draw the pan back, and simmer till done. (A pound of fish will probably need to simmer about fifteen minutes ; the exact time will depend upon the thickness.) It must not boil fast at any time. When done, lift it up, let it drain, and serve it at once with a sauce.

Sole on toast.—Take a small sole and lift the flesh from the bone to make four fillets. Trim these, and twist them neatly ; then put them into a saucepan with a gill of boiling water, a few drops of lemon juice, pepper and salt. Bring the water again to the boil, draw the pan back, and simmer gently for five minutes. Drain and lay each fillet on a square of toast, mix a little milk with the stock, and add a little chopped parsley ; pour a spoonful of sauce over each fillet, and serve.

5. **Poultry.**—Having passed from slops, jellies, etc., to fish, the invalid may return to ordinary diet, beginning, of course, with the more easily digested meats, such as chicken, partridge, and pheasant.

Chicken, boiled.—When well cooked this is a dainty dish, besides being very wholesome and digestible. The bird should be plucked and drawn with great care ; indeed, a chicken needs to be handled very gently, because the skin is so tender that it tears very easily. Truss it quite firmly, rub the breast with a cut lemon, and wrap the bird in a floured cloth, plunge it into hot water, and when it boils draw the pan back, and simmer gently till done, skimming occasionally. It will take three-quarters of an hour or longer, according to size, but the more slowly it is cooked the better it will be. It will be more tasty if an onion and a small bunch of herbs are put into the water with it. Before serving, a little sauce may be poured over it, and the rest may be sent to table in a boat. Fried bacon should be served with the dish.

Chicken, broiled.—It is a good plan to divide the bird in halves and cook the two portions on separate days. Put the half chicken in good position, and make it as flat as possible, so that the heat of the fire may reach every part equally, and also that there may be no danger of its sprawling in the dish. A little while before it is cooked, oil it all over, or brush it over with warm butter ; then put it on the gridiron over a clear fire, bones downwards, and keep it well basted. Turn it three or four times during the process of cooking, and begin to turn as soon as the gravy oozes out. Sprinkle with pepper and salt and serve. It will take about twenty-five minutes.

Pigeons, roast.—Take two young pigeons —house pigeons if they are to be had—and be careful that they are young and freshly killed; they quickly lose their flavour if kept. Put inside each a forcemeat ball made of bread-crumbs, a little butter, chopped parsley, pepper and salt. Truss firmly with the legs forward, the wings to the side and points turned over the back, and pass string round the skewers. Hang the birds back to back breast downwards, baste freely with good dripping or butter, and draw gradually nearer the fire. Ten minutes before taking them up, turn the birds so that the backs may be cooked. When the steam draws to the fire it is a sign that they are done. They will take from twenty to twenty-five minutes. Serve on a hot dish with a little gravy over them, and more in a tureen.

6. Drinks for Invalids.—Among the beverages suitable for invalids the following may be recommended :—

Apple water.—Pour a pint of boiling water over a couple of roasted apples; let it stand in a warm place for three hours. Strain and sweeten to taste.

Barley water.—Wash an ounce of pearl barley in cold water three or four times, or boil it for a few minutes. Place the washed barley in a pint and a half of water, with a bit of lemon peel and a little sugar. Allow it to simmer, stirring it constantly until it is of nice thickness, then strain it and add lemon-juice. If a slight flavour of lemon is preferred with a very little acid, put a slice of lemon with the barley in the water; sweeten to taste. Care must be taken not to make the drink too sweet for it will then cloy the palate and produce flatulence.

Blackberry cordial.—This home-made drink is valuable in hot weather as a preventive of diarrhœa. Squeeze enough blackberries to make a quart of juice, add a pound of loaf sugar, and let this dissolve, heating slowly. Add one teaspoonful of cloves, cinnamon, and nutmeg. Boil all together for twenty minutes. On removing from the fire add a wineglassful of brandy. Put into bottles while hot, and seal. Use a teaspoonful for a glassful of iced water.

Cream soda.—Boil together for a few minutes three pints of water and two pounds of white sugar, the juice of two lemons and two ounces of tartaric acid. Set it aside to cool. Beat the whites of three eggs to a stiff froth; slowly sift into this half a cupful of flour, and stir until smooth, then flavour with half an ounce of winter-green essence. When the syrup is nearly cool, stir in the eggs. When cold, pour into a stone jug which has been scalded until perfectly sweet, and keep in a cool place. For a drink, use two tablespoonfuls of this syrup for a glass of water, and just before drinking add a quarter of a teaspoonful of soda and stir well.

Egg drink.—Mix a tablespoonful of arrow-root to a smooth paste with cold water. Add two tablespoonfuls of white sugar and the whites of two eggs which have been whisked with a little water. Add boiling water to make up the quantity to three pints, boil up once quickly, and stir while it boils.

Egg gruel.—Beat an egg, add pepper and salt, and pour on a teacupful of boiling water, stirring briskly.

Egg, white of, with milk.—Beat the white of an egg, and mix with it a tumblerful of milk, a teaspoonful of brandy, and half a tumblerful of soda water. This drink is sometimes valuable in diarrhœa.

Fruit juice and soda water.—Express the juice from any sort of ripe, sound, fresh fruit, such as strawberries, raspberries, currants, oranges, apricots, peaches, or apples. The best way to do this is to put the fruit in a jar with a close-fitting lid, set the jar in a saucepan with boiling water round it, and allow to stew till the juice flows freely. The firmer fruits will need to have a small quantity of water stewed with them. A little sugar should be added to the juice according to its acidity. When the fruit is melted, drain the juice from it without squeezing it, put about two tablespoonfuls of the syrup into a tumbler, and fill the vessel with soda water. If a couple of tablespoonfuls of cream be used as well as the fruit, a delicious drink will be produced.

Lemonade.—Pare off the yellow rind of a fresh lemon, and be careful not to take any of the white pith, as it would make the lemonade bitter. Put the thin rind into a jug with the strained juice of two lemons and about an ounce of loaf sugar. Pour over all a pint and a half of boiling water, and let the liquid stand till cold. Strain and serve.

Oatmeal tea.—Add a tablespoonful of coarsely ground oatmeal to a pint of water, simmer gently for an hour, and replace the water evaporated.

Raspberry sharp.—Fill a two-quart glass jar with fresh red raspberries; pour over them cider vinegar until the jar is full. Screw the cover on and let stand one week, then scald and pour into a jelly-bag, and let drain ; to the juice add 1lb. of loaf sugar to every pint. Boil fast for twenty minutes, and skim when any scum arises ; while hot put into six bottles or glass jars. One spoonful in a glass of iced water makes a drink of delicious flavour.

Tea, milk.—This is made by using boiling milk instead of water when infusing the tea ; in this way is obtained all the pleasant flavour of the tea without the injurious ingredients, which are insoluble in milk.

Toast and water.—Toast a piece of crust of bread till it is quite brown or almost black, place it in a jug, pour some water upon it, and leave to stand for a short time.

CORNS.—A corn is an overgrowth of the outer layer of skin—the epidermis—caused by the pressure of or friction with tight or ill-fitting boots. It is distinguished from a callosity, a simple thickening and hardening of the skin, such as occurs on the heel, for example, by the presence of a central ingrowth. *Hard* corns usually form on the toes ; when the toes are doubled under by the use of short boots they appear on the prominent joints above or on the flat ends of the toes beneath. *Soft* corns, which are spongy and much more tender, are generally met with between the toes, their formation being encouraged by the moisture in this situation ; most often they are found on one or other side of the fourth toe, the one next to the little toe. The considerable pain which may be caused by corns is due principally to pressure of the thickened skin upon the ends of nerves ; it is often greater in moist and damp weather. Sometimes corns undergo inflammation, with the formation of " matter " (pus).

Treatment.—It is necessary, especially in the case of soft corns, that the feet should be kept clean and dry. Pressure from boots must be avoided, either by the use of a ring-shaped corn plaster, so applied that the corn is in the centre of the ring, or

by the use of specially made boots. For soft corns, a powder composed of salicylic acid (2 drachms) and boric acid (1 ounce) may be dusted between the affected toe and its neighbour, and a piece of boric-acid lint inserted to keep them apart. Hard corns may be treated with glacial acetic acid (1 or 2 drops applied at night with a brush), or salicylic collodion (salicylic acid $\frac{1}{2}$ drachm, extract of cannabis indica 5 grains, collodion to $\frac{1}{2}$ ounce) may be painted on daily for a week to soften the corn and facilitate its removal by cutting after soaking it in hot water. Inflamed corns should be treated with a compress of boric-acid lint moistened with warm water and covered with oil-silk. If pus has formed, a slight surgical operation may be necessary to give relief.

CORPUSCLES (*see* BLOOD AND LYMPH).

CORROSIVE POISONS (*see* POISONS AND POISONING).

CORROSIVE SUBLIMATE POISONING (*see* MERCURY, POISONING BY, ACUTE).

CORYZA (*see* CATARRH, NASAL).

COSTIVENESS (*see* CONSTIPATION).

COTTON-WOOL (*see* DRESSINGS AND STRAPPING FOR WOUNDS).

COUGH.—Cough is usually the result of irritation of the air-passages, as by cold air, an accumulation of phlegm, or the presence of a foreign body. One of the commonest causes is what is popularly known as a cold on the chest—that is to say, a slight attack of bronchitis. But all affections of the lungs, whether acute or chronic, including consumption, pleurisy, and asthma, are accompanied by cough. It may also be set up by the pressure, on the wind-pipe or the larynx, of an aneurysm, a goitre, or a tumour, or by enlarged tonsils, adenoids, inflammation of the pharynx or of the nasal mucous membrane, or nasal polypi. Cough may also be caused by conditions that affect the air-passages only indirectly. One form, for example, is due to heart disease; another, known as the stomach cough, often met with in dyspepsia, especially among children, is due probably to some indigestible matter in the stomach which presses upon the pneumogastric nerve, the great nerve which supplies both the stomach and the lungs. Cough may even, in the same way, be set up by intestinal trouble brought about by an overloaded bowel, or by worms. Yet another cause of cough is irritation of the ear by an accumulation of hardened wax. But the most curious of all causes of cough is hysteria, which is dependent on no discovered physical cause.

The character of a cough is some guide to its origin. In affections of the larynx—the voice-producing apparatus—it is *harsh, coarse* and *croupy*, or else *whispering*. In whooping-cough, advanced consumption, gangrene of the lung, pleurisy, etc., it is *paroxysmal*. If in children it occurs at night in paroxysms, it indicates adenoids, enlarged tonsils, or a long uvula—the " curtain " that hangs down from the soft palate at the back of the throat. A *hacking* cough, short, and frequently repeated, denotes early consumption of the lung, or simply a cold in the nose or throat. A *brassy, strident* cough is characteristic of laryngeal paralysis, and of aneurysm of the aorta—the great artery nearest the heart. The cough in hysteria is of a *barking* character; in pleurisy and pneumonia it is *short, restrained,* and *painful.*

Treatment.—Among the simple remedies used for coughs are medicated glycerin jujubes, Spanish liquorice, lozenges of potash, tannin, or borax (combined with menthol or eucalyptus), linseed tea, barley water, and black-currant jelly. For the cough due to relaxed throat, elongated uvula, or enlarged tonsils, it is desirable to apply an astringent such as glycerin of tannic acid, which should be painted over the affected surface with a brush two or three times a day. If local applications prove ineffectual it may be necessary to remove the tonsils, or to shorten the uvula, as the case may be. Gastric and intestinal coughs may be relieved by a good purge which clears the stomach and the bowel of offending matters. If the cough is due to cold on the chest it is necessary to observe whether it is dry, painful, and accompanied by soreness under the breast-bone, or loose and attended by a good deal of expectoration. In the former case a sedative medicine is required such as the following :

Paregoric elixir .... 2½ drachms
Oxymel of squill .... 2½ drachms
Sweet spirit of nitre...... 2½ drachms
Water to 8 ounces
Two tablespoonfuls (for children a teaspoonful) every four hours.

When the cough is loose and attended with free expectoration, stimulating mixtures are required, such as the following :

Carbonate of ammonia ... 40 grains
Tincture of senega .... 5 drachms
Syrup of squills.......... ½ ounce
Syrup of tolu............ 1 ounce
Chloroform water to 8 ounces.
Two tablespoonfuls every three or four hours.

Another good stimulating mixture is one containing antimonial wine as well as carbonate of ammonia :

Antimonial wine .... 40 minims
Carbonate of ammonia ... 40 grains
Syrup .... ½ ounce
Tincture of lemon........ 3 drachms
Water to 8 ounces.
Two tablespoonfuls every three hours during effervescence with a powder of citric acid, 10 grains.

If the throat is irritated, a mixture such as this will be found soothing :

Confection of hips ....100 grains
Powdered tragacanth..... 6 grains
Syrup of poppies .... 36 minims
Vinegar of squills .... 36 minims
Acetic acid.............. 2 minims
Ipecacuanha wine........ 30 minims
Boiling water to 1 ounce.

A teaspoonful every three or four hours.

The cough of chronic bronchitis may be relieved by the carbonate of ammonia mixture (p. 95), combined with an inhalation of Scotch pine oil or of pure terebene as in the following prescription :

Oil of Scotch pine (or pure
   terebene) .... 40 minims
Light carbonate of mag-
   nesia .... 20 grains
Water to 1 ounce.

A teaspoonful to be added to 1 pint of hot water at a temperature of 150° Fahr., and the steam inhaled for five to ten minutes. (Water of the specified temperature may be obtained by adding ⅔ pint of boiling to ⅓ pint of cold water.)

COUNTER - IRRITATION (*see* INFLAMMATION).

" COURSES " (*see* MENSTRUATION AND THE MENOPAUSE).

COW-POX (*see* VACCINATION).

CRAMP.—This is the popular name for what is medically known as involuntary tonic (i.e. continuous) contraction of muscle, an extremely painful affection which, fortunately, is of short duration, though it may recur. Any muscle may be affected, but those most often attacked are the muscles of the calves of the legs or those of the feet. Cramp is more likely to occur after fatigue, or when one is in a run-down condition, but it is sometimes due to exposure to cold, and is often associated with gout. It usually comes on during the night when a limb is moved or stretched ; the slightest movement is sometimes sufficient to induce an attack. The best way of cutting it short is to stretch the affected muscle, as by straightening the leg if its muscles are attacked, or by straightening the toes with the hand if the foot is affected. This requires a little resolution, but it is well worth the effort. Firm rubbing with the hand also relieves the pain. If one is below par, a tonic should be taken. If gout is present, it should receive the treatment described in the article on that subject. The cramp which occurs at night may in some cases be prevented by taking 10 grains of antipyrin on going to bed. For the cramp which sometimes occurs in pregnancy, *see* PREGNANCY, DISORDERS OF ; for occupational cramps, *see* WRITER'S CRAMP.

CRETINISM.—This form of arrested bodily and mental development is often met with in the valleys of mountainous districts, or in plains which are subject to inundations ; such cases are examples of *endemic* cretinism. Scattered, or *sporadic* cases, which are independent of locality, also occur. Both forms alike are due to failure of the thyroid gland to form its secretions properly. In the sporadic cases the defect in the gland is congenital ; in endemic cases the gland degenerates as the result of the action of some micro-organism, not yet identified, which is conveyed by drinking-water, and is destroyed by boiling. The marks of cretinism are unmistakable. The lower limbs are misshapen, the head is deformed, the nose flat and broad, the face large, the mouth, owing to enlargement of the tongue, is kept partly open, so that there is dribbling of saliva, the belly is prominent, growth stunted, the skin thick, wrinkled, and of a dirty yellow colour, and both hearing and speech are affected. In endemic cretinism the disease appears in earliest infancy, and may even be hereditary.

In sporadic cretinism it does not appear until the child is cutting his milk-teeth, or later.

Treatment.—In endemic cretinism the child should be removed to another region. In both forms great benefit is derived from administering extract of thyroid gland, especially in the case of quite young children. By this means the deficient secretion of the thyroid gland is supplemented. The treatment must be continued for the rest of life. If in endemic cretinism the child has reached the age of ten or twelve before thyroid treatment is instituted, it is comparatively inefficacious.

CROUP.—The subject of croup is involved in a good deal of confusion, for the name is applied to several different affections. We have already dealt in the article CHILD-CROWING with one of the affections for which the name is sometimes used; here we shall deal with two other conditions, which will be termed respectively *true* and *false croup.*

True or inflammatory croup.— This is a severe catarrh of the voice-box or larynx, with thick tenacious secretion and some spasm of the vocal cords. It attacks boys more frequently than girls, and is most common between the ages of one and seven.

Symptoms.—After a day or two's feverishness, with running at the nose and coughing, the breathing becomes noisy, the voice is almost lost, the cough becomes " brassy " and painful. The breathing grows more and more difficult, and the child has to be propped up in bed; the temperature may rise to 101° Fahr.; there is rapid pulse, the skin is moist, the forehead is bathed in sweat. Suffocation may appear to threaten; and in severe cases the patient may succumb to exhaustion. To avert suffocation, or to save the patient's strength from further exhaustion, it may become necessary to open the wind-pipe below the larynx (tracheotomy).

Treatment.—The patient should be kept in a temperature of not less than 60° nor more than 65° Fahr. both day and night. Heat may be applied to the throat by sponges or spongiopiline wrung out of hot water and frequently renewed, or cold water may be sprinkled upon the face and chest. In the case of older children a mustard plaster may be used, or tincture of iodine may be painted on the front of the throat. If the patient is strong, an emetic may be given as soon as obstruction to the breathing begins—say, 5 grains of powder of ipecacuanha in syrup of orange, repeated in ten minutes if vomiting does not occur to cause free expectoration and ease the breathing. The diet should be limited to warm milk and barley-water. The affection is unsuitable for domestic treatment, and careful watch must be kept for indications that tracheotomy is necessary.

False croup.—In this affection there is but slight catarrh of the larynx, and spasm of the vocal cords is the predominant symptom. It usually occurs in children above the age of two or three who have rickets or adenoids or enlarged tonsils, and appears to be in some measure hereditary.

Symptoms.—In the night, after having betrayed a slight hoarseness or cold in the head during the day, the child wakes up with a loud, barking cough, and the breathing begins to be difficult and noisy, while from time to time there are paroxysms of loud coughing. After a while the breathing becomes easier, the cough less harsh, and the child will fall asleep, waking up next morning with no symptom but slight hoarseness and a cough. During the next night, however, the attack is repeated, and may recur for three or four nights in succession. The difficulty of breathing and the distress the child suffers inevitably excite alarm, but the attacks very rarely have a fatal termination, and sooner or later, as he grows older, they will cease.

Treatment.—To ease the difficulty of breathing, ice may be placed at the back of the neck or hot sponges applied to the throat and face. If the spasms continue, an emetic of ipecacuanha, as advised for true croup, may be given. A steam kettle will also be found useful. Great care must be taken to prevent children subject to these attacks from catching cold, and the general health must receive attention. If adenoids are present, or the tonsils are enlarged, the condition should, of course, be corrected.

CRUTCH PARALYSIS (*see* PRESSURE PALSY).

CUPPING.—This form of counter-irritation consists in drawing blood to the surface by the application of cupping-glasses (Fig. 14), small glasses in which the air is rarefied by heat or is exhausted. If the skin is first scarified, the process is known as *wet cupping;* if not, it is termed *dry cupping.*

CURVATURE OF THE SPINE (*see* SPINAL CURVATURE).

CUT THROAT, TREATMENT OF (*see* HÆMORRHAGE).

CYANOSIS.—When, from either functional or organic disease, the heart fails in its work of pumping the blood through the body, and there is consequently an imperfect flow through the lungs, it follows that the blood receives from the lungs an insufficient supply of oxygen; it therefore remains blue instead of taking on the red colour characteristic of arterial blood, and in consequence the surface of the body is blue, as denoted by the word cyanosis. The same result is produced if the flow of blood through the lungs is impeded by disease in these organs, as in asthma and pneumonia. Cyanosis is met with in an extreme degree in infants born with malformed hearts, and such infants are said, in popular language, to suffer from " the blue disease." The symptom may be mitigated by

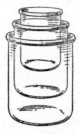

Fig. 14.—Cupping-glasses.

the inhalation of oxygen, the supply of this gas to the blood being thus artificially supplemented.

CYSTITIS (*see* BLADDER, INFLAMMATION OF).

CYSTS.—Of the many kinds of cysts, we shall deal in this article with three : (1) dermoid, (2) sebaceous, (3) hydatid cysts. Cysts of the eyelids are considered in the article EYELIDS, CYSTS OF.

1. **Dermoid cysts** are congenital, the result of a fault of development, and are lined with skin or mucous membrane. They most commonly contain material secreted by the sebaceous glands in the cyst-wall, from which fine hairs in some cases project, but sometimes they are found

to contain teeth, which are one of the appendages of the skin. The most common situation for dermoid cysts is the face. Unless they become inflamed they cause no pain. Treatment consists in cutting out the cysts, if they are not too numerous.

2. Sebaceous cysts (wens) result from an accumulation of sebaceous matter and shreds of scarf skin in the sebaceous glands, the glands of the hair-follicles. They most commonly occur on the scalp and face. They are usually doughy in consistence, but may be hard, are rounded in shape, though they may be flattened on the top, and may slowly grow to be as large as an orange. Unless they become inflamed they are painless ; when they undergo inflammation the skin is bright red, and the cyst sometimes suppurates and ulcerates. The treatment is to remove the cyst before it becomes inflamed.

3. Hydatid cysts are caused by a small tapeworm, *Tænia echinococcus*, which inhabits the intestines of the dog and enters the human system in the form of eggs that have been deposited on growing vegetables. The favourite situation for the cysts which develop from the eggs is the liver. If they give rise to no pain or inconvenience they should be let alone, in the hope that they may undergo spontaneous cure. In other cases various methods of treatment are employed. One consists in tapping the cyst and withdrawing the fluid by aspiration. In more serious cases it is often necessary to open the abdomen and withdraw the contents of the cyst by draining and irrigation, or to remove it altogether.

D

DANDRUFF.—Dandruff (pityriasis) is not an affection in itself, but a symptom of several other affections of the hairy parts of the body. It most frequently affects the scalp, where numbers of greasy white scales form. Sometimes there is more or less itching, but frequently the only sign of the affection to the patient is the shower of scales which collects on the collar of his coat or falls from his head when he brushes his hair. If the condition persists for a long time, much of the hair may be lost. In children dandruff is sometimes caused by their heads being kept too hot ; in adults, by continually sitting under a lamp, or by digestive troubles or constipation. *Treatment.*—The general health must be attended to. The head must not be over-brushed, nor should the brush used be hard, but the scalp should be kept perfectly clean, and both brush and comb frequently cleansed. The scalp should be washed with soap and water daily, and may then be rubbed with a lotion composed of the following ingredients :

Corrosive sublimate	3 grains
Alcohol 90%	3 ounces
Water and rose water equal parts to..............	2 pints

The hair-wash. Poison.

DAY BLINDNESS (*see* BLINDNESS).

DEAF-MUTISM.—If a child becomes totally deaf before the age of five or six, dumbness will follow the deafness, for, being unable to hear, he cannot in the ordinary way learn to speak ; such children are called deaf-mutes. Up to the age of about twelve months it is hardly possible to be sure whether total deafness is present or not, but if, having reached that age, a child who betrays no lack of intelligence has never attempted speech, the presumption is that this is owing to deafness. Fortunately, deaf children can not only be taught to speak by motions of the hands—the manual alphabet, but also by the oral method, by which they learn to read the movements of their teachers' lips and then to imitate them. A medium of communication being thus established, the deaf child can be taught to read and write, and can be educated to a fairly high standard.

DEAFNESS.—Loss of hearing, partial or complete, is a symptom of many affections of the ear, and it may occur in diseases not directly connected with that organ. Deafness may be present at birth, when both ears will be involved. Or it may be due to blocking of the ear-passages by wax, to the presence of foreign bodies, to inflammation of the lining membrane of the ear, to tumours or masses of fungus; in these cases it is one ear that is chiefly affected, and the trouble is more frequent in adults than in children. In old age the gristle of the ear sometimes collapses and blocks up the outer orifice. Not a few cases of deafness are dependent upon disease of the middle ear—the part inside the tympanic membrane (Plate VIII); the commonest of these diseases is inflammation, which may thicken or destroy the membrane, obstruct the cavity, or impede the movements of the little ear-bones (the ossicles) and fasten them together. Other causes of deafness are diseases of the excessively delicate nervous structures of the inner ear; these sometimes follow a severe attack of an infectious fever or of mumps, or they may be due to violent emotional disturbance, mental strain, or protracted anxiety. Nervous deafness, as it is called, may also be brought on by attacks of megrim (sick headache), or may follow in the train of Menière's disease (q.v.). Tumours of the brain, again, may destroy the sense of hearing, or it may be affected by injuries to the head.

A simple way of testing hearing is to ascertain the distance from one ear at which a watch must be held for the ticking to be audible, compared with the distance from the other ear or from the ear of a normal person. If the watch is placed in contact with the scalp the ticking is sometimes heard more plainly in the deaf than in the sound ear; it is then clear that the deafness is due to obstruction either in the outer passage or in the tube—the Eustachian tube—leading from the throat to the middle ear. But if the ticking is heard less plainly, or not at all, by the deaf ear, it follows that the nervous structures of the inner ear are at fault.

Treatment.—Whether or not a defect of hearing is remediable depends upon whether the cause can be removed. In cases in which the gristle of the ear collapses, a small silver tube may be worn to keep the walls of the canal apart. For defects due to such simple causes as the accumulation of wax and the presence of foreign bodies the remedy is obvious. In all cases arising from affections of the middle or inner ear the advice of a specialist must be sought. In cases of partial deafness ear-trumpets and various other devices are frequently of considerable service. If the tympanic membrane has been destroyed it may be replaced by an artificial drum, which the patient can learn to put into position himself.

DECAYED TEETH (*see* TEETH, DECAY OF).

DEFICIENCY DISEASES.—These diseases, forming at present only a small group, arise from deficiency or absence of one or other of the elements of a normal mixed diet. They are scurvy, many cases of beriberi, probably rickets, and possibly pellagra (*see* articles on these subjects). The element usually deficient or absent is a vitamin (*see* Vitamins, *under* Food).

DEFORMITIES, CONGENITAL (*see* Malformations, Congenital).

DELIRIANT POISONS(*see*Poison and Poisoning).

DELIRIUM.—This disturbance of consciousness is not a disease, but a symptom set up by inflammation or other morbid condition of the brain or its membranes, or by the presence in the blood of poisons, whether consisting of an accumulation of urea as in severe disease of the kidney, or formed by the action of germs as in the infectious fevers. It may also be caused by excessive consumption of certain drugs such as alcohol (*see* Alcoholism, Acute), Indian hemp and opium. Even in ordinary illnesses delirium may occur, usually at the time when the patient is waking from sleep ; this mild form is of no importance and gradually passes away with the return of health. In the more violent forms, those which accompany inflammation of the brain, mania, and high fever, the patient raves and shouts, and struggles violently against restraint. In the opposite form of delirium, met with in the later stages of long and exhausting illnesses, he lies unconscious, muttering to himself, and only notices what is going on around him to weave it into his dreams. This form is sometimes termed " muttering delirium," and is also known as the " typhoid state," from the frequency of its occurrence in the exhaustion stage of typhoid fever. In yet another of the many

forms of delirium, " busy delirium," the patient talks incessantly and incoherently, and is constantly arranging the bedclothes or picking at them or at anything within his reach.

DELIRIUM TREMENS (*see* Alcoholism, Acute).

DELUSIONS (*see* Insanity).

DEMENTIA (*see* Insanity).

DENGUE.—This disease, met with in many tropical and sub-tropical regions, usually occurs as a rapidly spreading epidemic. It is no doubt due to a germ, which is communicated by the bite of mosquitoes. It is characterized by fever, an eruption of red spots, severe aching pains, and prostration. It is very rarely fatal, but is apt to relapse and to be attended by serious complications.

DENTAL CARIES (*see* Teeth, Decay of).

DENTITION (*see* Teething and its Troubles).

DEODORANTS (*see* Disinfectants and Disinfection).

DERBYSHIRE NECK (*see* Goitre).

DERMIS (*see* Skin).

DERMOID CYSTS (*see* Cysts).

DHOBIE'S ITCH.—This is a popular designation in the East for a number of itching, ringworm-like diseases, but the term is most frequently applied to such diseases in the arm-pit or the crutch (*tinea cruris*). The common belief is that these affections, which are due to various kinds of parasites, are contracted from the clothes that have been to the dhobie or washerman ; hence the name. There is much inflammation of the skin and itching, and the consequent scratching frequently leads to the formation of boils or small abscesses. *Treatment.* —The affected part having been washed with soap and water, Vleminck's solution should be applied at night for three or four nights.

DIABETES INSIPIDUS.—Diabetes is a word of Greek origin which signifies " going through," and denotes the large quantity of urine which is secreted by or goes through the kidneys. The ordinary form of diabetes, of which the essential feature is the presence of sugar in the blood and urine, is formally termed *diabetes mellitus* (*see* the next article). Of diabetes insipidus the distinguishing characteristic is the excessive quantity of urine, which is free from sugar, and of low specific gravity—from 1001 to 1010.

Causes.—Excessive urine, technically termed *polyuria*, may be due to one of several distinct conditions : (1) a defect in the kidneys which incapacitates them from secreting concentrated urine, (2) diseases of the pituitary gland, situated below the brain, (3) an inflammation of the membranes of the brain due to syphilis, (4) the excessive consumption of fluid. Diabetes insipidus, unlike the ordinary form of diabetes, is more frequently met with in the young, and like the latter it is much more common in men than in women.

Symptoms.—The urine is not only excessive in quantity but unusually pale in colour and, though clear when first passed, soon becomes turbid. The patient suffers intensely from a thirst which he finds it impossible to quench, however much he may drink. As in ordinary diabetes, the skin is dry and rough and secretes little perspiration, and the tongue is red and glazed ; the mouth is coated with a sticky mucus. There is usually constipation, and the breath is foul.

Treatment.—Unless the condition is due to a habit of taking too much fluid, the patient should be allowed to drink freely, but should be cautioned to endeavour to control his thirst and to allay it as far as possible by rinsing out the mouth with water. Alcohol, tea and coffee should be prohibited, but no restriction need be placed upon food so long as it does not disagree. In the general treatment of the disease valerian is often employed, with or without bromide of ammonium and tincture of cannabis indica. Chills must be guarded against, and the general health carefully watched.

DIABETES MELLITUS.—The meaning of the term diabetes is explained in the preceding article, DIABETES INSIPIDUS. *Mellitus* means " honeyed " or " sweet " ; diabetes mellitus, therefore, is the form of diabetes which is characterized by the presence of sugar in the urine and in the blood, and it is the form which is usually meant when the word diabetes is used with no qualifying adjective. It should be premised that the presence of sugar in the urine is not necessarily an indication of diabetes. It may be merely a temporary circumstance which is explained by an excessive consumption of sugary foods and which ceases as soon as the diet is modified.

Cause.—It is now generally accepted that many cases of diabetes, though not all, are due essentially to a deficiency in the internal secretion of the pancreas. In addition to the pancreatic juice, which is carried by the pancreatic duct to the intestine, there to take its part in the process of digestion, the pancreas, like some other glands, forms what is called an *internal* secretion, which is taken up by the blood (*see* DUCTLESS GLANDS). In some persons this secretion is defective, and the consequence is that the sugar in the blood is not properly disposed of but remains there until it is filtered out by the kidneys and carried off in the urine. That this is the explanation of a large group of cases of diabetes is suggested by the fact that if this pancreatic secretion, obtained from oxen, and known as *insulin*, is administered in such cases, it causes a rapid reduction of the sugar in the urine and the blood. As to predisposing causes, diabetes is one of the affections in which hereditary influence appears to play a part. Rare in negroes, it is unusually frequent in Jews; in other races the disease appears to show a predilection for persons of fair complexion. It occurs more often in men than in women, is predominantly a disease of middle age, and, when it occurs in the young, usually runs a more rapid course. It is more common in the comfortable than in the poorer classes. The onset seems in not a few cases to be determined by a mental shock or nervous strain. Injuries to the brain or spinal cord are sometimes said to be a cause of diabetes, but other authorities contend that such injuries cause not true diabetes, but simply glycosuria —i.e. the temporary presence of sugar in the urine.

Symptoms.—The disease usually comes on insidiously. The urine is increased in quantity, though not usually to the same extent as in diabetes insipidus. It is clear and pale, but in many cases has a greenish tinge. Owing to the sugar it contains, the specific gravity is found on examination to be raised on an average to between 1030 and 1050. One indication of the disease is the peculiar odour of the urine—like that of apples or of new-mown grass. If the urine is excessive in quantity the patient suffers from extreme thirst. The appetite is voracious, but, however much food is consumed, there is so much loss of nourishment in the form of sugar that the patient loses weight and strength, and is easily fatigued. There is frequently great mental depression, with a good deal of irritability. The skin becomes dry and harsh, the secretion of sweat almost ceases, there is great liability to eruptions and boils, and gangrene may be set up by quite slight injuries, as for instance to one of the toes. The hair becomes thin and the nails brittle. In severe cases the tongue is raw and glazed, and occasionally is covered towards the root with black fur. The breath may have a sweet heavy odour, and the patient may be conscious of a sweet taste in the mouth. The bowels act very imperfectly, and the motions are hard and dry.

Enough has been said to show that diabetes is a serious affection, but if the patient has reached middle life there is ground for hoping that under proper treatment he may enjoy moderately good health for many years, and at last have the satisfaction of dying from some quite different disease.

Treatment. 1. *Medicinal.*—Until recently medicinal treatment in diabetes was of subordinate importance, but now that insulin can be given, that is so no longer. Insulin, as we have seen, is a pancreatic preparation which, in suitable cases of diabetes, enables the patient to take a moderate quantity of carbohydrate food—i.e. food containing sugar or starch. It does not actually cure the disease, and it is still necessary that the diet should be regulated, but it controls the symptoms and enables the patient to follow his ordinary avocation, and so marks a great advance in the treatment of diabetes. To diminish the acidity to which patients are liable, bicarbonate of soda is useful ; 15 grains may be taken in a wineglassful of water three times a day.

2. *Dietetic.*—Formerly the great aim of treatment was to prevent the entrance into the body of sugar, and greatly to limit the intake of starch, which is converted into sugar by the saliva and other digestive juices. Sugar, therefore, was entirely cut off, saccharin being used as a substitute. The daily allowance of milk, which is a sugar-containing fluid, was gradually reduced until it was taken only in tea and coffee, and finally it was replaced for those purposes by cream. The staff of life was tabooed, but a small quantity of potato was permitted. All the green vegetables were available, and virtually all animal foods, almost the only exceptions being liver and oysters. This regimen has now been considerably modified as a result of the discovery, made independently by Dr. Allen in America and Dr. Graham in London, of the value of alimentary rest as the foundation of a systematic re-education of the as- similative powers. This is known as the fasting treatment of diabetes. It may begin with two hunger days, in which the patient takes only bovril and broth, made without vegetables, and tea and coffee, with water or lemonade, sweetened if desired with saccharin. Then follow two vege- table-and-egg days, in which the patient is allowed five eggs per day, bovril or broth, or both, green vege- tables, tomatoes, butter, tea and coffee, and water or lemonade. Then meat or fish is added, then bacon with one egg less, then sardines with another egg cut out, then ham minus another

egg. This is what is known as the ladder diet, and it takes twelve days to reach the top rung. If at this time the patient is free from sugar, milk and bread are added to the menu, and gradually increased every other day until the limit of carbohydrate tolerance is found to be reached. If, on the other hand, the patient is not sugar-free when the top of the ladder is attained, the whole process is repeated. The patient, however, is not at the end of his hunger days when it is discovered just how much carbohydrate he can assimilate, for, in the discretion of his physician, two such days may be given at intervals —say once a month, the standard diet being then resumed.

The ladder diet, modifiable in de- tails, has given excellent results in the treatment of diabetes. In cases in which insulin is not contra-indicated, the ladder diet is combined with injections of this preparation, and then the hunger days may be dispensed with, except in obese patients, who may be all the better for a little starvation. If, when the patient has reached his standard diet, sugar re- appears, the symptom may in some cases be treated by increasing the dose of insulin. The dose may now and again be reduced in order to discover whether the patient's tolerance of carbohydrates has improved.

3. *Hygienic.* — Patients suffering from diabetes should be careful to avoid chills, to which, owing to defec- tive action of the skin, they are espec- ially liable. The action of the skin may be stimulated by a warm bath twice a week, or by a less frequent Russian or Turkish bath, and gentle exercise should be taken.

DIACHYLON PLASTER (*see* DRESSINGS AND STRAPPING FOR WOUNDS).

DIAGNOSIS.—This term signifies both the process by which the medical man discovers what disease his patient is suffering from, and the conclusion at which he arrives. The more familiar methods of diagnosis, such as taking the temperature, the pulse-rate and the rate of breathing, examining the tongue, etc., are referred to in other parts of this book, but a brief explanation of such of the more technical methods as are in common use may here be given.

Having made a careful inspection of his patient, the medical man avails himself of his sense of touch in the process which is termed **palpation ;** that is, he feels or manipulates the part of the body to which his attention is directed, in order to ascertain its condition or that of underlying organs. Thus, if a patient is suspected to be suffering from gall-stones the medical man can discover by his sense of touch that the gall-bladder is distended, and he may even be able to feel the gall-stones. Or if the case is believed to be one of cancer of the liver, that organ may be felt to be nodular, and even the depressions in the centre of the nodules may be detected.

Percussion consists in placing a finger or fingers of the left hand flat upon the chest and sharply tapping them with one or more of the fingers of the other hand ; or an instrument called a pleximeter is used ; the character of the sound produced in either of these ways being an indication of the condition of the underlying organ. For example, in lung disease the sound, instead of being resonant as in health, is dull, showing that the lung is solid or that its place has been taken by fluid.

In **auscultation** the doctor uses his unaided sense of hearing, or more frequently he employs an instrument known as a *stethoscope*, fitted with ivory end-pieces which he places in his ears. The stethoscope is indispensable in many affections, especially affections of the heart and blood-vessels and of the lungs. Thus in diseases of the circulatory system it enables certain abnormal sounds, such as those termed bruits, to be heard, while in lung disease any departure from the ordinary sound produced by the air as it passes through the lungs can be appreciated. If there is phlegm in the bronchial tubes the air will make a bubbling sound, varying with the thickness of the fluid ; if the tubes are contracted there will be a whistling sound. If, again, the lung is inflamed and solidified the sounds will be loud ; if fluid has accumulated between the lungs and the chest wall, as in pleurisy, the sound will be hardly heard at all or heard as in the distance.

Much light is thrown upon the nature of a large number of diseases by **microscopical examination.** In tuberculosis the presence of tubercle bacilli in the expectoration can be discovered; microscopical examination of the blood will reveal, among other things, whether there is a disproportion of the red or of the white cells, and, in malaria, the presence of the parasite which causes that disease. By microscopic examination of the urine the nature of any deposits in it, such as those which form calculi, can be distinguished, and in certain diseases of the kidney, casts of the tubes of that organ may be found. In the same way the presence of " matter " (pus) in the urine indicates inflammation of the kidney or bladder or some other part of the urinary tract.

The pulse.—Reference has been made to taking the pulse-rate as one of the familiar methods of diagnosis. But the pulse is examined not only to determine its frequency, but also its *regularity, force* and *tension,* and for these purposes ingenious instruments with formidable names which need not be quoted are used. An irregular pulse may indicate failure of the heart or some disturbance of the nerves which actuate or control its movements ; it is common also in certain forms of indigestion. A pulse of high tension, that is, a pulse which resists the pressure of the finger, may indicate disease of the kidney ; a pulse of low tension may be a symptom of heart-failure, and is often met with in the later stages of fevers, when the heart is weak and the blood-vessels are dilated.

Among modern discoveries in the art of medicine, perhaps the most important is that of the **X-rays.** Here we are concerned not with their value in the treatment of disease, but with their utility in diagnosis, which is already enormous and is constantly growing. Discovered in 1895 by the late Professor Röntgen, they are produced by electricity in a glass tube which has been partially exhausted of air, and their peculiar property is that, while able to pass through many opaque substances, they are unable to pass through metal, bone, etc., and consequently a shadow is cast. A shadow picture of the skeleton of a human body can thus be thrown on a screen, and broken bones, bony outgrowths, metal substances in the flesh or in the internal organs, stones in the kidney or the bladder, etc., become visible. The rays are also obstructed by other than hard substances. If, for instance, a meal of bread-and-milk and barium is eaten, the passage of the rays is obstructed by the barium, and by employing them at intervals the progress of the meal from the stomach to the rectum can be followed. Thus

the position and shape of the stomach, the efficiency of its muscular contractions, the position and size of the pylorus, through which the food passes into the intestines, the length of time the food remains in the stomach, and any peculiarity in the form or working of the intestine, can be determined. If, again, a liquid such as collargol, a form of silver in solution, or bromide of soda, is injected into the kidney, it offers obstruction to the rays, and in this way abnormal conditions of the kidney itself, or of the ureters, the tubes through which the urine descends into the bladder, can be detected.

Among the many special instruments used in diagnosis are the *cystoscope,* which enables the surgeon to inspect the interior of the bladder ; the *urethroscope,* which reveals the interior of the urethra ; the *ophthalmoscope,* by which the interior of the eye can be examined ; the *laryngoscope,* which reflects light down the wind-pipe so that a picture of the parts is seen in a mirror, and the *nasal speculum,* used for examining the interior of the nose. Similarly tubes are used by which the condition of the œsophagus (gullet) and of other parts of the alimentary canal can be discerned.

DIAPHORETICS (*see* Medicines, and how they are measured).

DIAPHYSIS (*see* Bones and Joints).

DIARRHŒA.—Diarrhœa is sometimes less a disease itself than a symptom of other diseases, such as dysentery, typhoid fever, and the later stages of consumption ; but here it will be considered only in the aspect of a distinct disorder. The form of diarrhœa which is known as epidemic or summer diarrhœa is dealt with in a separate article (*see* EPIDEMIC DIARRHŒA).

Causes.—Diarrhœa is sometimes brought on by exposure to damp and cold. Another group of cases can be explained by causes that act through the nervous system. The influence of disagreeable mental emotions on the intestines is very striking; a sudden panic will operate on the bowels of some persons as surely as a black draught, and much more rapidly. Probably everyone has experienced the aperient effect of the nervousness induced by some unusual ordeal, such as speaking in public, sitting for an examination, or even starting on a long journey. In this group of cases is usually placed the form of diarrhœa which is known as lientery, a word which means " smooth intestine "; the bowels in these cases are set in motion by the mere consumption of food, which, instead of remaining in the stomach until it is converted into chyme, at once passes into and is hurried along the intestines, appearing in the stools almost unchanged. But the most frequent cause of diarrhœa is the irritating and indigestible character of the food, or its excess in quantity. The food may disagree because it is contaminated or unsound, or it may be that the patient has what is called an idiosyncrasy to that particular food; that is to say, it may agree with most other people but disagrees with him. In one group of cases the patient suffers from what is called *morning diarrhœa*, the peculiarity of which is that he has two or three loose motions as soon as he gets up or immediately after breakfast, but is not further troubled in this way during the rest of the day.

Symptoms.—Diarrhœa is frequently accompanied by vomiting, and there is usually more or less pain. If the motions continue the patient soon suffers from exhaustion, has a feeble pulse and low temperature, and may be attacked with faintness. The urine is scanty, and the skin becomes dry. The attack may last only twenty-four or forty-eight hours, or in the absence of treatment several days, or in spite of treatment may become chronic.

Treatment.—In all the cases due to *dietary causes* it is important not to stop the diarrhœa until the irritating substances have been expelled from the intestine. The first thing to do is to take an aperient, such as a tablespoonful of castor oil, or a teaspoonful of Gregory's powder, or 5 grains of the compound rhubarb pill. The action of the bowels may be assisted by drinking freely of simple fluids such as milk-and-water, or barley-water; this will also relieve the severe thirst. If the patient complains of cold and pain a hot mustard bath may be given, or flannels wrung out of hot water and sprinkled with spirit of turpentine may be applied to the abdomen. If there are cramps the limbs may be rubbed with a stimulating liniment. If faintness comes on, small quantities of brandy and water may be given, and the patient should be kept in the recumbent position, or with the head slightly lower than the rest of the body.

The bowels having been thoroughly cleared, an attempt may be made to stop the diarrhœa. For this purpose an astringent such as sulphuric acid may be taken in the following form:

Aromatic sulphuric acid .. 80 minims
Tincture of lemon........ 2 drachms
Carbonate of bismuth .... 40 grains
Syrup .... ½ ounce
Water to 8 ounces.
Two tablespoonfuls every hour or two until the diarrhœa is relieved.

A favourite remedy is the chalk mixture of the British Pharmacopœia: two tablespoonfuls may be taken every two or three hours. Another favourite drug in diarrhœa is bismuth, which supplies a protective covering to the irritated mucous membrane of the intestine. It may be taken in the following form :

> Carbonate of bismuth .... 80 grains
> Bicarbonate of soda...... 80 grains
> Mucilage of gum .... ½ ounce
> Spirit of chloroform ..... 80 minims
> Peppermint water to 8 ounces.
> Two tablespoonfuls every two or three hours.

To each dose of this medicine, or of the chalk mixture of the British Pharmacopœia, if neither in itself suffices to check the diarrhœa, or if there is much pain, the doctor may add 10 minims of tincture of opium (laudanum).

In *nervous* and *lienteric diarrhœa* a mixture containing 5 grains of bromide of potash and 3 to 5 minims of tincture of belladonna, taken immediately before meals, will usually be efficacious in mild cases. If this is not effective the doctor may give tincture of opium.

For *morning diarrhœa* nothing more is necessary than that the patient should abstain from liquid after 6 o'clock in the afternoon.

In *chronic diarrhœa* the greatest attention must be paid to the diet. In obstinate cases the patient should live entirely for a time on milk, which should be boiled and diluted with Vichy or Apollinaris water ; 6 ounces of milk with 2 ounces of either of these waters may be taken every three hours for a time, and then, if there is no digestive trouble, every two hours. In cases in which the patient cannot take even diluted milk in large quantities, the milk may be peptonized. If this milk diet is adopted the patient should be confined to bed. It may be modified by the addition of raw meat, which should be divested of all fat and gristle, reduced to a pulp and flavoured with powdered sugar or currant jelly and taken two or three times a day. In some cases of chronic diarrhœa it is found that the patient does better on a diet of animal food, such as lightly cooked mutton, veal, or poultry.

Not merely, however, in chronic but in all forms of diarrhœa must the diet be carefully regulated. Until the looseness of the bowels is checked nourishment should be taken cold, or at most tepid, and in such forms as milk, gruel, and arrowroot, or weak chicken or mutton broths and beef tea.

Diarrhœa in children.—It is important that diarrhœa occurring in children, and especially in young children, should receive prompt treatment. The commonest cause of the complaint is food that is unsuitable or excessive in quantity ; it may be due in the case of children at the breast to the mother's indisposition or dietary indiscretions. But most of the cases occur in hand-fed children, cow's milk having a great tendency to irritate the stomach by curding and fermentation. With regard to what constitutes diarrhœa in children, it may be said that three or four actions of the bowels a day in a child of 3 months, and two or three a day in a child of 6 months, may be regarded as normal, but that anything beyond is excessive. In a healthy infant the motions are of a bright-yellow colour, while in diarrhœa they are apt to be pasty and greenish and to be mixed with curd. In mild cases, in which there are not more than four or five motions a day, the trouble may be relieved by peptonizing the milk or lessening the quantity, or partly substituting for it barley-water or weak arrowroot. In more severe cases the milk must for a few days be discontinued, its place being taken by small quantities of sweetened barley-water, arrowroot, and weak veal broth, given cold or at the most warm. At the beginning of treatment a mild aperient should be given in the form of 10-drop doses of castor oil mixed with syrup and given three or four times a day, or grey powder, a ½-grain tabloid twice a day. When the motions have become natural in number and colour an astringent should be given such as the mixture of which the formula appears on p. 46.

DIATHERMY (*see* ELECTRICAL TREATMENT).

DIATHESIS.—A term that indicates a physical condition which renders the body especially liable to some particular disease. This tendency—to use a simpler term—is frequently hereditary or congenital, as in gout, tuberculosis, asthma, affections of the organs of circulation, certain forms of kidney disease and nervous affections; but it may also be acquired, as the result of privation, intemperance, and many other inimical influences.

DICK TEST (*see* SCARLET FEVER).

DIET (*see* FOOD).

DIGESTION.—Digestion is the process by which food is prepared for absorption and assimilation by the tissues of the body. This process is performed while the food is passing through the alimentary canal (Fig. 15 and Plate VII), a tube beginning as the mouth and pharynx, continuing as the œsophagus (gullet), expanding into the stomach, contracting into the small intestine, expanding again into the large intestine, and terminating at the anus. Digestion begins in the mouth, where the food is divided by the teeth into small fragments so that the various digestive juices may act upon it more easily, and where also the saliva, the secretion of the salivary

glands (Fig. 16), partly digests starchy foods, which have to be converted into sugar. From the pharynx, at the back of the mouth, the food passes, by way of the gullet, into the stomach, where it is acted upon by the gastric juice, containing hydrochloric acid, pepsin, and rennin; with this it is thoroughly mixed by the movements

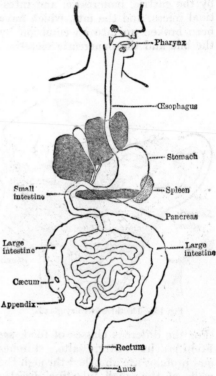

Fig. 15.—Diagram of the alimentary canal.

of the stomach. Alcohol, salts, a percentage of certain sugars, and a small proportion of meat are absorbed by the stomach; but much the greater part of the food passes through the sphincter called the pylorus into the small intestine, where it is acted upon not only by juices poured out by this part of the alimentary canal, but also by the secretion of the liver (bile) and of the pancreas. Before it has been long in the small intestine almost all that is absorbable is ready for absorption—the water, which required no change, the starches, which have been converted into soluble sugar by the salivary and pancreatic juices, the proteins, which have been split up into simpler chemical compounds—peptones and albumoses—by the gastric, pancreatic, and intestinal juices, and the fats, which have been broken up into an emulsion by the bile and the pancreatic secretion.

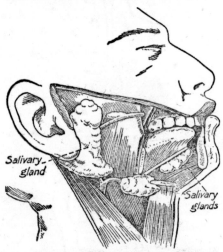

Fig. 16.—The three salivary glands.

(For the different classes of food, *see* Food.) The water, salts, starches and proteins are absorbed through the walls of the small intestine directly into the blood-vessels, and carried by them to the liver; the fats are removed by processes of the small intestines called villi, and are carried by a long tube (the thoracic duct) to the left side of the neck, where, mixed with the lymph which has exuded from blood-vessels, they enter a large vein and are so distributed by the blood-stream all over the body. The residue of the food passes on into the large intestine, where most of the

remaining fluid is absorbed, leaving little but solid waste products, which, mixed with multitudes of bacteria, are expelled as fæces from the rectum, the lowermost part of the bowel, through the anus.

DIGITALIS POISONING.—The drug known as digitalis, derived from foxglove leaves, is sometimes taken accidentally. The patient may lapse into unconsciousness and death quite suddenly. *Treatment.*—Give an emetic, and follow it up, as soon as vomiting has occurred, with draughts of hot strong tea or coffee, or half a teaspoonful of tannic or gallic acid in hot water. As the poison acts upon the heart, the patient should be kept lying down for some time after the symptoms have ceased, and should take stimulants in the form of sal-volatile and hot water, or hot gin or brandy and water.

DILATATION OF THE HEART (*see* Heart Disease).

DILATATION OF THE STOMACH (*see* Stomach, Dilatation of).

DIPHTHERIA.—Epidemics of this disease are more prevalent in winter than in summer, the mortality reaching its maximum in November or December. Formerly diphtheria was more a rural than an urban disease, but of late years it has been more prevalent in towns than in country districts. This change is doubtless an indirect result of compulsory education, the spread of the disease being promoted by the massing together of large numbers of children, many of whom, from defective nutrition and depressed health, are in such a condition as to be receptive of this as of other forms of infection. But diphtheria frequently appears not in epidemics but as isolated cases, which it is impossible to trace to any par

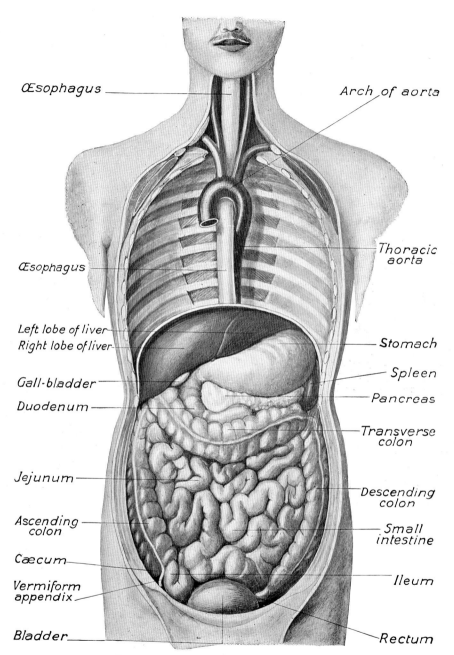

Œsophagus ⎯⎯⎯⎯⎯⎯

Arch of aorta

Œsophagus ⎯⎯⎯⎯⎯

Thoracic aorta

Left lobe of liver⎯
Right lobe of liver⎯

Stomach

Gall-bladder ⎯⎯

Spleen

Duodenum ⎯⎯⎯

Pancreas

Transverse colon

Jejunum ⎯⎯⎯

Descending colon

Ascending colon ⎯⎯

Small intestine

Cæcum⎯⎯

Vermiform appendix⎯

Ileum

Bladder⎯⎯

Rectum

PLATE VII. THE ORGANS OF DIGESTION, ETC.

ticular source of infection. After exposure to infection, a period of twelve days must elapse before the " suspect " can be regarded as having escaped the disease. A child who has " caught " the infection is not allowed to return to school until four weeks after the beginning of the illness, and only then if there are no discharges from the mouth, throat, or other parts, and no albumin in the urine, and if the diphtheria bacillus is absent from swabs of mucus from the throat and nose.

Cause.—The germ of the disease is the Klebs-Löffler bacillus, named after the bacteriologists who respectively discovered and isolated it. There is no evidence that the breath of the patient is infective, but by such acts as coughing, sneezing, and laughing the poison can undoubtedly be communicated, either directly to persons in the room, or by contaminating articles of furniture or wearing apparel, etc. The poison clings to such things with great tenacity. There is no clear evidence that it can be conveyed by water, but the culpability of milk is proved beyond a doubt ; either the milk may be contaminated by a person suffering from slight diphtheria, or possibly the cow may have been suffering from bovine diphtheria. Cats and dogs are subject to a contagious affection closely resembling diphtheria, and have conveyed it to children, in whom it appears as true diphtheria. The effluvia from drains are probably concerned in the dissemination of the disease, not directly, however, but indirectly, by causing a sore throat or inflammation of the nasal mucous membrane, etc., which aids the bacillus in its efforts to get a foothold, so to speak, in the mucous membrane. A damp soil, damp dwelling-houses, and deficient scaven-

ging are also predisposing causes. A method of discovering whether a person is susceptible to diphtheria was discovered in 1913. It is known as *Schick's test*, after its deviser. A tiny dose of diphtheria toxin is injected into the skin of a person who has been exposed to infection ; if no redness and hardness develop at the site of injection after twenty-four to forty-eight hours, the person may be regarded as not susceptible to the disease ; if the redness and hardness occur, he should be inoculated with diphtheria toxin-antitoxin in order to render him immune to the disease. The success of this method of prevention is emphatically vouched for by the Medical Research Council, who, in a report issued in 1927, announced that the Ministry of Health considered no further detailed inquiry to be necessary but would continue to urge local authorities to carry it out. It is hoped that by this means the prevalence of diphtheria, at present increasing, will be greatly diminished.

Incubation stage and symptoms. —As a rule, the interval between infection and the onset of the disease is only two or three days, but it may be not more than twenty-four hours, or as much as four days, or longer. The early symptoms often come on insidiously. The patient is conscious of soreness of throat, which may be slight. Usually, though not in all cases, a patch of " false membrane " forms on the affected part, most frequently the tonsil, and gradually spreads. It is of a dirty-grey or yellowish-white colour, and is firmly fixed to the mucous membrane, can only be separated with difficulty, and then leaves behind it a raw, bleeding surface. There is also fever, associated with drowsiness, irritability aching in the back and limbs, and digestive disturbance, but often such symptoms are not sufficiently severe to send the patient to bed. The lymphatic glands at the angle of the jaw and the sides of the neck become inflamed and enlarged. In favourable cases the symptoms abate after the fourth or fifth day, the false membrane comes away and does not grow again, the enlarged glands become smaller, the temperature sinks to normal, and by the ninth or tenth day convalescence may be established.

In less favourable cases the false membrane extends downwards into the larynx, or upwards into the nose. In the former case there is what is called diphtheritic or membranous croup, shown by the development of hoarseness, which grows gradually more severe until the patient can only speak in a whisper. This is a dangerous condition, for the obstruction may become so great as to cause suffocation. If the membrane spreads in the other direction, into the nose, it indicates a severe attack and much danger. The presence of albumin in the urine, due to inflammation of the kidneys set up by the poison in the blood, is a frequent complication of diphtheria; it occurs within the first ten days, and in most cases gradually passes off during convalescence. Vomiting is often an associated symptom. Paralysis may come on at any time, even weeks after the complaint seems to have quite disappeared; this complication, if limited to the throat, will gradually pass off as the disease subsides, but paralysis may appear in other parts, such as the legs and arms. As a rule it gradually passes off, though it may not finally disappear for many months.

Treatment.—The treatment of diphtheria has been revolutionized by the introduction of diphtheria *antitoxin*, one of the great triumphs of the serum method of treatment. The antitoxin is prepared by injecting doses of the diphtheria poison into an animal, usually a horse. On recovery from the complaint thus produced the animal is found to be " immune," or protected, against diphtheria, just as a human being is usually protected by an infectious fever from another attack of the same fever for a longer or shorter period; and if its blood-serum is injected into a person suffering from the disease, there are substances in it which act as an antidote to the poison, lessen the severity of the attack, and greatly increase the chance of recovery. It is important that the remedy should be used as early as possible; if only a suspicion of diphtheria arises the antitoxin should be given, for an unnecessary dose can do no harm, beyond possibly giving rise to itching or nettle-rash. Within twenty-four hours of the injection in a case of actual diphtheria, the throat trouble usually subsides, the fever grows less, and the general condition of the patient improves.

The room prepared for the patient should be well ventilated and kept at a temperature of 63° or 64° Fahr.; the air should be moistened by the vapour from a bronchitis kettle. The diet should be light and nutritious, and given every two hours during the day and every three hours at night. Milk is the best food; it must be supplied freely, and supplemented with farinaceous foods, beef tea, and meat soups. Plenty of fluid should be taken. Pieces of ice may be slowly sucked, and hot poultices and fomentations applied to the throat relieve the discomfort. If there is much exhaustion, or any sign of heart-failure, brandy in small quantities may be added to the food.

In children in whom the false membrane extends downwards into the larynx the bed should be surrounded by a tent and the enclosed space kept moistened with steam from the bronchitis kettle, fitted with a long tube. A spray may be used at intervals, consisting of glycerin of carbolic acid 6 drachms, bicarbonate of soda 60 grains, hot water 6 ounces.

If any of the complications mentioned above arise, the patient must remain in bed until recovery is fully established. Paralysed muscles should be treated with gentle massage and electricity.

Since antitoxin came into general use, *tracheotomy* is much less often necessary to save the patient from being suffocated by the extension downwards of the false membrane, but even now it sometimes has to be performed in diphtheria cases. It consists in making an opening into the wind-pipe and fixing in a tube (Fig. 17), which allows air to enter below the small and obstructed opening of the glottis—the space between the vocal cords. The nurse must be careful to keep the tube clean and free from obstruction. If the patient cannot take liquid food through the mouth, given with a spoon, nasal feeding may be employed. If all goes well, it may be possible to remove the tube by the third or fourth day.

DIPSOMANIA.—A dipsomaniac is one who, from time to time, feels an impulse to excessive alcoholic indulgence which he is unable to control, just as in other cases an irresistible impulse to the commission of some absurd or criminal act is felt. The impulse having been yielded to, the patient returns to his normal habits, and may even be horrified at the recollection of his fall, until the impulse arises again. The attack is preceded by irritability, depression, loss of appetite, and failure

of attention. The chief hope lies in giving the patient treatment by suggestion (hypnotism) and in inducing him, when he becomes conscious of the preliminary symptoms, to place himself under a control which will prevent him from having access to drink.

DISEASE, CAUSES OF.—The causes of disease—in medical phraseology their etiology—are divided into two great groups—(1) *predisposing* and (2) *exciting* causes. Predisposing causes are those which render a person especially liable to the attack of the exciting cause—which is sometimes

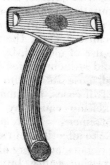

Fig. 17.—Tracheotomy tube.

alternatively known as the determining cause. Among **predisposing causes** is *heredity*. The influence of this factor in the production of disease is involved in much obscurity, and all that need be said about it here is that what is transmitted from parent to child is in most cases a tendency to a particular disease rather than the disease itself. The diseases in which heredity can most clearly be traced are certain nervous and arterial affections. Perhaps the most easily recognized of the predisposing causes is *previous disease ;* thus, one attack of pneumonia or of bronchitis is likely to be followed by others. Yet other predisposing causes are age, sex, climate, and occupation, but the most prolific of them all may be summed up in the words *bad hygiene,* a phrase which includes, among other things, bad ventilation, overcrowding, contaminated water, defective drainage, insufficient food or clothing, alcoholic intemperance, and excess of all kinds. Of **exciting causes** of disease, the most important are *germs* and *parasites.* The list of germ diseases includes tuberculosis and infectious fevers, and is gradually being extended with the development of more and more refined methods of research (*see* GERMS). It is not necessary to attempt an enumeration of all the exciting causes of disease, but it may be pointed out that the same agent may act both as a predisposing and as an exciting cause. Thus, the habitually excessive use of alcohol, by impairing vitality and reducing defensive power, may predispose its victim to a great variety of diseases, and may also act as an exciting cause by producing delirium tremens. Heat, again, may predispose to affections of the liver and digestive organs, and may also operate as an exciting cause by producing heat-stroke.

DISEASE, CLASSIFICATION OF.—There are various methods of classifying disease. One method depends upon the distribution of the particular disease. Thus, an affection which is always more or less prevalent in a given region, as, for instance, one of the forms of goitre, which haunts damp, sunless valleys, is said to be *endemic* to that region. If a disease spreads rapidly and widely it is said to be *epidemic,* and if it should spread over a large part of the world it is spoken of as *pandemic.* It is clear from this that the same disease may be endemic, epidemic and pandemic. More or less opposed to all these terms is the term *sporadic,* which is used

when a disease occurs in isolated cases; thus, cerebro-spinal meningitis (spotted fever) is apt to occur in this apparently casual kind of way. Diseases are also classified according to their intensity and duration; if a disease comes on suddenly, is accompanied by severe symptoms, and runs a rapid course, it is said to be *acute,* or, if the symptoms are of more moderate severity, *sub-acute;* if, however, it is slow, protracted, and accompanied by no violent symptoms, it is said to be *chronic.* Here, again, it is obvious that the same disease may have both an acute and a chronic stage, as, for instance, bronchitis, which may begin with an acute attack that subsides into the chronic form. Another classification divides diseases into *organic* and *functional,* the former group consisting of diseases in which the structure of the affected part undergoes definite change, and the latter of disorders which simply affect the working of an organ without inflicting traceable damage upon its structure. Examples of these two kinds of disease in the same organ are valvular disease of the heart, in which the valves of the heart have undergone permanent deterioration, and palpitation, which in many cases is due merely to nervous or other temporary disturbance. A disease, again, may be either *general* or *local;* that is, it may affect the whole body, or only some special organ or part. The infectious fevers, for example, are general diseases; eczema is a local disease which is usually limited to some part or parts of the skin. Yet another form of classification divides diseases into *hereditary, congenital,* and *acquired* groups. The first of these terms is applied to diseases which are actually transmitted from parent to child—hæmophilia (q.v.) for instance; the second, to diseases which, though present at birth, are not necessarily inherited—for example, the deformity known as club-foot; the third, to diseases that develop at some time during post-natal life quite apart from hereditary influence, such as an infectious fever. Finally, it may be pointed out that literally a *contagious* is not precisely the same as an *infectious* disease. A contagious disease is communicated by actual contact with the patient or with a secretion or discharge from the body. In an infectious disease, on the other hand, such as influenza, no direct contact is necessary; the infection may, for example, be borne by the air. This distinction, however, means little more than that contact is direct in one case and indirect in the other; and the term infectious covers both kinds of transmission. *Notifiable* diseases are infectious diseases which medical practitioners are bound to notify to the Sanitary Authority (*see* NOTIFICATION OF DISEASES).

DISEASE, STAGES OF.—The course run by many diseases can be divided into fairly definite stages. The first of these stages is termed the *onset*, which is frequently gradual, but may be sudden as in the case of a paralytic "stroke." Usually, following exposure to an infection, there is an interval, of varying length, which is known as the *incubation period*. After this comes the period of *invasion*, in which the symptoms of the disease appear. In the case of eruptive fevers a characteristic rash now comes out; this is termed the stage of *eruption*. The disease then reaches its climax, and the patient either dies or begins to recover. In the latter case the disease enters the stage of *decline*, which may be sudden as in pneumonia, or gradual as usually in cases of typhoid fever. If the disease abates

suddenly, the decline is by *crisis*; if gradually, the decline is by *lysis*, a term of Greek origin signifying a loosening. The final stage is that of *convalescence*, in which the patient tends to return to his normal state of health. A disease may, however, leave behind it what are termed *sequelæ*, which may persist for a longer or shorter time and then disappear, as in the case of a cough following bronchitis, or may remain permanently, as in the organic disease of the heart which is often set up by rheumatic fever.

DISINFECTANTS AND DISINFECTION.—Disinfectants are substances which destroy infective germs; hence they are also called germicides. They are to be distinguished from antiseptics (q.v.) which merely arrest the development of germs, and still more from deodorants, which only neutralize disagreeable smells. Some substances may be used either as disinfectants or as antiseptics, according to the strength in which they are prepared.

Disinfection of the hands.—Wash them in a 1-in-40 carbolic acid solution, or a 1-in-20 solution if the skin is not tender.

Disinfection of discharges.—In a case of infectious disease all the patient's discharges must be disinfected. The excreta and disinfectant should not at once be poured down a drain but should stand for about half an hour. Efficient disinfectants are chloride of lime ($\frac{1}{4}$lb. to the gallon of water), potassium permanganate (1 in 100), carbolic acid (5 per cent.), corrosive sublimate (1 in 1,000), cyllin, and izal. Corrosive sublimate (perchloride of mercury) is one of the most reliable of all disinfectants. It is, of course, a deadly poison—all disinfectants are poisons

—and the bottle containing it should be labelled " Poison " and should also be coloured, so that the sublimate may not deteriorate under the influence of light. Tuberculous sputum should be disinfected by a 5-per-cent. carbolic-acid solution.

Disinfection of mattresses, bed-clothes, clothing, carpets, etc.—Such articles as these are best disinfected by steam. Hot air, which was once used for the purpose, only kills germs when it is so hot that the fabrics are in danger of being scorched. The steam is passed into the disinfecting chamber and the articles are exposed within cylinders to either saturated or super-heated steam. If this method is not available, the things should be soaked in a 5-per-cent. carbolic or chloride of lime solution, and then thoroughly washed. Letters and books, too, may be disinfected by steam. Things that have leather coverings should be baked in an oven, or may be put into a cupboard and disinfected by formaldehyde.

Room disinfection.—During occupation the floor must daily be wiped over with a broom covered with a piece of cloth that has been dipped in some such disinfectant as lysol—one teaspoonful to a pint or more of warm water, and the same solution may be occasionally sprinkled on the floor. A disinfectant should be placed in all the utensils used in the room, and a quantity should be kept outside the room in a tub, bath or pail, and the bedclothes and the patient's night garments, handkerchiefs, etc., steeped in it for eight hours before being sent to the wash. No dish, spoon, or tumbler should be sent out of the room until it has been scalded with boiling water. Before the patient leaves the sick room he should have a disinfectant bath or be washed all over with a disinfectant, and then

wrapped in a blanket or dressing gown and taken to the room he is to occupy, where he must put on fresh night-wear or underclothing as the case may be.

The room he has left—floor, walls and furniture—must now be thoroughly cleansed with soap and water. After cases of measles and German measles (rubella) this, followed by leaving the doors and windows wide open for a few hours, is all that is needed. After other infectious diseases the room, after soap-and-water cleansing, should be washed with a solution such as that mentioned above. It may then be prepared for gaseous disinfection—fumigation as it is commonly called. The blankets should be thrown one by one over the end of the bed, or over the open door of a wardrobe ; rugs should be thrown over chairs, the mattress set on its edge, all cupboard doors opened, all drawers taken out and stood on end against the wall. The register of the grate must be closed, or the mouth of the chimney stopped up with straw or canvas, the windows must be closed and latched, and pieces of paper pasted over the edges, where air might enter, and also over the key-hole. Water is sprinkled over the floor and walls, a damp atmosphere being conducive to gaseous disinfection, and the room should be warmed and kept at a temperature of between 50° and 70° Fahr. One of the best gaseous disinfectants is formalin, applied with a Lister's Formaldehyde Fumigator, which is made in three sizes to suit the size of the room. Placed on a fireproof plate and lighted, it is left in the room for at least four hours, preferably for all night. The room is then unsealed and thoroughly aired, the doors and windows being left wide open for at least twelve hours.

An older method of disinfecting by

means of sulphur is still sometimes used. Not less than 3lb. should be burnt for every thousand cubic feet of space (to measure a room, *see* VENTILATION). The rolls of sulphur, broken up into small pieces the size of marbles, are placed on a tray supported by, say, a pair of tongs laid across a pail or foot-bath that contains a few pints of water. The pail or foot-bath should be in the centre of the room, but if it is a large room several must be used, and placed in different parts of it. Not only should the sulphur be burnt over water, but the walls should be sprayed with water, for unless the air is damp, sulphuric acid gas will not be formed and the germs will not be destroyed. As soon as the sulphur is alight the room must be closed up, the door locked, the key removed, and the key-hole and door edges pasted up.

The room must be left undisturbed for twenty-four hours, and then unsealed, and the doors and windows should be left wide open for at least twelve, and preferably for twenty-four hours. It is well to strip off the wall paper and limewash the walls, and it should remain empty and exposed to full ventilation for a week before being repapered. The floor and skirting must be scrubbed, and the furniture and fixtures cleansed with a cloth that has been dipped in the carbolic-acid solution. Dry dusting or sweeping is inadmissible; it is just the way to give any germs that may still be living their chance of doing further mischief. The disinfection of bedding, carpets, etc., has already been described.

Disinfection of a room during or after tuberculosis.—The National Association for the Prevention of Consumption has formulated rules for the disinfection of a room which is in occupation by a tuberculous patient,

and recommends that this should be done two or three times a year, and again, of course, before the room is used for ordinary purposes. These are the rules :

1. Gaseous disinfection of rooms, or "fumigation" as it is termed, by whatever method it is practised is inefficient in such cases.
2. In order to remove and destroy the dried infective discharges, the disinfectant must be applied directly to the infected surfaces of the room.
3. The disinfectant may be applied by washing, brushing, or spraying.
4. Amongst other chemical solutions used for this purpose a solution of chloride of lime (1 to 2 per cent.) has proved satisfactory and efficient.
5. In view of the well-established fact that it is the dust from dried discharges which is chiefly infective, emphasis must be laid upon the importance of thorough and wet cleansing of infected rooms.
6. Bedding, carpets, curtains, wearing apparel, and all similar articles belonging to or used by the patient, which cannot be thoroughly washed, should be disinfected in an efficient steam disinfector.
7. After all necessary measures of disinfection have been carried out, the essential principle governing the subsequent control of a case of consumption is that all discharges, of whatever kind (especially expectoration from the lungs), should under no circumstances be allowed to become dry.

If the room is clean, and there has been no direct soiling of walls or floors with sputum, it is not necessary to use the chloride of lime solution, and Esmarch's method of disinfection will suffice. The wall-paper is well rubbed with bread-crumb or with dough ; floors, painted walls, and woodwork are washed with boiling water, and ceilings lime-washed. Bedding, articles of clothing, etc., are washed with boiling water or disinfected by steam. If this method is adopted it is necessary to make sure that all dust is removed from the walls, especially from the corners.

DISLOCATION.—Dislocation may be defined as a displacement of a bone at a joint—either *partial* or *complete*, according as to whether the surfaces of the bones are or are not entirely separated. If the dislocated end of the bone comes through the skin the dislocation is said to be *compound*.

A joint may be dislocated by muscular action, as sometimes happens to the lower jaw, which may be " put out " in yawning. But a much commoner cause is external violence, which may be direct, i.e. applied to the joint itself, or indirect, i.e. applied to some other part of the body. An example of the former is furnished by dislocation of the patella or knee-cap as the result of striking the knee against, say, a piece of furniture. An example of the latter is dislocation of the shoulder as the result of a fall on the hand.

The pain of dislocation is often of a sickening character, and may induce a feeling of faintness. The joint is fixed, and its usual movements are possible neither to the patient nor to a bystander. The joint-end of the displaced bone is felt in a new position, and there is an effusion of blood into and around the joint, which causes swelling. Whether the case is one of fracture or of dislocation, it is equally necessary that the greatest care be taken in attempting any movement of the bone to determine which condition is present.

If a joint has once been dislocated it is prone to slip out again, and in some joints, such as the patella (the knee-cap), the patient learns how to reduce the dislocation himself, but except in such cases as these the reduction is often attended with much difficulty, and should not be attempted by unskilled persons. Until surgical aid arrives cold-water cloths or ice may be applied to the joint, and the arm—if the arm is in question—should

be supported in a large sling ; a leg should be supported with a splint or by keeping the patient lying down in whatever attitude he may find most comfortable. If he is collapsed he must be kept warm and given some simple drink. If the dislocation is compound the end of the protruding bone must be covered with lint or a clean handkerchief wrung out of boiled water.

Dislocated shoulder.—The shoulder is dislocated as frequently as all the other joints put together. The deformity caused by its dislocation is very obvious, the head of the arm-bone forming a distinct projection, while the shoulder is flattened, or may even be hollowed out. If the accident occurs out of doors the clothing should, if uncomfortable, be eased and the arm, left in whatever position the patient finds least painful, should be secured to the body by bandages so as to prevent movement of the joint, an extemporized pad having been applied between the elbow and the side of the body. As soon as the patient reaches shelter the clothing should be removed, if necessary by cutting, so that the injured shoulder is bared. He should then lie down and the limb be maintained in the position which he finds most comfortable, the pain being eased by cold or hot applications as he may prefer. Nothing more need be done pending the doctor's arrival.

Dislocated elbow.—This joint is often dislocated, and the most common form which the accident takes is that in which the bones of the forearm are carried backwards so that the olecranon or " funny-bone " distinctly projects. First-aid treatment consists in supporting the arm on a splint formed of two pieces of flat wood tied together, bandages being then applied around the splint and arm both above and below the elbow-joint, and the whole supported in an arm-sling.

Dislocated Jaw.—The result of this dislocation is that the patient is unable to close his mouth and can only speak or swallow with extreme difficulty. In order to steady the part until the doctor arrives a hand-kerchief should be placed with its centre over the tip of the chin and tied on the top of the head. After the dislocation has been reduced the four-tailed bandage (*see* p. 267) should be applied, and for a few days the patient should abstain from talking or from eating solid food.

Dislocated hip.—When this serious accident happens nothing can be done in the way of first aid except to keep the part absolutely at rest and endeavour to relieve the pain by hot fomentations.

Dislocated patella.—If the patient has suffered from this accident before he may have learnt how to reduce the dislocation himself by bending and then straightening the limb, or by pushing the knee-cap into its place when the knee is straight. If not, the limb should be kept at rest by bandages or splints in the position he finds most comfortable and cold-water dressings applied.

Dislocated digits.—The finger-joint is sometimes reduced by the patient himself by means of a steady pull on the finger, when the joint may return into position with a snap. But if this is not done within a minute or two after the accident, skilled aid will be required. A dislocated thumb demands the exercise of much more force, and reduction should only be attempted by a medical man. Meantime nothing need be done except to relieve the pain by wrapping the thumb in a wet cloth.

DISPLACEMENTS OF THE WOMB (*see* Womb, Displacements of).

DISSEMINATED SCLEROSIS.—In this disease there are hardened patches of inflammation, or of scarring following inflammation, in the brain or spinal cord, caused probably by a germ. The germ may possibly be that of one of the infective diseases, such as whooping-cough or influenza, and it may have lain dormant for years until it wakes up to do its baneful work. The disease usually " comes on " between the ages of 20 and 35, but it may begin as early as 15 or as late as 50. It sets up a long train of paralytic and other symptoms, affecting the limbs, the eyes, the speech, the bladder, etc. Those who have read Barbellion's " Journal of a Disappointed Man " will recall his graphic description, founded on his own experience, of the behaviour of his legs under the influence of the spasmodic paralysis which is one of the symptoms of this disease. No specific has been found for it. The patient may survive for many years, but in rare instances there is a fatal termination in a few months. The drug most used in treatment is arsenic.

DISTURBED SLEEP IN CHILDREN (*see* Sleep, Disturbed).

DIURETICS (*see* Medicines, and how they are measured).

DIVER'S PALSY.—Divers and others who have to work in compressed air are liable to this affection, which is known also as caisson disease. It is caused, not by the compressed air in the caisson or diving-suit, but by a too rapid decompression on returning to the surface. The symptoms are pains in the limbs and joints, headache, giddiness, and vomiting, and in bad cases collapse and various forms of paralysis. The remedy is to recompress the air the patient is to breathe, and decompress it again much more gradually. In many cases the patient is himself again in a few days.

DOUCHES.—The douche consists essentially of a jet of water played upon the body, or some particular part of it, through a pipe connected with a cistern, etc., the effect being to set up vibration in the structures treated. It is much used in chronic rheumatic affections and as a nervous stimulant, etc. In the *massage douche* the body is massaged while a stream of water is directed upon it from a hose-pipe. This form of massage is especially beneficial in cases of stiff muscles or joints. Of the *Scottish douche*, first used by a Savoy physician as a form of shower-bath which he had seen practised at Edinburgh, the special feature is the application alternately of hot and cold streams to the same part of the body. In the familiar *needle douche* the body is usually played upon by warm jets of water which are gradually cooled ; it is employed as a stimulant of the nerves. In the *underwater douche*, while the patient is immersed in water, jets are directed upon the joints or the abdomen or some other region, the effect being similar to that of deep massage. The *Plombières douche* is used to clear the large intestine of accumulations of fæces, etc., and to soothe the irritated mucous membrane, a rubber tube being inserted into the rectum and some variety of natural mineral water propelled through it. Douches are also frequently used for the vagina (*see* INJECTIONS).

DRAW-SHEET (*see* NURSING, DOMESTIC).

DRESSINGS AND STRAPPING FOR WOUNDS.—The material most used as a **dressing** or covering for wounds is *lint*, which is smooth on the side to be applied to the wound, and fluffy on the other side. Ordinary lint is white, boric lint is coloured pink. Another familiar dressing is *gauze*, which is used as an absorbent of discharge, and as a packing for wounds so that they may not close before the deeper parts have healed. Plain gauze is white, cyanide gauze mauve, iodoform gauze yellow. Gauze may also be medicated with various other drugs. *Absorbent cotton-wool*—ordinary cotton-wool that has been freed from its natural oil—is not applied next to the wound, but is placed over other dressings to absorb discharge or equalize pressure, to keep out germs, to serve as a padding for splints, etc. Plain cotton-wool is white, boric pink, iodoform yellow, double cyanide mauve, sal alembroth (ammonio-mercuric chloride) blue. These and other forms of cotton-wool are used for swabbing out wounds and as a covering for powders that are dusted on wounds, etc. *Gamgee tissue* consists of layers of cotton-wool interposed between layers of gauze. *Sphagnum moss*, consisting of stems and leaves of various bog mosses, cleansed and dried, is a highly absorbent deodorant. It is used loose to absorb fæcal and urinary discharges, or in pads as a substitute for cotton-wool. It may be medicated with mercuric chloride. *Surgeons' tow*, made up of the finer fibres of teased flax, is used for collecting fæcal and other discharges. *Cellulose wadding* (Tillmann's dressing), composed of fine layers of wood fibre, is somewhat less absorbent than cotton-wool but is cheaper. In an emergency, pieces of linen, cotton, silk, muslin, etc., may be used for dressings, but they must first be sterilized by boiling. If some regulation dressing is not kept in the home, as it ought to be, a supply of these improvised dressings, sterilized in advance, ought to be at hand. If nothing else is available, clean note-paper may be applied to a wound as a covering, and if heated before the fire until lightly scorched it will be sufficiently sterile. The material commonly used for *impervious dressings*, to prevent absorption of moisture by the bandage or other outer covering, is oil-silk, which is green. Gutta percha tissue, jaconet, and battista are used for the same purpose.

Various kinds of **strapping** are in use to bring together the edges of wounds, to retain dressings, etc.; it is usually made of loosely woven cotton, calico, or flannel in widths of 1 to 6 inches. Sometimes it is medicated. In place of bandages, adhesive rubber plaster tape may be employed. If strapping is applied to a hairy part the skin must first be shaved. *Mead's plaster* can be used without previous heating; *diachylon* (or lead) *plaster* must be warmed. In removing plaster, both edges should be raised at once, equally and slowly; if any of it should stick to the skin it can be removed with olive oil or turpentine.

DROPSY.—When the serous or watery part of the blood oozes through the walls of the blood-vessels in abnormal quantity it accumulates in the loose tissue beneath the skin or in one of the cavities of the body; this is the condition known as dropsy. If the accumulation is beneath the skin the condition is known as *œdema* or *anasarca;* if in the chest, as *pleural effusion* or *hydrothorax;* if in the abdominal cavity, as *ascites;* if in the scrotum (the bag containing the testicles), as *hydrocele.* The excessive oozing is frequently due to obstruction of the blood-vessels, or to slowness of the blood-stream owing to disease of the heart, or to the circulation of poisons which injuriously affect the walls of the vessels, as in inflammation of the kidney. If the cause is inadequate propulsion of the blood-stream by the heart, the dropsy first affects the feet, and especially in the later part of the day; if the cause is disease of the kidney, the eyelids are usually first affected. Dropsy affecting the surface of the body is recognized without difficulty. The skin is smooth and more or less tense; it may be white, or dull-red, or purple, and if pressure is applied with the finger the swollen part " pits "—that is, a depression is made which only disappears gradually as the displaced fluid flows back.

Treatment.—If there is a great accumulation of fluid in the abdomen (ascites), or in the scrotum, it may be drawn off by the surgical operation known as tapping; in dropsy of the legs, the water may be withdrawn by means of small silver tubes inserted under the skin or by other means. Other palliative measures consist in the administration of drugs which increase the flow of urine (diuretics), or which set up perspiration (diaphoretics), or which carry off the fluid through the bowels (purgatives).

DROWNING (*see* Respiration, Artificial).

DRUG HABITS (*see* Stimulants; Narcotics and Hypnotics).

DRUGS (*see* Medicines, and how they are measured).

DUCTLESS GLANDS.—Many glands are furnished with ducts which carry away their secretions. Thus, the ducts of the salivary glands discharge the saliva into the mouth, and those of the liver convey the bile to the gall-bladder and the alimentary canal. But there are some glands that have no ducts, and in these cases the secretions, called internal or endocrine secretions, return to the blood either directly, or indirectly through the lymph-stream. Examples of ductless glands are the thyroid (Fig. 24, page 178), situated just below " Adam's apple " in the throat; the thymus, lying behind the breast-bone; the suprarenals, above the kidneys; and the pituitary, at the base of the brain. Until about the middle of the last century nothing was known of the uses of internal secretions, but it has since been discovered that they act as physiological stimuli of extraordinary potency, and are indispensable to the development and proper working of the body. The importance of these hormones, as they are called, has been learnt chiefly from what happens when they are insufficient, or are present in excess, or are perverted. Thus, if the thyroid secretion is scanty, the patient suffers from myxœdema (q.v.); if it is excessive, Graves's disease (q.v.) is set up. If the suprarenal glands are attacked by tuberculosis, etc., the result is Addison's disease (q.v.). If the pituitary secretion is in excess there is enlargement of parts of the body (acromegaly, q.v.), or overgrowth of the whole body (gigantism, q.v.); if it is deficient, the body fails to develop (infantilism, q.v.). Experimental study of the ductless glands has thrown light upon several important diseases and suggested effectual means of treatment; but there is still much to be learnt about their relations to each other and the functions of their secretions. It should be added that many of the glands that *are* furnished with ducts form internal secretions, in addition to the more obvious secretions which the ducts carry away. Thus the liver forms not only bile but glycogen, which appears in the blood-stream as sugar; the pancreas, in addition to the pancreatic juice, which takes part in the process of digestion, secretes a substance which in the form of insulin, derived from the same gland in oxen, is employed in the treatment of diabetes; and the testicles form not only the seminal fluid but an internal secretion which stimulates the development of male characteristics.

DUMBNESS (*see* DEAF-MUTISM).

DUODENUM, ULCER OF (*see* STOMACH, ULCER OF).

DUPUYTREN'S CONTRACTURE (*see* FINGERS, CONTRACTED).

DYSENTERY.—This term covers a group of affections characterized by inflammation of the large intestine, griping, straining at stool, and the passage of frequent but scanty motions containing mucus or mucus mixed with blood. Dysentery is endemic in many tropical and subtropical regions. In Britain and on the Continent it is rare, and occurs chiefly in the form of small epidemics in lunatic asylums, or in barracks or camps, where numbers of people are crowded together. Dysenteric disease is caused by quite a number of different micro-organisms, of which the most important are those that set up the form known as bacillary or epidemic dysentery, and the form styled amœbic dysentery, due to an amœba, the *Entamœba histolytica*. The predisposing causes are lowered vitality, chills, intestinal catarrh, malaria, the eating of irritating or unsound food, scurvy, etc.

Treatment.—The medicinal treatment of dysentery should begin with a dose of castor oil and laudanum.

In *amœbic* dysentery the drug which has long been used is ipecacuanha, but experience has proved that its alkaloid, emetine, is a much more effective remedy than the crude drug; it is injected beneath the skin or given through the mouth. In the *bacillary* form of dysentery the most efficacious drug is sulphate of soda. Among other drugs used in the treatment of dysentery are sulphate of magnesium, perchloride of mercury, and calomel, and the last of these is sometimes combined with opium and ipecacuanha. The intense straining may be relieved by an enema of 30 drops of laudanum in a wineglassful of thin starch. In cases in which there is high fever with constitutional disturbance, anti-dysenteric serum is given.

In *chronic* dysentery the chief reliance should be placed upon medicated injections into the bowel. Other measures are the systematic washing out of the bowel once a day with warm boric-acid water, or milk, or linseed infusion, or weak solutions of alum or tannin, etc., while internally small doses of castor oil once a day, fresh, ripe bael fruit, or a course of Vichy water may be taken. Some authorities recommend a diet of grapes only, or of milk only, or of beef only.

DYSMENORRHŒA.—When the monthly periods are attended by actual pain, as distinct from mere discomfort, the condition is termed dysmenorrhœa. It may be of several kinds. In *obstructive* dysmenorrhœa the passages through which the blood has to pass on its way to the vagina are narrowed, so that active contractions of the muscular walls of the womb are necessary to force it along. In *membranous* dysmenorrhœa the lining membrane of the womb is discharged not in small particles, but in large flakes, or entire casts, which can only be forced through the passages by violent contraction of the walls of the uterus. The pain of membranous dysmenorrhœa is felt in the lower abdomen, groins, and pelvis before the appearance of the discharge. It is of a bearing-down, forcing character, and is accompanied by a sensation of weight and fullness in the bowel, with straining at stool or when water is passed. It grows worse as the flow sets in, and, lasting perhaps for twenty-four to forty-eight hours, ceases as soon as the membrane has been passed, but may return when another piece is on its way. In bad cases the patient's health is undermined by the constantly recurring severe pain, and symptoms of hysteria may develop. Another form of this trouble is *congestive* dysmenorrhœa, in which the increased flow of blood to the genital organs during menstruation is excessive. The pain, relieved by lying down, is often most intense, not in the centre of the lower part of the abdomen, where the womb lies, but on one or the other side (especially the left side), in the region of the ovaries. Severe as it is, it is not so excessive as the pain of *spasmodic* dysmenorrhœa, which comes on suddenly with the commencement of the flow, and is due to violent paroxysmal contractions of the walls of the womb. *Neuralgic* dysmenorrhœa, chiefly affecting highly-strung women and girls when they are run down, is accompanied by attacks of the same kind of pain in other parts of the body. First felt in the pelvis a day or two before the flow begins, it spreads to the groins and down the legs, while at the same time the patient complains of neuralgic headache, has attacks of vomiting, and may become hysterical. In *ovarian* dysmenorrhœa the pain is limited to the region of the ovaries and is similar to that of the congestive variety. Its precise cause is not known, but it may be due to an inflamed state of the ovaries which interferes with the functioning of these organs. It is possible that the pain which some women feel each month *between* the menstrual periods is due to the same cause.

Treatment.—The treatment of a condition due to such diversified causes can only be generally indicated in these pages. During an attack the patient should remain in bed in the recumbent position, but in spasmodic dysmenorrhœa the violence of the pain may compel her to walk about or place herself in whatever attitude gives most ease. Warmth in any form is comforting ; the patient may sit in a hip-bath as hot as can be borne, lie in a hot bath, take a hot mustard-and-water foot-bath, apply hot linseed poultices to the abdomen, or lie in bed embracing a hot bottle. Drugs such as antipyrin, phenacetin, and aspirin, in 10-grain doses, tend to mitigate the pain. In spasmodic dysmenorrhœa a capsule of apiol (common parsley) containing 3 minims may be taken night and morning for three or four days at the time of the period, or guaiacum resin, 10 grains in a tablespoonful of honey three times a day. In the congestive variety, douches, as hot as can be borne, should be used night and morning between the periods, and a glycerin suppository introduced into the vagina at bed-time. In neuralgic dysmenorrhœa, bromide - of - potash tablets in 10-grain to 20-grain doses, are useful. Great care must in all cases be taken of the general health ; the patient should have plenty of fresh air and a reasonable amount of exercise with as much nourishing food as she can take. The digestive organs and the bowels should be kept in good working order, and everything must be avoided that might check menstruation, such as exposure to cold, excessive exercise, unsuitable food, mental disturbance, and, in the married, over-indulgence. In some cases relief is obtained by dilating the neck of the womb or scraping the interior of the cavity (curetting).

DYSPEPSIA (*see* INDIGESTION).

DYSPNŒA (*see* BREATHING, DIFFI-CULTY OF).

E

EAR (*see* Plate VIII, facing page 140).—The ear is divided into three parts, the external, the middle and the internal ear. The **external ear,** called also the pinna or concha, is so shaped as to collect the waves of sound and bring them to a focus at the aperture of the ear, the entrance to the *external auditory meatus.* This canal is 1¼in. long, composed partly of cartilage and partly of bone, which leads inwards and slightly forwards to the delicate membrane which closes in the passage, and is often called the drum. It really, however, is the membrane of the drum (membrana tympani), for the drum itself is the cavity of the middle ear. A channel, the *Eustachian tube,* leads from each side of the middle ear to the pharynx (the back of the mouth), and through this flows air to equalize the pressure upon the tympanic membrane from without. When sound-waves travel through the external meatus and impinge upon the membrane, this vibrates and sets in motion certain structures in the **middle ear.** They consist of a chain of three small bones (ossicles), the *malleus* (hammer), the *incus* (anvil), and the *stapes* (stirrup). The handle of the hammer is fixed to the tympanic membrane, the bar of the stirrup to a membrane at the other end of the middle ear, and the intermediate ossicle, the anvil, is articulated to them both. By means of these little bones vibrations of the tympanic membrane are communicated to lymph in the **internal ear,** and so to filaments of the auditory nerve. The internal ear consists of the *cochlea* and the *semicircular canals*, the latter of which are concerned with the maintenance of equilibrium. Hence it is that disease of the internal ear sometimes causes extreme giddiness (*see* MENIÈRE'S DISEASE).

EAR, ABSCESSES AND BOILS IN.—" Gatherings " which cause acute pain are not infrequent in the ear-passage near the orifice. They are due to the action of microbes. Predisposing causes are eczema, a discharge from the ear, and a low state of the general health. *Treatment.*— The itching should be treated with zinc ointment. At a later stage hot fomentations should be used, and the following antiseptic ointment may be applied on long plugs of cotton-wool inserted into the orifice, viz. menthol 2 grains, iodoform 4 grains, lanolin 2 drachms, vaselin 2 drachms. The pain may be allayed by drops of warm oil with laudanum. If the boil is large the intense pain may demand that the medical attendant should incise it. If the patient is stout and full-blooded—for boils occur in such persons as well as in those who are run down in health—the diet should be restricted and rather free action of the bowels secured.

EAR, DISCHARGE FROM.— There may be " running " from the ear (*otorrhœa*) owing to the breaking of an abscess or boil in the outer pas-

sage, or to a cold, or to eczema, etc. Whatever the cause, the discharge must be kept clean and free from smell; the passage should therefore be washed out night and morning with a lotion consisting of warm water made a faint purple with Condy's fluid, or of a teaspoonful of boric acid in a tumblerful of warm water. This should be syringed into the ear just as warm water is, as described under EAR, WAX IN, and it is even more important than in that condition that the syringing should be done quite gently. It is also important that the discharge should not be blocked up with plugs of cotton-wool; if used at all, these should be frequently changed, as soon as they are wetted. In some cases the discharge is the result of an inflammation of the middle ear—that is, of the cavity of the " drum "; in other cases it is due to disease of the surrounding bone. Both of these are serious affections quite unsuitable for domestic treatment (*see* EAR, MIDDLE, INFLAMMATION OF).

EAR, FOREIGN BODIES IN (*see* FOREIGN BODIES).

EAR, MIDDLE, INFLAMMATION OF.—The middle ear lies between the external and internal ears (*see* EAR and Plate VIII, facing p. 140). It communicates with the outer air by the Eustachian tube, which runs inwards and downwards to the throat; and the roof of the middle ear is only separated from the brain cavity by a thin layer of bone. It will be understood that inflammation may readily extend from the throat along the Eustachian tube, and thus so simple an affection as sore throat may develop into inflammation of the middle ear (*otitis media*), which in turn may easily set up the still graver affection known as meningitis—that is, inflammation of the membranes of the brain (*see* MENINGITIS); or the facial nerve may be involved, with resulting paralysis of the face (*see* FACIAL PARALYSIS); or the mastoid cells may be implicated (*see* MASTOID DISEASE). Inflammation of the middle ear is not infrequently a complication of influenza, mumps, diphtheria, tuberculosis, or pneumonia, and especially of scarlet fever; in children it may also be caused by adenoids. The symptoms are acute and throbbing pain in the ear and the head, aggravated by blowing the nose or by swallowing; there may also be noises in the ear and some amount of deafness. If in one of these cases there is discharge from the ear, it means that accumulated matter has broken through the " drum."

Treatment.—This consists in the application of moist heat; thus the affected ear may be kept covered by a hot camomile-flower compress, or a hot-water india-rubber bottle may be used. The patient should be put upon light diet, and an aperient administered. Should discharge occur, the canal of the ear should be gently syringed with boric-acid lotion (a teaspoonful of the acid to a tumblerful of warm water) every two or three hours, and in the intervals cotton-wool, frequently changed, should be worn in the ear to soak up the fluid. A ruptured tympanic membrane may heal in a week or ten days; on the other hand the discharge may become chronic, and it is in such cases that there is most danger of the hearing being affected or of the other complications that we have mentioned arising. As soon as middle-ear inflammation is suspected medical aid should be summoned.

EAR, NOISES IN.—Tinnitus, to use the medical term for noises in

the ear, may mean little or may mean much. It may be due to causes so simple as the taking of drugs such as quinine and salicylate of soda, the accumulation of wax in the outer canal, or the blocking, by a cold, of the Eustachian tube, so that the passage of air from the mouth to the middle ear is obstructed; or it may be caused by affections of the middle ear or of the delicate nervous structures of the inner ear (*see* EAR). The noises may resemble many different sounds, such as hissing, buzzing, humming, the ringing of bells, or the sound of voices.

Treatment.—If the noises are caused by an accumulation of wax the ear should be syringed as described under EAR, WAX IN; if to obstruction of the Eustachian tube, the doctor may force air along the tube into the middle ear. The mouth is closed, the nose pinched between the finger and thumb, and the cheeks are blown out while a mouthful of water is swallowed. If the obstruction cannot be overcome in this way the doctor may use a Politzer's bag (Fig. 18). In these cases of obstruction of the Eustachian tube, glycothymoline may be used as a gargle every three or four hours and as a nasal douche night and morning, a tablespoonful being mixed with five tablespoonfuls of warm water. Where tinnitus is caused by affections of the nervous structures of the ear, little can be done to relieve it, but the patient may try the effect of taking 10 to 15 grains of bromide of potash three times a day. If the condition is set up by inflammation of the middle ear the treatment must be that described under EAR, MIDDLE, INFLAMMATION OF.

EAR, RUPTURE OF DRUM OF. —The tympanic membrane, which

divides the external from the middle ear (*see* EAR), and is popularly known as the drum, may be ruptured without permanent damage to the sense of hearing. The injury may be caused by a blow or fall on the head, by the explosion of a gun, by a box on the ears, by removing accumulated wax with a sharp instrument, by too forcible syringing, or by violent sneezing or vomiting ; or it may occur in inflammation of the middle ear in cases in which the accumulated discharge perforates the membrane in order to escape. At the moment of rupture the patient has the sensation of hearing a loud sound and feels a sickening kind of pain, and these symptoms are often followed by faintness, discharge of blood from the ear, earache, deafness, and tinnitus (noises in the ear) in various forms ; when he blows his nose or sneezes, air issues from the ear.

Treatment.—If the injury is caused by an explosion or a blow, the nervous structures of the ear may be damaged, and there may be persistent deafness, but in ordinary cases of rupture nothing more is usually necessary than rest, and protection of the orifice of the ear with a plug of sterilized cotton-wool. No syringing should be done, nor should oil be dropped into the ear, as is sometimes done. If, however, there is a discharge, the doctor will apply treatment such as that described for the perforation that occurs in middle-ear disease (*see* EAR, MIDDLE, INFLAMMATION OF).

EAR, WAX IN.—The cerumen which is formed by small glands in the ear-passage may accumulate to excess, as for instance after a cold in the ear, and may become dry and hard. For a time it may cause no inconvenience, but if it should press

against the "drum" it may prevent that membrane from vibrating and so may cause deafness. The patient also in many cases is troubled with noises in the ear, and he may suffer from giddiness and from a persistent dry cough caused by irritation of nerves which are pressed upon by the hardened wax. The deafness, when it occurs, may come on quite suddenly from some slight movement

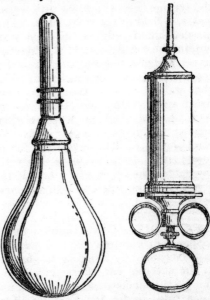

Fig. 18.—Politzer's bag.   Fig. 19.—Ear syringe.

of the wax or from the entrance of moisture which causes the wax to expand.

Treatment.—At bed-time, from an ordinary teaspoon which has been warmed by being dipped in hot water, a few drops of warm olive oil or glycerin should be dropped into the ear, the head being laid on one side ; the liquid may be kept from running out by the insertion of a small plug of cotton-wool. The wax having thus been softened, the ear should be syringed. Great care and gentleness must be exercised if this is done by an inexperienced person, for violent syringing might tear the drum ; and only three or four syringefuls should be used at a sitting. A towel is placed over the shoulders of the patient, who presses firmly against his head below the ear a small basin or jug to receive the water as it runs out of the ear. The ear is drawn upwards and backwards with the left hand so as to straighten the passage, while the syringe (Fig. 19), filled with warm water, is held in the right hand. The nozzle should only be inserted just within the orifice, and the stream directed slightly upwards against the roof of the canal. The wax having been thus washed out, the canal should be dried with cotton-wool fixed on a cotton-holder, and as a precaution against catching cold a plug of cotton-wool should be left in the ear for a few hours. If there is a mattery discharge the syringing should be done even more gently than in ordinary cases.

EARACHE.—This trouble, more frequent in children than in adults, may be caused by a boil or an abscess in the external ear, or by inflammation of the mucous membrane set up by a cold, or by the presence of a " foreign body," or by inflammation of the middle ear ; or it may be due to causes extraneous to the ear, such as a decayed tooth or neuralgia. Neuralgic cases may be distinguished from those due to inflammation by the sudden onset of the pain, which does not usually vary in severity, and comes and goes capriciously ; moreover, unlike the earache due to inflammation, it is unaccompanied by a rise in temperature. *Treatment.*— In neuralgic cases a nerve tonic should be taken (*see under* NEURALGIA). If the trouble is due to a decayed tooth a visit should, of course, be paid to

the dentist. If there is a boil or an abscess the treatment should be that described under EAR, ABSCESSES AND BOILS IN. In many cases of earache, relief may be obtained by the use of a poultice in the form of camomile flowers placed in a small muslin bag which is dipped in boiling water, wrung out dry, laid over the ear and covered up with oil-silk. Or the ear may be covered with a hot fomentation sprinkled with laudanum and renewed every hour or two, or it may be rubbed all round with a mixture of equal parts of belladonna and glycerin. The pain is often assuaged by dropping into the ear equal parts of warm olive oil and laudanum. The laudanum must be prescribed by a doctor.

ECCHYMOSIS.—This term usually denotes the escape of blood from blood-vessels into the tissues underneath the skin, as in a bruise (*see* BRUISES). One of the most noticeable forms of ecchymosis is that which appears as a bright-red patch on the white of the eye, caused by bleeding under the conjunctiva—the membrane lining the eye and the inner surface of the eyelids—owing to the rupture of a small blood-vessel, frequently as the result of violent coughing or sneezing or vomiting. This is called subconjunctival ecchymosis (Frontispiece, Fig. 6). Nothing more need be done than to bathe the closed eye with cold water ; even if left to itself the patch will disappear in the course of a few days.

ECLAMPSIA (*see* PREGNANCY, DISORDERS OF).

ECTROPION (*see* EYELIDS, INVERSION AND EVERSION OF).

ECZEMA.—This most common of all skin affections assumes a bewildering variety of forms, but essentially it is an inflammation of the skin in which there is an oozing-out of the watery part of the blood, which forms tiny blisters known as vesicles. In most cases the fluid is discharged on the surface, but not in all, for if it oozes into the deeper layers of the skin it may not succeed in finding its way out.

Causes.—An attack of eczema may be provoked by any one of a large number of external agents. In some cases the condition is set up by handling certain kinds of sawdust, or mustard or eucalyptus leaves, or daffodils, or even the common orange; in others, by contact with hair-dyes and other cosmetics, or dyes for cloths, or sugar dust, or stains and polishes for wood; yet another common cause of eczema is the use of soap. Inasmuch as such substances as these can be handled with impunity by most persons, it follows that they can only set up an eczematous irritation in those whose skin has a special susceptibility. The susceptibility may be due to profuse perspiration which accumulates in the folds of the body and undergoes decomposition, or to excess of the oily fluid which is secreted by the sebaceous glands of the skin, so that the ducts which bring the fluid to the surface become obstructed and irritation is thus set up. In some persons the skin is irritable because of defective circulation; in old age, on account of diminished nutrition; or poisons may be formed in the stomach and intestines and be carried by the blood to the skin, there to set up irritation. In one group of cases the affection originates in nervous disturbance, as from worry, or strain, or shock. It is not possible, indeed, in the space available, to enumerate all the causes of eczema, but it may be added that some cases are probably due to the action of microbes.

Symptoms.—The first signs of an attack are usually itching and burning; the part where these sensations are felt grows red, and soon there appear upon it a number of minute blisters. The itching grows worse and the usual signs of inflammation appear—swelling, redness, heat and pain. The blisters, at first no larger than a pin's head, grow, and often run together, and finally burst or are broken by scratching which the itching provokes, when a clear, somewhat sticky fluid oozes out. Other vesicles are formed and keep up the discharge, but sooner or later crusts or scales are formed. In many cases fresh crops of blisters appear around the edges of the older patches, and new centres appear elsewhere, and in this way, in bad cases, almost the whole surface of the body may be involved. In chronic cases the skin becomes hard and thick, and where there is much movement, as at the joints, around the mouth, the anus, and the genital organs, deep fissures may occur. In cases that have not become chronic, when the crusts have disappeared the surface is covered with a new outer skin, which is shed in scales that become thinner and smaller until at last healing is completed and no trace of the eczema is left except a brownish stain. Sometimes there is a predominance of what are called papules— spots which instead of containing fluid like vesicles, are solid. As the result of the scratching, the skin may be inoculated with micro-organisms and painful boils may develop; not infrequently, too, the lymph-glands near the affected part become inflamed. The worst feature of eczema, as a rule, is the itching. This varies in degree in different cases, but is sometimes so intense as to be almost unendurable. There is usually little pain, except from boils and from the fissures that may form where the skin cannot be kept at rest. Nothing is more uncertain than the course of an attack of eczema. It may be of quite brief duration, may persist for weeks, or may be prolonged until it becomes chronic ; but, whether its course is long or short, there is a pronounced tendency to recurrence.

Treatment.—The first thing to do in the *local* treatment of eczema is to remove all crusts and scales, which may be done by softening them with a weak solution of bicarbonate of soda, or by olive oil applied on strips of lint. In *acute* cases involving a large area of skin the pain may be relieved by the use of warm lotions on lint or linen covered with oil-silk ; for this purpose dilute lead lotion, or calamine lotion, or boric-acid lotion (a dessert-spoonful to a pint of water), or thin starch, is suitable. The affected parts may be covered with a sedative ointment smeared thickly on lint, such as a drachm of solution of subacetate of lead to an ounce of vaselin. As the irritation subsides, a stronger ointment may be used, such as one composed of equal parts of zinc and boric-acid ointment. The itching may be relieved by a lotion of carbolic acid (1 drachm) and glycerin (2 drachms) to 8 ounces of water. In cases in which the eczema is both acute and extensive the patient should take to his bed so that his skin may be kept at a uniform temperature. The diet should be simple and easily digestible, and stimulants should be avoided, but tea may be taken unless it should provoke indigestion. If the bowels fail to act regularly they should be stimulated by an aperient such as a glass of mineral water in the morning. Not only should the use of soap be avoided, but water should be applied to the skin as little as possible, and only in

the form of rain- or boiled water which has been softened by adding to it bran or oatmeal.

In *chronic* eczema more stimulating measures must be employed such as the use of tar ointment, oil of cade ointment, or a zinc and sulphur ointment—equal parts. In these chronic cases it may be necessary for the medical man to employ one agent after another before he finds one that produces much effect, for they are often extremely refractory to treatment.

In eczema no great emportance is to be attached to *internal* treatment. Where there is much nervous disturbance the doctor may order sleeping drugs ; in somewhat less severe cases a simple sedative may suffice, such as 10-grain doses of bromide of potash. If there is prostration, quinine is indicated. In chronic cases benefit is sometimes derived from arsenic—3 minims of the solution in water thrice a day after food—or from phosphorus or strychnine.

In **children,** and especially in infants, eczema is even more common than in adults. Teething is believed to be in a measure responsible for some cases ; there can be no doubt that indigestion and diarrhœa are other contributory causes ; and it has been observed that eczema in children is frequently associated with asthma. In some cases, too, eczema follows vaccination, beginning at the " spots," just as in those of older growth it sometimes starts in an operation wound which is healing.

Treatment.—The skin, where eczema appears, should not be washed, but should be cleansed by dabbing it over with a piece of cotton-wool soaked in warm milk and water. In eczema of the scalp a very weak sulphur ointment should be applied in the form of 4 grains of precipitated sulphur to 1 ounce of benzoated lard. An excellent lotion for the early stage is one consisting of 2 drachms of calamine powder, 3 drachms of hazeline, and ½ drachm of boric acid to an ounce of water ; in the later stage an ointment may be applied consisting of 1 drachm of oxide of zinc, 2 drachms of tar ointment, 2 drachms of rosewater ointment, and 4 drachms of lanolin. The bowels, if their action is defective, should be carefully regulated by, say, a grain of grey powder twice a week for a child of one year. In all cases the diet must receive attention. If the child is breast-fed the mother must abstain from stimulating foods and drinks, and if her health is below par she must be careful to take a sufficiency of simple nutritious food. In the case of bottle-fed children, the motions should be examined, and if lumps of milk curd are found in them a starch-free infant food should be substituted for milk.

ELECTRICAL TREATMENT.—

Electricity is employed in medicine in many different forms—as galvanism, faradism, the alternating current, static electricity, the high-frequency current, and radiation. The following forms are of special interest and may be briefly described :

Diathermy.—By this method, which is a special adaptation of the high-frequency current, heat is generated in the tissues owing to the resistance they offer to the passage of the electric current ; thus their temperature and that of the blood flowing through them is raised. Diathermy is used in the treatment of chill, diseases of the breathing organs, sciatica and neuralgia, frostbite and trench-foot, etc. It is also employed to destroy cancers and other tumours without causing bleeding.

Radiant heat.—Here the electrical current is converted into heat for external application, the patient or the part affected being placed in a reflecting case furnished with many electric lights. The affections treated in this way are chronic inflammation of the joints and muscular rheumatism, impaired nutrition, etc.

Light treatment. — The ultra-violet rays are used in what is known as *artificial sunlight*, which is considered in the article SUNLIGHT TREATMENT. A somewhat similar adaptation of electricity, known as the *Finsen light*, is used in the treatment of lupus vulgaris, etc.

X-rays.—Of all the medical applications of electricity the X-rays have the widest field of usefulness. Besides being extensively used diagnostically (*see under* DIAGNOSIS) they are of great service in a large number of skin diseases, and are also useful as palliatives in more serious diseases such as cancer and rodent ulcer.

Electrolysis.—In this method of treatment, known also as cataphoresis and ionic medication, electricity is used to break up drugs into positive and negative elements (ions) and introduce them into the tissues. In this way superfluous hairs, small moles, and port-wine stains can be destroyed, the pain of neuralgia, sciatica, and inflammation of the joints relieved, warts got rid of, fibrous tissues softened, local anæsthesia produced, and septic conditions neutralized.

ELECTROLYSIS (*see* ELECTRICAL TREATMENT).

ELEPHANTIASIS (*see* FILARIASIS).

EMBOLISM (*see* ARTERIES, DISEASES OF).

EMBROCATIONS (*see* LINIMENTS).

EMETICS.—The chief uses of emetics are to relieve an overloaded stomach, to secure the ejection of poisons, and to assist breathing by promoting the removal of phlegm which is obstructing the bronchial tubes. In cases of poisoning, emetics must on no account be resorted to if the lips, tongue and throat are stained and burnt, or if the patient has been reduced to unconsciousness; in the latter case the emetic itself or the matter vomited from the stomach might pass into the air-passages and cause suffocation. The simplest of all emetic measures is to tickle the throat with a feather, or to insert a finger into the throat and move it to and fro. Emetics which are always at hand are common salt—two tablespoonfuls in a tumblerful of tepid water; and mustard water—a tablespoonful of mustard in a tumblerful of water; another easily accessible emetic is alum powder—a tablespoonful in water. Among drugs which are used to produce vomiting is ipecacuanha, half a teaspoonful of the powder in water, or one or two tablespoonfuls of the wine in water; for children a teaspoonful of the wine is the proper dose, followed after a ten minutes' interval by a second dose, and if necessary, at the same interval or intervals, by a third or fourth. Another effective emetic drug is apomorphine, the adult dose consisting of two $\frac{1}{15}$ grain tabloids by the mouth.

EMPHYSEMA.—Emphysema is a dignified name for the condition which in horses is known as "broken wind." Cavities are formed in the lungs as the result of air-cells breaking into one another consequent upon strain set up by the playing of large wind instruments, by the difficulty of breathing which attends bronchitis and asthma, or by violent coughing. The condition also occurs as a senile change when the chest-walls lose their elasticity. The chief symptom is great and growing shortness of breath. Treatment consists in careful attention to the general health and in the use of tonics.

EMPYEMA.—This is an occasional complication of pleurisy and pleuropneumonia, especially in children under ten, in whom nearly half the cases occur. In these diseases, as the result of inflammation of the pleura, the membrane that lines the lungs, and also lines the walls of the chest, there is an accumulation of watery fluid (pleurisy) in the space between the two surfaces of the membrane, and in some cases this fluid becomes "mattery" in character, from the action of germs, and may gradually become converted into thick pus. The same condition sometimes arises in tuberculosis of the lungs, as well as in other diseases of the chest. The fluid may be removed with an aspirator, but it usually re-forms, and the surgeon then has to open the chest and insert a tube through which the pus drains out.

ENCEPHALITIS LETHARGICA.—Under MENINGITIS, SUPPURATIVE, it is explained that inflammation of the membranes of the brain is called meningitis, and that inflammation of the brain itself is called encephalitis. The latter condition may arise by extension from the former, or after injuries to the scalp, etc., but sometimes it occurs as an independent infection, and it is then known as encephalitis lethargica or as epidemic encephalitis. Popularly, it is often called sleepy sickness, an unfortunate name that may be confused with "sleeping sickness," a term that has long been used to denote the terminal stage of a tropical disease (*see* TRYPANOSOMIASIS). Encephalitis lethargica, first reported in this country in 1918, is undoubtedly a germ disease, though the micro-organism which causes it has not yet been definitely identified. The disease attacks persons of all ages, it appears to be more an urban than a rural disease, and the majority of cases occur in the early months of the year. Some authorities believe that the germ finds entrance to the body through the upper air-passages ; in some cases it appears first to attack the conjunctiva, the membrane lining the eye and eyelids, causing inflammation of that membrane—conjunctivitis. The symptoms vary greatly. One of them is paralysis, which may occur in different forms—among them, double vision. In some cases lethargy is a prominent feature ; in others, it is insignificant. Some attacks are slight and clear up in a few days ; others are severe and protracted, and may leave behind them permanent paralysis, or may end in death. Sometimes the nervous symptoms are preceded or accompanied by a sore throat, by disorder of the stomach and intestines, or by hiccough, and occasionally there is a rash not unlike that of measles or of scarlet fever. About half the cases end fatally. Little can be done in the way of treatment except to endeavour to mitigate the symptoms. In some cases, especially in the young, the disease leaves behind it mental and moral deterioration and other grave sequels.

ENDEMIC DISEASES (*see* DISEASE, CLASSIFICATION OF).

ENDOCARDITIS (*see* HEART DISEASE).

ENDOCRINE GLANDS (*see* DUCTLESS GLANDS).

ENEMATA (*see* INJECTIONS).

ENGLISH CHOLERA (*see* EPIDEMIC DIARRHŒA).

ENLARGED GLANDS (*see* ADENITIS).

ENLARGED PROSTATE (*see* PROSTATE GLAND, ENLARGED).

ENLARGED TONSILS (*see* TONSILS, ENLARGED).

ENTERIC FEVER (*see* TYPHOID FEVER).

ENTERITIS (*see* BOWELS, INFLAMMATION OF).

ENTROPION (*see* EYELIDS, INVERSION AND EVERSION OF).

EPIDEMIC CEREBRO-SPINAL MENINGITIS (*see* CEREBRO-SPINAL FEVER).

EPIDEMIC DIARRHŒA.—This is the official name of a disease which has a string of popular aliases, such as *summer diarrhœa, choleraic diarrhœa, English cholera,* and, when it occurs in young children, *infantile cholera.* To attach to it the designation of cholera, even with a qualifying adjective, is misleading, for while it is no doubt a germ disease, the germ is certainly not the comma bacillus, which is generally accepted as the cause of cholera. It is much the most fatal of the infective diseases of infancy. The greatest mortality from it is in the first year of life, but children appear to be most liable to attack in the second year ; it also accounts for a large proportion of deaths at the other extreme of life. It may occur at any season, but is far more prevalent in the height of summer than at any other time. The temperature of the soil is a truer guide to its incidence than the temperature of the air, for the summer rise of mortality from this disease does not begin until the earth-temperature 4 feet below the surface is about 56° Fahr., however high the atmospheric temperature may be. The microbe responsible for this form of diarrhœa is conveyed in or encouraged to its baleful activities by contaminated food, one proof of which is the fact that breast-fed infants are remarkably exempt from attack. In the transmission of the disease the house-fly plays a leading part, and among the influences that favour it are bad ventilation, impure air, lack of cleanliness, and maternal neglect. It is much more a disease of large towns than of rural districts, and some towns are scarcely ever entirely free from it.

Symptoms.—The onset is usually quite sudden, with violent purging and vomiting. The patient suffers severely from thirst, and still more from colicky pains and from cramps in the limbs. The pulse becomes feeble, the temperature falls, the voice fails, and the patient may look as though about to die ; but with suitable treatment, which must be carried out by a doctor, he in most cases recovers, unless very young or very old.

In *children* the disease runs much the same course as in older patients, though the effects are more serious and alarming. The child soon begins to look worn, is restless and irritable, and often cries out with pain, at the same time drawing up the legs. Presently the face becomes pinched and ashy and the nose thin, the eyes are deeply sunken and partly closed, the muscles wasted. Thirst increases until it is insatiable, the urine is scanty, and the belly flabby, so that it can be pinched up like a sheet ; the extremities, and even the tongue, are cold, the child grows drowsy, and

gives scarcely any sign of consciousness. At this stage the vomiting may cease, but the diarrhœa may continue and the disease go on to a fatal termination, death being heralded by quick breathing, collapse, and possibly convulsions. Should the case take a favourable turn, the diarrhœa ceases, colour returns to the face, and the child begins once more to take notice. Fatal cases usually run a course of from seven to ten days, or less in very young infants ; in cases which recover it may be three weeks or longer before the health is fully recovered. In many children the disease bequeaths a legacy of anæmia or dropsy, or of chronic disease of the bowels and wasting.

Treatment.—The first thing the doctor will do is to endeavour to expel irritating matters from the bowels by means of an aperient. When the severe symptoms have subsided, he will probably have resort to a sedative and astringent mixture. Thirst may be mitigated and the bowels flushed with soda-water and milk, chicken-broth, barley-water, or some such simple drink. The cramps may be relieved by rubbing the affected limbs with dry ginger or with chloroform liniment, while in the stage of collapse hot poultices and fomentations are applied to the abdomen, and brandy-and-water may be given in small quantities.

In *children*, as soon as the attack begins, milk and milky fluids should be replaced by barley-water or egg-water. Castor oil in doses of half to one teaspoonful is required to clear the stomach and bowels, unless to the diarrhœa is added a good deal of sickness, when calomel is better. As soon as the motions are free from undigested curd an attempt should be made to check the vomiting and the diarrhœa. It may be necessary to administer some form of opium. Milk must not be given for some time after the attack is over ; its place may be taken by whey, buttermilk, meat juice and meat broths.

EPIDEMIC DISEASE(*see*DISEASE, CLASSIFICATION OF).

EPIDERMIS (*see* SKIN).

EPILEPSY.—The popular name for this condition is " falling sickness," because the patient, when taken with a fit, falls to the ground. Epileptic attacks may be placed in two distinct categories, *major* epilepsy or *grand mal*, and *minor* epilepsy or *petit mal*. In both alike there are strange premonitory symptoms called *auræ*. In major epilepsy these premonitory symptoms are followed by a convulsive fit or a series of convulsive fits. In minor epilepsy, on the other hand, after the warning symptoms the patient may be conscious of nothing but strange sensations which he may describe as " faints " or " turns," or of rather violent attacks of giddiness, or there may be a momentary loss of consciousness. Sometimes, however, the loss of consciousness may last a few minutes, though without preventing the patient from continuing the occupation of the moment ; even if walking or running, he will continue to walk or run although his mind is a perfect blank. When consciousness returns the patient has no recollection of what has occurred.

The essential cause of epilepsy is not understood, except, indeed, a small proportion of cases which are due to injury to the brain. It is clear, however, that epilepsy is in many cases hereditary in the sense that one or both the parents of the patient have suffered from some mental disease, or at least from nervous instability. In all these numerous cases the patient, therefore, begins life with a delicately poised nervous system, which may be thrown out of balance by causes by which normal persons would not be seriously affected, such as eye trouble, polypi of the nose, adenoids, digestive disturbance, the irritation of intestinal worms, the troubles of teething, fright, fits of anger, alcoholic excess. In the majority of cases the first attack of epilepsy occurs in early life.

Symptoms. (1) *Premonitory.*—An *aura* means " a breath of wind," and the term was applied to these premonitory symptoms because the most familiar of them is a sensation of " something passing up the arm or leg," as might a current of air. Visual and auditory auræ may take the form of flashes of light, of loss of vision, of images of various kinds, or of noises and whistlings. These auræ of sight and hearing are not usually unpleasant, but those of taste and smell appear always to be so. The warning may also consist of twitching of limbs. But the most interesting of these auræ are those which are purely mental, such as strange dreamy states of mind which are not at all disagreeable, and the peculiar sensations termed reminiscences, which are experienced by many people who are not affected by epilepsy, and have been described by Oliver Wendell Holmes and Tennyson among other writers. The patient has a strange, mystical sense that the scene which he is witnessing or in which he is taking part has occurred before at some remote period, and as each incident is evolved it comes home to him as familiar. The aura, whatever its nature, may last for a few seconds only, but sometimes it is of longer duration and the patient is able to put himself into a position of safety by lying down, while in some cases he violence during the night, and the attack may thus continue to recur for about five days to a fortnight. The local condition is accompanied by symptoms of fever, there is rise of temperature with chilliness, and sometimes a violent shivering fit, the patient loses his appetite and suffers from thirst, the tongue is furred, the bowels are constipated, the urine is high-coloured and scanty, and becomes thick and reddish on standing. When at last the attack passes off, the joint is left stiff and painful, and the skin over it swollen and peeling. Presently, with or without massage, or the application of radiant heat, or of tincture of iodine, the swelling and stiffness disappear, but sooner or later a second attack may be expected, and then others.

Treatment of acute gout.—The foot should be raised a little above the level of the body on a comfortable cushion or pillow; it should be covered with a " cradle " to take off the weight of the bedclothes, and the joint should be wrapped in cotton-wool saturated with the following lotion, mixed with an equal quantity of hot water :

Carbonate of soda .... 3 drachms
Belladonna liniment........ 2 ounces
Tincture of opium .... 2 ounces
Water to 8 ounces.

When the pain has subsided, gentle friction with the hand, or rubbing with belladonna and chloroform liniment, may be employed to reduce swelling and stiffness. The drug most frequently taken for acute gout is colchicum, which has been used for this affection for many hundreds of years. A suitable form is the following :

Wine of colchicum ....3½ drachms
Carbonate of magnesia .....80 grains
Cinnamon water to 8 ounces.
Two tablespoonfuls at bed time.

This medicine should be continued for a few days until the symptoms subside. If the bowels do not act freely, 5 grains of the compound rhubarb pill may be taken.

The diet should at first be limited to milk and milk foods, with a little toast or stale bread or biscuit. Barley water and toast water may be taken freely; stimulants must be strictly tabooed, except in those of enfeebled constitutions, when the milk may be laced with a little whisky or brandy; in these cases the milk diet may be reinforced with whipped eggs. As the symptoms pass off, beef tea, soups, and eggs beaten up in milk may be allowed. The return to ordinary fare must be careful and gradual.

Chronic gout.—This is a sequel of the acute form of the disease. At first one or two joints are usually affected, but after a time the tendency is for other joints, and especially those of the hand, to be involved. The result, in the case of the hand, is that after a time the knuckles become much deformed and their movements are impeded. The knobs which appear on the knuckles are due to the formation of so-called " chalk-stones," which are really composed of biurate of soda, deposited in and around the joints by the blood. The skin over the protuberances becomes stretched, and is liable to inflammation and injury; when this occurs the concretions—*tophi* they are termed— are exposed and come away as a gritty material mixed with discharge. Small tophi are sometimes met with in the margins of the ear, and are a sign of a tendency to gout in persons who may never have had an actual attack.

Irregular gout.—This form of gout may manifest itself in a great many ways, such as violent vomiting of bile, acute attacks of cramp in may prevent the fit by adopting one of the measures described later.

(2) *The fit.*—An epileptic fit frequently begins with a loud scream or yell. The patient falls like a log, breathing ceases, the body becomes rigid, and the back may be arched, and frothy fluid appear at the lips. After a few seconds a little twitching is seen, and the fixed spasm gives place to violent convulsive movements. After two or three minutes the convulsions gradually subside, and the patient either, if circumstances allow, has a long sleep, or gets up and in a more or less dazed condition goes about his business. In some cases there is a succession of fits with hardly any appreciable intervals of consciousness between; this is the condition termed *status epilepticus*, in which death sometimes occurs from exhaustion.

As already remarked, the premonitory symptoms may usher in an attack either of major or of minor epilepsy. In both forms alike the patient may lapse into a state of what is called *automatism*, in which he acts without the least knowledge of what he is doing. Thus he may do something quite innocent, such as walking for hours and finding himself on coming to his senses miles from his intended destination, or he may commit a crime of which he is entirely unconscious and of which, therefore, he has no recollection. Epilepsy is sometimes associated with extraordinary mental and nervous energy, as in Julius Cæsar, Mahomet, Peter the Great, and Napoleon, who were all epileptics, but in the great majority of cases, if the attacks continue, the nervous system manifestly suffers, the patients becoming low-spirited and querulous or excitable, losing their memory, finding great difficulty in applying themselves to work, and finally in very severe cases sinking into a state of imbecility. The fits rarely disappear spontaneously, but in some cases the disease is permanently arrested as the result of treatment. Cases beginning in later life are more amenable to treatment than those arising during the later years of childhood, and the more infrequently the attacks occur the better is the outlook.

Treatment. (1) *Preventive.*—In some cases, by adopting one of many measures as soon as the warning symptoms appear, the epileptic fit may be averted. Some patients are able to effect this by mere power of will aided by the exercise of muscular force, as by grasping an object tightly and clenching the teeth. When the aura takes the form of muscular contraction the patient should try the effect of holding the affected part straight and stretching the affected muscles. Thus, if by a contraction of the muscles of the neck the chin is drawn towards one shoulder the head should be rapidly turned towards the other shoulder; or if the muscles of the forearm contract, the forearm should be forcibly straightened with the hand of the other arm. When a peculiar sensation passes up a limb the threatened fit may be averted by tying a handkerchief or bandage tightly round, or by tying and untying it several times in quick succession. Sniffing strong salts, or taking snuff or, if the aura consists in a sense of discomfort in the stomach, swallowing a dose of sal volatile or of spirit of chloroform or of spirit of ether, may be tried. Other methods that are sometimes successful are the sudden dashing of cold water in the face, plunging the hands into hot water, reading loud and fast, and pressing or striking any part of the body where the muscles become rigid.

(2) *Treatment of the fit.*—If possible, the patient should be placed on some soft, flat surface, such as a rug, clear of any article of furniture which he might strike during the convulsions. A piece of stout india-rubber tubing, or the handle of a tooth-brush wrapped in a cloth, should be placed between the back teeth to prevent the tongue from being bitten, and should be firmly held so that it may not slip down the throat. When once the fit has come on it is a mistake to throw cold water on the patient, but the window should be widely opened so that there may be abundant fresh air. As soon as the fit is over he should be lifted on to a bed and not be disturbed in the sleep which usually follows.

(3) *Medicinal treatment.*—The most valuable drugs in the treatment of epilepsy are the bromides of potash, soda, and ammonia. The dose must be suited to the individual case, for some patients can tolerate larger quantities of the bromides than others, but the doctor will probably begin with small doses and gradually increase the quantity until he discovers how much is needed to ward off the attacks. In some cases the regular use of the bromides gives rise to a rash, as well as to disagreeable constitutional symptoms. When this happens the doses should be reduced or suspended and the bromide should be combined with a small dose of arsenic in the form of Fowler's solution. It is believed by some French authorities that by eliminating salt from the diet the effect of the bromides is greatly increased, so that small doses become as effective as, in ordinary cases, larger doses are. This method may be worth a trial in cases in which an eruption is easily provoked by the use of bromides. When no ill effects arise the bromide treatment should be persevered in without interruption until the patient has been free from fits for two years.

(4) *Dietetic and hygienic treatment.*—The food should be nutritious but quite simple and free from anything likely to irritate the stomach or cause indigestion. Alcohol and coffee, especially alcohol, should be entirely avoided, but most patients are able without detriment to take weak tea. The bowels must be very carefully regulated with mild aperients, for constipation is not seldom found to provoke attacks. A quiet, regular life free from violent exertion or excitement should be followed, if possible in the country. No occupation is more suitable to an epileptic than that of gardening. The régime at colonies such as that at Chalfont in Buckinghamshire, where the patient spends the greater part of his time in the open air, is carefully watched so that the treatment may be adapted to his special needs, and is encouraged to take gymnastic exercises, and where all salutary influences are brought to bear upon him, has proved to be very successful. The education of epileptic children need not be neglected, but the greatest care should be taken to avoid anything in the nature of mental strain. The patient should be warmly but not heavily clad, should take a daily bath, and should form the habit of going to bed early so that he may have plenty of sleep.

EPIPHORA.—When the lachrymal or tear-gland secretes fluid too rapidly, or when the ducts which convey the fluid from the inner corner of the eye to the nose become obstructed, as from inflammation, there is an overflow of tears, which run down the cheek. This condition is known popularly as " watery eye " and medically as epiphora. When the lachrymal sac, in the inner angle of the eye, or the nasal ducts (*see* Fig. 20, p. 141), are inflamed, the fluid, instead of running down over the cheeks, forms a swelling on the inner side of the eye. If the trouble is in the lachrymal sac an abscess may form ; the eyelids become red and swollen, the eye cannot be opened, and if the abscess is left to itself the " matter " will burst through the skin.

Treatment.—If the lids of the eye are thickened from protracted or repeated inflammation, it may be necessary for the surgeon to slit up the ducts. If the trouble is due to a turning-out (eversion) of the lid, as sometimes occurs in old people, the lower lid may be painted with flexile collodion, which tightens up the skin, or may be supported with a small strip of isinglass plaster. In the early stage, inflammation may be relieved by frequent bathing with warm boric-acid lotion (a teaspoonful of boric acid to a pint of water), and by instilling into the eye, every three hours, two or three drops of a solution of argyrol (10 grains) in distilled water (a tablespoonful). If the lachrymal sac is swollen, the contents should be gently pressed into the nose every two or three hours, before each application of the drops. A warm compress of lint soaked in the boric-acid lotion, and covered with oiled silk, should also be applied. But whenever the lachrymal sac or the nasal ducts are affected, it is better to call in a medical man than to rely upon domestic treatment.

EPIPHYSIS (*see* BONES AND JOINTS).

EPIPHYSITIS (*see* BONE, DISEASES OF).

EPISTAXIS (*see* NOSE BLEEDING).

ERUCTATIONS (*see* FLATULENCE).

ERUPTIONS IN THE COMMONER FEVERS.—In what are called the eruptive fevers it is often impossible to determine from what affection the patient is suffering until the rash has begun to appear. One indication is furnished by the *situation* of the rash at the beginning. In chicken-pox it usually appears on the trunk ; in measles, in crescents on the face or forehead ; in smallpox, on the face, neck and wrists ; in scarlet fever, on the neck, front of chest, etc. ; in typhoid fever, on the abdomen and trunk ; in typhus on the chest and abdomen. Significance attaches, too, to the *time* at which the rash comes out relatively to the appearance of the first symptoms of illness. In chicken-pox the rash shows on the first day, so that if twenty-four hours have elapsed after the first symptoms of illness without an eruption appearing, this disease can be ruled out. The same is usually true of German measles, although in some cases the rash does not appear until the second, or even the third day of the illness. In scarlet fever the rash appears on the second day, in cerebro-spinal meningitis (" spotted fever ") on the second to the fourth, in smallpox on the third, in measles on the fourth, in typhus from the fourth to the seventh, in typhoid on the sixth or seventh. A third aid to the diagnosis of an eruptive fever is to be found in the *character* of the rash. Cerebrospinal meningitis begins with rose-coloured spots or hæmorrhagic patches; chicken-pox with small rose spots that become blisters ; German measles with tiny red spots that run together into patches ; scarlet fever with minute red dots surrounded by a paler area, but the rash soon becomes bright red and diffuse ; smallpox, with scattered, hard, shotty pimples that turn first into blisters and then become "mattery"; typhus fever with red spots, either separate or grouped, which after two or three days become darker, like a mulberry (hence the term "mulberry rash"); measles has red, slightly raised spots that form crescents or patches; typhoid fever, small rose-coloured spots.

ERYSIPELAS.—This inflammatory infection of the skin and adjacent mucous membranes is known as *the rose*, from the redness of the affected part, and as *St. Anthony's fire*, from the belief that the relics of this saint were capable of curing it. It is caused by a germ of the streptococcus group, which usually, if not always, effects entrance through a breach of the skin or mucous membrane, as in accidental or surgical wounds, cracks, fissures, etc.; the breach may be so small as to escape observation.

Incubation stage and symptoms. —The usual incubation period is from one to three days, but it may be rather longer. The inflammation of the skin or mucous membrane may be preceded or accompanied by constitutional symptoms—a high temperature, a shivering fit, which may be violent enough to be termed a rigor, headache, vomiting, loss of appetite, and general malaise. The temperature remains high as long as the surface inflammation continues to spread; it is subject to morning and evening remissions. The eruption begins with an elevation of the surface, shining, swollen, and hot to the touch, with a raised border, which is generally scarlet. In that variety of the affection which is known as *erysipelas migrans*, wandering erysipelas, several parts of the body are successively and, it would seem, independently attacked. In about a week, but in some cases much longer, the inflammation ceases to spread; by this time the face—if it is the face that is attacked—may be greatly swollen. Sore throat and an eruption on the lips are frequent manifestations, and the neighbouring lymph-glands may be involved. In the healthy the complaint usually runs a mild course, but in the delicate, and in those who suffer from kidney disease or who are alcoholic, the symptoms may be serious.

Treatment.—The patient must take to bed, the bowels be well opened, and a light diet of milk, beaten-up eggs, clear soups and broths, instituted. The headache may be relieved by the application to the head of an ice-bag or by bathing it with iced water; restlessness soothed and delirium checked by sponging the body with warm water. If there are signs of failing strength, stimulants must be administered. Salicylate of soda, in 10-grain doses every four hours, is also to be recommended. The inflamed skin may be dusted over with boric-acid powder or oxide of zinc, and then covered with a thin layer of cotton-wool. A soothing application for the face is lead-and-opium lotion, in which lint should be soaked and applied in the form of a mask, holes being cut for the eyes, nose and mouth. If the mouth or throat is involved, lotions of boric acid (a teaspoonful to a tumblerful of warm water) or Condy's fluid (of a faint purple) should be frequently used as a mouth wash and gargle; ice should be sucked, and a hot fomentation applied round the throat.

Serums and vaccines have been used in the treatment of this affection. The serums have proved disappointing, but a vaccine made from germs taken from the patient may be tried when there are frequent relapses, and also in chronic cases of wandering erysipelas.

ERYTHEMA.—This is the term applied to a superficial redness of the skin, disappearing on pressure. In the simpler forms of erythema there is no inflammation. Patches of redness, at first scarlet, afterwards pinkish in hue, appear, most often on the face, or on surfaces of the skin which are in contact with each other or are exposed to friction. After a day or two, or longer, the redness gradually fades, with slight scaling. In the severer forms of erythema the flow of blood through the affected part is obstructed until stagnation takes place, and then inflammation is set up. Among these inflammatory forms is *erythema intertrigo* (*see* CHAFING), *erythema pernio* (*see* CHILBLAIN), *frostbite* (q.v.), *erythema multiforme*, so called from the many different forms the eruption may take, and *erythema nodosum*. This last type of erythema is often associated with rheumatism, is much more common in girls than in boys, and is rare after the age of twenty. The patient feels ill and complains of rheumatic-like pains in or around the joints, especially of the lower limbs.

Attacks of erythema may be due to cold or heat, or to contact with coarse flannel, or dirty underclothing, or vegetable or chemical substances. Or the irritation may arise in the digestive or other internal organs and be reflected to the skin.

Treatment.—For the simple forms of erythema nothing is necessary but to remove, or avoid, the cause of the irritation. In the acute stage of erythema nodosum rest in bed with elevation of the affected limbs is desirable. The best drug is salicylate of soda, 5 to 15 grains three times a day, according to the patient's age. A quinine and iron tonic (p. 42) will be found serviceable during convalescence. The spots may be treated with a compress of warm lead lotion; they should never be opened.

ETHER (*see* ANÆSTHESIA).

ETHYL CHLORIDE (*see* ANÆSTHESIA).

EUSTACHIAN TUBE (*see* EAR).

EXERCISES, REMEDIAL. — Exercises for the alleviation or cure of deformities, injuries, and various diseases have been in use for many years, but the system received a great impetus from the War. At first they consisted of active movements only i.e. movements carried out by the patient's voluntary effort, with or without resistance, but now they include also passive movements, which are performed by an operator with the patient's body. Among the disorders in which exercises have justified themselves are spinal curvatures, wry neck, congenital dislocation and other affections of the hip-joint, knock-knee, and club-foot. They are also of service in such nervous diseases as locomotor ataxy, disseminated sclerosis, one-sided paralysis, paralysis of the lower limbs, and affections of the surface nerves. The injuries in which exercises are beneficial are those followed by contractures and those leading to weakness of muscles.

EXOPHTHALMIC GOITRE (*see* GRAVES'S DISEASE).

EYE (Plate VIII).—The eyeball, spherical in shape, is about 1in. in diameter; it is protected by the bones of the orbit, except in front, where it is covered by the eyelids. The *lachrymal gland*, which secretes the tears, is situated in the orbit, on the outer and upper side of the eyeball (Fig. 20). It has ducts which open on the under-surface of the upper lid. The tears are collected on the inner side of the eyeball into two small channels—the canaliculi

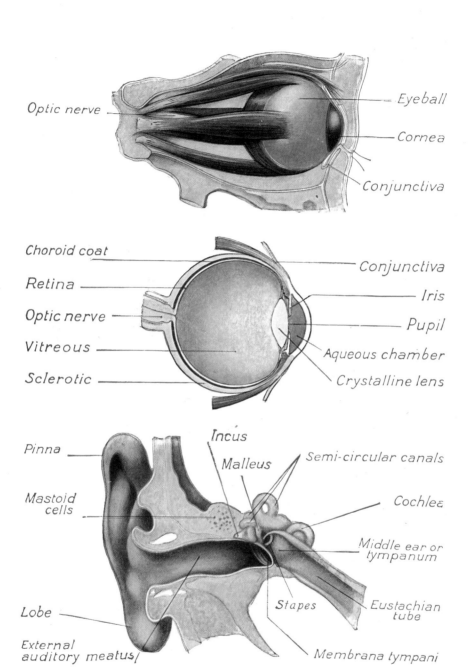

Optic nerve — Eyeball

Cornea

Conjunctiva

Choroid coat — Conjunctiva

Retina — Iris

Optic nerve — Pupil

Vitreous — Aqueous chamber

Sclerotic — Crystalline lens

Incus

Pinna — Malleus — Semi-circular canals

Mastoid cells — Cochlea

Middle ear or tympanum

Lobe — Stapes — Eustachian tube

External auditory meatus — Membrana tympani

PLATE VIII. THE EYE AND THE EAR.

—which open, one on the upper, the other on the lower lid (Fig. 20). Thence, the ducts lead into a sac at the side of the root of the nose, and so into the nasal duct (Fig. 20). If the secretion is excessive or the ducts are blocked, the tears escape over the lower lid and run down the cheek.

In looking at the eye, one sees a coloured part (the *iris*) occupying the centre of the globe, and a white part (the *sclerotic*) all round. The sclerotic is a thick fibrous coat which covers the whole eyeball, except that behind it is pierced by the optic nerve, and that in front, over the iris, it is modified into a transparent structure called the *cornea*, which may be said to cover the front of the eyeball as a glass covers the dial of a watch. Externally, the sclerotic and the cornea are lined by a transparent mucous membrane — the *conjunctiva*, which also lines the inner side of the eyelids; its office is to keep the surface of the eye moist, and allow the eyelids to move easily on the front of the eyeball. Inside the sclerotic, and therefore not visible, is a second coat, the *choroid*, which contains the blood-vessels of the eye, and is deeply pigmented so as to make of the eye a dark chamber. This also, like the sclerotic, is pierced at the back of the eyeball by the optic nerve. Inside the choroid coat again is the *retina* ; this is an expansion of the optic nerve, and is the sense-organ of sight. These, then, are the coats of the eye—the sclerotic, the choroid, and the retina.

Immediately behind the cornea is a space which is known as the *aqueous chamber*, containing a thin watery fluid (the *aqueous humour*). This chamber is partially divided into two by a muscular curtain, which has already been referred to as the iris. In the middle of the iris is an aperture, the *pupil*, which becomes larger or smaller as the iris dilates or contracts under the influence of light falling upon the eye. Behind the iris lies the *crystalline lens*, convex both in front and behind, which focuses the rays of light upon the retina, as the lens of a camera focuses them on a film. Behind the lens is a much larger chamber than

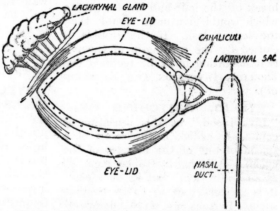

Fig. 20.—Diagram of the lachrymal gland and ducts, etc.

the aqueous, containing a clear, jelly-like substance, the *vitreous humour*.

When a ray of light falls upon the eye, its path lies through the cornea, across the aqueous chamber, and through the pupil. Thence it traverses the lens, the vitreous chamber, and so reaches the back of the eyeball, where it impinges upon the retina. The image there imprinted is conveyed to the brain by the *optic nerve*. The place where the optic nerve enters the eye is known as the *optic disc*, and is the *blind spot* of the eye, while the part of the retina which is the seat of most acute vision, the *yellow spot* (macula lutea), is a little to the inner side of the disc.

EYE, FOREIGN BODIES IN (*see* FOREIGN BODIES).

EYELASHES, INGROWING.— This condition (*trichiasis*) is a sequel of chronic inflammation of the edges of the eyelids (*see* BLEAR EYE.) One or several hairs are turned towards the eyeball, causing constant irritation of the cornea, the transparent part of the eyeball, with profuse watering. The treatment is to pull out the misguided lashes with a fine pair of forceps, care being taken to apply steady traction so as not to break off the hair and leave a stump which would give more trouble than the longer lash. If the trouble is caused by the turning-in of the lid, that condition must be rectified (*see* EYELIDS, INVERSION AND EVERSION OF).

EYELID, TWITCHING OF.— " Live blood," as this sensation is commonly called, is the result of a spasm of one of the muscles of the eyelid. It is hardly to be regarded as an " affection," but in some cases it is so persistent as to be troublesome. Persons of a nervous temperament are especially liable to it. When it is the result of some digestive disturbance, or of threadworms, a few doses of aperient medicine should be taken, preparatory to a tonic ; if it is caused by worry or overwork, the tonic should be taken without the aperient.

EYELID, UPPER, DROOPING OF.—Falling of the upper eyelid (*ptosis*), which cannot be raised, is due to paralysis of the cranial nerve that supplies the muscle by which this eyelid is elevated, and treatment must be directed to the cause of the paralysis. When ptosis is congenital it may be due to a birth injury, or to failure of the muscle to develop properly.

EYELIDS, CYSTS OF.—At the base of the eyelashes are a number of glands, the Meibomian glands, which secrete an oily fluid that is discharged through ducts which open on the edges of the lids. If a duct becomes blocked the secretion accumulates and a little swelling or cyst is formed which may not only irritate the eye but may itself become inflamed, leading to the formation of an abscess, visible on the inner surface of the lid as a yellow spot. The lower lid is more frequently affected in this way than the upper. The abscess may be subdued by hot fomentations or may break spontaneously, but it is better that it should be incised by the doctor and the hardened secretion expelled.

EYELIDS, INVERSION AND EVERSION OF.—In children, especially those who suffer from conjunctivitis—inflammation of the membrane that covers the front part of the eyeball and the inner surface of the lids—the eyelids sometimes turn inwards (*inversion, entropion*) from frequent contraction of the muscle that governs their movements. The condition may be remedied by painting the lid with contractile collodion, by which it will be drawn outwards to its normal position, but it may be necessary to insert temporary stitches to keep the lids in proper position. Inversion of the eyelids in the aged may require the removal of a horizontal strip of skin and muscle from the region of the lashes.

The turning-out of the eyelids (*eversion, ectropion*) is often due to chronic conjunctivitis. In some cases it is sufficient to treat the conjunctivitis (q.v.), but in others a small operation is necessary.

EYES, SPOTS BEFORE.—The medical name for this condition, which is more common in short-sighted than in normal-sighted persons, is *muscæ volitantes*, or " floating flies." The " spots " usually take the form of thin, filmy threads, dots, or circles, which float before the vision after any sudden movement of the eyes, and gradually settle down when the eyes are kept still. They are seen when the eyes are shut as well as when they are open. The peculiarity of the spots is that they never prevent even the smallest object from being seen. They often excite apprehension of serious eye trouble, but in point of fact they are quite negligible, being due simply to irregularities in the structure of the vitreous humour of the eye—the jelly-like fluid which is contained in the chamber behind the crystalline lens, and gives to the eyeball its roundness. No treatment is necessary, but if the patient is inconvenienced, or worried with fears, coloured glasses may be worn. If spots before the eyes, instead of being temporary and occasional as described, are permanent and are always seen in the same place, they may indicate that the lens is becoming opaque (cataract), or that there is an opaque patch on the cornea, or that the iris is adherent to the front of the lens as a result of past iritis. Such cases require treatment at the hands of an oculist.

EYESTRAIN.—This is the designation for fatigue of the muscles and nerves of the eye. It may arise in many different ways, but most often from some slight error of refraction (*see* REFRACTION AND ACCOMMODATION, ERRORS OF), and it is especially felt when the health is below par. In some cases eyestrain is caused by the wearing of unsuitable glasses. The symptoms are eyeache, headache—most frequent about the forehead—both of them worse towards the end of the day, watery eyes, and heaviness of the lids. The patient should lose no time in having his eyes examined by an oculist, who will prescribe glasses that will rid him of the trouble.

F

FACIAL NEURALGIA (*see* NEURALGIA).

FACIAL PARALYSIS (BELL'S PALSY).—The facial nerve originates in the under part of the brain, passes through a canal in the skull, and spreads over the side of the face from a point immediately in front of the ear. It may be paralysed by compression from a tumour, or by disease, in or at the base of the brain, or by disease of its bony canal, or as the result of wounds in the face. A common cause is exposure to cold, especially from sitting opposite an open window in a train, the immediate result being inflammation of the sheath of the nerve within the bony canal, accompanied by an exudation that compresses the fibres of the nerve. The affection is sometimes known as Bell's palsy, after Sir Charles Bell, a famous surgeon at the Middlesex Hospital. The affected side of the face becomes expressionless and mask-like ; the skin is smooth, all wrinkles being effaced ; the eye cannot be closed, and waters ; the corner of the mouth droops, and fluid cannot be retained ; the face is drawn to the opposite, the sound side ; on the affected side the patient can neither laugh nor frown. The tongue on the affected side may be deprived of the sense of taste. All these symptoms may come on within twenty-four hours of exposure to cold.

Where exposure to cold is the cause the symptoms frequently disappear in two or three weeks, although some slight loss of power may persist for months. In cases due to tumours, cure depends, of course, upon the possibility of removing the new growth; in cases due to wounds which sever the nerve, upon suturing the nerve-trunk.

Treatment.—The regular application of the galvanic current will help to maintain the nutrition of the facial muscles against the time when impulses will once more be able to travel along the nerve. Poultices and fomentations may also be applied, and counter-irritation, in the form of blisters, of liniment, or of gentle friction with some stimulating embrocation. Iodide of potash, 2 or 3 grains in a tablespoonful of water three times a day, is useful in many cases. Later a course of tonics may be taken to improve the general health and the tone of the affected muscles. If at the end of six months there are no signs of improvement, the medical attendant may consider the propriety of an operation designed to establish connexion between the facial and one of the other nerves. In many cases, however, the deformity and inconvenience caused by facial paralysis are too slight to make this operation worth while.

FAINTING.—The condition of partial or complete unconsciousness termed a fainting fit, or syncope, is due to a variety of causes—mental causes such as fear, fright, or a sudden reception of emotion-stirring news; or physical causes such as hæmorrhage, heart disease, starvation, fatigue, exposure to severe cold or to the hot, close atmosphere of ill-ventilated rooms. Treatment consists essentially in restoring to the brain its normal supply of blood. To this end, the clothing round the neck, chest and abdomen having been loosened, the patient should be laid down on a couch or bed and the head lowered a little beneath the level of the body by being allowed to hang over the edge, supported by the helper's hands; or if the patient is in the sitting posture, her head should be gently depressed between her knees for a few seconds. Contributory measures are sprinkling cold water on the face, or fanning it, slapping the hands, applying smelling salts to the nostrils, and, when the patient has recovered sufficiently to swallow, *but not before*, administering sal-volatile and water, or a little brandy. If the room is hot, fresh air should if possible be admitted, and, in any case, as soon as possible the patient should be helped out of it. A fainting fit may sometimes be averted by stooping as to tie a shoe-lace.

FALLING OF THE WOMB (*see* WOMB, DISPLACEMENTS OF).

FALLING SICKNESS (*see* EPILEPSY).

FALSE CROUP (*see* CROUP).

FARADISM.—One of the forms of electricity used in electrical treatment (q.v.).

FAST (*see* FOOD).

FAVUS.—Common in the East End of London a generation or so ago, this skin disease is now very rare in England, but less rare in Scotland. It is infective in only a low degree, and one member of a family may suffer from it without communicating it to others. A low state of health and insanitary conditions are the chief predisposing causes. The exciting cause is a fungus, which in some cases is " caught " from the mouse. The site it most prefers is the scalp.

The disease begins as a tiny yellow point or a scaly spot which enlarges into a disc, sulphur-yellow in colour. The lesion usually takes several months to mature, when it comes away. In severe cases several discs run together, forming crusted patches which may be of considerable extent. The only symptoms are slight itching or discomfort. The crusts should be removed by a thorough soaking with carbolized oil. The head, if that is the seat of the disease, should be washed with soft soap, and the scalp then X-rayed in sections until all the hairs have fallen out. Drugs of the same kind as those used in ringworm (q.v.) can now be rubbed in.

FEEDING OF INFANTS AND YOUNG CHILDREN (*see* INFANTS AND YOUNG CHILDREN, FEEDING OF).

FEET, SWEATING.—For this disagreeable condition boric acid should be freely used. Every night and morning the feet should be washed in warm water to which a tablespoonful of the powder has been added for each pint. The powder should also be sprinkled into the boots and socks before they are put on, and if the perspiration is very free, oxide of zinc may be added—1 part in 4. The socks should be frequently changed ; the boots should be light, and should never be of patent leather, and two or three pairs should be kept and worn in turn ; they may be fitted with cork soles, which should be washed occasionally in boric-acid lotion. The bowels should be kept regular, and anything that is wrong with the general health corrected. To check the excessive sweating a tabloid containing 5 minims of tincture of belladonna may be taken three times a day.

FEVER.—The raised temperature which is the chief sign of fever or pyrexia may be of various degrees. If the clinical thermometer registers 100·4° Fahr. to 101·1°, the fever is *slight ;* if 101·3° to 103·1°, *moderate ;* beyond this it is *severe,* and if it reaches or exceeds 106° it is termed *hyperpyrexia.* As a rule a persistent temperature of 107° is fatal, though cases are on record in which patients with a higher temperature have survived. A view of the essential nature of fever which is not wanting in plausibility is that which regards it as an effort on the part of Nature to protect the organism from the bacterial or other noxious influences to which it is exposed. If this theory is true, it must be admitted that Nature in many cases acts with excess of zeal.

Causes.—The usual cause of fever is the action of bacterial poisons. But there are sundry other agents which may produce various degrees of fever ; the injection into the veins of so innocuous a fluid as distilled water is one of them.

Fever is said to be *continuous* when the temperature remains high for some time without marked variation ; *remittent,* when it rises and falls without ever becoming normal ; *intermittent,* when it falls to normal for a time and again rises high ; *relapsing,* when the normal intervals are more prolonged. A *specific* fever is one that is due to the action of a specific germ ; an *infectious* fever, one that is transmitted from one person to another by poison particles ; an *eruptive* fever, one in which a characteristic rash comes out. The same fever may be, of course, at once specific, infectious and eruptive—measles, for example.

Treatment.—The first thing a fever patient should do is to get to bed, for fever is most exhausting ; moreover, he will then avoid the injurious results of exposure to cold. He will need little inducement to take to his bed, for he is sure to feel weak and ill. If the temperature should rise until the hyperpyrexial stage is reached, cold may have to be applied. The body may be sponged all over, beginning with water at 90° Fahr., which is gradually reduced to 70° or less. Or the patient is put bodily into water at the temperature of his body, and the water gradually cooled by the addition of cold and then iced water, and finally of solid ice. The cooling of the water may be accelerated by running off the hot water or bailing it out. This drastic treatment should never be given except under skilled supervision, for, unless carefully watched, the patient may collapse under it. The same caution must be given in the case of the *wet pack*, which is described in the article on that subject. The doctor may order drugs such as antipyrin or phenacetin, and if the heart shows signs of weakness, digitalis or strychnine may be prescribed. Purgatives are useful in reducing the temperature and carrying off waste material; salts, such as Epsom or Glauber's salts, are more suitable than vegetable purgatives, such as rhubarb or castor oil.

Diet.—In fever there is at once great body waste and much difficulty in taking solid food, owing to digestive disturbance and loss of appetite. The old plan of " starving a fever " was a mistake which in many cases must have had fatal results. Obviously the right thing to do is to *feed* a fever, but to feed it with nutritious fluids, with which the patient must be plied frequently, but in small quantities. The most useful articles of diet are beef tea, mutton, chicken, or veal broth, arrowroot gruel, eggs, milk and jellies; to the beef tea vermicelli may be added; to the mutton broth, rice

or bits of toast. Eggs in custard or beaten up with milk or wine, and blancmange made of isinglass are also suitable. Meat extracts are serviceable, but they should be taken sparingly, for they are stimulating rather than nutritious. Milk is almost indispensable, but as digestion is enfeebled it should be diluted with about one-third its quantity of barley water, soda water, or plain water. Or it may be peptonized (*see* p. 91), or lime water may be added to it in the proportion of two tablespoonfuls to a tumblerful. Plenty of fluid should be given, not only to assuage thirst but also to flush waste material out of the body. Plain water, toast water, barley water, cold weak tea and home-made lemonade are all suitable drinks, but they must be given in small quantities at a time, otherwise diarrhœa may be induced. Ice may be added, or broken into small pieces and slowly sucked. In some cases, particularly in young children and old people, stimulants are necessary, but they should only be given under medical orders and their effect carefully watched. There is little to choose between good brandy and good whisky. Champagne is valuable in severe exhaustion, as it is also in convalescence. Gin is indicated in cases in which the kidneys need stimulating.

FIBROMAS (*see* TUMOURS).

FIGURE-OF-EIGHT BANDAGES (*see* BANDAGES).

FILARIASIS.—This term covers the diseases produced in tropical and sub-tropical countries by the action of tiny blood-worms called filariæ, and especially by the one that is named *Filaria bancrofti*, after the Queensland parasitologist who first discovered it. This parasite is introduced into the body by the bite of a mosquito, and takes up its abode in the lymphatic vessels, where it breeds and sets free swarms of young filariæ, which find their way into the blood. The ill the adult worms do arises from the obstruction they cause in the lymphatic vessels and glands, either by their mere presence or by setting up inflammation, the result being that the affected vessels become varicose, or that œdema (dropsy) is set up ; or both these effects may be produced. It is to the late Sir Patrick Manson that we owe most of our knowledge of filariæ and the many diseases they produce, and it was his discovery that the filaria is imbibed from human blood by the mosquito and is in turn communicated by that insect to man that led him to formulate the theory that the mosquito plays a corresponding part—that of the intermediate host— in the dissemination of malaria, a theory which was proved to be true by the researches of Sir Ronald Ross and other investigators. Among the diseases coming under the head of filariasis are *lymph scrotum*, in which the skin of the scrotum—the bag containing the testicles—is enormously enlarged ; *chyluria*, in which the contents of lymphatic vessels escape with the urine ; *elephantiasis*, in which the affected part—it may be the leg, or the arm, or some other part—swells to an enormous size. As a rule, the most suitable treatment consists in rest in bed, the avoidance of fatty foods, including milk, and the administration of gentle aperients. In lymph scrotum and elephantiasis the affected part may become so heavy that operation may have to be resorted to.

FILTRATION OF WATER.—This method of purifying water may easily lead to a delusive sense of security. The charcoal filters in common use strain out very few of the micro-organisms which the water may contain, and if not regularly cleansed they make things worse by polluting the water with the micro-organisms which they have accumulated. The Pasteur-Chamberland and Berkefeld filters are in a different category : they do strain out a good many bacteria ; but even they require brushing and sterilizing from time to time. If the water is muddy, the mud and slime should first be removed by sand filters or by precipitation with alum. The surest method of purifying water is to boil it for at least ten minutes ; this will not only destroy all the harmful micro-organisms it may contain, but will render it soft. To neutralize the resulting flatness and tastelessness of the water it may be aerated by being shaken vigorously in an open vessel or unstoppered bottle only partly filled.

FINGERS, CHAPPED (*see* CHAPPED HANDS AND LIPS).

FINGERS, CONTRACTED.— Many men who are past the age of thirty suffer from a contraction of one or more fingers of one or both hands—most often the ring finger, but sometimes the little finger, and occasionally the index finger. The deformity, which is called *Dupuytren's contraction*, is often associated with gout, and in some cases appears to be favoured by the frequent clutching in the hand of a stick or a tool. The patient first notices a thickening in the palm just above the base of the ring finger ; over this spot the skin may be tender or crinkled. Before long he finds that he has lost the power to stretch out this finger to the full extent, and gradually it and the little finger are drawn more and more into the palm. In some cases pains are felt in the hand that shoot up the arm ; in others all that the patient complains of is that he no longer has the full use of his hand. Something can be done to hinder the progress of the deformity at an early stage by massage and by wearing a special splint at night. But the contraction tends to grow worse, and at last the hand becomes almost useless as well as disfigured. The remedy is an operation by which the shortened tissues are completely removed, followed by massage and exercises.

FINSEN LIGHT (*see* ELECTRICAL TREATMENT).

FIRST-AID (*see* DISLOCATION ; FRACTURES ; HÆMORRHAGE ; POISONS AND POISONING, etc.).

FISSURE AND FISTULA, ANAL.—An anal fissure is a small crack or sore just inside the orifice of the bowel ; a fistula is a suppurating tract in the same region which opens on to the skin of the anus at one end and into the bowel at the other end.

A **fissure** occurs most frequently in nervous and delicate women, usually as the result of chronic constipation ; the skin of the orifice is torn by the hard motions, and healing is prevented by the stretching which takes place when the bowels move and by the contraction of the muscle which keeps the orifice closed. Treatment consists in administering laxatives and injecting oil into the bowel, so that the motions may be soft, in applying cocaine ointment so that no pain may be felt when the bowels move, and in rubbing in a calomel or resin ointment to promote healing of the fissure. In many cases these measures are successful ; if after about a month the fissure has not healed, operation should be resorted to.

An anal **fistula** is almost always due to an abscess which has burst and never completely healed. There may be comparatively little discharge, or both wind and (in rare cases) motions may find their way through the external opening or openings, and there is more or less suppuration. Operation is the only effective treatment.

FITS (*see* CONVULSIONS ; EPILEPSY ; FAINTING).

FLAT WARTS (*see* WARTS).

FLAT-FOOT.—In infancy, or later during the active stages of growth, especially after a debilitating illness or prolonged rest in bed, the muscles or ligaments of the arch of the foot may give way, producing the condition known as flat-foot. Prominent among the causes to which it is due are bad habits of standing and walking, such as standing at ease with almost the whole weight of the body thrown on to one foot, and walking with the toes turned out too much. Flat-foot is often associated with knock-knee, and one deformity may induce the other ; lateral curvature of the spine often leads to flat-foot ; and a disease or injury of one leg that necessitates uneven walking may cause flat-foot in the opposite limb. The deformity may be identified by making the child stand on each foot in turn, when the arch will be seen to have given way more or less, in some cases to such an extent that the inner ankle almost touches the ground. The patient complains of pain, especially along the outer side of the foot, and along the inner part of the sole, and sometimes extending up the calf ; it is much worse after standing and walking, and in bad cases the child may be afraid to attempt either. Very bad cases are incurable when the condition is once well established, and even in cases of less severity it may be eighteen months before treatment effects a permanent cure. In its early stages, however, flat-foot yields to simple measures. Faulty habits of standing and walking must be corrected. Moderate exercise of all kinds is beneficial, as promoting the general health. Among special exercises, the best is walking on tip-toe, with the toes turned in as much as possible, and walking on the outer edge of the feet, with the soles turned inwards and forwards. Massage of the muscles of the leg is useful; the foot should be daily douched with cold water, and hot, dry, friction then applied; the stockings should be warm, and garters discarded. Special boots, made without heels, fitted with a wedge-shaped pad corresponding to the arch of the foot, and stiffened at the " waist," should be worn. In more severe cases it is necessary to insist upon the wearing of an outer leg-iron.

FLATULENCE.—The popular phrase for this condition is " wind in the stomach," but in many cases the excess of gas is in the intestine rather than in the stomach. Whether the flatulence is stomachic or intestinal, the causes are much the same. In both, (1) the gas may be the result of excessive fermentation or putrefaction of food, owing to digestive deficiency or to bacterial action; or (2) it may be simply swallowed; or (3) the normal absorption of gas may be defective. The second of these causes—the swallowing of air—accounts for more cases of stomachic than of intestinal flatulence. Air is swallowed in the act of eructation—that is, belching. The patient belches because he has an uncomfortable sensation in the stomach, which he thinks to be due to wind, and instead of relieving himself of gas he swallows it. He swallows it also with the

saliva, which is always frothy with air; and when there is an excessive secretion of saliva, as occurs in some stomachic disorders and in mouth troubles, a large quantity of air gradually accumulates in the stomach. If air accumulates in the stomach when this organ is empty of food, some of it may pass into the intestine, where it may either be absorbed or may escape through the anus. When the flatulence is chiefly in the intestine the condition is termed *tympanites* (from *tympanum*, a drum), for the abdomen may become tight and resonant like a drum.

Symptoms.—Wind in the *stomach* gives rise to a sensation of fullness, and the diaphragm, the great muscle which separates the chest from the abdomen, may be pushed up and cause not only palpitation but pain, and these may be interpreted as symptoms of heart disease; difficulty in breathing may also be present. *Intestinal* flatulence produces not only a sensation of fullness but rumbling sounds, and may set up colicky pains, for the distended bowel tends to undergo violent and spasmodic contractions. Many cases of abdominal distension which are purely nervous are mistaken for cases of flatulence; the distension is caused by spasm of the diaphragm; it comes on suddenly, and disappears no less suddenly, and without any escape of gas, and if the patient is examined under X-rays it is seen that no excess of gas is present.

Treatment.—In so far as flatulence is due to the swallowing of air, the patient should be directed to avoid belching; when he feels the impulse to this act, he should open his mouth, or clench his teeth upon a cork, when it will be impossible for him to swallow air, though any excess of gas present in the stomach will not be prevented from escaping. In other cases, large draughts of hot water are useful ; or sal-volatile (30 to 40 minims), spirit of chloroform (20 minims), or spirit of ether (30 minims), may be taken in half a wineglassful of water. If the flatulence is accompanied by acid eructations a couple of soda-mint tabloids, which contain peppermint and bicarbonate of ammonia as well as soda, may be taken, and two more an hour later if necessary. Another useful drug in these forms of dyspepsia is bismuth, which may be taken in the form of lozenges, or in the following draught :

> Solution of bismuth and citrate
>   of ammonia .... 1 drachm
> Bicarbonate of soda..........10 grains
> Spirit of chloroform ....20 minims
> Infusion of calumba to 1 ounce.
> Make a draught. To be taken an hour before food three times a day.

Charcoal will be found to absorb gases ; a teaspoonful of the freshly-prepared powder may be taken as a dose, or it may be employed in the form of biscuits or lozenges. When the wind is in the lower part of the bowel an enema may be given—a pint of warm water containing a teaspoonful of spirit of turpentine or ten drops of oil of rue. To clear the intestines of substances that are evolving gas, a suitable aperient is two grains of calomel in tabloid form at night, followed by a dose of Epsom salts next morning. As to diet, it may be found desirable to avoid, or to take less, starch and sugar, or fruits, or green vegetables, or tea, or soup, as the case may be, to substitute toast for bread, and to take very little fluid with meals.

FLEA-BITES (*see* STINGS AND BITES).

" FLOATING FLIES " (*see* EYES, SPOTS BEFORE).

FLOATING KIDNEY (*see* MOVABLE KIDNEY).

FLUSHING.—This common and very troublesome condition may be distinguished from blushing (q.v.) in that it is not mainly an expression of emotional disturbance, though it may be intensified and maintained by emotion. It may be associated with many different conditions—menstruation, or the cessation of menstruation, pregnancy, suckling, dyspepsia, anæmia, defective circulation, alcoholic excess, etc. It may start in the head and take a downward course, may begin in the lower regions and ascend to the head, may travel both upward and downward, or may be felt simultaneously in a number of different parts. It may be either heralded or, as more frequently occurs, succeeded by a cold stage. There is, therefore, no lack of variety about it, and the same may be said of the symptoms that may accompany or follow it—nausea or actual vomiting, faintness, a sense of suffocation, giddiness, numbness, tremors, noises in the ears, and palpitation. It will be sufficient to describe the flushing that attends the change of life, and that form of it which is associated with dyspepsia. The former usually affects women of forty-five to fifty. The sensations start from some particular spot, such as the pit of the stomach, and radiate thence ; when they reach the face it becomes scarlet. The patient may perspire so profusely as to run the risk of catching cold from the wetting of her clothing. The flushing due to indigestion usually comes on soon after a meal, when the face, particularly the nose, grows hot and red. It is usually accompanied by other symptoms of indigestion, which need not here be described. Both sexes are liable to it, but women more than men. If it should frequently recur, it may cause a permanent reddening of the nose and cheeks.

Treatment.—Flushing, whatever the special cause, is so intimately associated with the nervous system that a sedative is in most cases suitable. Two 5-grain tablets of bromide of potash in a wineglassful of water may be taken three times a day. If constipation is present, a glass of mineral water may be drunk first thing in the morning. In some cases it will be found helpful to stimulate the skin two or three times a week by hot baths at a temperature of 100° to 104° Fahr. for fifteen minutes at bed-time. Alcohol should be tabooed, and the strictest moderation observed in tea and coffee. Meat should be taken sparingly, and not more than once a day; condiments and spices should be avoided; vegetables and fruit may be eaten freely. Open-air exercise is desirable, and a quiet, even life, devoid of excitement, is the ideal to aim at.

FOLLICULAR CONJUNCTIVITIS (*see* Conjunctivitis).

FOMENTATIONS.—A fomentation, or stupe, is the application of moist heat, to allay pain, to prevent or subdue inflammation, or to promote the pointing of an abscess. Pieces of flannel, or of an old soft blanket, cut the required size, or better still a piece of spongiopiline, are suitable materials for the purpose. Besides the material itself, a basin, a large towel, and a piece of waterproof are required. Lay the towel across the basin with the flannel in its centre; over the flannel pour boiling water until it is well soaked; then wrap it up in the towel, and twist the ends of the towel in opposite directions until the flannel is wrung dry; take it out

of the towel, unfold it and apply it as hot as it can be borne, covering it with the waterproof and securing the whole with a bandage. If the fomentation is a large one, the wringing will require the strength of two persons, who must, of course, twist against each other. Or a wringer made with a yard and a half of strong coarse calico 18in. wide, doubled, and stitched like a small roller towel, may be used, two sticks being put through the ends of the wringer and twisted in opposite directions. After use the wringer should be dried, so that it may not be damp and cold when next used.

In making an *opium* fomentation the flannel should be wrung out first and then sprinkled with about 30 minims of laudanum; the quantity, however, will be specified by the doctor. For *poppy-head* fomentations four ounces of dried poppy-heads are taken and the seeds emptied out; the shells are boiled in three pints of water for a quarter of an hour; the decoction is then strained and the flannel wrung out of it. A *camomile-flower* fomentation is made in the same way. If a *belladonna* fomentation is ordered, the affected part is painted with a thick coating of belladonna and glycerin and then covered with a piece of white lint or flannel wrung out of boiling water, and this in turn is covered with a piece of pink mackintosh and a layer of cotton-wool and bandaged on. The only difference in the preparation of a *turpentine*, as distinct from an ordinary stupe or fomentation is that before boiling water is poured on, the flannel is sprinkled evenly with turpentine— usually one drachm. The flannel must be well saturated with the boiling water. A *boric-acid* fomentation is used to prevent or allay inflammation of open wounds. A piece of lint of a suitable size should be doubled up and dipped into a hot solution of boric acid and applied to the part, and covered up in the usual way. Instead of plain lint, boric lint, which is pink in colour, may be used ; this is already saturated with the acid, and nothing need be done except to dip it into hot water and apply it.

FOOD.—The three great classes of nutrient materials are proteins, carbohydrates, and fats. *Protein* contains nitrogen, and a food in which protein is present is therefore called nitrogenous, while all other foods are termed non - nitrogenous. Nitrogenous foods, and they alone, have the power of building up and repairing tissue ; non-nitrogenous foods only produce energy. Nitrogenous foods also produce energy, but their chief use is as tissue-builders. If all foods were definitely nitrogenous or non-nitrogenous, the formation of a dietary would be a very simple matter. But Nature has a great weakness for complexity, and so we find that in most of the common articles of food nitrogenous and non-nitrogenous elements are combined, as for example in meat, bread, rice, potatoes, peas and nuts. The *carbohydrates* include sugars and starches, and are for the most part of vegetable origin ; *fats* occur both in the animal and in the vegetable kingdom, and carbohydrates and fats alike are readily combustible in the body. Formerly it was considered that most of the muscular energy of the body was produced by the combustion of proteins, and that the combustion of carbohydrates and fats went largely to maintain the bodily temperature, but more recent investigations tend to show that we may get all the energy we need from carbohydrates and fats, and that protein is only required for tissue-building.

Vitamins.—Certain mysterious food elements which are essential to growth and health are known alternatively as vitamins, because of their importance to life (*vita*, Latin—life), and as accessory food factors. Their chemical nature has not yet been definitely ascertained, and little is known of them except from the effects of their presence in or absence from foods. Those at present recognized are three in number. The first of them is termed *fat-soluble A*, and is the growth factor. It is found in green leaves, and in milk, cream and butter, yolk of egg, beef tea, fish oils and peanut oil. The deficiency of this substance in the diet of children is believed to be one of the causes of rickets (q.v.). The second vitamin, known as *water-soluble B*, exists in greatest amount in eggs and in seeds, especially the seeds of the pulses—peas, beans, lentils, etc. But in cereals, such as wheat and rice, it is confined to the germ and the layer immediately beneath the pericarp (husk). The deficiency of this factor in diet leads to the development of the disease known as beriberi (q.v.) in those whose food consists largely of over-milled rice. Yeast and commercial yeast extract (marmite) are very rich in this vitamin, and it is present also in considerable amount in milk (but not in butter), liver, brain, pancreas and fish-roe, while it is contained to a less extent in many green vegetables, in potatoes, in fish, and in kidneys. The third vitamin, *water-soluble C*, is found in fresh vegetables and fruit, and especially oranges, lemons, cabbage, swedes, turnips, and lettuces. It is the absence of this factor in diet which causes scurvy (q.v.). It will be seen that accessory food factors are present in many animal foods, but in every case the original source of them is the vegetable kingdom.

FOOD-POISONING.—Food-poisoning was formerly thought to be caused by the presence of chemical substances called ptomaines, produced by putrefaction, and cases of food-poisoning are still sometimes so described. Now, however, it is taught that the usual cause of food-poisoning is infection with bacteria. The agent of food-poisoning may be fish, shell-fish, tinned fish, meat—especially sausages and tinned meat—vegetables and fruit, or milk. Sausages are a frequent source of danger because, by the process of mincing, meat becomes especially liable to contamination, because it is easy for the taste of unwholesome meat to be disguised by the flavouring, and because they are often eaten uncooked or but slightly cooked. In some cases of poisoning by sausages or potted meat the germ is not one of the ordinary germs of food-poisoning, but one which bears the name of *Bacillus botulinus* : in such cases the disease is known as botulism. It was almost unknown in these islands until a group of cases occurred in Scotland in the summer of 1922. It should be understood that cooking is not an adequate safeguard against food-poisoning, because, although the germ may be destroyed by the heat, it may have produced toxins which are unaffected by heat. The only safeguard, therefore, is to avoid contaminated food. When food has to be stored, it should, of course, be stored in proper safes, where it can be kept cool and free from contamination.

Symptoms.—The effects of eating impure food may begin in a few hours, or not until after three or four days. The time depends partly upon the amount of poison and partly upon the condition of the stomach ; if the stomach is empty at the time the food is taken, the symptoms will arise earlier. When they do arise, the onset is sudden. There is severe abdominal pain, with a rise of temperature. The tongue is furred, vomiting and purging are often present, heart-weakness may supervene and the patient may collapse. Sometimes the attack is ushered in by a shivering fit. In severe cases cramps may occur in the calves of the legs, and the patient may become cold and blue owing to the enfeebled circulation. A rash also may appear. In mild cases the symptoms clear up in a few days.

Treatment.—This can only be properly carried out by a medical man, who will prescribe the drugs required to allay the irritation and control the diarrhœa, etc. The pain in the abdomen may be relieved by hot applications, but where it is severe the doctor will probably inject morphia ; he may also have to inject saline. In all cases rest in bed is desirable. The diet should consist of liquids such as water, white of egg, chicken broth and whey.

FOREIGN BODIES.—Dirt was once defined as matter in the wrong place, and a foreign body may be defined as an object in the wrong place. The wrong places are usually the passages or cavities of the body, but a broken fragment of a needle in the flesh, or a fish-hook which has pierced the skin, is also classified as a foreign body.

Foreign bodies in the nose.—It sometimes happens that objects, such as beads, inserted in the nostrils by children in sport, become fixed. To remove the obstacle the unaffected nostril should be closed by pressure with the finger, and the child should then blow through the obstructed nostril. Or sneezing should be induced by sniffing a pinch of snuff up the open nostril. Or recourse may be had to syringing, the water being injected into the unblocked nostril, when, if the patient leans forward and keeps the mouth open, it will run round the back of the nose and down the other nostril and may wash out the foreign body.

Foreign bodies in the ear.— Although there is no truth in the common notion that earwigs are given to creeping into the ear, it does occasionally happen that a small insect finds its way into the ear and causes some pain and irritation, and more alarm. The child's head should be placed in the horizontal position and warm water gently poured into the ear, when the insect will probably be floated out of the cavity. Or the ear may be filled with warm olive oil, which is kept from running out by means of a plug of cotton-wool; this will drown the insect and bring it to the surface. Another plan is gently to inject warm water into the ear with a syringe, as described in the article, EAR, WAX IN. Objects similar to those mentioned in connexion with the nose are frequently introduced into the ear by children. For such things as stones and beads, syringing may be employed, but this method is unsuitable for peas, beans, seeds, etc., which may swell when soaked in water. In these cases it is better to send for the doctor, who will perform the extraction with an instrument. No unskilled person should ever try by the use of instruments to extract objects from the ear, for there is danger of injuring the membrane dividing the outer from the middle ear.

Foreign bodies in the eye.— From its position the eye is the organ most exposed to invasion by foreign bodies, such as insects, or pieces of grit, etc., which may be blown into it by the wind. Sometimes they can be got rid of by drawing one eyelid over the other. Usually a flow of tears is produced, and this may be increased by closing the unaffected eye and rubbing it, while carefully avoiding rubbing the affected eye; in many cases this suffices to wash out the intruder. If a fragment of coal, etc., as from a locomotive, should be imbedded in the cornea—the transparent part of the eye—the doctor should be sent for, nothing meanwhile being done except to place a few drops of olive oil in the turned-down lower lid and to keep the eyeball from movement by gently applying to it a pad of cotton-wool fixed with a bandage. It often happens that after a foreign body has been removed from the eye the irritation does not at once cease and it seems to the patient that the intruder is still there. In such cases the eye may be gently moistened with olive oil applied with a camel's-hair brush.

Foreign bodies in the gullet.— Occasionally a foreign body, such as a fish-bone or a coin, will lodge in the œsophagus, the tube leading from the mouth to the stomach. It may at once set up irritation, but in some cases it remains a long time without causing symptoms. Sooner or later, however, the foreign body is almost sure to cause ulceration, and it may then perforate the tube and probably damage one of the large blood-vessels in the vicinity. The object most likely to cause trouble is a tooth-plate. Smaller and rounder objects which lodge in the gullet may sometimes be carried on into the stomach by swallowing a large mouthful of well-masticated bread. If this plan does not answer, the doctor should be sent for. The toy bicycle shown in the illustration (Plate IX) was removed from the gullet by operation after it had been cut in two.

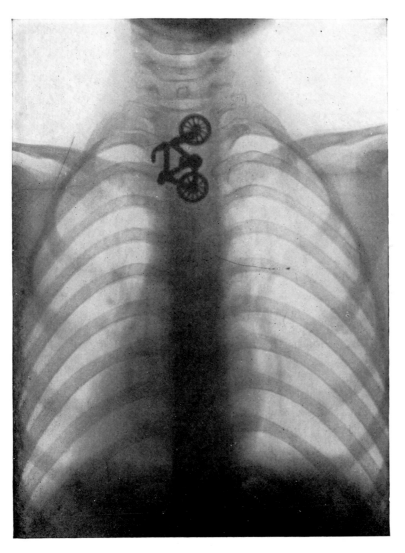

PLATE IX. TOY BICYCLE IMPACTED IN THE GULLET.

Foreign bodies in the stomach. —In most cases such things as coins or pins and needles which are accidentally swallowed and find their way into the stomach will pass through the intestines without treatment. The aim should be to envelop the foreign body in such food as porridge or mashed potatoes; no aperient should be given for some days, so that the object may have a chance of escaping spontaneously. The motions should be examined to see whether it has been passed.

Foreign bodies in the larynx and windpipe.—If coughing fails to remove the obstruction the patient should be struck on the back with the open hand, and if a child, may be held head downwards before being so struck. Another way of removing the obstruction is for the finger to be passed down the throat to dislodge it. If, when the object has been removed, respiration is still suspended, cold water should be dashed on the chest, and if this is ineffectual, artificial respiration must be employed. These measures failing, the doctor will remove the object with instruments, or open the larynx or the windpipe.

FOUR-TAILED BANDAGE (*see* BANDAGES).

FRACTURES.—In youth and middle age fractured bones are more

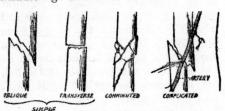
Fig. 21.—Types of fracture.

common in males than in females, owing to the greater exposure of the former to violence. In old age, how-

ever, the proportions are reversed, for in elderly women the bones undergo atrophy to a greater extent than in men of the same age.

Varieties of fracture (Fig. 21).— In a *simple* fracture the bone is broken in two, with but slight injury to the surrounding parts, and without the skin being penetrated.

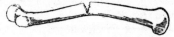
Fig. 22.—Greenstick fracture.

In a *comminuted* fracture the bone is broken or crushed into several or many pieces.

In a *complicated* fracture, surrounding structures, such as blood-vessels and nerves, or an organ such as the lung, may be seriously injured.

In a *compound* fracture the skin over the seat of the fracture is torn, usually by the protrusion of one end of the broken bone, so that it is possible for air and poisons to enter the wound.

In a *multiple* fracture the bone is broken in several places, or more than one bone is broken at the same time.

In a *greenstick* fracture (Fig. 22) the bone is bent and splintered, but not completely broken. This variety of fracture is frequent in the case of children, whose bones are not yet fully formed, and especially in rickety children.

In an *impacted* fracture the bone is completely broken, but the ends are driven into one another.

More than one of these varieties of fracture may be present in the same case. Thus, in a compound fracture the bone may not only penetrate the skin, but, before it does so, may injure a blood vessel or some other neighbouring structure; this is termed a *compound complicated* fracture.

Causes of fracture.—1. Many fractures are due to *direct violence*, such as a severe blow, the crush of a wheel, or the impact of a bullet.

2. When a fracture is due to *indirect violence* the impact is applied at some distance from the spot at which the bone is broken. Thus, in alighting on the feet from a height, the bones of the leg, the thigh-bone, the pelvis, or even the skull may be broken, while the bones of the feet escape fracture, the force being transmitted to the bone which is actually injured.

3. Many fractures are due to *violent muscular action*, as when a horseman breaks his collar-bone in striking his horse a back-handed blow. But the bone most frequently affected in this way is the knee-cap, for if the large muscles of the thigh, which are fixed to it, are suddenly contracted when the knee-joint is somewhat bent, as in avoiding a false step, this bone is easily broken in two.

Signs and symptoms of fracture. —When a bone is broken there are usually several indications of what has happened, though they are not all present in every case. Sometimes, however, the diagnosis of a fracture is very difficult; in such cases the patient should be treated as though a fracture were present. If none has occurred no harm will have been done by the over-precaution, whereas the consequences of neglecting a fracture might be serious.

1. *Unnatural position of the limb*.— If a limb is broken it will lie in an abnormal position. Thus, if both bones of the leg are broken, the foot by its own weight may fall outwards and lie on its side, while the knee-cap remains in the middle line.

2. *Shortening of the limb*.—The broken limb may be obviously shorter than the other, owing to the fractured

ends over-riding as the result of contraction of the muscles.

3. *Deformity*.—At the seat of the fracture there will be a bend or angle, or some other abnormality of form.

4. *Irregularity of outline*.—In bones immediately beneath the skin, such as the shin-bone, the collar-bone, and the lower jaw, the break may be felt by running the finger along the length of the bone, when a depression, a lump, or a sharp projection is felt. This sign is much less apparent in deep-set bones such as the thigh-bone.

5. *Increased mobility*.—When a limb is fractured, unless it is a greenstick or an impacted fracture, the limb may fall about like a flail, the fracture really constituting a joint.

6. *Swelling*.—In most fractures, owing to the over-riding of the fragments, the contraction of the muscles, and the effusion of blood, there is enlargement at the site of the injury.

7. *Discoloration*.—In fractures due to direct violence, discoloration at the seat of the injury will be seen almost immediately. If the violence in indirect, this discoloration may be delayed for hours, or even days.

8. *Crepitus*.—Except in impacted fractures, in which the bones are immovable, in greenstick fractures, in which they are not entirely divided, and in fractures in which the fragments of bone are widely separated, as in a broken knee-cap, a peculiar grating may be both felt and heard when the surfaces of the broken bone are rubbed together by moving the limb. This sign of fracture must be felt for with the greatest gentleness, for it causes the patient great pain, and serious injury would be done by rough movements.

9. *Pain and loss of power*.—When a bone is broken pain is caused by the slightest movement of the part. There is also loss of power over the

part, due to pain, injury to muscles, and breach of continuity in the bone. These two indications are, however, less diagnostic of fractures than some of the others that have been mentioned, since they may be present in injuries in which no bone is broken. It should be remembered too, that in parts, such as the leg and the fore-arm, where there are two bones, and only one is broken, the loss of power may not be obvious.

How fractures are repaired.— The union of the broken bone is, of course, the work of Nature, and all that treatment can do is to protect the process from interruption or disturbance. Before describing the first-aid treatment of fractures we may very briefly and generally explain how Nature does her work. As a result of inflammation of the wounded parts, broken bones are surrounded by a glutinous material termed lymph, which forms a sheath on the fracture, thickest opposite the break, and tapering off in both directions. This substance is gradually hardened by the deposit in it of particles of new bone, and it is thus converted into *callus*, which continues to grow harder until it is identical in composition with bone. In course of time the callus covering the bone on either side of the fracture is absorbed, leaving only that which unites the separated ends of the bone, and in time the bone is stronger here than in any other part. One of the reasons why movement is to be avoided is that it provokes an excessive formation of callus. In cases in which the broken ends of the bone are widely separated and cannot be kept together, as in the knee-cap, union is brought about by the formation of fibrous tissue instead of callus. In these cases no new bone is formed, the fibrous tissue taking its place.

General first-aid treatment of fractures.—A fracture is almost always indicated by pallor of the face, coldness of the skin, and possibly shivering. In such cases the patient must be covered up at once, and as soon as possible supplied with a hot drink—tea, coffee, milk or soup. If he is faint, give him a little sal-volatile.

The great thing to aim at is to avoid movement of the injured part. Movement, unless of the gentlest kind, will not only cause the patient acute pain, but may produce spasm of the muscles and so increase the displacement of the bone, may injure blood-vessels and cause dangerous hæmorrhage, or may drive the broken ends of the bone through the skin and so convert a simple into a compound fracture —a thing to be avoided at all costs, for, while a simple fracture is not a dangerous accident, a compound fracture is always serious, involving the risk of blood-poisoning. The utmost gentleness must therefore be exercised, whether in taking off the clothes, or moving a limb, or moving the patient. It is better to slit up the seams of the sleeves or legs of garments, and tear open the shirt and vest, rather than remove the clothing bodily. If the fracture is compound the bleeding must be stopped as quickly as possible (*see* the article on HÆMORRHAGE), and the wound washed with a clean piece of linen or lint dipped in boiled water, and then covered with a dressing of the same material soaked in carbolic lotion 1 in 40, the dressing in turn being covered with oil-silk or, if this is not available, enveloped in a thick layer of cotton-wool, fixed by a bandage. In simple and comminuted fractures a handkerchief, or a piece of lint or linen, dipped in cold water, or an ice-bag may be placed on the seat of the fracture. If the thigh-bone, the leg-bones, the pelvis, or the spine are broken, the patient must on no account be moved from where he falls, even in a crowded thoroughfare; the traffic must be held up until the limb has been immobilized by the application of splints. If the patient is indoors he must not even be lifted on to a couch or bed until this has been done. As we read in the British Red Cross Society "First-Aid Manual," perhaps the only situations in which moving a patient without first fixing the limb is justifiable are when he is threatened by flames in a burning house, or lying in a railway track between the rails and a train is approaching.

The immobility which is the most important point in the first-aid treatment of fractures is secured by the application of splints, which must be sufficiently long to extend from beyond the joint above to beyond the joint below the fractured bone. Thus if the forearm is broken, the splint must extend from above the elbow to below the wrist; if the thigh-bone, from above the hip to below the knee; if the leg, from above the knee to below the ankle. The bandages by which splints are secured to the limb or body should never be applied at the seat of the fracture, unless it is a compound fracture (*see* BANDAGES). How splints may be improvised is described in the article SPLINTS. They should not be removed until the medical man has seen the patient.

Special fractures.—We may now consider the first-aid treatment of fractures of the chief bones, taking them in alphabetical order.

Ankle.—One of the most frequent fractures at the ankle is that which is known as *Pott's fracture*, after a famous surgeon at St. Bartholomew's Hospital. It consists of a break of the smaller of the two leg-bones—the fibula—3 inches or so above the ankle-joint, and of the end of the other bone—the tibia—and causes a good deal of deformity, the foot being turned outwards and upwards. *Treatment.*—No attempt should be made to remedy this deformity by force; all that it is safe to do in this direction is to put the foot in as near the natural position as it will readily come to. The boot should be cut off and a splint applied from the knee to below the foot, either on the inner or the outer side, and fixed in position with several bandages.

Arm-bone.—If the humerus is broken at its **upper end** near the shoulder-joint, the condition may be very difficult to recognize. *Treatment.*—Apply a broad-fold bandage over the injury and round the arm and body, tie off at the top of the shoulder on the sound side, place a pad of cotton-wool in the armpit, and on the sound side also, and support the arm in a narrow sling.

Fractures in the **shaft** of the arm-bone are easy to recognize, the arm hanging helpless, the limb being shortened between the shoulder and the elbow, and crepitus being distinct. *Treatment.*—Bend the forearm to a right angle, and apply to the four sides of the arm four narrow splints, long enough to stretch from the shoulder to the elbow; those on the inner and outer sides are the most important, and should be of especially firm material, while care must be taken that the one on the inner side is not so long as to impede the circulation at the elbow. The splints should be fixed by two narrow triangular bandages, one round the upper end above the fracture, the other below it. The hand and wrist are then supported in a narrow arm sling.

Collar-bone.—Of all the bones in the human body, the clavicle is the one most frequently broken, generally from indirect violence, such as falls on the shoulder or hand or arm, but sometimes from direct violence, and sometimes also from muscular contraction. *Treatment.*— Place a pad about the size of a man's fist in the armpit of the injured side ; bend up the forearm, cross it over the chest with the palm of the hand turned towards the chest and the point of the elbow held well back ; support the arm in a large sling ; finally fix it to the side of the body by applying a broad-fold bandage immediately over and upon the elbow, carrying the ends horizontally round the chest, so as to lever out the arm at the shoulder-joint with the pad as the fulcrum.

Forearm and wrist.—In the forearm there are two bones, the radius and the ulna. If only one should be broken, the uninjured bone prevents displacement, and this sign of fracture is therefore absent. If, however, a little gentle pressure is applied to the two bones simultaneously, pain will be complained of at the seat of the breakage, and perhaps crepitus will be felt. *Treatment.*—Support the limb by two splints running along the front and back of the hand and forearm, and extending from the elbow to the tips of the fingers in front (taking care not to compress the artery at the elbow) and from the elbow to the wrist at the back. Bend the forearm up across the chest with the palm turned inwards and the hand raised above the elbow. Secure the splints by bandages above and below the fracture and support the arm in a large sling.

One of the commonest fractures of the forearm is that which is known as **Colles's fracture,** after an eminent Irish surgeon who flourished in the early part of the nineteenth century. It consists of a fracture of the radius, the outer of the two bones, at its lower end. It is an impacted fracture, and on this account the injury is frequently supposed at first to be a sprain. If, however, the hand is carefully looked at, it will be seen to be tilted towards the thumb, which is on the radial side of the arm. It will also be noticed that the seat of pain is not at the wrist, but just above. *Treatment.*—For this, as for other fractures at the wrist, a large sling is all that is necessary for first-aid treatment, but if there is much pain, a soft splint may be lightly applied along the front of the hand and forearm.

Hand and fingers.—When the hand is crushed, the bones in the palm are frequently broken. This accident sometimes happens in boxing, especially to the bone of the ring finger. *Treatment.*—Cover with some soft material a straight splint 3 or 4 inches wide and a foot long. Place it along the palm and front of the arm, fixing it with bandages above the wrist and round the hand, and then supporting the whole in a large arm sling. If only a single finger is broken, apply a narrow splint along its palm surface, keeping this in position by a narrow strip of linen, or a piece of tape, and support the hand in a sling.

Haunch-bone.—The pelvis may be fractured by a fall from a height, by the passage of a heavy wheel over the body, by crushing between the buffers of railway carriages, or indirectly by a fall on the feet. The danger of such fractures is that some of the organs within the pelvis, such as the bladder or the intestines, may be injured. *Treatment.*—With the patient lying on his back, pass a broad-fold bandage round the pelvis, tightening it only just enough to afford support and give relief; then pass beneath the patient, disturbing him as little as possible, a blanket or rug, and so lift him on to a stretcher so that he may be carried home or to a hospital.

Jaws.—The **upper** jaw is seldom broken; when this accident happens the accident may be recognized from the irregularity of the upper teeth, or by feeling a crack in the bone through the cheek. No bandage is necessary unless the upper teeth are irregular; in that case the jaws should be bandaged together as in fracture of the lower jaw.

The **lower** jaw is broken more often than any other bone in the skull, usually as the result of a blow or a fall on the chin. The signs of fracture are unmistakable: the patient will be unable to speak distinctly or move the jaw, and if the fingers are passed along it, irregularity and perhaps grating will be felt; the teeth will be irregular, and probably blood will issue from the mouth owing to the tearing of the gums. *Treatment.*—Raise the jaw gently into its natural position and fix it against the upper jaw with a soft handkerchief or a narrow triangular bandage, or a four-tailed bandage, passed under the chin and over the top of the head. If the bandage is long enough it can be made firmer by placing the centre of it to one side of the chin, carrying the ends up the side of the head, crossing them just above one ear, passing the ends round the head, and tying them on the side of the head opposite the crossing. If yet more support is needed, place a second bandage over the point of the chin, carry its two ends round and tie them together at the back of the neck, and finally tie them to the ends of the first bandage.

Knee-cap.—When the patella is fractured by direct violence, as by falling upon the bone, it is usually broken into a number of pieces, but more often it is fractured by muscular contraction. This accident is frequently the result of a slip in going upstairs; the powerful muscles of the thigh are thrown into action to prevent the threatened fall, and the strain upon the knee-cap while the knee is bent is so severe as to break the bone. Not seldom the effort to recover the balance when one knee-cap is broken leads to fracture of the other also. *Treatment.*—To prevent the fragments of bone from separating, the leg should be kept perfectly straight, and a firm splint applied along the back of it, so that it may not bend. The splint may consist of an umbrella or board stretched along the whole length of the limb, and securely fixed to the limb by bandages. Or the broken fragments may be kept together by applying a figure-of-eight bandage. Lay the centre of this above the broken bone, pass the two ends round the limb and cross them behind, carry them to the front and cross them below the knee-cap, then take them round the leg and tie with a reef-knot at one side. Cold should be applied to the knee-joint to prevent it from swelling, and the foot should be supported on a box or some other object.

Leg-bones.—As in the case of the forearm, either one or both of the bones of the leg—the tibia and the fibula—may be broken. When the tibia is fractured the injury is easy to recognize, as it is also, of course, when both bones are fractured, for by running the finger along the shin an irregularity can be felt. When, however, the fibula alone is broken, it may only be possible to detect the injury by grasping the leg firmly and pressing on the bone, when pain will be felt, and perhaps grating heard.

Treatment.—Get two splints long enough to reach from above the knee to below the foot, one for each side of the leg, and fix them with bandages on each side of the fracture, above the knee and round the foot, the bandage above the knee being first adjusted and the foot being then gently pulled into its natural position before the other bandages are tied. Then tie both legs together with several bandages. If a wound is present the clothes must be removed, and the wound washed and covered with a dressing; in the absence of a wound the splints may be applied outside the clothing. If the boot can be easily taken off, as by cutting up the sides or the back, this should be done, but it is better to leave it alone than to cause the slightest displacement of the limb.

Ribs.—The ribs may be broken either by direct violence, as from a kick or blow, or by indirect violence, as when the chest is squeezed between railway-carriage buffers and the bones are broken at some distance from the seat of impact. If only one or two ribs are broken, those above and below will keep the chest-walls rigid, and there is less danger, therefore, of the lung being pierced by broken bone than when a number of them are fractured. A wound of the lung is the complication most to be feared. With a broken rib the patient at once feels a stabbing pain in the side, and has a " catch " when he takes a deep breath. These symptoms might be caused simply by a bruise, but if they are due to fracture the pain will be relieved by pressure of the hand. Moreover, if the hand is placed over the seat of pain and the patient takes a deep breath, the broken surfaces of the bone may be felt grating together. When the fracture is complicated by a wound of the lung there will be a painful cough and spitting of bright, frothy blood. *Treatment.* —(*a*) If the lung is injured no bandage should be applied round the chest lest the injury be aggravated by driving the broken ends of the rib still farther into the lung. The clothing should be loosened, the patient laid down inclining towards but not actually lying on the injured side, and ice given him to suck. Ice may also be laid upon the wound. The room should be well ventilated. (*b*) If the lung is uninjured, apply a broad-fold bandage round the chest with the centre over the seat of pain. Bring the ends round the chest to the other side and tie them towards the front of the sound side of the chest, in a line with the nipple. Apply a second bandage so as to overlap the lower half of the first, and let the knot come just below the knot of the other. Pull the second bandage tight enough to allow of shallow breathing without much discomfort. Support the forearm on the injured side in a large sling.

Shoulder-blade.—A fracture of the scapula is an infrequent occurrence, but this bone is sometimes broken by a very heavy blow as from the buffer of a railway carriage; usually the ribs also are broken and other serious injuries sustained. The arm is helpless and hangs as a dead weight by the side. *Treatment.*— Remove the clothing and put a layer of cotton-wool or other soft material in the armpit on both sides. Wind a broad triangular bandage round the chest and tie the knot below the armpit on the uninjured side. Then support the arm in a large sling and enjoin the avoidance of all movements.

Skull.—When the *vault* of the skull is fractured a wound of the scalp may be present and expose the broken bone. In such cases the diagnosis is easy. If the fracture involves the *orbit*, the bony cavity of the eye, an extensive black eye and a discoloration of the eye-ball may appear. A fracture at the *base* of the skull is shown by bleeding from the ears or from the nose ; the blood from the nose may run down into the stomach and be vomited. A fracture of the base of the skull may also be indicated by the discharge of a clear watery fluid from the ear, which escapes through the crack in the bony framework of the ear ; this means that the tympanic membrane (*see* EAR), is ruptured. What is to be feared in all fractures of the skull is injury to the brain or its covering membranes. The brain may be only shaken, or it may be lacerated. One curious effect of severe blows on the head is that while the patient can recall without difficulty all that happened up to a certain period—in some cases an hour, in other cases half an hour—before the accident, his memory then becomes a blank up to the moment when he recovered consciousness. Why the loss of memory should thus, so to speak, antedate the injury which causes it is not known. *Treatment.*—Having sent for a doctor, put the patient in as easy a position as possible, with his head slightly raised, loosen any tight clothing around his throat and chest so that he may have freedom of breathing, and see that he has plenty of air. If the wound in the head is bleeding, stop the hæmorrhage, wash the wound, and cover it with a clean dressing. If he is unconscious, be careful not to give any nourishment by the mouth, or he may be choked. If he has to be taken home or to a hospital, keep him in the recumbent position and apply cold to the head. At home, see that the room is darkened and that he is kept absolutely quiet. Continue cold applications to the head while applying hot-water bottles to the feet, taking care that the bottles are not too hot.

Spine.—The danger of fracture of the vertebral column is that the spinal cord may be injured. The symptoms vary according to the situation of the fracture. If it is high up in the neck, death may be instantaneous from paralysis of the muscles of respiration ; if a little lower down, all the body below the seat of the fracture will be paralysed, only movements of the head will be possible, and the skin will lose sensation ; if in the middle of the back, the muscles of the lower extremities and of the wall of the abdomen will be paralysed, and the contents of the bladder may dribble away. Fractures of the spine may be caused through falling from a height on to the back across a bar, by a heavy weight falling on the head, or by the head being bent forcibly backwards. *Treatment.*—It is better to leave the patient alone until a doctor arrives. If this is not possible, the greatest care must be taken to move the body, or even the limbs, as little as possible. The patient should be laid flat on his back on the ground, with the body as straight as possible, and a blanket, rug, or horse-cloth gradually passed beneath him from the head downwards so that he may be lifted by means of it. A gate, or hurdle, or door should then be put by his side and he should be lifted on to it by five people—one at each side of the head, one at each side of the pelvis, and one supporting the back. He should be covered warmly to counteract the shock from which he will be suffering, but no stimulant should be given unless he should be actually in danger of death, for this would tend to increase bleeding into the spinal cord. Those who carry the patient should not walk in step.

Thigh-bone.—Fracture of the upper part of the femur most often occurs in elderly people, and may be due to so slight a cause as missing a step on the stairs. Fracture nearer the middle of the bone is caused by great violence, either direct or indirect. Fractures of this bone are easily recognized : the injured leg is shorter than the other, and the foot in most cases falls outwards by its own weight and lies on its outer side. *Treatment.*—The patient must lie where he falls until the injured limb has been rendered immobile by splints. Tie the two feet together with a broad-fold bandage, or a couple of handkerchiefs knotted together. The splint must reach from the arm-pit to just beyond the foot ; a broomstick, a rifle, or a couple of billiard cues (the thick end of one against the tapering end of the other) may be used. The splint must be laid against the outer side of the trunk and limb on the injured side of the body, and tied firmly by bandages applied round the chest and hip. Then grasp the foot with both hands and steadily and gradually pull it down to the same length as the sound foot. An umbrella, a walking-stick, or a thin board must be applied to the inner side of the thigh and fixed to the limb with three or four more bandages.

FRAMBŒSIA (*see* YAWS).

FRECKLES.—The small coloured spots which bear this name are sometimes present at birth, but usually they first appear about the age of ten. Favourite situations are the face, especially the cheeks and round the nose, and the back of the hand ; sometimes they occur on covered parts. They have some resemblance in shape and size to a lentil ; hence the condition is known medically as *lentigo.* The chief exciting cause is sunlight ; a fair, delicate skin acts as a predisposing cause. Freckles are generally most distinct in summer, and fade more or less in winter. When, as sometimes happens, they develop in adults or in elderly persons, the cause is probably impaired nutrition of the skin. The only way of treating freckles would be to remove them by blistering, but they would probably return, and, as a rule, they are much better left alone.

FREEZING, TREATMENT BY (*see* CARBONIC ACID SNOW, TREATMENT BY).

FREQUENCY OF MICTURITION (*see* MICTURITION, FREQUENT).

FROSTBITE.—Frostbite may be regarded as a more advanced stage of the same process as chilblain. In temperate climates the process seldom goes so far as to cause death of the structures affected. A rapid restoration of warmth is to be avoided, for the effect would be to send a rush of blood to the part, with resulting inflammation and gangrene. The patient should not have hot drinks, should not go near a fire, should not even enter a warm room. The part should be rubbed gently in a cold room, with snow if possible, then with water at ordinary temperature, then with vaselined hands. As the local circulation tends to be re-established the part should be wrapped up in cotton-wool or flannel. It will become hot and painful as the blood begins to circulate again in it ; it should then be raised so that blood may flow out of it. Inflammation, if it occurs, should be relieved by warm compresses of boric lint which are sprinkled with, say, tincture of belladonna and covered with oil-silk. Cases in which gangrene supervenes require surgical treatment.

FUNCTIONAL DISEASE (*see* DISEASE, CLASSIFICATION OF).

FUNGI (*see* GERMS).

FUNGI, POISONING BY.—When poisonous mushrooms are eaten, violent pain is felt in the stomach about half an hour afterwards, and is quickly followed by vomiting and diarrhœa. In bad cases, unless treatment is applied, mental excitement supervenes, and is gradually replaced by loss of consciousness. In fatal cases death is due to heart-failure. *Treatment.*—Give an emetic (*see* EMETICS), and, as soon as this has acted, an ounce of castor oil. Apply warmth to the extremities and the abdomen, and administer stimulants.

FURRED TONGUE (*see* TONGUE, APPEARANCE OF, IN DISEASE).

FURUNCULOSIS (*see* BOILS AND CARBUNCLES).

G

GALLOPING CONSUMPTION (*see* CONSUMPTION).

GALL-STONES.—Gall-stones may be formed either in the gall-bladder, as more frequently happens, or in the liver ducts. So long as the flow of bile is normal, gall-stones are not formed, but when the bile becomes stagnant, formation of gall-stones may take place—in some cases, probably, as the result of the action of microbes, which tend to become virulent in stagnant bile. Sedentary habits, since they favour stagnation of bile, may therefore be regarded as a predisposing cause of gall-stones. Other predisposing causes are believed to be excessive eating, especially of animal food, eating at too frequent intervals, and the taking of too little liquid, so that the secretions of the body are not adequately diluted.

Gall-stones may occur singly, or in considerable numbers. When solitary they are usually round or oval or pear-shaped; when there are several they may have polished facets as the result of pressure and friction. In size they vary from a small seed to a large mass several inches in circumference. Their weight is inconsiderable; when fresh they are heavier than bile or water, but when dried they readily float. In colour they vary from a pearly white to a deep black, but usually they are of a reddish-brown tint. They are composed chiefly of the substance known as cholesterol, mixed with the colouring matter of the bile and with thick mucus.

Symptoms.—A stone may be present in the gall-bladder without causing symptoms, but if it should escape into, or be formed in, the ducts, which are scarcely larger than a goose quill, and are lined by an exquisitely sensitive mucous membrane, the patient is attacked with biliary colic, one of the most agonizing of all pains. The pain usually starts with a shooting, burning, or stabbing sensation in the upper part of the abdomen on the right side, and slowly spreads downwards to the navel and upwards to the right shoulder. It is accompanied by shivering, fever, and vomiting. The attack may continue for several days, or may last for two or three hours only. When the concretion is carried into the bowels the pain ceases, and with it the other symptoms. The stone may not be voided from the body for some days; meanwhile it should be sought for in the motions.

Treatment.—As soon as an attack of biliary colic occurs, the doctor should be sent for. Meanwhile a hot bath should be got ready and the patient put into it, or a large and quite hot linseed poultice, or a hot fomentation, applied to the seat of the pain. If ether, inhaled from a handkerchief upon which 20 drops have been placed, does not subdue the pain, the doctor will probably inject morphine, possibly combined with atropine. The patient should be encouraged to drink large draughts of hot water in which bicarbonate of soda and salicylate of soda have been dissolved—60 grains of the one and 20 grains of the other to a pint of water. It may at first be vomited, but it should be persevered with until it is retained, and repeated at frequent intervals until the attack is at an end. It not only acts as an internal fomentation, but dilutes and stimulates the flow of bile.

If, from the occurrence of jaundice, the recurrence of pain at intervals, and other symptoms, it is evident that gall-stones remain in the ducts or in the gall-bladder, and medical treatment fails to give relief, the question of operation will have to be considered. Whether an operation is performed or not, those who are subject to gall-stones should carefully follow the course about to be outlined, in the hope of avoiding trouble in future. A moderate amount of active exercise should be taken, and plenty of diluted alkaline drinks, such as Apollinaris or Vichy water, on an empty stomach. The digestion should be kept in order, and constipation carefully guarded against. Diet should be strictly moderate. All rich, strongly flavoured foods must be avoided. Bread should be eaten sparingly, and sugar and farinaceous foods taken only in very small quantities. Fresh green vegetables, salads, and ripe fruits may be used freely. The only form in which alcohol is permissible is that of a light wine such as hock or moselle, mixed with mineral water. The regimen here prescribed may be supplemented by courses of Carlsbad water.

GALVANISM.—One of the forms of electricity used in electrical treatment (q.v.).

GAMGEE TISSUE (*see* DRESSINGS AND STRAPPING FOR WOUNDS).

GANGLION.—In the pathological as distinct from the anatomical sense of the word, a ganglion is a cyst in the capsule of a joint, or in a tendon. These swellings are most frequently met with on the back of the wrist, but they also occur in the region of the ankle and the knee. Often met with in pianists, typists, and women who wring clothes, they seem to be the result of a slight but prolonged overstrain of a joint or a tendon. If they give no trouble, they may be left alone ; but if they cause pain or weakness, or are unsightly, a little operation should be performed.

GANGRENE.—Mortification, to use the popular term for this condition, is, as the word implies, the *death* of a part of the body. It is the sequel of a number of quite different disorders, but the largest group of cases is that in which the condition is the result of circulatory disturbances. These disturbances may be due to disease of the heart or of the blood-vessels, to the formation of bloodclot by which a blood-vessel is blocked, to pressure on blood-vessels by tumours or by fractured bones, to degeneration of blood-vessels as in senile decay, or to spasm of the smaller arteries as in Raynaud's disease. In this group of cases comes the form of gangrene, still prevalent in certain parts of Europe, which is due to the prolonged consumption of bread made from rye that is affected with the parasite known as *Claviceps purpurea.*

Treatment.—This varies, of course, with the condition to which the gangrene is primarily due, but the main objects to be kept in view are the protection of the affected part from bacterial and other poisons by the most rigid cleanliness and by the use of chemically prepared dressings, the application of warmth by hot-water bottles and other means, and the maintenance of the patient's strength by nourishment and stimulants. In suitable cases the affected part is amputated.

GARGLES.—Gargles are used to cleanse or soothe the throat, or to brace up its tissues when they are relaxed. Probably few persons succeed in acquiring the knack of so using them that the fluid is brought into contact with the back and sides of the throat, as it ought to be. The following prescriptions will be found useful :

Antiseptic and Soothing Gargle
Carbolic acid ....50 grains
Purified borax ....60 grains
Bromide of potash ....60 grains
Spirit of peppermint .... ½ ounce
Glycerin to 4 ounces.
A teaspoonful in half a tumblerful of tepid water.

Soothing Gargle
Chlorate of potash.........1½ drachms
Boric acid ....1½ drachms
Compound tincture of lavender ....1 drachm
Water to 8 ounces.
To be used with an equal quantity of tepid water.

Astringent Gargle for Relaxed Sore Throat
Alum ....60 grains
Tannic acid ....80 grains
Distilled water to 10 ounces.

Gargle for Ulcerated Throat
Tincture of myrrh .... 3 drachms
Honey .... 3 drachms
Acid infusion of roses to 8 ounces.
To be warmed before use.

Stimulating Gargle in Chronic Sore Throat
Tincture of capsicum ......80 minims
Dilute acetic acid ....25 minims
Water to 8 ounces

Gargle in Affections of the Tonsils
Salicylic acid .... ½ drachm
Chloride of soda .... 5 drachms
Bicarbonate of soda........1½ ounces
A teaspoonful in a tumblerful of tepid water

GAS, POISONING BY.—Since the introduction into warfare of asphyxiating and torturing gases, this expression has acquired a new signficance, but in this work the subject is dealt with in its earlier and more limited sense. The form of gas poisoning most frequently met with in civil life is that due to coal gas—carbon monoxide and carbon dioxide (carbonic acid) gas. Cases of death from the gas of burning charcoal or of coke (carbon monoxide) are usually suicidal. The gas which collects in sewers (sulphuretted hydrogen) is also poisonous. The gas expired from the lungs, carbonic acid gas, if sufficiently concentrated, may cause insensibility, although it is not a fatal poison. *Treatment.*—To enter a room filled with coal or charcoal gas, the mouth should be covered with a handkerchief soaked in vinegar and water, and the window must at once be opened or broken to admit air. In the case of coal gas, no candle or lamp must, of course, be taken into the room. The patient must at once be carried into the fresh air, the clothing loosened if sufficiently tight to impede breathing, and respiration stimulated by slapping the face and chest with a wet towel or dashing cold water over them. In bad cases artificial respiration may be necessary, as described under RESPIRATION, ARTIFICIAL.

GASTRIC CATARRH (*see* GASTRITIS, ACUTE).

GASTRIC FEVER (*see* Bowels, Inflammation of; Typhoid Fever).

GASTRIC JUICE (*see* Digestion).

GASTRIC ULCER (*see* Stomach, Ulcer of).

GASTRITIS, ACUTE. — Acute gastritis, or gastric catarrh as it is also called, is often *secondary* to some abdominal or other disease, such as appendicitis, or to some infectious disease, such as influenza or scarlet fever, or to some disease of the nervous system, etc. Here we shall consider it as a *primary* affection caused as a rule by some dietary error—too much food, or coarse and indigestible food, or food soaked with fat or rich sauces, or food that is partly decomposed, or food against which the patient has an idiosyncrasy. Another exciting cause is the habitual and excessive use of strong drink, especially spirits. The affection may also be induced by chills, and in highly strung persons it may even be set up by emotions such as fear, anger and anxiety.

Symptoms.—The tongue is coated, the breath foul, appetite is lost, there is heartburn with sour eructations, flatulence is present, with tenderness at the pit of the stomach, and in severe cases there is pain as well as tenderness, with vomiting. The bowels may be constipated or there may be diarrhœa. The patient is depressed, and complains of bad headache, and coldness of the hands and feet.

Treatment.—Vomiting must not be checked too early, and in some cases should even be encouraged by giving large draughts of warm water, and finally a glass of hot water containing a teaspoonful of bicarbonate of soda. If vomiting has not occurred at all, the patient should irritate the back of the throat by touching it with the finger, or should take an emetic (*see* Emetics). The bowels should be cleared of irritating contents. For adults a 3-grain dose of calomel may be placed at the back of the tongue and washed down with a little hot water, and this should be followed in the morning by a dose of Epsom salts or some aperient mineral water. To children, 10 to 20 grains of compound rhubarb powder should be given. In some cases it becomes necessary to check the vomiting. In such cases, especially if there is much thirst, without pain in the stomach, an effervescent drink is serviceable such as the following :

Bicarbonate of soda........ 3 drachms
Cherry-laurel water .... 4 drachms
Water to 8 ounces.
Get eight powders, each containing 8 grains of tartaric acid, dissolve one powder in a tablespoonful of water, add this to two tablespoonfuls of the mixture, and take while effervescing, every hour or two.

No food should be taken for twelve to eighteen hours, but if there is severe thirst small pieces of ice may be sucked. When food is allowed again, it must be in small quantities and at short intervals, and in fluid form, such as milk and soda water equal parts, barley water, beef tea, chicken, mutton or veal broth. Afterwards the patient may go on to arrowroot, well-cooked sago, tapioca, or bread-and-milk, and then gradually return to more solid fare.

GASTRITIS, CHRONIC.— Chronic gastric catarrh may be the sequel of an acute attack, or it may be a symptom of some other disease, but most often it is due to long-continued errors in diet, and especially to the abuse of alcoholic beverages and of tobacco. The symptoms are similar to those of acute gastritis. Treatment is chiefly dietetic. The following is the diet recommended by Sir W. H

Willcox in " The Dictionary of Practical Medicine " :

The meals should be light, and taken at regular times. Excess of starchy food and indigestible articles, such as pastry, and food containing much fat, such as grilled food, are to be avoided. Alcohol and tobacco must be prohibited. When there is gastric fermentation associated with flatulence, it is well for the meals to be taken dry with a minimum of liquid, a glass of hot water or milk being taken two hours after a meal, e.g. at 11 a.m. and 5 p.m., and also in the early morning and at bedtime. In cases associated with general weakness, loss of weight, and malaise, complete rest in bed is essential, and the diet should consist of milk or citrated milk (2 gr. of citrate of soda to the ounce) given at two-hour intervals, 6-8 oz. at a time. As the gastric symptoms disappear a modified Weir-Mitchell treatment may be instituted. When solid food can be taken the dietary may be made up of boiled or poached eggs, boiled or steamed fish (sole, plaice, cod, turbot, halibut, fresh herring), chicken, tender mutton, cream cheese, clear soup or beef tea, milk, weak tea, toast, rusks, stale bread, mashed potatoes, purée of spinach, custard or thin milk puddings, and jellies. Fruit is best taken cooked, though fresh orange or grape juice may be allowed.

GASTRO - ENTERITIS. — In gastro-enteritis, not merely the stomach, as in gastritis, but also the intestines are the seat of inflammation and catarrh. It is especially an affection of children, and is usually due to the consumption of bad food. The symptoms are vomiting and diarrhœa, acute pain in the abdomen, fever, and tendency to collapse. The treatment is the same as for epidemic diarrhœa, q.v.

GAUZE (*see* DRESSINGS AND STRAPPING FOR WOUNDS).

GENERAL PARALYSIS OF THE INSANE.—This terrible disease, known also as dementia paralytica, usually appears between the ages of thirty-five and fifty-five. Until recently it was believed to be an indirect sequel of syphilis, but it is now known to be a direct, though long-deferred manifestation of that disease. In some cases the symptoms of general paralysis manifest themselves a few years after infection with syphilis, while in others they may be delayed for twenty or twenty-five years ; the average interval is about ten or twelve years. Although usually a disease of middle age, general paralysis sometimes appears in the young ; in these cases the patients are victims of the congenital form of syphilis. The changes caused by this disease in the brain take the form of a general progressive wasting until the patient becomes bed-ridden, and at last lives a merely vegetative life. He must be put under proper care and control, and individual symptoms dealt with as they arise. In this latest and worse stage of syphilis salvarsan and mercury have proved to be of little service. In carefully selected cases benefit has been derived from inoculating the patient with a mild form of malaria.

GENU VALGUM (*see* KNOCK-KNEE).

GERMAN MEASLES.—This fever bears some resemblance to measles, but is much less infectious. In some epidemics German measles also resembles mild scarlet fever. Its differentiation from measles and from scarlet fever was mainly the work of German physicians, who termed it *Rötheln*. It is also known as *epidemic roseola* and as *rubella*, from the redness of the spots constituting the eruption. The disease, which often occurs in widespread epidemics, has a low mortality, nor are there usually complications or after-effects. The patient should be isolated for at least three weeks after the appearance of the rash ; and for persons who have been exposed to infection, a quarantine of twenty-one days should be enforced. The disease is more frequent at the age of puberty than in either children or adults, but the latter are not infrequently attacked.

Incubation stage and symptoms.—The incubation period is generally about two and a half weeks. The patient may then complain of lassitude, fullness in the head, aching pains in the back and limbs, chilliness, and slight sore throat. In a day or two, or sooner, the rash appears. An important and early sign of German measles, especially in children, is enlargement of the glands of the neck, which may be tender also, and give rise to a certain amount of stiff-neck. There is little or no catarrh, but the eyes may be suffused and the eyelids swollen and irritable. The throat is red, the tonsils are full and smooth, but there is never any ulceration. The rash, which first appears on the face, and is most profuse, as a rule, on the neck, chest and back, the front of the arms and the back of the thighs, usually consists of patches of a rose-red colour which shade away into the colour of the skin. The patches often join together, but do not produce the fine uniform redness seen in scarlet fever. The eruption is generally most intense on the second day, but has mostly faded by the third or fourth day. Feverishness may be entirely absent; when it is present, the temperature returns to normal with the disappearance of the rash.

Treatment.—The patient must be isolated, and should stay in bed during the eruptive stage. The diet may be the same as that recommended for measles (p. 240), and the medicine that prescribed for chicken-pox (p. 70). The disappearance of the eruption may be expedited by warm baths and friction. During convalescence a tonic should be given. The room must be disinfected.

GERMS.—The infectious diseases, including the different fevers, are now known to be due to minute forms of life, each of which produces its own disease and no other. In many instances the organism has been identified; in others, as for example smallpox and measles, identification has not yet been accomplished, but the fact that such diseases are infectious, and their general correspondence with other diseases in which the germ has been isolated, make it evident that they are caused by germs.

The chief groups of disease germs are bacteria, fungi, and protozoa, the first and second belonging to the vegetable, and the third to the animal kingdom.

1. Bacteria.—This is the largest of the three groups of disease-germs. Our knowledge of bacteria dates from about the middle of the last century. Even before the Christian era it was thought by some that diseases were possibly caused by forms of life so minute as to be invisible, but this was mere speculation, and it was only when Pasteur, the great French chemist, discovered by his brilliant researches between 1850 and 1860 that putrefaction and fermentation were both due to bacteria that this new world was opened to the mind of man. One result of Pasteur's discovery was that the late Lord Lister, at that time professor of surgery at Glasgow, applied himself to the task of devising means of preserving surgical wounds from the invasion of harmful organisms, and thus founded the system of antiseptic surgery. Not long before Pasteur began his experiments, Davaine observed the presence of rod-like structures in the blood of animals dead of anthrax, but without identifying them with the cause of the disease. In the light of Pasteur's discovery he returned to the subject (1863), and showed that blood, when introduced into healthy animals, was only capable of causing the disease when these rods, now known as bacilli, were present in it. That this was the first bacterium to be discovered is explained by the fact of its being the largest of such germs. Even now, however, the proof that the germs were the cause of the disease was not complete. There was the possibility that the

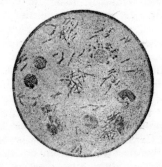

Fig. 23.—A rod-shaped germ, the bacillus of tuberculosis, in sputum ; highly magnified.

disease was transmitted, not by them, but by some other maleficent substance in the blood which was invisible. Thirteen years later, Robert Koch, the great German bacteriologist, grew successive generations of the germs on suitable material, and showed that the disease could be caused by inoculation of these "cultures," as they are called. The case, then, was at last proved so far as the bacillus of anthrax was concerned : it, and it alone, was the cause of the disease. Not long afterwards Koch himself discovered the bacterium of tuberculosis (Fig. 23), and since then many other disease-germs have been identified.

A bacterium may be described as a minute vegetable organism which multiplies by division. Thus, one bacterium divides into two, and these grow until each is as large as the original organism. Each of the two bacteria then undergoes division, so that now there are four bacteria. The next division results in the production of eight bacteria, and so on. Bacteria are so small that it would require from ten to fifteen thousand placed end to end to form a line an inch long. Their rapidity of growth is equally remarkable. Under favourable conditions division may take place once every twenty or thirty minutes, and if this rate were kept up continuously, a single germ would give rise in the course of forty-eight hours to a colony of thirty billions. Nature seems determined to give bacteria every chance of survival. When the conditions of life are unfavourable to multiplication, certain bacteria form bodies that are called spores, which are to some extent similar to the seeds of plants, and are much more resistant to antagonistic influences than the bacteria themselves, partly because they are covered with a thick double membrane. As soon as the spore gains access to materials which favour its growth—it may be years after it was formed, it develops into an ordinary bacterium, which then is able to multiply in the ordinary way. Bacteria are grouped into classes according to the shape they assume. Thus there are *bacilli* (Fig. 23) which appear as more or less straight rods ; *vibrios, spirilla,* and *spirochætes,* which are curved rods ; and *cocci,* which are rounded organisms. The bacilli may occur in pairs, when they are called diplobacilli, or in chains —streptobacilli. The cocci may also be arranged in pairs—diplococci ; or in chains—streptococci ; or they may occur in bunches—staphylococci. Among the bacilli are the germs of tuberculosis, diphtheria, typhoid fever, and lockjaw ; among the curved rods are the germs of syphilis, yellow fever and relapsing fever ; among the rounded organisms are the germs of pneumonia, spotted fever, and gonorrhœa.

DISTRIBUTION.—Bacteria are so widely distributed that they might almost be said to be omnipresent. They are met with on the surface of all objects, living or dead, and are present in air, soil and water. As one graphic writer has said, " We swallow and breathe them in countless multitudes. A pint of milk contains innumerable multitudes of them. Cream, butter and many other substances swarm with them. . . . Our mouths and our nostrils harbour hundreds of them. It is calculated that each inhabitant of London inhales, on an average, fourteen thousand microbes an hour." Fortunately many of them are harmless, and some positively useful, as, for instance, those that give aroma to tobacco and flavour to cheese and butter, and those which act as scavengers by decomposing dead organic matter and resolving it into its elements.

In the *air* the presence of bacteria is, so to speak, accidental ; it is not their natural habitat, but they are carried up into it in dust, or are discharged from the mouth and air-passages of man and the lower animals in coughing, speaking, or sneezing. The bacteria met with in *water* find their way there in the sewage discharged into rivers, or are washed down from the soil by rain. In water they are exposed to the destructive power of sunlight and other antagonistic influences. Many harmful germs are to be found in *soil*, which is con-

stantly being polluted by the germ-laden dejections of men and animals. Among the germs which flourish in the soil is the tetanus bacillus ; hence the liability to lockjaw when an accidental wound is contaminated with dust or mud.

The skin of the human body harbours many harmful bacteria, especially the parts that are moist and warm, such as the armpits and the groins. The mouth, the nose, and other cavities which communicate with the surface of the body abound with bacteria, both harmless and harmful. Thus, the germ which causes pneumonia is quite commonly present in the saliva of healthy people, and that of diphtheria is often found in the throats of those who nurse diphtheria patients, though not themselves affected. It should be pointed out that normally bacteria only live on the surface of the body, or in cavities into which they can find their way from the exterior. The actual tissues of the body, and also its secretions—blood, the urine, the bile, the milk—are free from them unless they have obtained entrance to the body from without, either through the skin or mucous membranes, the air-passages, or the alimentary canal. Infection through intact skin and mucous membrane is unusual, and in the vast majority of instances the germ finds its way in through some lesion, so slight it may be that the patient is unconscious of it. One mode of skin penetration is by the bites of insects. Thus the germ of plague is communicated by the bites of the rat-flea, and that of typhus fever by lice.

TOXINS.—The harm wrought by bacteria in man and the lower animals is due chiefly to the action of the poisons (toxins) which they form. Those poisons are remarkable for their intensity ; thus, the poison of the bacillus of tetanus (lockjaw) may be several hundred times as powerful in its action as strychnine.

ANTISEPTICS.—As already mentioned, sunlight is destructive to bacteria ; so also are extreme degrees of heat. In most cases cold merely arrests the development of germs, without killing them. Certain chemical substances — antiseptics—are highly inimical to germs ; these include carbolic acid, mercury, and iodine.

2. Fungi.—Like the bacteria, the fungi belong to the vegetable kingdom, and the two groups were not at first separated. One of the differences between fungi and bacteria are that the former do not multiply by division, but only by spores. Among fungi which attack man are the organisms of ringworm, favus, and actinomycosis. Like bacteria and protozoa, they can be grown in successive generations on suitable media.

3. Protozoa.—Protozoa, as the term implies (*zoon*, animal), belong to the lowest class of the animal kingdom, but for the most part what has been said of bacteria applies also to them. They include the microbes of malaria and sleeping sickness.

GIGANTISM.—As is explained in the article ACROMEGALY, the growth of the body depends upon the secretion of a gland at the base of the brain, known as the pituitary gland or hypophysis. If this gland secretes in excess in early life, there is general overgrowth of the body, and so we have the condition which is called giantism or gigantism. Sir John Bland - Sutton, in his work on " Tumours," points out that the most striking feature of giants, apart from their height, is the enormous size of their hands. They are usually short-lived.

GIDDINESS.—Vertigo, as this condition is termed medically, is a symptom rather than a disease in itself. It takes two different forms. In one, while the patient feels uncertain of being able to maintain his equilibrium, the objects around him are stationary ; in the other, surrounding objects assume abnormal positions, the patterns on wall-paper, for instance, seeming to chase each other round the room. It varies in degree from a mere " swimming in the head " to a condition in which the patient has to cling to something for support. It is most often caused by ear trouble —for the semicircular canals which form part of the internal ear are concerned in the maintenance of equilibrium (*see* MENIÈRE'S DISEASE). Giddiness may also be due to inflammation of the middle ear, or even to a thing so simple as an accumulation of wax in the external canal of the ear. It may, however, be a symptom of epilepsy, and of various other affections of the brain, especially those involving the cerebellum (little brain). Or it may arise from mere slight derangements of the stomach and liver, or from circulatory disorders. Anything which causes a deficient supply of healthy blood to the brain will be attended by giddiness ; this explains the giddiness which may be felt when one rises from a stooping posture, the circulation of blood through the brain being affected by the change of position. Giddiness may be caused, too, by poisons in the blood, as in alcoholism and excessive smoking. Finally, there are certain affections of the eyes which are attended by this symptom. Treatment must, of course, be directed to the condition of which the giddiness is a symptom.

GIN-DRINKER'S LIVER (*see* CIRRHOSIS OF THE LIVER).

GLANDERS.—This disease is caused by a germ (*Bacillus mallei*), and is almost always conveyed to man from the horse in discharge from the nostrils or from ulcers ; it therefore occurs most frequently in coachmen, grooms, stablemen, and veterinary surgeons, though occasionally it is communicated from man to man. If the infection is very mild, the disease may be confined to the spot where it was inoculated, but usually the infection sooner or later becomes generalized. In acute cases general infection ends in death within a few weeks ; in chronic cases the outlook is much more hopeful. The sore at the point of inoculation should be excised, if possible, and the wound cauterized. Little more can be done, except to alleviate symptoms as they arise and maintain the patient's strength by rest, diet, stimulants, and drugs such as quinine. Nasal and other cavities from which discharges come should be douched with disinfectants such as permanganate of potash and iodine. Abscesses and fistulæ should be treated surgically. In some cases injection of a vaccine (mallein) under the skin appears to be beneficial.

GLANDS (*see* BLOOD AND LYMPH ; and DUCTLESS GLANDS).

GLAUCOMA.—This term (derived from the Greek *glaukos*, sea-green) at first denoted an affection of the eye in which there was a greenish opaque appearance behind the pupil. It now covers all affections in which there is a morbid increase of the fluids natural to the eye-ball, with the result that the nerves of the eye are compressed and the circulation in the eye is interfered with. It is a disease of middle and old age. Both eyes are usually attacked, though seldom at the same time. Long-sighted persons are especially prone to it ; the very short-sighted are immune. It may be brought on by acute and prolonged mental depression, by exposure to cold, by over-eating, by excessive fatigue, or by general disturbance of the circulation. A frequent early symptom is an occasional attack of dimness of sight, and the appearance of coloured rings or haloes when looking at a light. At first the attacks of dimness and attendant symptoms pass off, but they tend to become more frequent and last longer, and finally, unless skilled treatment is applied, the sight is permanently impaired.

Treatment.—The only medical treatment that is appropriate is to use eserine drops twice daily to produce contraction of the pupil, at the same time giving the eyes absolute rest, and endeavouring to improve the general health. Belladonna (or atropine) drops, which cause the pupil to expand, must on no account be used. Nor must reliance be placed even upon eserine, except to afford temporary relief. Many patients have lost their sight irretrievably from not having been treated surgically in time. In all but a few cases the condition can be permanently relieved by operation.

GLEET (*see* GONORRHŒA).

GLIOMAS (*see* TUMOURS).

GLOSSITIS (*see* TONGUE, INFLAMMATION OF).

GNAT-BITES (*see* STINGS AND BITES).

GOITRE.—This affection consists in an enlargement of the thyroid gland, which is situated at the front of the windpipe, close to " Adam's apple." It may take the form of a localized tumour, known as an adenoma ; but more often it is a diffuse enlargement the result of drinking water that has been infected with a germ which has not yet been identified. In this latter form it occurs chiefly in the higher valleys of mountainous regions. From its prevalence in the valleys of Derbyshire it is sometimes termed " Derbyshire neck." It is not, however, more frequent in Derbyshire valleys than in valleys in other districts or countries, nor is it confined to valleys. The symptoms are mostly caused by pressure of the enlarged gland on the gullet, the windpipe, and other surrounding parts, with the result that there may be difficulty in swallowing, or in breathing. The affection is amenable to treatment. When it takes the adenomatous form the growth should be removed. When it occurs in goitrous regions the patient should migrate elsewhere, or, if this is impossible, should abstain from water which has not been boiled ; the X-rays may be tried, or a vaccine administered ; if such measures as these fail, an operation may have to be performed. Goitre is often associated with the form of idiocy known as cretinism (q.v.). The serious form of thyroid-gland enlargement known as exophthalmic goitre, or Graves's disease, is described under the latter heading.

GONORRHŒA.—Gonorrhœa is an inflammation of the mucous membranes of the genito-urinary organs, either male or female, due to the action of a germ called the gonococcus, and almost invariably " caught " in sexual intercourse, the only exceptions being that the disease is sometimes conveyed by contact with a towel or some other infected object. Painful rather than serious if promptly treated, it may, if neglected, lead to very grave consequences.

Symptoms.—The incubation period of gonorrhœa, i.e. the time between infection and the onset of symptoms, is, on an average, from three to five days. A sensation of heat and itching in the urethra or water passage is then experienced, the orifice becomes red and swollen, and a discharge exudes which at first is thin and whitish, but in a few days becomes thick and greenish-yellow. It is accompanied by intense smarting and scalding, especially during or after the passing of water. If properly treated the attack comes to an end in from three weeks to six months, but if treatment is delayed, or is not of the right kind, the disease may pass into the chronic stage, known as *gleet*. Everything depends upon the germs being destroyed before they have passed into the deeper parts of the urethra, or, in the cases of women, to the womb and other organs in the neighbourhood of the vagina. In men the complications which may be set up by persistent gonorrhœa include inflammation of the prostate gland, the testicles, the bladder, and the kidneys, as well as of the glands of the groin, which swell and suppurate (" buboes "). Further, the germ may find its way into the blood-stream and set up an acute blood-poisoning ; or it may settle in the joints, causing a form of inflammation known as gonorrhœal rheumatism ; or it may attack the tendons and muscles and give rise to lumbago, sciatica, etc. In women the complications of chronic gonorrhœa are somewhat similar to those in men ; in them it is a frequent cause of sterility.

Treatment.—From the beginning the aim must be to destroy the germs before they penetrate to the deeper parts. Some special preparation of nitrate of silver, such as a weak solution of protargol or argyrol, is injected into the male urethra as soon as the case comes under treatment, except where the inflammation is so acute that it may be necessary to wait until this has partly subsided. Alcohol in all forms must be avoided, but an abundance of bland fluids should be drunk, and the patient be put on a light diet. When the inflammation is reduced and the discharges are diminished, a more astringent injection may be used, such as permanganate of potash in the morning and at mid-day, and nitrate of silver in the evening. If the disease once passes into the chronic stage, prolonged treatment will be required, and even with the most skilful treatment the patient will have to endure a great deal of pain. In women treatment proceeds on the same general lines as in men ; but the use of antiseptic douches is now regarded by some authorities as dangerous, because the germs may thus be carried to the neck of the womb. Instead, local applications of some preparation of silver nitrate may be employed.

GOUT.—The acute form of this disease is much less often met with than it was even a few years ago. A predisposition to gout may be hereditary. But an inherited tendency to gout by no means implies that the disease will develop ; in the great majority of cases that will depend upon the mode of life of the individual. Habits which are chiefly responsible for gout are the abuse of malt liquors and wines, the excessive consumption of rich and indigestible food, insufficient exercise, and the imperfect elimination which is the result of constipation. Except in the subjects of an inherited predisposition, the disease rarely develops before the age of thirty-five. Quite apart from bad habits, gout may be induced by lead-poisoning.

It has usually been taught that gout depends upon the excessive formation of uric acid—that the disease is a manifestation of uric-acid poisoning. This view has of late years been challenged, and it is now held by some authorities that the excess of uric acid is merely a symptom and not a cause, and that the disease is really a form of blood-poisoning originating in the stomach and intestines. Those who hold this view point to the undoubted fact that the administration of purgatives at the beginning of an attack causes a rapid diminution of the symptoms, and that the drugs that have so long been in favour in the treatment of gout tend to check intestinal putrefaction and empty the bowels. As to whether germs are responsible for the disease, there is difference in opinion. In the view, held by some authorities, that the poison is bacterial there is certainly no antecedent improbability, seeing that the intestine swarms with bacteria which under appropriate conditions become harmful to their host. But the whole question of the cause of gout must be regarded as unsettled.

We have been dealing so far with the more permanent causes of gout, but it must be added that an attack may be precipitated by an eating or drinking bout, by violent emotion, by worry, by exposure to cold, or by strains or sprains of joints.

Gout may take (1) the acute form, (2) the chronic form, (3) the irregular or suppressed form.

1. *Acute gout.*—A seizure of acute gout most frequently begins in the early hours of the morning with severe pain, generally in the great toe. The toe swells and the skin reddens, and the joint is excruciatingly painful. During the day the pain is less acute, but comes on again with renewed

the stomach, palpitation and rapid pulse—or, on the other hand, a slow pulse with faintness—neuritis, sciatica and neuralgia, asthma, bronchial catarrh, severe headaches, inflamed eyes and throat, eczema, redness and itching of the nose, stones in the kidneys, and chronic Bright's disease. A special variety of irregular gout is known as *retrocedent* gout, a term which denotes the course of events when an attack of acute gout suddenly subsides and is followed by the development of the disease in an internal organ such as the stomach, intestine, heart, or liver. If the disease rapidly shifts from point to point it is called *flying* gout.

Treatment of chronic and irregular gout.—Colchicum may be given in the following form :

    Colchicum wine............ 80 minims
    Iodide of potash .... 24 grains
    Bicarbonate of potash .....120 grains
    Carbonate of lithia .... 24 grains
    Chloroform water to 8 ounces.
Two tablespoonfuls three times a day.

Another valuable drug in these forms of gout is guaiacum ; it may be obtained in 5-grain capsules, two of which should be taken two or three times a day. This is a chief ingredient of the medicine known as " Chelsea Pensioner." Another popular remedy is that known as " Nun Powders," from the fact that they are prepared at the pharmacy of the Benedictine Sisters at Pistoja, in Tuscany.

In ordinary cases, however, the treatment of chronic and irregular gout is largely a matter of diet and regular life, even more than of drug treatment. Rigid moderation in the use of animal food and of sweet and starchy foods must be observed. In most cases the patient will be better without alcohol, but if a little stimulant is required, it may be taken in the form of claret, hock, or some other light dry wine, or as good whisky, freely diluted with potash or lithia water. Of fluids generally the patient should drink freely, so as to wash out the waste material from the body.

GRAND MAL (*see* Epilepsy).

GRANULAR OPHTHALMIA (*see* Trachoma, under Conjunctivitis).

GRAVEL (*see* Stone in the Bladder).

GRAVES'S DISEASE.—This singular affection is known as Basedow's or Graves's disease, after the physicians who first described it, and it is also styled exophthalmic goitre—*goitre* because the thyroid gland, in the neck, is enlarged, *exophthalmic* because a noticeable symptom in many cases, though not in all, is a protrusion of the eyeballs.

Causes.—The affection is much more common in women than in men, the proportion being at least ten to one. As a rule the symptoms do not appear before the age of fifteen, or after the age of fifty. Enlargement of the thyroid gland is an invariable symptom, and it is believed that the essential cause of the disease is an excessive or otherwise abnormal secretion on the part of this gland, which is situated just below and beside " Adam's apple," as shown in Fig. 24.

Symptoms.—Besides enlargement of the thyroid gland and protrusion of the eyeballs, other characteristic symptoms are rapid action of the heart, with paroxysms of palpitation, and a generalized trembling ; but one or other of the symptoms may be absent. In severe cases there is difficulty in breathing, which is not due entirely to pressure of the enlarged thyroid gland on the windpipe. The patient is nervous, excitable, suffers from depression, and as a rule is extremely irritable. Often there is painful flushing, the skin is moist from excessive perspiration, and there may be patches of brown staining. Anæmia is a frequent symptom; not seldom the digestive system is disordered, and vomiting and diarrhœa may be present.

Treatment.—The disease rarely ends in death, and in many cases it tends to recovery, which in some

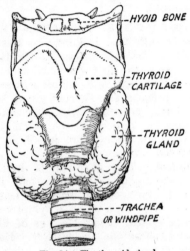

Fig. 24.—The thyroid gland.

cases is complete, while in others one or more of the symptoms may not entirely disappear. In a few instances the symptoms, gradually subsiding, are finally replaced by those of myxœdema (q.v.), a sequel which suggests that the thyroid gland, after a long period of overactivity, becomes exhausted and fails to act. The drugs which are most used in this disease are digitalis to control the action of the heart, iron to remedy the anæmia, bromide of potash or of soda to soothe the nervous system, and arsenic as a general tonic. In some cases treatment by radium, in others by X-rays,

has been beneficial. Serum treatment has not found general acceptance. Much depends upon rest, good nursing, and diet. The patient should take much repose in the recumbent position; and if she is able to bear it, gentle massage should be administered. If there is much wasting, and the nervous symptoms are prominent, the Weir-Mitchell "rest cure" is appropriate. Change of air and scene is desirable, and when the weather is suitable, as much time as possible should be spent in the open air. The diet must be nutritious, bland, and light. The patient should be encouraged to drink as much milk as possible, while tea, coffee, and all forms of alcohol must be given up. In carefully selected cases the removal of a part of the thyroid gland has yielded good results.

GREENSTICK FRACTURES (*see* Fractures).

GREY HAIR.—Greyness of the hair (*canities*), though usually a manifestation of old age, may occur quite early in life. In some cases premature greyness is hereditary; it may also be caused by disease, or long-continued nervous exhaustion, while under the influence of acute grief the hair may become grey, or even white, suddenly, as in the historic case of Marie Antoinette. In some cases, as when greyness is due to an attack of neuralgia, it disappears with the condition which caused it, and when it is the result of ill-health, some improvement, at any rate, may be expected from tonics and a nutritious diet. In other cases, and when the condition is caused by old age, there is no remedy except the use of hair-dyes, which are better avoided.

" GRIPES " (*see* Colic; Flatulence).

"GROWING PAINS" (*see* RHEU-MATISM, ACUTE).

GUINEA - WORM DISEASE.— The guinea-worm (*Dracunculus medinensis*) is met with in certain parts of India, in Persia, Arabia, and tropical Africa, especially on the West Coast, and in a certain region of Brazil. The mischief is done by the female worm, which, having been swallowed, bores its way through the tissues of the body until it reaches one of its favourite situations—usually just beneath the skin of the legs, but in some cases the skin of the arm or elsewhere. At this spot there is constant discharge of a milky fluid, which contains myriads of embryo worms. In from fifteen to twenty days the discharge stops, the worm having ceased to produce its young, and it may then work its way out. If so, a little gentle traction may be employed to assist the process. Cure may be expedited by simple surgical measures.

GULLET, FOREIGN BODIES IN (*see* FOREIGN BODIES).

GULLET, STRICTURE OF.— The œsophagus (Fig. 15, p. 109), the tube through which food passes from the mouth to the stomach, sometimes becomes inflamed as the result of injury caused by a foreign body such as a tooth-plate which has slipped down the throat, but more frequently from the swallowing of boiling water or caustic poisons such as carbolic acid, with the result that at the site of the injury, and above and below, the gullet is transformed into a tough unyielding tube. In other cases the stricture is caused by spasm in nervous children or neurotic adults, by congenital malformations, or by the pressure of a tumour. The patient gradually becomes conscious of a difficulty in swallowing—at first only when he attempts to swallow a larger lump of food than usual, but after a time he finds himself unable to swallow any solid food at all, and finally the same difficulty may be experienced even with liquids. Treatment consists in gradually widening the narrowed channel, and keeping it open, by passing a bougie. In severe cases operation may be necessary.

GUM RASH (*see* URTICARIA).

GUMS, DISEASED (*see* PYORRHŒA ALVEOLARIS).

GUMS, SPONGY (*see* BREATH, OFFENSIVE).

GUMBOIL.— The real cause of this painful affection is the action of microbes, which usually gain access through the decayed part of a tooth, and pass down to the root and provoke inflammation in the deeper parts of the socket, with the result that an abscess is formed. Usually the abscess discharges on to the gum, but in some cases the matter finds its way to the surface of the cheek and leaves a disfiguring scar. It is seldom worth while to wait until the abscess bursts ; as soon as matter has formed, it should be let out by the prick of the dentist's or doctor's knife, which can be done without causing pain if cocaine is applied to the part. The mouth should then be frequently rinsed out with an antiseptic lotion such as permanganate of potash. A threatening gumboil may sometimes be checked by inserting a small piece of breadcrumb soaked in quite hot water between the gum and the cheek.

H

HÆMATEMESIS (*see* BLOOD-SPITTING).

HÆMOPHILIA.— There are some people, called "bleeders," in whom profuse hæmorrhage, which it is very difficult to stop, may be caused by a slight injury, or the extraction of a tooth or any other simple surgical operation, or may even arise spontaneously. The condition is sometimes met with in hysterical women, and in persons suffering from scurvy, jaundice, and some other affections. There is a tendency to regard all cases of abnormal bleeding as coming under the head of hæmophilia, but the term should be limited to cases in which the disorder is hereditary. Hæmophilia, so regarded, is a most interesting affection because it is transmitted by females who do not suffer from it themselves. Let us take a case of a man who is a " bleeder " : his sons do not inherit the disease, but one, or several, or all of his daughters, though not " bleeders " themselves, may pass on the disease to *their* sons, though sometimes a generation may be skipped. The nature of the disease is not yet understood. Some have conjectured that it arises from a peculiarity in the composition of the blood which prevents the normal formation of blood-clot ; others have supposed it to be due to an abnormality of the arteries which causes the blood-pressure to be exceptionally high ; but all this is little more than conjecture. Another curious feature is that the tendency to excessive bleeding is not constant, often becomes less as age advances, and may entirely disappear.

Treatment.—The drugs which have the property of checking hæmorrhage in ordinary cases should be tried one after another. But this is essentially one of those affections in which prevention is all important. Children who inherit the disease should be most carefully guarded against all the common accidents of childhood, and obviously operation should never be resorted to unless without it death would be inevitable. Daughters of fathers who suffer from hæmophilia should avoid marriage ; this applies also to " bleeders " themselves.

HÆMOPTYSIS (*see* BLOOD-SPITTING).

HÆMORRHAGE.—In approaching this subject it is well to remind ourselves that the blood is pumped by the heart into strong elastic tubes called arteries, which become smaller and smaller until they shrink into the capillaries (Fig. 9, p. 39). From the capillaries the blood passes into tiny veins (venules) which become larger and larger as they approach the heart, into the right side of which the blood is poured, having completed its circuit of the body (*see* BLOOD, CIRCULATION OF). Hæmorrhage is said to be arterial, capillary, or venous according as to whether the blood comes from the arteries, the capillaries, or the veins. In *arterial* hæmorrhage the blood, of a bright scarlet colour, issues from the end of the vessel nearer the heart, and spurts out in jets corresponding with the beats of the heart. In *capillary* hæmorrhage the blood, also scarlet in colour, oozes slowly from the cut or torn surface of the wound. In *venous* hæmorrhage the blood is of a dark-blue colour, flows in a steady stream, not in spurts, and issues from the end of the vessel farther from the heart.

If the blood escapes to the surface of the body, the hæmorrhage is said to be *external*. If into one of the cavities of the body, as, for instance, the abdomen, it is termed *internal*.

Treatment of the effects of hæmorrhage.—The effects of hæmorrhage, as distinct from the arrest of bleeding, are dealt with by unfastening the clothing around the neck, chest, and abdomen, raising the lower limbs so that the blood may flow to the head, opening doors and windows to ensure free circulation of air, and giving ice to suck and cold

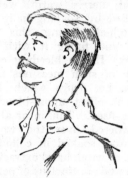

Fig. 25.—Digital compression of the left carotid artery.

water to sip (unless the stomach is wounded). Cold water may be sprinkled on the face and chest, and the patient may be allowed to inhale smelling salts. But no alcoholic stimulant must be given, for the effect would be to increase the heart's action, and so encourage the bleeding. If the loss of blood is very considerable, two pints of warm saline may be injected into the lower bowel—one teaspoonful of common table salt for each pint of water, which should be raised to a temperature of about 100° Fahr.

Natural arrest of hæmorrhage. —In the absence of artificial aid, bleeding tends to cease partly owing to the clotting of the blood (coagulation), and partly, in the case of arterial bleeding, owing to a tendency in the arteries to contract and shrink when cut. This natural arrest of hæmorrhage is aided by a weakened action of the heart, as more and more blood is lost.

Arrest of hæmorrhage by pressure.—First-aid treatment of arte-

rial or venous hæmorrhage consists in the application of pressure in various forms. The simplest form is that known as *digital compression*, in which fingers and thumb are applied either to the bleeding-point or to the artery close to it, but on the side nearer to the heart. As a rule it is better not to apply the pressure to the bleeding-point itself, lest poison should be introduced into the wound. Fig. 25 shows digital compression applied to the left carotid artery, in the neck. Another method is that in which use is made of a *pad and bandage*. The pad, made of several layers of lint, or of a handkerchief folded small, is laid on the bleeding-point, and kept in position by a bandage—say a handkerchief, or strap, or brace—which encircles the part, and is tied firmly, so as to press the pad tightly on the bleeding-point. In the case of the axillary artery in the armpit, the popliteal at the back of the knee, and the brachial artery at the bend of the elbow, the pressure may take the form which is known as *pad and flexion* (Fig. 26). Thus, in the case of the elbow the arm is bent so that the hand touches the shoulder, the pad

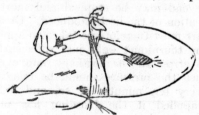

Fig. 26.—Pad and flexion method of arresting hæmorrhage applied to brachial artery.

is inserted between the arm and the forearm, at the bend of the elbow, so as to press upon the artery, and the arm is then drawn close to the forearm by a bandage carried from the armpit to the wrist. But the most effective method of applying pressure to an artery is that of the *tourniquet*, an apparatus consisting essentially of a band to encircle the limb, with or without a pad over the artery, and a rod for tightening the bandage by twisting. Surgical tourniquets take different forms, and need not be described here, as we are concerned rather with improvised tourniquets. For these a pencil (Fig. 27), a penholder, a poker, a key, or a stick, anything in short that can be inserted in the knot so that the bandage may be twisted, is suitable. It must be remembered that great force of compression can be exerted by means of a tourniquet, and that if it is twisted

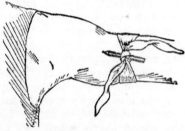

Fig. 27.—Pencil used as tourniquet to stop bleeding from the brachial artery.

too tightly, or is maintained in position too long, the circulation in the part beyond may be stopped and mortification of the limb produced. Great care must therefore be taken to apply the tourniquet only just sufficiently to arrest the hæmorrhage, and even then the pressure should be relaxed every ten minutes or so, and only reapplied if the bleeding has not ceased. As a general rule, resort should only be had to a tourniquet in first-aid when it is found impossible to arrest hæmorrhage by the other modes of compression, or when many injured persons have to be attended to by a single helper. Before it is applied the skin should be shielded by a piece of flannel or lint or a handkerchief, etc.

Arrest of capillary hæmorrhage.—Exposure of a wound to the air for a time is often sufficient to arrest bleeding from the capillaries. If not, the wound should be douched with iced or quite cold water, or very hot (not merely warm) water may be applied by soaking in it a clean handkerchief, laying this on the wound, and fixing it with a tight bandage. If the bleeding continues in spite of such measures as these, styptics, i.e. drugs which have an astringent effect upon blood-vessels, must be used. Tannin or alum may be powdered over the wound, or cotton-wool soaked in collodion laid upon it, or witch hazel extract dabbed on with wool, or tincture of perchloride of iron and water—equal parts— poured into it. Such measures as these, however, should if possible be avoided as liable to interfere with healing, and the same remark applies with still greater force to the use of cobwebs, which are positively dangerous.

Situation of the chief arteries and veins.—The course of the principal *arteries* is shown in Plate X, and the points at which pressure can most effectually be applied to them are indicated by arrows. It will be noticed that the pressure-points are so chosen that the artery may be pressed against a bone. The large *veins* follow the same course as the arteries, and bear the same names, except in the case of the vein accompanying the carotid artery in the neck, which is called the jugular vein.

Hæmorrhage from the thigh.— Apply a pad and bandage over the bleeding-point, or compress the femoral artery at the point where it passes over the haunch-bone (Plate X), grasping the limb with the two hands and placing the thumbs one upon the other over the artery, while

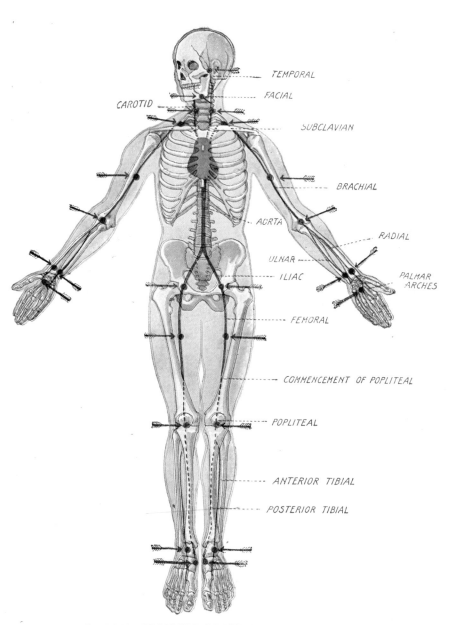

TEMPORAL

FACIAL

CAROTID

SUBCLAVIAN

BRACHIAL

AORTA

RADIAL

ULNAR

ILIAC

PALMAR
ARCHES

FEMORAL

COMMENCEMENT OF POPLITEAL

POPLITEAL

ANTERIOR TIBIAL

POSTERIOR TIBIAL

PLATE X. PRESSURE POINTS OF THE MAIN ARTERIES.

the fingers at the back use counter-pressure. Another method is to bend up the thigh against the abdomen and fix it there with a bandage passed round both the thigh and the body. Or a tourniquet may be applied with a knot or pad in the course of the artery.

Hæmorrhage from the leg and foot.—A bleeding wound in the *leg* should first be treated with a pad and bandage. If the hæmorrhage continues, a pad about the size of a hen's egg should be placed in the hollow of the knee, and the leg then bent up against the thigh and fixed with a bandage. This is also the method for dealing with bleeding from the popliteal artery in the ham. In the *foot*, bleeding from the sole may be treated by pressure with the fingers placed just below the inner ankle, or by a pad and bandage. If the bleeding does not cease, the pad should be placed in the hollow of the knee and the leg bent up and tied firmly to the thigh. If the bleeding is from the front of the foot, place the pad over the wound, or upon the artery which passes over the ankle-joint from the leg.

Hæmorrhage from the arm.—To arrest bleeding from the upper part of the arm (including the armpit), the subclavian artery (Plate X) may be compressed, or direct pressure may be applied to the armpit. In compressing the subclavian artery, use the right hand for the left artery, and the left hand for the right. Having bared the patient's neck and shoulder, stand on the injured side, grasp the neck in the hand by pushing the thumb down into the hollow behind the collar-bone at about its centre, and the fingers at the back, and with the thumb apply pressure backwards and downwards to the artery as it crosses the upper rib.

If the wound is in the armpit, roll up a firm pad the size of an orange, press it well into the hollow under the arm, and fix it with a bandage, the centre of which should be placed over the pad, while the ends are carried up and crossed over the shoulder and then carried across the back and chest to the opposite armpit, where they are tied. Then bind the arm to the side by a broad bandage encircling the lower part of the arm and the body. If the hæmorrhage still persists, the subclavian artery must be compressed as described above.

If the wound is in the lower part of the arm, towards the elbow, pressure may be applied to the bleeding-point, or the brachial artery may be compressed by the fingers. As the artery is near the surface, it is easily felt. Stand at the side of the patient, extend his arm straight outwards with the palm upwards, and grasp it from the back, bringing the ends (not the tips) of the fingers over the artery. Or, standing in front of the patient, grasp the arm with the thumb on its inner side, and press the thumb over the artery. If the pressure is properly applied, the pulse at the wrist will be stopped.

Hæmorrhage from the forearm and hand.—Hæmorrhage from the *forearm* may be stopped by applying a pad over the wound and fixing it with a firm bandage, or by two other methods which have already been described, viz. compressing the brachial artery (*see* above), or bending the elbow-joint (*see* p. 181). In bleeding from the *hand*, pressure may be applied simultaneously to the radial and ulnar arteries at a point about one inch above the wrist (Fig. 28 and Plate X). The wrist is grasped with both hands, the pressure being applied by the thumbs. Or instead of the thumbs, small oblong pads may be used, which are fixed in position by a tight bandage passed two or three times round the wrist. The wounds in the hand which bleed most freely are those in the palm, by which the palmar arch (Plate X) is cut. The best method of applying pressure here is to place a small pad of lint over the wound, to cover this with a second and larger piece, and then to apply a third and fourth piece, each being rather larger than the one beneath, until a thick cone-shaped pad is formed, the whole being then fixed by a tight bandage.

Hæmorrhage from the neck.— When there is great bleeding from the

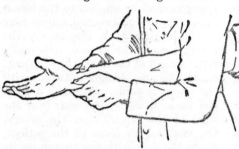

Fig. 28.—Digital compression of the ulnar and radial arteries.

neck it is most often from the carotid artery (Plate X). It is this artery which is injured in attempts at suicide by cutting the throat, and it is the artery on the left side that is the more often injured. The emergency is a very trying one. It is not possible to apply a bandage or a tourniquet to the neck with sufficient force to arrest the bleeding, because the patient would be suffocated by pressure upon the windpipe. The only thing to do is to push the thumb deep into the wound, directing the pressure backwards and inwards towards the back of the windpipe, where bony support from the spinal column is obtained, at the same time grasping the neck with the fingers so as to exert

counter-pressure (Fig. 25). In this manœuvre care must be taken to avoid compression of the windpipe. The pressure must be maintained until a medical man arrives, and if there is long delay it may be necessary for several persons in succession to take up the task, which makes great demands upon strength and endurance.

Hæmorrhage of the smaller arteries of the neck can be dealt with by pressure of the finger, followed by the application of a pad and bandage, care being taken not so to tighten the bandage as to cause difficulty in breathing.

Hæmorrhage from the head.— In hæmorrhage from the temporal artery (Plate X) the thumb must be pressed upon the bleeding-point and kept there until a pad and bandage are ready to take its place. Having laid the pad on the wound, place the centre of a narrow-fold bandage (*see* Band-ages) on the opposite side of the head, and carry it round the head and forehead, keeping it low down to the brows. Twist the ends together over the pad, then carry one over the head, the other under the chin, and tie off on the temple of the sound side. Bleeding from the *facial* artery or its branches to the lips and chin can best be stopped by pressure on the bleeding-point. It may also be lessened by pressure on the artery (Plate X) as it crosses the edge of the lower jaw 1½ inches from the angle. In bleeding from the *cheek and lips* the artery should be compressed between the finger in the mouth and the thumb outside on the face. Hæmorrhage from *gums and tooth socket* after the extraction of a tooth is sometimes difficult to stop. If washing out the mouth freely with ice-cold water is without effect, pressure must be applied. Take a long wedge-shaped piece of lint, wet the pointed end with oil of turpentine, press it into the socket, and refold it upon itself so as to make a firm pad large enough to fill the space between the bleeding-point and the teeth of the other jaw. The mouth is then closed, and pressure maintained by the other jaw. If the pressure is inadequate, a piece of cork may be laid on the top of the pad. A bandage is tied under the chin and over the head to maintain sufficient and equable pressure. For hæmorrhage from the nose, see NOSE-BLEEDING.

HÆMORRHOIDS (*see* PILES).

HAIR, CARE OF.—Care of the hair resolves itself chiefly into cleanliness, which should be secured even more by brushing than by washing. Among those who have studied the question, there is a general agreement that the frequent application of water to the hair is not favourable to its growth. In men it is sufficient if the head is washed once every week, and in women with long hair, once a fortnight, a pure soap or simple shampoo powder being used for the purpose. In both men and women the hair should be brushed regularly night and morning. "Use a soft brush and use it gently," was a maxim of the late Dr. Allan Jamieson, of Edinburgh. If dandruff is present, the scurf should not be removed by the use of hard brushes, for it reforms faster than ever if removed in this way. When scurfy matter forms on the heads of infants and young children, it must be removed by soap and water, never by a comb ; and combs of the small-toothed variety should never be used, either for children or by adults. Hair should be cut about once a fortnight, and if it is worn long, somewhat oftener, otherwise the ends are liable

to split. The custom of singeing the hair, which was prevalent a few years ago, has now gone out of vogue. It was never anything but a superstition, based upon a groundless belief that the hair is a tube provided with microscopical blood-vessels which bleed invisibly when cut. The less hair-dressing that is used, the better. In some persons, however, the hair is dry from lack of the oily secretion of the sebaceous glands, so that the use of a simple dressing, such as the following, is desirable.

Castor oil .... 2 drachms
Almond oil................14 drachms
Glycerin .... 6 drachms
Jockey Club perfume.......1½ drachms
Rectified spirit .... 4 ounces

HAIRINESS.—Overgrowth of hair (*hirsuties*) may take the form either of an abnormal growth on some hairless region, as on the upper lip or chin of women, or of an exaggeration of the natural growth of hairy parts. The tendency in many cases is hereditary, and is often associated with some anomaly of the teeth. Sometimes overgrowth of hair follows severe illness, and it is often the accompaniment of menstrual irregularities. It is only in slight cases that treatment can be successfully applied. In some cases superfluous hairs can be destroyed by electricity, but this method is not applicable when there is an undergrowth of fine hair. The only alternative is shaving. Plucking out hairs with tweezers is useless as well as painful, for they grow thicker and stronger than before. Depilatories also do more harm than good. When the condition is a symptom of uterine trouble, this must, of course, receive attention.

HALLUCINATIONS (*see* INSANITY).

HAMMER-TOE.—In this condition one of the toes, nearly always the second toe, is so deformed as to have suggested a rough resemblance to a hammer. Sometimes the deformity is present at birth, but usually it is due to the wearing of ill-fitting boots. The results are pain in walking, often aggravated by the presence of corns. In slight cases the deformity may be corrected by manipulation and by the use of strapping inside the shoe, and wearing a splint during the night. Other cases must be treated by operation.

HANDS, CHAPPED (*see* CHAPPED HANDS AND LIPS).

HANGNAIL.—The best way of treating the little shred of separate skin which sometimes occurs at the border of the nail is to cut it off and apply a little boric-acid ointment, or paint with tincture of iodine. If this is done, the little wound will quickly heal up.

HARD CHANCRE (*see* SYPHILIS).

HARE-LIP.—This is the commonest malformation of the face, which is estimated to occur in one out of every 2,400 infants. Like cleft palate, with which it often co-exists, it is an error of development, the separate parts from which the child's face is developed before birth failing to unite properly. The condition is sometimes hereditary, and the tendency is generally transmitted by the mother. In a few cases the furrow is in the middle of the upper lip, as in the hare, but much more often it is on one side, usually on the left side, while in some cases it is on both sides. Male children are more subject to the deformity than female. The defect varies from a slight dent in the red of the lip to a deep fissure extending to the nostril. *Treatment.*—The fissure

can be closed by an operation. If the child is feeble and badly nourished, operation must be postponed until its health has improved. In the case of normal infants, many surgeons prefer to operate during the second month of life. In slight cases, however, in which the child can suckle without difficulty, it may be considered better to wait until weaning time. If the cleft is large, feeding should be carried on by means of a glass nipple shield, fitted with a large rubber teat to fill the gap in the lip.

HARVEST - BUG BITES (*see* STINGS AND BITES).

HAY FEVER.—This troublesome affection, known also as hay asthma, is due in many cases to irritation of the mucous membrane of the nose by the pollen of various grasses and cereals. Hence its frequency between the middle of May and the beginning of July. The little pollen sacs, borne by the wind, are inhaled, settle on the nasal mucous membrane, burst and scatter minute granules over the surface; "hence these tears." Precisely the same effect may be induced by the perfume of roses or other flowers, the exhalations of horses, cats, rabbits, guinea-pigs, or by the dust of wood pavements, while in another group of cases the same symptoms are produced by a draught, by passing from shade into bright sunlight or vice versa, or even looking at a bright surface. In all cases alike it must be assumed that the mucous membrane of the nose is abnormally sensitive. Neurotic persons are especially liable to hay fever, and it prevails most among the educated and refined. It is most common between the ages of twenty and thirty, and is said to occur more frequently in men than in women and children.

Symptoms.—Without the slightest

warning, it may be on getting out of bed in the morning, a sensation of tickling or dryness in the nose, and perhaps in the eye, is felt, an attack of violent sneezing follows, and the nose runs with a watery, irritating fluid, the eyes water, and the head begins to ache from spread of the inflammation to the cavities in the frontal bone. The nose soon becomes stuffed up from swelling of the mucous membrane, the eyes blood-shot and swollen, the tears trickle down the cheeks from the blocking of the ducts leading to the nose. As in a cold, the inflammation may spread backwards from the nose and mouth to the throat, or to the ears, causing partial deafness, or it may extend downwards to the bronchial tubes and bring on an attack of asthma. If the attack is left untreated it may persist for four or five weeks, returning when the patient is again exposed to the same irritation.

Treatment.—The irritated mucous membrane may be soothed by the following inhalation, the steam being drawn up into the nostrils through a folded handkerchief placed over the mouth of the vessel.

Oil of pine .... 2 drachms
Compound   tincture of
   benzoin .... 1 ounce
Light carbonate of magnesia 1 drachm
Rose water .... 1 ounce
Glycerin to 3 ounces.
Half an ounce to one pint of water in the inhaler.

The inhalation of menthol and euca-lyptus has also been found beneficial. The pain in the eyes may be relieved by a boric-acid lotion and the wearing of smoked glasses, and if light is painful, as it often is, the patient should rest in a darkened room. The general nervous irritation may be soothed by phenacetin or antipyrin or aspirin. In some cases an antitoxin

known as pollantin has been used with good results. A small drop of pollan-tin may be placed in the eyes at the beginning of an attack as an experi-ment. Inoculation with a pollen vaccine has also been tried, and it is claimed for this agent that it confers immunity to the disease for at least a year. A preventive measure which answers in some cases is that of anoint-ing the inside of both nostrils with zinc ointment. If the irritation is due to pollen the patient may go to the seaside, choosing a place protected from land winds by high cliffs. High mountain stations may also afford immunity, while many patients find that they enjoy most freedom from the affection in the centre of a large town.

HEADACHE.—Headache is less a disease in itself than a symptom of several different diseases ; but it is so common and troublesome a con-dition that not only must it receive separate consideration, but a good deal of space must be devoted to it. In this place we shall not consider it in so far as it is a manifestation of organic nervous disease—that is, disease of the brain or its membranes. Headaches from less serious causes may, for the sake of clearness, be broken up into five different groups —(1) megrim, (2) toxæmic headache, (3) congestive headache, (4) rheu-matic headache, (5) anæmic headache. Another type of headache, the neu-ralgic, which includes the headache caused by eyestrain, is touched upon in the article on NEURALGIA. This classification must not be interpreted too rigidly, for there is not a little overlapping between the different groups.

1. *Megrim.*—This is the kind of headache which is usually spoken of as " sick headache," though other forms of headache also produce

vomiting. "Megrim" is a popular rendering of "migraine," and this in turn is derived from "hemicrania," which literally means "half the skull," the pain being in many cases limited to one side of the head. A peculiarity of the attacks is that in many patients they occur at regular intervals—on the same day, it may be, every two or three or four weeks. Thus we know of a patient in whom they nearly always occurred at intervals of three or four weeks on a Sunday. In the symptoms which precede and accompany the attacks there is great diversity. In some cases the attack is heralded by a sensation of cold and chilliness, much more frequently it is ushered in by disturbances of vision—scintillating circles like "wheels of fireworks," bright spots of light, or instead of these appearances, or in addition to them, vision is blurred and indistinct, and only part of an object seen; there may also be hallucinations. Hearing or speech may be affected, or there may be cramp or spasms of muscles, or sensations of numbness, tingling or pricking. At the same time there may be stupor, or mental confusion, or a state of excitement. In some cases nothing follows these symptoms but perhaps a slight feeling of fullness in the head, but much more often they are followed, after varying intervals, by headache, which may be very severe, though it is not invariably so. It may be limited to a small area—the eye, the temple, or the forehead, whence it may gradually spread. As the pain becomes worse the patient feels sick, and at last may vomit. The act of vomiting, though it aggravates the pain for a time, in many cases is followed by a feeling of relief. The attack may last only a few hours, and only in rare cases does it persist for more than twenty-four hours. Usually the patient feels exceptionally well when the attack passes off—the result, no doubt, of abstention from food, and of the vomiting, but in some cases, especially those in which there is little or no headache, there are indications of a slight nervous shock. This suggests a comparison with epilepsy, an attack of which leaves behind it a feeling of nervous shock; but a more striking resemblance is to be found in the sensations which precede the two conditions. There would appear to be some relation between megrim and epilepsy, but precisely what that relation is has not yet been ascertained.

Causes.—The theory which seems best to explain the premonitory symptoms of megrim is that spasms of the blood-vessels occur, which interfere with the supply of blood to the brain, and that this temporary cerebral anæmia is followed by an excessive flow of blood. An antecedent cause may be the absorption of poisons from the intestines. Fortunately megrim tends to disappear after middle age.

Treatment.—As soon as the premonitory symptoms occur a teaspoonful of sal-volatile or a cup of hot strong tea or coffee may be taken in the hope of warding off the threatened attack. If, in spite of this, the attack develops, a tablet containing phenacetin and caffeine may be taken. Another useful remedy is aspirin, one or two 5-grain tablets for a dose, which may be repeated in two hours' time. Or caffeine may be taken with bromide of potash—one teaspoonful of the effervescing citrate, or combined with antipyrin in the form of migranin (dose 10 grains). Guarana gives relief in some cases—10 grains with 5 grains of salicylate of soda, the dose to be repeated in half an hour.

Treatment between the attacks

must take the form chiefly of attending to diet. In many cases a contributory cause of the attacks is overfeeding, or the consumption of indigestible and over-rich food. No malt liquors or sweet wines should be drunk, and in most cases the patient will be better without alcohol at all. Worry and excitement should be avoided, for there is undoubtedly a nervous element in megrim. Regular exercise in the open air is desirable, and in cases in which there is a tendency to constipation, the bowels should occasionally be cleared out with an aperient.

2. *Toxæmic headache.*—It has already been pointed out that megrim may be due primarily to the absorption of poisons from the intestines, and it may very well be that most headaches are more or less due to poisons circulating in the blood. Headaches caused by the poison of gout, of malaria, of advanced kidney disease, or of lead poisoning need only be mentioned, for those conditions are considered in other articles. Dyspeptic or " bilious " headaches are described under the head of BILIOUSNESS.

3. *Congestive headache.* — Congestive headaches are to be distinguished from other forms of headache by flushing of the face, throbbing of the blood-vessels of the head, giddiness, and the fact that the pain is dull and heavy rather than acute as in megrim. The attack may be brought about by excitement, excessive mental exertion, worry, over-eating, or the abuse of alcohol or of tobacco. In some cases these headaches may be due to so slight a cause as the wearing of a tight collar which obstructs the return of blood from the head. They are also met with in some cases of heart or lung disease. For treatment the feet should be placed in hot mustard and water, and cold applied to the head. In some cases a mustard plaster to the nape of the neck is beneficial. Blue pill and black draught form a suitable aperient, or, instead, a grain of calomel may be taken at bedtime and a dose of Epsom salts the next morning. Between the attacks the mode of life should be that recommended in the article on BILIOUSNESS, with a little emphasis laid upon the diet, which should be spare as well as simple.

4. *Rheumatic headache.*—From this kind of headache women above middle age are the chief sufferers. The pain, which is intermittent, starts at the back of the head, and radiates over the head and sometimes also into the neck ; it is increased by exposure to cold and chill. A distinctive feature of this headache is that at the back of the head and neck small nodules which are very tender to pressure can be felt in the tissues beneath the skin. Treatment consists chiefly in massage of the neck and back of the head, beginning with very gentle rubbing of the nodules, and becoming firmer as the tenderness disappears. Large hot poultices should also be applied to the back of the head and neck three times a day.

5. *Anæmic and neurasthenic headache.* — Anæmic headaches, whether or not neurasthenia (extreme nervous weakness) is associated with the anæmia, are due mainly to impoverishment of the blood, which results in impaired nutrition of the nerves. It is believed also that the insufficient elimination of poisons is one of the causes of these headaches. They may be induced by fatigue, or by over-indulgence in alcohol. The pain may be felt in the forehead or the back of the head, but is most often felt at the top, and often is so acute that it seems to the patient as if a

nail were being driven downwards into the head—*clavus hystericus* (hysterical nail) this symptom is termed in medical literature. The pain, usually more or less continuous, is relieved by lying down with the head rather below the level of the body, so as to promote the flow of blood through the brain. In this group of cases a nerve stimulant is usually beneficial, such as tea or coffee or sal-volatile. One or two tablets of phenacetin, of antipyrin, or of aspirin may be given. For general treatment the best drug is iron (*see* ANÆMIA), to which arsenic or strychnine may be added. Where the anæmia is accompanied by neurasthenia the rest cure (q.v.), complete or partial, is suitable.

HEALING (*see* WOUNDS).

HEARING, DEFECTS OF (*see* DEAFNESS).

HEART (*see* BLOOD, CIRCULATION OF).

HEART DISEASE.—In this article we shall consider *organic* diseases of the heart—diseases, that is, in which the organ is structurally damaged or deteriorated. Functional disorders of the heart form the subject of the next article. The structure and working of the heart are described in the article BLOOD, CIRCULATION OF.

In most cases heart disease, when not congenital—and in congenital cases the little patient seldom lives long—is the result of acute rheumatism—rheumatic fever as it is popularly called, though some cases are due to other diseases, such as scarlet fever, measles, and blood-poisoning. But heart disease may also be caused by the severe strain which athletes and some manual labourers undergo, while in old age it may come on from degenerative changes that represent a lifetime's wear and tear.

When heart disease has its origin in acute rheumatism or an infectious fever it takes the form of inflammation, set up by the poisons formed by the germs of the disease. The double membrane enclosing the heart may be involved—*pericarditis;* or the muscular substance of the heart—*myocarditis;* or the membrane lining the interior of the heart—*endocarditis*.

Pericarditis usually appears within a few days of the onset of the antecedent fever, its advent being announced by a rise of temperature. It may be prolonged into chronic pericarditis. Acute pericarditis requires little treatment additional to that demanded by the fever in which it usually originates. Absolute rest must be insisted upon, for even rising to the sitting posture is dangerous. To mitigate the pain, leeches may be applied to the heart region, or counter-irritation by poultices or iodine may be employed. If heart-failure threatens, alcohol must be given, and the doctor may administer ether, ammonia, strychnine, or digitalis. If sleeplessness is pronounced, he may order a hypnotic. If the effusion from the inflamed membrane is very considerable, it may have to be removed by the surgeon. In the later stages, every means must be employed to maintain the physical strength and keep the stomach and bowels in working order. When the patient begins to mend, he must still keep to his bed. Tonics will be required, and massage is indicated to stimulate the circulation, improve the appetite, and brace up the general physical tone. For the victims of *chronic* pericarditis little can be done beyond caring for the general health, seeing that all strain is avoided, and giving stimulants when heart-failure threatens.

Myocarditis.—In this affection the heart muscle usually becomes inflamed by extension from its membranes. In some cases the irregular heart-beat which occurs takes the form of *auricular fibrillation*, in which the auricles (*see* CIRCULATION OF THE BLOOD) fail to contract and remain distended in a state of tremor, while the ventricles beat very irregularly ; in others there is *auricular flutter*, in which the auricle contracts so rapidly as quite to outpace the ventricle. The disease runs a rapid course, from a few hours to about a week. Many cases have a fatal termination. Treatment runs on the same lines as in pericarditis. The great danger is cardiac failure.

Endocarditis.—There is little pain or fever unless the valves of the heart are seriously involved, as in many cases they are. Except in congenital cases, it is the valves of the left side of the heart that become diseased. In many cases the damage to the valves is automatically *compensated*, to use the medical expression. As the result of having extra work to do in pumping the blood through the diseased valve, the muscle of the heart grows thicker and stronger. When compensation is thus established the circulation is maintained as efficiently as though the valves were healthy. In some cases, unfortunately, there being no reserve power to draw upon, compensation is impossible, and then the heart, overworked and exhausted, becomes flabby, undergoes dilatation, and a train of serious symptoms is set up, among them pain, palpitation, shortness of breath, and dropsy. Treatment is similar to that of the other forms of inflammation of the heart. Rest in bed should continue for three months, if possible, exercise must be resumed very gradually, and the patient must be content in future to avoid all forcible exertion. Diet, baths, drugs, and regular exercise must

all be pressed into the service in the hope of establishing compensation.

Heart weakness. — The only other form of organic heart disease which need be dealt with in these pages is that of heart weakness. It may be due to high fever in such diseases as typhus, diphtheria, septicæmia, and influenza, in which the heart is damaged by powerful poisons. Other causes are exhausting illness, and the fatty degeneration which sometimes comes on in old age. The signs of a weak heart are cold hands and feet, feeble pulse, general debility, a tendency to faint, and breathlessness on exertion. Treatment must aim at strengthening the heart by toning up the general health. Nourishing and sufficient but not excessive food, gentle exercise in the open air, avoidance of physical or mental strain, and tonics such as iron and strychnine are the most important features of the régime.

For angina pectoris, *see* the article on that subject.

HEART, FUNCTIONAL DISORDERS OF.—In this group of cardiac affections the heart is structurally sound, but its working is deranged by some abnormal condition of the blood or by influences unfavourably affecting its nerve supply. Two of the manifestations of functional heart disorder, *palpitation* and *fainting*, are considered in separate articles.

Causes.—Functional heart trouble may be due primarily to unsuitable or insufficient or excessive food, or to any other condition, such as gout, which prejudicially affects the blood. Many cases are explained by the intemperate use of alcohol or tobacco, or tea or coffee ; others by indigestion, setting up flatulence or over-acidity, or by chronic diarrhœa, or constipation, or intestinal worms, or by lung or liver or kidney disease. In another group of cases excessive, long-continued physical exertion, or violent emotional disturbance, is responsible for the trouble.

Symptoms.—Besides palpitation, pain in the region of the heart, sometimes radiating over the left side of the body and down the left arm, and either sharp and sudden or dull and protracted, is a frequent symptom. The pulse-rate may be more, or less, rapid than normal, or the beats may be irregular, or intermittent, as described in the article on the Pulse, or "murmurs" may be heard through the stethoscope as in valvular disease. These various symptoms are common both to functional disorder and to organic disease of the heart, but if they can be traced to any of the causes mentioned above it may be assumed that they are functional only.

Treatment.—This must be directed to the cause of the symptoms. The diet must be regulated, the rules of hygiene generally must be respected, excitement must be avoided, the patient must take a long rest if there has been over-exertion, constipation or diarrhœa must be corrected, the digestion set right. If anæmia is present, iron is required. (*See also* PALPITATION OF THE HEART.)

A few words may be added by way of reassuring those who are disturbed by the fear that they have heart disease. More needless apprehension is felt on this score, probably, than on any other. The symptoms that give birth to the anxiety may be manifestations, as we have seen, of mere functional disorder. Moreover, pain felt in the heart region may have nothing to do with the heart; any one of a number of other causes may be responsible for it. Thus, the muscles of the chest may be strained,

or there may be soreness set up by violent coughing, or the chest muscles may ache because they are flabby, the patient being in a low state of health, or the pain may be rheumatic, or may be caused simply by flatulence. In itself, therefore, pain in the region of the heart need occasion no anxiety, though the patent will do well to satisfy himself, by skilled examination, that the trouble is not organic.

HEART, PALPITATION OF (*see* PALPITATION OF THE HEART).

HEARTBURN.—Heartburn is the curious name given to a familiar condition which is due to excess of acid in the stomach, the acid being that of the gastric juice, which may, however, be mixed with acids resulting from the decomposition of food. Medically the affection is called *pyrosis*. A sensation of heat is felt in the stomach, and spreads up the gullet, and a scalding acid may rise into the mouth. The patient should take 15 to 30 grains of bicarbonate of soda in half a teacupful of hot water. Two or three soda-mint tablets may also be taken at bedtime dissolved in a wineglassful of hot water, especially if the discomfort hinders sleep. But to remove the cause of heartburn the diet must be so regulated as to reduce fat, sugar and starch to a minimum, and tobacco and alcohol should be avoided altogether or indulged in very sparingly. When heartburn occurs in advanced pregnancy, as it frequently does, the eating of lettuce often gives relief.

HEATSTROKE AND SUNSTROKE.—The effects of exposure to high temperature in the shade are known as heatstroke; those of exposure to the direct rays of the sun, as sunstroke. The ability of the healthy human body to adapt itself to high temperatures is remarkable.

In the tropics men work out of doors in temperatures of 100° Fahr., or even 120°, with impunity. In other parts of the world such industries as glass blowing and sugar boiling are carried on at temperatures far above these, while the stokers of steamships, especially in the tropics, sometimes work for hours in a temperature of over 150° Fahr. This, however, presupposes a state of sound health. If a man indulges freely in alcohol, or habitually eats too much, or is oppressed by too heavy clothing, or is exposed to a damp atmosphere which checks perspiration, his capacity for withstanding an abnormally high temperature is seriously diminished.

Heatstroke.—The patient may suddenly become insensible and die without recovering consciousness. Or the attack may come on gradually with drowsiness, pains in the muscles, headache, quick, shallow breathing, a sensation of tightness round the chest, nausea, and vomiting. These symptoms grow rapidly worse, the face is flushed and red, the pulse rapid, and, with or without an intervening phase of delirium, unconsciousness sets in. *Treatment.*—The head should be shaved, and a bag containing pieces of ice applied to it ; the body should be wrapped in a wet sheet, or ice water poured in a fine stream from a height of three or four feet on to the head and spine. If the temperature falls two or three degrees as the result of these measures they must be discontinued, and the patient wrapped in blankets, with hot-water bottles to his feet to encourage free perspiration. If he is able to swallow, quinine may be given in 5-grain doses every three hours. The bowels should be cleared with a large soap-and-water enema,

or three grains of calomel powder may be given. Later, mustard poultices may be applied to the feet and calves, and a blister to the nape of the neck. When the patient is able to take light food, it must be given frequently, and in small quantities. All exertion must be avoided.

Sunstroke.—The attack comes on with dimness of sight, giddiness, severe faintness, and exhaustion. The patient may lapse into unconsciousness and die, but in the majority of cases there is a gradual return to health, although for a time there may be severe headache and exhaustion. *Treatment.*—Remove the sufferer to a cool and shady place, lay him on his back, loosen any garments that may be tight, sprinkle water over the face and chest, apply smelling salts to the nostrils and, if the patient is conscious, give a tea-spoonful of sal-volatile, or some brandy and water.

Whenever exposure to high temperature, whether indoors or out of doors, is unavoidable, special precautions should be taken. The clothing should be as light as possible, and loose fitting, and the undergarments of thin wool ; the head should be protected from the sun by a wide-brimmed, well ventilated, pith cap, which shields the neck and temples as well as the top of the head.

HELIOTHERAPY (*see* Sunlight Treatment).

HEMIPLEGIA (*see* Apoplexy).

HEREDITARY DISEASE (*see* Disease, Classification of).

HERNIA (*see* Rupture).

HERPES ZOSTER (*see* Shingles).

HICCOUGH. — This condition is caused by irritation of the diaphragm, the large muscle separating the chest from the abdomen. It occurs not infrequently in drunkards; in others, it may be induced by eating spiced or peppery foods, or taking hot drinks. Some people have an attack if they begin to eat without drinking. As a rule, hiccough arises from such simple causes as these, but it may also occur after abdominal operations, or as a symptom of peritonitis, or in extreme exhaustion. In ordinary hiccough the best thing to do is to put the diaphragm on the stretch, as by trying to count a hundred without taking breath. Some persons find relief by swallowing a mouthful of water with the fingers stuffed well into the ears; in others, a sudden shock, such as is caused by an unexpected shout, may have the desired effect. In the hiccough of drunkards an hourly dose, for three or four hours, of tincture of nux vomica and tincture of capsicum, 5 minims of each in a tablespoonful of water, is often beneficial. A popular remedy for hiccough generally is sipping a tumblerful of hot water in which a teaspoonful of mustard has been dissolved.

HIGH-FREQUENCY CURRENT (*see* ELECTRICAL TREATMENT).

HILL DIARRHŒA.—This is a curious form of flatulent indigestion and diarrhœa which is chiefly prevalent among Europeans visiting hill regions of tropical countries after residence in the hot lowlands. The patient is attacked regularly every morning, at some time between 3 and 5 o'clock, with urgent diarrhœa. By about 11 o'clock the symptoms cease, and the patient is not further troubled until the early hours of the following morning. *Treatment* consists in a pure milk diet, with rest and warm clothing, and the administration of a half a teaspoonful of solution of perchloride of mercury in

water, about a quarter of an hour after meals, followed by 12 grains of pepsin two hours later.

HIP-DISEASE.—Inflammation of the hip-joint, which is known as hip-disease, is usually tuberculous. It is almost confined to children; such children are usually delicate from birth, and in many cases the disease can be traced to an injury, which may be quite slight in character. Many patients do not live to grow up, succumbing to other forms of tuberculosis, or to illness of other kinds; but with the improved methods of treatment now employed the prospects are much more favourable than they were, and not merely are the lives of the patients preserved, but there is very little deformity resulting from the disease. The symptoms begin insidiously. The child complains rather of being tired than of pain, and is noticed to walk with a slight limp. Appetite is capricious, the patient becomes pale and peevish, and his sleep may be disturbed. These symptoms come and go, but after a time are more constant. One of the most unmistakable of them is limitation of the movement of the joint. The position of the limb then undergoes alteration; in most cases the thigh is bent upwards and drawn away from its fellow, while the foot is turned outwards; the limb is also shortened, though it appears to be longer than the other. Wasting of the muscles of the buttock and thigh is observed. By this time pain, which may have been absent at the onset of the symptoms, is complained of, not only in the hip-joint, but in some cases on the inner side of the knee. As the child is about to go to sleep there often occur what are called "starting pains," caused by a spasm of the muscles. *Treatment* consists in complete rest, the use of splints to fix the limb, and the employment of weights and various mechanical appliances to extend it. It is necessarily a very protracted treatment, which may have to be carried out over a period of five years, or even longer. As far as possible the patient should live in the open air. In cases that have gone too far for this treatment, operation may be necessary to remove the diseased bone, while in still severer cases, fortunately not common, amputation may have to be resorted to.

HIRSUTIES (*see* HAIRINESS).

HOARSENESS.—This condition is not an affection in itself, but a symptom of such disorders as laryngitis, "clergyman's sore throat," bronchitis, etc. It is dealt with in the articles on these diseases, but some tabloids which are useful for the voice may here be mentioned. One of the best of them is the potash, borax and cocaine tabloid, which can be kept under the tongue and allowed slowly to dissolve. If the throat is dry, the compound benzoic acid tabloid will encourage the secretion of mucus. Menthol and eucalyptus jujubes will be found to have a soothing effect. Inhalations such as eucalyptus oil, compound tincture of benzoin, or chloride of ammonium, are among the best ways of treating hoarseness. (*See* INHALATIONS.)

HOBNAIL LIVER (*see* CIRRHOSIS OF THE LIVER).

HODGKIN'S DISEASE.—This mysterious disease, called also lymphadenoma, is fortunately rare. It consists in an enlargement of lymphatic glands, together with anæmia ; and in many cases there is enlargement also of the spleen and the liver. Of the cause of the disease little is known. The drugs which have given the best

results are arsenic and phosphorus, and especially the former.

HOLLOW FOOT (*see* CLUB-FOOT).

HOOKWORM DISEASE (*see* MINER'S ANÆMIA).

HOSPITAL SORE THROAT (*see* SORE THROAT).

HOT PACK (*see* WET PACK).

HOT-AIR BATHS (*see* BATHS).

HOUSEMAID'S KNEE (*see* BURSÆ).

" HUMP-BACK " (*see* SPINAL CURVATURE, ANGULAR).

HYDATID CYST (*see* CYSTS).

HYDROCELE. — Hydroceles are caused by an accumulation of liquid in the scrotum, the pouch containing the testicles. They are most often met with in elderly men, especially those who have lived in the tropics, but they may occur at any age, even in quite young boys. The condition may be caused by chronic inflammation of the testicle. The scrotum should be supported by a suspensory bandage, and painted with tincture of iodine. If the swelling increases it may have to be " tapped." If the fluid should continue to accumulate after repeated tappings, the medical attendant may advise an operation.

HYDROCEPHALUS. — This condition, " water on the brain," may originate in meningitis (*see* MENINGITIS, TUBERCULOUS), or may be due to a tumour of the brain. It is usually present at birth, when it may cause trouble in the delivery of the child, owing to enlargement of the head, or it may first appear when the child is a few weeks or months old. In some cases it is a manifestation of congenital syphilis. The cavities within the brain are distended with fluid, and as this increases, the bones of the skull, which have not yet become joined together, are forced farther apart, and may be thinned. Hydrocephalus can easily be distinguished from rickets : in the former, the head is globular, and bulges in all directions, while in rickets it is square and flat at the top, and the edges where the bones join are thickened. In some cases the mind is not appreciably affected ; in others its development is permanently arrested. Most of the patients do not live to grow up. On the other hand there are cases in which the fluid ceases to accumulate and is absorbed, and the skull assumes almost the normal shape, although larger than ordinary.

HYDROCHLORIC-ACID POISONING.—Hydrochloric acid, or spirit of salt, is a caustic, which stains the mouth and throat with a white coating, while clothing is stained bright red. No emetic should be given. Recourse must be had to alkaline substances which will neutralize the acid, such as fluid magnesia, or lime water, which may be given with milk or gruel, or chalk, which may be obtained from the ceiling, or carbonate of soda. Milk, beaten-up eggs, and olive oil may also be given. The alkalis must be given in small doses, frequently repeated ; if given in large doses, a large volume of carbonic acid gas might be produced and thus dangerous distension of the stomach might be caused.

HYDROCYANIC - ACID POISONING (*see* PRUSSIC-ACID POISONING).

HYDRONEPHROSIS.—If the flow of urine from a kidney is obstructed by a stone (calculus) or other cause, the water will accumulate in the basin-shaped cavity of the kidney (the pelvis) and distend it ; this is what is called hydronephrosis. The pelvis of a kidney thus affected may be invaded by pus-forming germs ; if so, the hydronephrosis becomes a pyonephrosis. The obstruction should be removed by operation.

HYDROPATHY (*see* BATHS ; MINERAL WATERS).

HYDROPHOBIA.—This disease, also known as *rabies*, has been virtually exorcised from this country, where formerly it was not uncommon. Its suppression was effected by a protracted muzzling of dogs, supplemented by provisions for regulating the importation of dogs from other countries. It never arises spontaneously, but is always transmitted by a previous case, whether in an animal or a human being. It is a disease to which animals generally, and not merely dogs, are subject, and it has been met with in most parts of the world.

Cause.—Hydrophobia is undoubtedly due to a microbe, of which the poison attacks the nervous system. The affection is nearly always transmitted by the saliva. The interval between the occurrence of the bite and the onset of symptoms is on an average six weeks, but it may be very much longer, while in children bitten in the face it may be as short as one week. Bites about the head, face, or hands are more fatal than in other parts, owing to their being less protected by clothing—which in many cases prevents the infected saliva from entering the wound—and abundantly supplied with nerves.

Symptoms.—The patient first feels pricking sensations in the region of the bite ; he then becomes depressed and restless, suffers from severe headache, has hallucinations of hearing and smelling, and his sleep is disturbed by nightmares. In some cases the depression gives place to excitement and loquacity. From two to five days afterwards he finds pain and difficulty in swallowing ; any attempt at eating or drinking produces a painful spasm of the throat, while even the mere sight of liquid may cause his jaws to clench and his breathing for the moment to stop. It is this symptom which has given rise to the designation " hydrophobia." The spasms may also be caused by a current of air, an unexpected noise, a brilliant light, or a strong odour. This condition, with intervals of apparent relief, lasts for two or three days, and is succeeded by paralysis which, after from six to twelve hours, leads to collapse and death ; or instead of the paralysis, the breathing may be affected and the patient die of suffocation. In some cases the spasmodic stage is very short, and paralysis at once sets in. The disease seldom lasts longer than six days.

When the disease has once developed there is little hope, but fortunately by the inoculation treatment originated by Pasteur in 1885, and since improved, it can be successfully averted during the period of incubation, the poison deposited in the wound being destroyed before it reaches the central nerves. A bite from an animal suspected to be rabid should be allowed to bleed freely and then be cauterized, say with pure carbolic acid. If the animal is proved to be rabid, the inoculation treatment should be given.

HYDROTHERAPY (*see* BATHS ; MINERAL WATERS).

HYPERMETROPIA (*see* SIGHT, DEFECTS OF).

HYPERPIESIS (*see* BLOOD-PRESSURE).

HYPERPYREXIA (*see* FEVER).

HYPNOTICS (*see* NARCOTICS AND HYPNOTICS).

HYPNOTISM. — Hypnotism, a state of mind in which the patient becomes extraordinarily susceptible to " suggestion " conveyed to him by the operator, is now a recognized branch of medical treatment. On the one hand, it has been associated with much false theory, and more charlatanism ; on the other hand, it has had to encounter a good deal of prejudice in medical circles. It may be that a satisfactory theory of hypnotism has still to be framed, but medical science now welcomes its aid in the treatment of cases which are peculiarly refractory to ordinary methods. One of the most remarkable effects of hypnotism is in the production of anæsthesia. The patient retains consciousness, but becomes insensible to the pain even of a major operation, such as the amputation of a limb. The first medical men to use hypnotism —or mesmerism, as it was then called —for this purpose were Dr. John Elliotson and Dr. James Esdaile, the one at University College Hospital, in London, the other in Calcutta, and afterwards at Perth in his native country. To Dr. Esdaile's success emphatic testimony was borne by Dr. Webb, of the Calcutta Medical Hospital. " In the Mesmeric Hospital in this city," he said, "the most dreadful operations are daily performed without pain. . . . I cannot recall without astonishment the extirpation of a cancerous eye while the man looked at me unflinchingly with the other one. In another case, the patient looked dreamily on with halfclosed eyes the whole time, even while I examined the malignant tumour I had removed, and then, having satisfied myself, concluded the operation." About the time that Elliotson and Esdaile were using hypnotism to make operations painless, Simpson discovered chloroform, and the availability of this and other anæsthetics, both general and local, has made it unnecessary to use hypnotism for the production of anæsthesia. But it has a large field of usefulness in those curious mental and nervous cases in which there is no discoverable organic disease. Hysteria, neurasthenia, insomnia, mental depression, obsessions, such as the fear of being in closed or in open spaces, and functional disorders of the digestive and other organs, are amenable to its influence. Hypnotic treatment should be sought only from a person with proper medical qualifications, who can judge whether the case is suitable, and can be relied upon not to abuse the *rapport* which must be established between practitioner and patient if the treatment is to be successful.

HYPOCHONDRIASIS.—A hypochondriac is sometimes supposed to be one who suffers from an extreme degree of general depression, but in medical literature the term denotes one who is morbidly concerned about the state of his health. Hypochondriasis may be looked upon as a form of nervous instability, and insanity, or some other form of nervous disorder, may often be traced in the family history. If this tendency to brood upon quite imaginary or trivial ailments is not checked, the patient may go on to invent monstrous explanations of trifling sensations, such as that he has snakes in his stomach. In most cases the only foundation in fact for his morbid anxiety is some such affection as indigestion, which is maintained and aggravated by his state of mind. The remedy is to be found in cheerful companionship by which his attention may be drawn off

from himself and his interest in what is going on around him stimulated. Endeavours must be made to dissuade him from taking drugs, except under medical direction.

HYSTERIA.—This affection is almost limited to the female sex, but is occasionally met with in highly-strung men and boys. The emotional Latin races are more liable to it than the comparatively phlegmatic Anglo-Saxon; it is also exceptionally prevalent among Jews. There are no traceable lesions in the brain or spinal cord or nerves to account for the symptoms, and the disease is therefore classified as functional, not organic. Its exact nature is not understood, but that it is a true disease, beyond the control of the patient, except in a very slight degree, cannot be denied. It often appears at the time when the child is growing into the woman. One of the influences that conduce to its development is defective moral training. Other influences that favour hysteria are lack of exercise, over-study, and the reading of exciting literature. Hysteria may be brought on by emotional shock, in the form of love disappointment, the strain of nursing, grief, or fright. It may also follow accidents, injuries, and serious illness. Formerly it was thought to be a manifestation of disease of the female sexual organs—hence the name, from the Greek *hustera*, the womb, and while this is not usually the fact, it does happen in a few cases that disease of these organs leads to hysteria.

Symptoms.—These are of the most extraordinary and varied nature; there are few affections, indeed, of which some feature or other is not mimicked by hysteria. Thus, a common symptom is pseudo-paralysis, which may affect the whole of one side, as in hemiplegia, or the whole of the lower part of the body, as in paraplegia, or only an arm, or a leg, or a group of muscles may be put out of action. There may be spasmodic contractions of the body muscles, or the eye or the tongue may be similarly affected. The limbs may be violently contracted, or so stiffened that it is impossible to bend them. Or a condition of catalepsy may arise, the limbs being fixed for an indefinite period in any position in which they are placed. The patient, again, may lose sensation in some part of the body, or, on the other hand, sensation may be abnormally acute in certain parts, and tenderness and pain be complained of. The pain may take very various forms, as, for instance, the sensation of a nail being driven in over the eyebrow, or it may simulate the pain of headache, of rheumatism, or of angina pectoris. A common sensation in hysteria is that of a lump rising in the throat (*globus hystericus*) and producing a feeling of suffocation. The sense of taste, of smell, or of hearing may be temporarily lost, and the voice may be reduced to a whisper. The patient may be untruthful and suspicious, and her morbid craving for sympathy may be such that she will inflict wounds upon herself in order to excite pity and concern. The will is weakened, and she is the prey of every passing whim and impulse.

At times the manifestation of hysteria takes the form of a violent fit, which is known as *hysterics*. The patient screams, falls on the sofa or to the ground, and is seized with convulsions; in turn she screams, cries, groans, and talks unintelligibly. Her responsibility for these proceedings is probably but small, yet it is clear that they are not quite without method. Thus, the patient never falls so as to hurt herself, never bites her tongue, and never injures herself by her violent gesticulations. It will be noticed, too, that the attacks only occur when she is in the presence of others, whom she wishes to move to sympathy or alarm. Nor is she completely unconscious. If, for instance, it is suggested that she should be douched with cold water, she will make it clear that the remedy is not to her liking.

Treatment.—In mild cases, especially in children, little more is necessary than to encourage healthy habits and wholesome exercise and attend to the general health, giving tonics if the patient is run down. In more pronounced cases it is often desirable that the patient be removed from the care of over-sympathetic relatives and have a complete change of scene and surroundings. In such cases the Weir-Mitchell treatment is often beneficial; the patient is kept in bed, sees no one but her nurse, is fed with plenty of easily digested food, and takes passive exercise in the form of massage. In all cases alike the power of reasoned persuasion should be brought to bear, with a view to developing the patient's self-control. Hypnotism has sometimes been employed with success, but this is a remedy which should only be applied by responsible persons. For a " fit " of hysterics the best thing to do is to loosen any tight garments, place the patient on a bed or couch, and leave her to herself. If this is done the convulsions will soon cease. Smelling salts may be applied, but a more effective stimulant is the dashing of cold water in the face, especially as the patient disapproves of it; sometimes the mere mention of it is sufficient to cut short an attack. A measure that is often found to be effectual is to prevent the patient from breathing for a few seconds by compressing the nose and mouth; she struggles to free herself from the

IDIOCY.—This condition may be defined as an imperfect development of the brain resulting in gross mental deficiency. The term "imbecility" denotes mental deficiency of a less pronounced kind. The defect in the brain may be present at birth, may result from injury to the head during birth, or may be due to malnutrition or to disease. The development of the body, as well as of the mind, usually goes awry. The head may be smaller or larger than normal, the teeth defective, the skin coarse and thick, the muscles flaccid, the bones specially liable to fracture, the circulation feeble. Frequently also there are physiological defects, the senses of sight, smell, and hearing being blunted or perverted, and speech being usually defective. Treatment consists in special methods of mental and moral training, in the strict observance of all the rules of health, and in endeavours to modify whatever physical defects are present.

ILLUSIONS (*see* INSANITY).

IMBECILITY (*see* IDIOCY).

IMMUNITY.—The theory of immunity, or resistance to disease, forms a singularly interesting branch of medical science. It has been built up on the fact, observed in quite early times, that in the case of certain diseases one attack serves as a protection against subsequent infection. The first application of this knowledge in the civilized world was the practice, instituted by Jenner, of inducing cowpox, by means of vaccination, as a protection against smallpox, the former disease being probably the

restraint, is thus obliged to make deep inspirations, and this may bring the convulsions to an end.

same as the latter, but milder in degree, because the cow is more resistant to it than man. No further progress was made in this direction until it was discovered that infectious diseases are due to minute living germs (*see* GERMS). Discoveries as to the life-history and toxins (poisons) of these germs followed, and gradually a conception of the real nature of resistance to infectious disease was formed.

We borrow the following lucid exposition of the theory of immunity from the late Sir Malcolm Morris's "Story of English Public Health":

"There is, to begin with, a natural immunity to infectious disease, and this natural immunity may be either racial or individual. Thus, man is immune to swine fever, and the lower animals are immune to leprosy. These are instances of *racial* immunity. To give an example of *individual* immunity: two persons are exposed to the same amount of infection, say of scarlet fever, and while one 'takes' the infection, the other escapes it, the latter being immune —it may be only temporarily—to that disease.

"So much for natural immunity. Acquired immunity may be the result of a previous attack of a disease, or may be induced artificially by inoculation with the causal germ or its poisons. In both cases alike the system is stimulated to the production of antagonistic substances, known as *antibodies*, which act as antidotes. This is the *active* form of acquired immunity, and it is so called because a person who acquires immunity in either of these ways, i.e. by a previous attack or by inoculation, creates his own antibodies or antidotes. In the *passive* form of acquired immunity the work is done for him—that is to say, the antibodies are furnished by the serum of animals that have themselves been actively immunized by inoculation with the germ or its poisons, and he is injected with these antibodies so that they may reinforce his own defensive powers. An example of passive immunity is that resulting from the use of diphtheria antitoxin, consisting of serum from the blood of horses that have been inoculated with the poisons of the diphtheria bacillus in order that they may create antibodies for the benefit of human sufferers.

" The substances used to produce active immunity are termed *vaccines*, and the process by which they are introduced into the system is known as vaccination or inoculation. The substances by which passive immunity is effected are called *serums* or *antitoxins*. An antitoxin is really a serum, but, as the name implies, it is only efficacious against the *poisons* of a germ, while other serums are capable of destroying the germs themselves. The latter, therefore, are *bactericidal* serums, whilst antitoxins are *antitoxic* serums."

Although there is still much to learn in connexion with immunity, this department of medicine has undergone enormous expansion, and has achieved triumphs of great practical importance in smallpox, diphtheria, typhoid fever, plague, cholera, hydrophobia, tetanus, and other diseases. (*See* VACCINE AND SERUM TREATMENT.)

IMPACTED FRACTURES (*see* FRACTURES).

IMPERFORATE ANUS.—Some children are born with no opening through which the contents of the bowel can be discharged. If, therefore, a baby has no action of the bowels within twenty-four hours of birth, the anus should be carefully examined and, if necessary, an operation performed.

IMPETIGO.—The skin affection known as contagious impetigo consists in the eruption of small red spots on which small blisters appear that soon become filled with pus, and then break, discharging a fluid that dries up and forms scabs. If the patient, much more often a child than an adult, can be kept from " picking " the blisters or crusts, the eruption will probably disappear in the course

of a few weeks, but in many cases it is prolonged indefinitely by repeated reinoculations with the finger-nails. The affection may also be communicated from one part of the body to another by contaminated garments. Impetigo is caused by germs which are especially liable to attack delicate and ill-fed children. The affected parts and the surrounding skin should be washed with a lotion of a teaspoonful of boric acid to a tumblerful of warm water, and the scabs softened with carbolized oil or a weak carbolic lotion (1 in 100) and then removed. To prevent scratching, the parts should be covered with sulphur ointment and vaselin or with white precipitate ointment. Injections of collosol manganese are beneficial. Weakly and ill-nourished children should take a course of cod-liver oil and, if possible, should have a change of air. For adults, tonics such as quinine are suitable.

INCONTINENCE OF URINE (*see* URINE, INCONTINENCE OF; BED-WETTING).

INCUBATION PERIODS.—The time which elapses between the entrance of a germ into the body and the onset of symptoms is known as the incubation period. The average incubation periods of the more common fevers are as follows :

Disease	*Incubation period*
Chicken-pox	10—16 days
Diphtheria	2—4 ,,
Erysipelas	1—3 ,,
German measles	14—17 ,,
Influenza	1—5 ,,
Measles	10—14 ,,
Mumps	18—21 ,,
Relapsing fever	2—10 ,,
Scarlet fever	2—3 ,,
Smallpox	12—14 ,,
Typhoid	10—21 ,,
Whooping-cough	10—14 ,,

INDIGESTION.—Is there any difference between indigestion and dyspepsia ? Essentially there is none. The one expression is of Latin, the other of Greek derivation, but they mean the same thing. In common usage, however, " indigestion " generally denotes slight and temporary, and " dyspepsia " severer and more obdurate derangement of the digestive function. There are some who will never use a simple word when a less simple one will do as well, especially when they have to give a name to their own ailments. And " dyspepsia " sounds more important and dignified than " indigestion " !

Indigestion is often not a substantive affection, but a mere symptom of some quite different disease. The digestion is greatly disordered, for example, in fevers, and in grave organic disease of the stomach, such as gastric ulcer or gastric cancer. With indigestion arising from gross disease we are not concerned in this article, but only with such cases of disordered digestion as can be treated more or less directly.

Cause.—For most of our digestive troubles we have ourselves chiefly to thank. Many people, from lack of time or because they do not restrain themselves from eating ravenously, " bolt " their food, and probably few masticate it sufficiently. When it is swallowed in lumps it is not properly mixed with saliva, which digests starchy foods and converts them into sugar, nor is it divided finely enough for the gastric juice secreted by the stomach to act upon it ; thus digestion is delayed and fermentation in the stomach may set up. In some cases food is not masticated sufficiently because of dental difficulties. Worse still, the mouth may be septic, and the food may be polluted with germs from decayed teeth, or from the teeth sockets (*see* PYORRHŒA ALVEOLARIS). Or the food may be poisoned before it is eaten, from having been kept too long, or from lack of cleanliness in keeping or handling it. But food may cause indigestion from no fault in itself but because the consumer has what is called an idiosyncrasy—that is, a special susceptibility—in relation to it. Some people cannot eat strawberries without suffering for the indulgence, others cannot eat a banana without feeling " headachy." Food, again, may be indigestible from bad cooking. It may be toughened by being overdone ; in frying it may be so coated with fat as to be almost impervious to the saliva and the digestive juices. It may be deprived of its flavour or even made unpleasant, and thus the digestive glands may not be stimulated to pour out their secretions.

Further, indigestion may arise not from any fault in the kind of food, or in its condition or preparation, but because of deficiency or excess in the quantity. Some are prone to eat too little and they suffer from indigestion because their digestive organs, in common with their organs generally, are enfeebled. On the other hand, many of us eat too much, especially too much animal food. A man who has got into the habit of eating large meals may feel hungry after a moderate one, but if he gradually diminishes the quantity he will come to feel satisfied without eating to excess. Many, again, without overburdening the stomach at any one time, eat too frequently, so that during the day the stomach is never at rest and never empty. On the other hand, the intervals between meals may be too long, as when little or no food is taken between breakfast and a late dinner. In such cases one " overstays one's appetite," and severe and intractable indigestion may be set up.

Indigestion may also be induced by painful emotions such as anxiety or fright, or even by moroseness and bad temper. Hence the rationale of eating the chief meal of the day in pleasant surroundings and agreeable company, avoiding controversial topics or topics that would put a strain upon the mental faculties. It is a mistake also to engage in either physical or mental exertion after any but a light meal. In order to do its work properly the stomach at these times needs an extra supply of blood ; this it will not get if the brain or the muscles are strenuously exercised, and the result will be indigestion. Further, if one has had to engage in a long spell of work before the chief meal and is fatigued, it is well that there should be an interval of rest—say half an hour—before sitting down to the table.

Symptoms.—The sensations induced by indigestion may be so slight as a mere sense of weight or fullness, or so severe as attacks of colic. If pain comes on before a meal, and is accompanied by a craving for food, it is a reminder that the stomach is empty. If it does not come on until some hours after food is taken, it probably denotes delayed digestion, with fermentation and, perhaps, an excess of acid gastric juice. Heartburn, waterbrash, eructations, hiccough, flatulence, nausea and sickness are common symptoms. The patient usually has distaste, if not repugnance, for food. There may be headache, the tongue is furred, the breath offensive, the bowels are either constipated or loose, the complexion is muddy. The nose may be red and pimply, and there may be a nettlerash. In many cases the patient is alarmed by finding that he has palpi-

tation of the heart, but this is not a sign of heart disease, and is due merely to flatulent distension of the stomach and acidity. He may complain of a feeling of tightness in the chest, or of giddiness. In bad cases he is not only irritable and depressed, but may waste and lose strength, so that the least exertion causes fatigue.

Treatment.—In all cases in which indigestion is not the result of serious organic disease an attempt should be made to determine to what error of diet or of habit it is due. This decided, correction of the error should not be difficult. If the food is " bolted," the habit of deliberate eating must be formed. If the gums are diseased, the doctor must be visited. If teeth have been lost, they should be replaced ; if decayed, they should be stopped or extracted. Constipation, if present, must be relieved ; it will be well to take an aperient to start with and then to rely rather upon food which has enough unassimilable residue to stimulate the bowels (*see* CONSTIPATION). A good plan is to drink in sips a glass of quite hot water while dressing in the morning, when the stomach is empty of food, so as to wash out any mucus that may have accumulated ; and many find this beneficial also before the chief meal of the day.

The food of dyspeptics should be simple in kind and easily digested, and all rich, or highly seasoned, or very sweet dishes should be excluded. Pastry and preserves and jams are liable to set up acidity and fermentation. Fried and twice-cooked meat, and fish and meat that have been salted, cured, or preserved are difficult to digest, and so also are new bread, wholemeal bread, muffins and crumpets, and buttered toast. Breakfast may consist of a boiled egg or boiled fish and stale bread or toast with very little butter, washed down with quite weak China tea, or cocoa or hot milk-and-water; lunch, of lean roast mutton or chicken, mashed potato and spinach, dry toast or stale bread; afternoon tea, of lightly buttered bread and weak China tea; dinner, of half a dozen spoonfuls of clear soup, fish, or lean meat or game, well-cooked green vegetables, stale bread or dry toast, milk pudding and stewed fruit. Among fish, salmon and mullet are usually found indigestible, and even turbot is not so suitable for dyspeptics as sole, whiting, halibut and brill. If toast is taken, one must remember that it requires more mastication than bread. Raw vegetables should be avoided, and pickled vegetables are still more undesirable. If even weak tea disagrees it must, of course, be given up. Milk is an excellent beverage, both hot and cold; it may be diluted, according to taste, with seltzer water or barley water or lime water. If alcohol is taken with meals—it should not be taken at any other times—it must be in strictest moderation. Sound sherry or diluted whisky are the forms most suitable in these cases. As a rule, malt liquors are contra-indicated, but in some cases a glass of bitter or of lager beer may be taken with impunity and even with benefit. Tobacco, again, if used at all, must be used moderately.

Plenty of fresh air, and free exercise not carried to the point of fatigue, are beneficial, but in acute attacks rest in bed may be required. Chronic dyspeptics who suffer from depression of spirits and are over-anxious about their health may be benefited by travel.

To tone up the stomach and improve the general health the following mixture may be recommended :

Sulphate of quinine .... 8 grains
Dilute   nitro - hydrochloric
    acid .... 80 minims
Syrup of orange .... 3 drachms
Water to 8 ounces.

Two tablespoonfuls three times a day, 20 minutes before meals.

If the appetite needs stimulation, a suitable mixture is :

Dilute hydrochloric acid ....80 minims
Dilute hydrocyanic acid ....20 minims
Compound tincture of gentian 4 drachms
Spirit of chloroform ....80 minims
Peppermint water to 8 ounces.

Two tablespoonfuls three times a day, 20 minutes before meals.

In the indigestion of debility a nux-vomica mixture is indicated, such as this :

Tincture of nux vomica.....80 minims
Carbonate of bismuth ......80 minims
Mucilage of gum .... 4 drachms
Tincture of orange ....2½ drachms
Chloroform water to 8 ounces.

Two tablespoonfuls three times a day, 10 minutes before meals.

If anæmia is present, tabloids containing iron, arsenic and strychnia may be taken.

If the pain comes on from two to four hours after meals and is associated with heartburn and acid eructations, the patient is possibly of gouty tendency, and may be advised to clear the bowels with a pill consisting of two grains of blue pill and three grains of colocynth and hyoscamus pill, taken at night, and a dose of aperient mineral water in the morning, and then to begin the following mixture :

Solution   of   bismuth   and
    citrate of ammonia....... 8 drachms
Bicarbonate of soda ....80 grains
Spirit of chloroform .... 2 drachms
Infusion of calumba to 8 ounces.

Two tablespoonfuls three times a day, an hour before food.

If the digestion is very slow, it is probably due to the gastric juice being insufficiently active, a fault which may be corrected by the following mixture :

Tincture of nox vomica..... 2 drachms
Tincture of calumba ...... 3 drachms
Dilute hydrochloric acid ... 1 drachm
Tincture of capsicum.......20 minims
Pepsin ....40 grains
Compound infusion of orange peel to
    8 ounces.
Two teaspoonfuls three times a day, an hour
before meals.

Indigestion in infants has been touched upon in the article INFANTS AND YOUNG CHILDREN, FEEDING OF, but something must here be said about indigestion *in children*. This is usually due to hasty eating or to unsuitable food, but causes such as chill or excessive exercise may come into the account. The child complains of pain at the pit of the stomach, which may be swollen and tender, of drowsiness and headache. Partly-digested food may be returned to the mouth, and there may be retching and vomiting. When the stomach has been relieved by vomiting he may fall asleep and wake feeling much better, but diarrhœa, with colicky pains and rumblings, may ensue, undigested food having passed into the intestine, which it irritates. If the stomach is much distended, treatment may begin with an emetic—for young children 5 grains of powdered ipecacuanha, the dose repeated in ten minutes; for older children, 10 grains, repeated in a quarter of an hour. A dose of castor oil, or of calomel (half a grain to a grain, according to age) may then be given to clear the intestine, and later a sedative mixture :

Bicarbonate of soda........36 grains
Carbonate of magnesia .....36 grains
Syrup of ginger............ 1 drachm
Dill-water to 1½ ounces.
Two teaspoonfuls every four hours.

INFANT, NEW-BORN, CARE OF (*see* LYING-IN PERIOD, MANAGEMENT OF).

INFANTILE CHOLERA (*see* EPIDEMIC DIARRHŒA).

INFANTILE PARALYSIS.—This infectious disease is technically known as *acute poliomyelitis*, the latter word signifying inflammation of the grey matter of the spinal cord. It is predominantly a disease of infancy, but may occur up to the age of ten, and adults are not absolutely exempt from it. The germ is found in the secretions of the nose and throat and intestines, and is probably conveyed by kissing, sneezing, coughing, and spitting, possibly also by articles soiled with a patient's discharges. The germ can be " carried " by healthy persons who, though they do not suffer themselves, are centres of infection. The disease may occur in scattered cases (sporadically) or in epidemics, which are more frequent in summer and autumn. Possibly exposure to cold when over-heated, and fatigue from too much walking in young children, may act as predisposing causes.

Symptoms.—After the incubation period, which is believed to vary from seven to fourteen days, the child suddenly becomes fretful, restless, and feverish ; the temperature may rise as high as 104° Fahr., and with it there may be sickness and diarrhœa. In some cases there is inflammation of the brain as well as of the spinal cord, and delirium and convulsions may ensue, and the head be spasmodically drawn backwards, as in meningitis. The child is evidently in pain, and shows great disinclination to be touched or moved. After a day or two, in a typical case, the mother or nurse notices that one or more of the limbs are not being freely used, and examination then reveals the presence of paralysis, which is at its worst in the course of the first few days. The lower limbs are affected more frequently than the upper. Only one limb, or a few muscles in different parts of the body, may be affected, or nearly all the muscles may be involved, in which case the child can neither sit up nor even hold the head erect, can only breathe feebly, and may be unable to cry. After a few days the stage of fever and development of paralysis may come to an end, the fever passing off and the other symptoms remaining stationary for several weeks, when some or all of the muscles begin gradually to regain power. The recovery of power may continue up to the end of a year from the onset of the illness ; after this, apart from treatment, there is little hope of further improvement. Fortunately, there are cases in which the illness consists almost entirely of fever and the accompanying constitutional symptoms ; in such cases no fear of permanent paralysis need be entertained. Infantile paralysis is attended by a rather considerable mortality, which differs in different epidemics, being as low as 2 per cent. in some and as high as 20 per cent. in others. The disease is more likely to end fatally in adults than in children.

Treatment.—As the infectiousness of infantile paralysis has hardly yet been brought home to the general public, the necessity for isolating the patient must here be insisted upon. In the first stage of the disease nothing more can be done than to keep the bowels open and to give such drugs as aspirin or phenacetin to subdue the fever. The child must, of course, be kept in bed, and the affected limbs should be wrapped up in cotton-wool to maintain an even temperature, while mustard plasters may be applied to the spine. The diet should be limited to fluid and consist chiefly of milk. When the fever is gone the diet may be strengthened, and cod-liver oil with extract of malt given.

After about a fortnight, massage and galvanism may be started, to promote the nutrition of the muscles until the nervous system has begun to return to its duties, and endeavours may be made by passive movements of the limb and the application of splints to prevent deformities and contractures. The greatest care and perseverance are required, and the treatment must be persisted in as long as there is the least chance of further improvement. When there is no more progress to be hoped for, the orthopædic surgeon may be able to lessen any serious deformity that may be present.

INFANTILISM.—This is the name given to cases of retarded growth in which the patient, so far as physical development goes, either remains permanently a child or becomes an adult in miniature. It may be due to the defective secretion of certain glands such as the pituitary and thyroid glands, or to disease of the heart, or kidney, or liver, etc.

INFANTS AND YOUNG CHILDREN, FEEDING OF.—That infants should be fed at the breast is obviously Nature's intention, and not with impunity can her plans be set at naught. The vast majority of infants that perish during the first year of life are hand-fed. Those who are breast-fed not only have a much better chance of escaping digestive disorder and infectious disease, but are likely to enjoy a superior vitality in the years that follow infancy.

The mother's milk is not usually secreted during the first day or two after the birth, but in most cases the child can afford to begin its independent existence with a fast, for it enters the world with the intestines full of a substance known, from its superficial resemblance to poppy juice, as meconium, and until this has been passed in the motions it has no urgent need of food. If, however, it cries and seems hungry, it may have a mixture of milk and water—one part of milk to two parts of water, sweetened and warmed. The sooner the mother can allow it to take the breast, the better. At first it should be fed every two hours, from each breast alternately, and then somewhat less frequently, but the mother must be on her guard against giving the breast too often during the night : an infant's stomach ought not to be kept constantly at work, if indigestion is to be avoided, and the mother should be careful to secure for herself several hours' consecutive sleep. The child should be weaned during the ninth month (*see* WEANING).

Substitutes for human milk.—The best of these substitutes is asses' or goats' milk. The former is very easy to digest, but too weak for any but temporary use unless extra fat and protein are added. Goats' milk is about on the same level of nutrition as cows' milk, but it has the advantage of being much less likely to contain the germs of tuberculosis, for the goat is virtually immune from that disease, while the cow is not. Cows' milk contains about the same proportion of fat as human milk, considerably less sugar, and about twice as much protein. This excess of protein makes dilution necessary in order that the milk may be digested. The dilution should be as 2 to 1 (that is, two parts water to one part milk) in the first month, 1 to 1 in the second month, 1 to 2 in the third, 1 to 3 in the fourth, and 1 to 5 in the fifth month ; after this undiluted milk may be given. Barley water, oatmeal water, or arrowroot water may be employed instead of plain water for the dilution of milk, but not until after the seventh month, for until then infants cannot digest the starch these waters contain.

In exceptional circumstances in which neither goats' not cows' milk is available, partly desiccated (that is condensed) milk or wholly desiccated (dried) milk is the best substitute, but these forms of milk are not suitable for prolonged use. If condensed milk is used, it should be unsweetened.

Quantity of milk.—The amount of milk an infant needs each twenty-four hours differs with the weight of the child. On an average, the daily quantity of good milk containing the full 4 per cent. of cream is about one-eighth of the child's body-weight ; but this proportion may need to be increased to one-seventh in some cases and diminished to one-ninth in others. The proportion, whatever it is, will remain the same, but the *quantity* of milk will, of course, increase with the augmentation of the body-weight.

Number of meals.—The food should be divided into ten meals a day for the first month, nine meals for the second month, eight meals for the third and fourth months, seven meals for the fifth, sixth and seventh months, and six meals afterwards. Not more than one meal should be given during the night, and night feeding should be discontinued altogether as soon as possible. It is a great mistake to feed the child whenever it cries ; this is very frequently the explanation of the regurgitation, followed by vomiting, from which many infants suffer.

Test of good feeding.—Speaking generally, the best test of the suitability of food, both as to quantity and quality, for the individual infant is its gain in weight. Roughly, the weight at birth should be doubled at the end of the fifth month and trebled at the end of the first year. The increase in the first and second months should be 6 to 7 oz. a week ; in the third and fourth months, 5 to 6 oz. ; in the fifth and sixth months, 3½ to 4½ oz. ; in the seventh and eighth months, 2½ to 3½ oz. ; in the ninth to the twelfth month, 2 to 3½ oz. ; and during the second year, ½ lb. a month.

Sterilization of milk.—To prevent the germs of tuberculosis and other diseases from being conveyed to the child by the milk, it should be sterilized—that is, boiled for thirty minutes. The only serious drawback to sterilization is that this process destroys certain food elements, called *vitamins*, which are essential to growth and health (*see under* FOOD). To compensate for this deficiency a little orange or grape juice should be given daily. Pasteurization of food is a modified form of sterilization which consists in heating milk to a temperature of about 156° Fahr., which is 56 degrees below boiling-point. This, however, is not a sufficient safeguard against infection with germs.

At least three times a day the child's mouth should be washed out with a piece of clean boiled linen dipped in weak boric-acid lotion. At the age of six months the glands which secrete the saliva are active, and the mouth-washing need then only be done night and morning.

Peptonized milk.—In cases of wasting it may be necessary to peptonize the milk and so predigest it (*see* Milk, Peptonized, *under* COOKERY, INVALID). This, however, should be regarded as a temporary expedient, to be gradually discontinued as the child's digestion and condition improve. Peptonized food can be flavoured with lemon juice, two teaspoonfuls to four ounces of milk.

Unsuitability of starch for infants.—It has already been hinted that starch should not be included in the food until after the seventh month, for it is only then that the child begins to secrete the ferments that convert starch into sugar, and this function is not thoroughly performed until about the end of the second year. Proprietary foods that contain starch are therefore unsuitable in the early months of infant life : the child may get fat upon them, but the fat may be only a mask for rickets. After the seventh month a little starch, in the form of a proprietary food that contains it, may be added to the milk once or twice a day. The best foods are those malted and other preparations in which the starch is predigested. After the ninth month the diet may include bread, barley water, and (daily) 2 or 3 teaspoonfuls of beef juice and ½ to 2 oz. of orange juice.

After infancy.—From 2 to 5 years of age the daily allowance of good milk should be at least two pints, and during the next two years, at least one pint. Children at this time usually get quite enough starch and sugar, but not enough protein and fat. The protein so necessary to tissue-building may be given in the form not merely of meat, but of eggs, fish, red gravy, plasmon, haricot beans and lentils ; the fat, in the form of butter and cream.

INFANTS, HYGIENE OF.—A great deal of the infant mortality in this country, still much too high, is due primarily to ignorance on the part of the mother as to the treatment her child needs. It is necessary, therefore, in a work such as the present, to give some consideration to the subject of infant management.

Food and feeding has already been considered (*see* INFANTS AND YOUNG CHILDREN, FEEDING OF), teething is dealt with in the article on that subject, and we may begin the present article with some remarks on *cleanliness*. It ought not to be necessary to say that the infant, after the first week of life, should have a bath night and morning. The evening bath should be at a temperature of 100° to 101° Fahr.; the temperature of that given in the morning may be gradually lowered until it is 80° Fahr. Soft water should, if possible, be used, and superfatted soap. At the age of two months a beginning should be made with the process of bracing up the skin to resist chills: a sponge wrung out of water colder than that of the bath may be rapidly passed over the chest and back, and after the bath the child may be left unclothed for a few minutes and encouraged to kick about. The mouth should be washed out daily with a piece of linen applied with the finger, and as the teeth come, a soft tooth-brush should be brought into use.

In the choice of *clothing* the aim must be to prevent the body-heat from escaping too freely, but without causing obvious perspiration. A long vest of woven or knitted wool should be provided, reaching from the shoulders to below the hips, with sleeves as far as the wrists, or at any rate the elbows. The sensitive abdominal organs should be protected from chill by a knitted or woven binder, which should always be worn until the child is two or three years old. The napkin should be made of cotton-wool tissue, which can be burnt after use. The only outer garments necessary are a flannel petticoat and a thin woollen frock extending five or six inches below the feet, to keep out draughts. But when the child is taken out of doors in a perambulator, wraps, of course, will be required, and in cold weather a hot-water

bottle should be placed near the feet. Shetland shawls are much better than cloaks. As the infant grows and takes delight in kicking, the clothes can be shortened, but the legs and thighs must be kept well covered with knitted drawers placed over the napkin and firmly attached to the binder.

Few mothers sufficiently recognize the importance of keeping infants well supplied with *fresh air*. Even in well-ventilated rooms the air should be changed every three or four hours by opening the doors and windows for a few minutes. If the child in its cot is entirely covered while this is done there will be no danger of a chill being taken. The child should gradually be made to breathe cold air—not through the mouth, but through the nose, so that the air may be warmed before it reaches the lungs. The child should be trained to keep its mouth shut, both when asleep and when awake. While seeing that there is a proper supply of fresh air, the mother must, of course, be careful to keep the child warm. Its limbs should never feel cold to the touch, and, if necessary, well protected hot-water bottles should be placed in the cot. A week after birth a room temperature of 55° to 60° Fahr. is high enough.

If the baby is healthy it will spend nearly all its time in *sleep*, except when it is feeding. An occasional fit of crying is a thing to be desired, because it expands the lungs. After a few weeks there will be longer intervals of wakefulness. The custom of rocking a child to sleep is ridiculous, if not harmful. After being fed, it should be laid on its right side, never on its back, lest it be choked by regurgitation of the food. An infant should never sleep with its mother or any other grown-up person, for, apart from the danger of overlying, it is impossible for the child to breathe fresh air with its head below the bedclothes.

Finally, it may be pointed out that many mothers, in their natural eagerness to see signs of dawning intelligence, make the mistake of over-stimulating the nervous system of their children. There can be no doubt that if there were less " fussing " of infants there would be fewer cases of nervous instability. In its first weeks or months of life the child should live as placid an existence as possible, and the mother who is constantly trying to make her child coo and smile and recognize things, unwittingly sacrifices its welfare to her own pleasure. The intelligence and affections of a normal child may be left to develop without any intentional stimulation.

INFECTIOUS DISEASE (*see* DISEASE, CLASSIFICATION OF).

INFLAMMATION.—This is the name given to the series of changes that occurs in greater or less degree whenever any structure in the body is irritated or injured, whether by violence, as in a fractured bone or dislocated joint, by an incised wound, by burns and scalds, by the action of chemicals, or by disease germs. Of these various causes of inflammation, that which is due to germs is by far the most serious. It is also the most frequent, and in many instances germs come in to complicate and aggravate the inflammation which originates in other ways. Inflammation in which disease germs are at work is called *septic*, i.e. poisoned ; that in which they have no part, *aseptic*—free from poison.

The various agents mentioned above are the *exciting causes* of inflammation. There are also *predisposing causes*,

which comprise all the conditions that lower vitality and so lessen the individual's power of resistance to noxious influences. One of the commonest of these predisposing causes is cold, which for the time being may depress the local or general vitality, or both, and so give their chance to any microbes of disease we carry about with us or may happen to encounter.

Inflammation, it should be understood, is not a mere destructive process, but also serves the end of repairing the mischief that has been done. It is made up both of destruction and of repair, and though these two processes are separated in thought, they are essentially one. If the inflammation is very severe, the destructive process is in the ascendant ; but the process of repair is never entirely absent, and in some cases is more important than the process of destruction.

Signs and symptoms.—The classical signs of inflammation, so called because they were familiar to the physicians of the ancient world, are redness, heat, swelling and pain. A fifth sign now recognized is impairment or loss of function, the proper working of the part affected being interfered with by its inflamed state. After a time, inflammation tends to cause general, or constitutional, symptoms, which are summed up in the word fever.

Treatment of acute inflammation.—We shall consider first what must be done in cases in which no germs are present—*simple* or *aseptic* inflammation. The first step is *to remove the cause*. Whether this takes the form of a piece of grit in the eye, of indigestible food in the stomach, of stone in the bladder, or what not, it must be got rid of. The next requisite is *rest*. An inflamed eye, for example, should be protected from the light by a covering, an inflamed limb should be raised and supported to allow the excess of blood to drain out. Another way of relieving the inflamed part of blood is to make an incision, or to apply leeches. Or the blood may be driven out of the vessels by making them contract under the application of *cold*, in the form of a compress (*see* COMPRESSES), or of a waterproof bag filled with ice. Or cold may be applied as an evaporating lotion— an ounce of strong solution of sugar of lead, and half a pint of methylated spirit of wine to three parts of distilled or rain water ; in this, two or three folds of a piece of lint or linen are soaked, laid upon the inflamed part, exposed to the air, and kept constantly wet. The rapid evaporation will abstract the heat from the part, just as the evaporation of sweat abstracts heat from the body generally, and so the inflammation will tend to subside. The same end may be secured by the application of *heat*. Moist heat is more convenient than dry heat (hot flannel), but the latter is to be preferred in colic and neuralgia. Moist heat may be applied as poultices, fomentations, or compresses, and a sedative such as laudanum, tincture of belladonna, or aconite liniment may be added. As to whether heat or cold is the better means of subduing inflammation, no absolute rule can be laid down, but cold is better when the tissues of the part are loose and swelling can take place freely, and also in the case of sprained joints, while heat is more efficacious when " matter " is forming and the part is hot and throbbing.

In the early stage of *septic* inflammation the treatment is the same as for simple inflammation. When pus has formed, an incision is made to let out the matter and a tube or piece of gauze is introduced so that any further pus may readily come to the surface and escape. Fomentations should then be applied to hasten the removal of the products of inflammation by stimulating the flow of blood and the healthy action of the tissues. If a limb is inflamed, instead of applying fomentations it is better to immerse the inflamed part in a hot bath of diluted antiseptic solution which can be kept at about the same temperature by adding more solution from time to time.

Treatment of chronic inflammation. — Chronic inflammation is usually the result of an acute attack that has been imperfectly cured. *Counter-irritation* is employed in the form of blisters, or tinctures, or ointments, in addition to the measures recommended for simple inflammation. Blisters (q.v.) are most serviceable for inflamed joints ; the tincture in most frequent use is the tincture of iodine, which should be painted thoroughly over the part with a brush ; a useful ointment for counter-irritation is the compound ointment of mercury, " Scott's dressing," which should be thickly spread on slips of lint about $1\frac{1}{2}$ inches wide, and long enough to go well round the limb. The slips are applied diagonally round a limb and then covered with strips of lead strapping. Another kind of treatment consists in the application of *pressure*, with the view of causing the absorption of the exudate before it can be converted into fibrous tissue and so set up the condition known as fibrosis. The limb may be strapped from below upwards with lead plaster, or elastic bandages may be used—Martin's bandages, which are plain india-rubber, elastic-web bandages, or stockinette bandages ; the latter of these, having in them no india-rubber, can be washed. They are put on evenly with spiral turns round the limb (*see* BANDAGES). Pressure may be supplemented by *massage*, combined with *passive movements* to break down adhesions that may be forming. *Hydropathy* and *electrical treatment* are also beneficial.

INFLAMMATION OF THE BLADDER (*see* BLADDER, INFLAM- MAT ON OF).

INFLAMMATION OF THE BOWELS (*see* BOWELS, INFLAMMA- TION OF).

INFLAMMATION OF THE BRAIN (*see* MENINGITIS, SUPPURA- TIVE and ENCEPHALITIS LETHARGICA).

INFLAMMATION OF THE KIDNEY (*see* BRIGHT'S DISEASE).

INFLAMMATION OF THE LIVER (*see* LIVER ABSCESS; CIRRHOSIS OF THE LIVER).

INFLAMMATION OF THE LUNGS (*see* PNEUMONIA).

INFLAMMATION OF THE PLEURA (*see* PLEURISY).

INFLAMMATION OF THE STOMACH (*see* GASTRITIS).

INFLAMMATION OF THE TONSILS (*see* TONSILLITIS, ACUTE).

INFLAMMATION OF VEINS (*see* PHLEBITIS).

INFLUENZA. — When influenza raged in this country in 1889–90, it was regarded by many as a new disease, for there had been no previous epidemic in Great Britain since 1847–8. It is, however, one of the historic diseases, which can be traced back at least as far as the early years of the sixteenth century. Painful as are the symptoms, it is usually more serious in its after-effects than in its immediate results, especially in those who are already weakened by previous disease, or are prone to bronchitis or pneu-

monia; but a curious feature of the severe epidemic of 1918–19 was that it was strong young adults rather than the aged or the weakly who succumbed. It has been found to recur epidemi- cally at intervals of thirty-three weeks, but, fortunately, it seldom comes in a severe form. The epidemic of 1927 was a distinctly severe one, the deaths from this cause in England and Wales in the first quarter of the year number- ing 17,931. The disease leaves in its train a degree of prostration altogether disproportionate to the severity of the illness. This is one of the reasons why, so far from conferring any degree of immunity upon the patient, it inflicts upon him a strong predis- position to contract the disease again. Influenza is undoubtedly a germ disease. A microbe which is named *Bacillus influenzæ* would appear to be chiefly responsible, but other germs are also culpable.

Symptoms.—After an incubation period varying from a few hours to four or five days the patient, in an average case, feels severe aching pains in the eyes, head, and back, and is feverish. The disease may especially attack either the breathing organs, or the stomach and intestines, or the nervous system. In the first of the three groups all the symptoms of a common cold will be present, and the inflammation may spread upwards from the throat and nose to the ear, or downwards to the bronchial tubes and the lungs. In the second group there may be a good deal of pain in the abdomen, with violent vomiting and diarrhœa. In the third group the headache which is seldom absent from any case of influenza may be intense, and delirium, or widely- diffused neuralgia or neuritis, or paralytic symptoms may develop. Sometimes the heart is affected. The prostration which is so frequently a sequel of influenza is often accompanied by great depression of spirits.

Treatment.—The first thing for the patient to do is to take to his bed, where he should remain until the temperature has been normal for at least four days. He should be isolated, and, for the sake of those who have to wait upon him, as well as in his own interests, the sickroom should be well ventilated, though he must not, of course, be exposed to draughts. The medical man may give hourly doses of salicin for the first twelve hours and then every two hours for the following twelve hours, or phenol, a quarter to half a grain every hour or two until the urine becomes dark brown, in the hope of aborting the illness. If this should fail, the pains in the back and limbs must be attacked. The following mixture will be beneficial:

Salicylate of soda	96 grains
Bicarbonate of potash	120 grains
Bromide of potash	80 grains
Oil of lemon	8 minims
Chloroform water to 8 ounces.	

Two tablespoonfuls every four or six hours.

If there is much restlessness and insomnia, 10 grains of compound ipecacuanha powder and 10 grains of trional may be given for the first night or two. If the expectorated mucus is very thick, a glass of hot milk containing half a teaspoonful of bicarbonate of soda should be taken the last thing at night. If bronchopneumonia develops, it must be treated like an ordinary case of that disease. Warm applications to the chest, such as antiphlogistine, and stimulating liniments are comforting. In cases where there are gastric symptoms, such as pain and vomiting, powders containing bicarbonate of soda, magnesia, and salicylate of bismuth may be taken. While the fever lasts the diet must be limited to liquids, but these should be administered freely and in nourishing forms, such as milk and milk foods, egg-flip, light meat soups, etc. If there is much thirst, home-made lemonade will be a welcome beverage. As soon as the temperature has become normal, a gradual return to solid food may be permitted. If at this stage there is much depression and prostration, a little alcoholic stimulant is desirable, such as a glass of good sound port wine twice a day. During convalescence the quinine and iron mixture (p. 42) will be found useful. The patient must not be in a hurry to go out of doors, and when he does venture forth must be careful to avoid chills. One of the best preventives of a second attack is ammoniated tincture of quinine, a teaspoonful three times a day in half a wineglassful of soda water.

INGROWING EYELASHES (*see* Eyelashes, Ingrowing).

INGROWING TOENAIL (*see* Nails, Diseases of).

INGUINAL HERNIA (*see* Rupture).

INHALATIONS.—The application of drugs to the mucous membrane of the nose, mouth, throat, windpipe, bronchial tubes and, to a limited degree, to the lungs, is a method employed (1) to promote the removal of expectoration from the air-tubes, as in bronchitis, (2) to neutralize the odour of offensive expectoration, (3) to soothe irritable conditions of the air-passages, (4) to relieve spasm, or nervous irritability, as in asthma, (5) to dry up secretion and produce an astringent effect. Some drugs, such as chloroform and ether, give off vapours at the ordinary temperature of the air, but usually a small quantity of the substance has to be put into boiling water, when its vapour is inhaled with the steam. Steam alone is also used as an inhalation.

Inhalations may take the form of medicated cigarettes, of pastilles, or of sprays. But most commonly the drug and boiling water are placed in a vessel (Fig. 29) with a spout and short tube, the patient putting his mouth to the tube and so breathing in the steam; or this may be inhaled by holding the head over a jug. If the inhalation is intended for the nose only, it is drawn up the nostrils and then driven

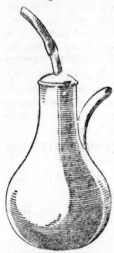

down them, but if for the larynx or the lungs, deep breaths have to be taken through the nose and mouth. Each inhalation may occupy about five minutes, and may be repeated at hourly or less frequent intervals. After an inhalation the patient should not go out of doors for at least half an hour. Among special

Fig. 29.—Inhaler.

inhalers is one used for chloride of ammonium, the fumes of which are beneficial in chronic inflammatory conditions of the throat and bronchial tubes with thick, tenacious expectoration. Sometimes the inhalation is dropped on the pad or sponge of a respirator. The inhalations given below will be found of service in the conditions indicated in the headlines:

For Chronic Laryngitis and Bronchitis and for Consumption

Oil of Scotch pine..........40 minims
   Or pinol ....40 minims
   Or terebene ....40 minims
Light carbonate of magnesia 20 grains
Water to 1 ounce.
A teaspoonful to be added to a pint of water at a temperature of 140° Fahr.

For Nasal Catarrh, Asthma, etc.

Oil of eucalyptus ....20 minims
Light carbonate of magnesia 10 grains
Water to 1 ounce.
A teaspoonful to be added to a pint of water at a temperature of 140° Fahr.

One of the simplest inhalations in nasal catarrh, which will be found useful when the nose is blocked up by the inflamed mucous membrane, is obtained by pouring a little friar's balsam into a jug of steaming water.

INJECTIONS.—Injections are made into the rectum—the lower part of the intestine—to produce an action of the bowels, to check diarrhœa, to relieve pain and flatulence, or to administer nourishment in cases where it cannot be taken through the mouth. Injections, medicated or non-medicated, are also made into the vagina in various conditions of the female sexual organs. Besides these more ordinary kinds of injection, saline fluid is passed into the rectum to counteract shock in serious surgical operations, or to neutralize the effect of severe hæmorrhage, and drugs, including serums and vaccines, are introduced under the skin—*hypodermic* or *subcutaneous* injections; or into the veins—*intravenous* injections; or into the muscles—*intramuscular* injections; or into the spinal cord—*intrathecal* injections. Into the details of these and other injections the performance of which demands technical skill, we need not enter in these pages.

Aperient injections.—These injections, now often called enemata, and formerly clysters, are employed where an immediate action of the bowels is desirable, or where aperient medicines cannot be taken through the mouth and it is desired to unload the lower part only of the bowels.

The syringe ordinarily used is Higginson's (Fig. 30), consisting of an india-rubber ball which, when worked by squeezing, acts as a force pump, with two tubes, and a valve so arranged that liquids enter by the one tube and leave by the other. At one end of the tube is a nozzle; the other end is placed in the vessel containing the injection, which should be at a temperature of 100° Fahr. A simple and common injection takes the form of a pint to a pint and a half of soapsuds and water. One and a half to two ounces of soft soap, warmed by being placed near the fire, may be rubbed down with a little water into a creamy substance and the rest of the water added. Or ordinary yellow soap may

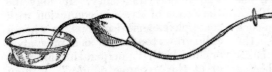

Fig. 30.—Higginson's syringe.

be finely shredded, and melted by pouring over it boiling water and letting it stand in a warm place. In obstinate cases 3 or 4 ounces of olive oil may be injected two or three hours before the soap-and-water with the view of softening the contents of the bowel, or an ounce of castor oil may be added to the soap-and-water, or a sulphate-of-magnesia enema may be made by adding an ounce of Epsom salts and an ounce of olive oil to 15 ounces of water in which 3 drachms of starch have been boiled. The best aperient injection for children is glycerin, given warm with a special syringe which holds from 2 drachms to an ounce. If the aperient injections described above are given to children, only a portion of the injection may be used—4 to 6 ounces, and for a baby one ounce is enough.

To receive an injection the patient should lie on the left side with the back towards the nurse, and close enough to the edge of the bed for part of the body to project over it. The head should be kept low by removing the pillow, which, folded in half, should be placed under the hips so as to elevate them, and covered with some waterproof material. Before the syringe is used, air must be expelled from it; this may be done by placing the metal end of it in the fluid and working the ball until there is a steady flow of fluid through the nozzle. Having been well oiled, the nozzle is gently introduced into the orifice and the fluid slowly injected. After the withdrawal of the nozzle the buttocks should be pressed together for a few minutes to help the patient to retain the injection as long as possible. The direction of the bowel is towards the left side and backwards, and the tube should, therefore, be pointed towards the left hip-bone. No force must be used, lest the tube should injure the bowel.

Vaginal injections. — Vaginal douches, as injections into the vagina are more commonly called, are given to cleanse the mucous membrane of the passage and wash away any accumulated discharge, to relieve inflammation and act as an astringent, to remove the thickening and swelling left after a severe attack of inflammation, and to check hæmorrhage. The fluid may consist simply of water, either hot or cold, or of medicated water, the latter being usually raised to a temperature of about 100° Fahr. The temperature of douches of hot water may be 105°, 110°, or even 115°. The last temperature will at first be felt to be almost unbearable, but after a few douches have been given the patient becomes accustomed to it.

For very hot douches a special nozzle is used with a double channel, and with a rim to close the orifice of the vagina so that the hot water has to return through one of the two channels, and is thus prevented from coming into contact with the skin, which is more sensitive to heat than is the mucous membrane. The openings through which the fluid is discharged are at the sides of the nozzle, and not at the end, so that there may be no risk of the fluid being driven into the womb. The patient may use either a Higginson syringe (*see* above) with a vaginal tube fixed to it, or a douche-can—a metal or earthenware vessel holding from one to two quarts which is hung on the wall or placed on a table about 3 feet above the level of the patient's body. To it is fixed a tube ending in a stop-cock and nozzle. In giving a douche the tap is turned on until the tube is emptied of air and the fluid begins to flow; it is then turned off until the nozzle has been inserted into the vagina, when the fluid is allowed to run until the can is nearly empty— nearly, but not quite, for if the nozzle is not withdrawn while there is still water in the douche-can, air may enter.

The patient lies on her back on a circular bed-pan or bed-bath, the hips being thus raised above the level of the shoulders. If the douche is self-administered, the nozzle, soaked in carbolic lotion (1 in 40), warmed, and lubricated with carbolized vaselin, is carried under one knee and gently passed backwards and upwards. The fluid must be allowed to run in slowly and gently; if too much force is employed pain may be caused, or inflammation set up, or air may be driven into the womb and the Fallopian tubes. After use the entire apparatus must be carefully cleansed before being put away, lest it become infected with germs.

Among *soothing* injections for the vagina are decoction of poppy-heads, weak starch, linseed tea, boric acid (a tablespoonful to a pint of water), and subacetate of lead (a tablespoonful to a pint of water). For *astringent* injections, alum (one or two teaspoonfuls to a pint of water), decoction of oak bark (with an equal quantity of water), chloride of zinc (5 to 10 grains to a pint of water), are suitable. Warm water should be used.

INJURIES (*see* WOUNDS).

INSANITY.—The causes of insanity are very various. The condition may be present at birth, as in idiocy and imbecility. It may be the result of stress in connexion with some physiological process, as when a child grows too fast, or as in pregnancy or child-birth (" puerperal insanities "), or at the " change of life." It may also be caused by the poisons of other diseases, such as the infectious fevers, consumption and syphilis, or it may be due to alcoholism, starvation, accident and shock, worry, exhaustion and overwork. Yet other causes of insanity are cerebral tumours, apoplexy, injury to the brain, and senile decay. But probably the most important of all the factors in the production of insanity is *heredity*. In the family history of many of the patients there is a record either of insanity or of nervous instability. It is not insanity, as such, that is transmitted, but a *tendency* to insanity. Whether or not the tendency develops will depend upon the strain to which the possessor of it is exposed in his passage through life.

Idiocy, general paralysis of the insane, and puerperal insanity are dealt with separately; in this place we shall very briefly consider Mania,

Melancholia, Recurrent Mania and Melancholia, Delusional Insanity, Stupor, and Dementia.

Mania.—Mania may be roughly defined as insanity characterized by mental exaltation. In the milder forms the memory is but little affected, and perception becomes keener and more rapid, but the reasoning faculty is impaired, the patient is talkative and boastful, and sometimes mischievous, is irritable and restless, and is intolerant of control or guidance. In many cases the patient is ecstatically happy, but there are rapid transitions to moods of irritability and antagonism.

Melancholia.—This, one of the most common forms of insanity, comes on gradually, and is often a sequel to an exhausting illness or a severe mental shock. In some respects it is the antithesis of mania. Instead of ecstatic happiness, the patient's mood is one of profound depression, and the mind is not abnormally active, but sluggish. In the milder stages there may be nothing more than a feeling of despondency accompanied by a vague sense of fear, with confusion of thought, impairment of memory, inability to come to conclusions or to take action, and a pronounced tendency to sleeplessness. In more advanced cases the patient may have delusions of various kinds. In all forms of melancholia there is a proneness to suicide or self-mutilation.

Recurrent mania and melancholia.—In this form of insanity there may be "lucid intervals" lasting from a few days to years. Attacks of mania or of melancholia follow each other, but in some cases an attack of the one is succeeded by an attack of the other, the alternation being regularly maintained : this is called *manic-depressive insanity*. The patient may be the victim of a great variety of foolish notions, or they may be confined to a single subject (*monomania*). In the former he gradually becomes irritable and suspects all those around him of having designs upon his life or well-being.

In the more limited forms of **delusional insanity** the patient may believe that he is constantly being experimented upon by scientists, or that he has been placed by Act of Parliament in a condition in which it is possible for everyone to mesmerize him, etc. Patients of this class need very careful watching lest they attempt crimes of violence.

Stupor.—This condition may be regarded as intermediate between mania and melancholia ; in many cases it is a transition stage from one to the other. In one form the stupor is termed *resistive*, an impulse to any action, such as dressing or undressing, being immediately countered by an opposite impulse. In the other form of stupor the patient does not seem so much to resist impulses to action as to be destitute of all power to act. In both forms the patient may become cataleptic (*see* CATALEPSY), or he may suddenly become rational for a time, or the stupor may give place to maniacal frenzy in which murder or suicide may be committed.

Dementia.—This form of insanity may be temporary or permanent. *Temporary* dementia may be the result of alcoholism or of addiction to drugs, or a sequel of severe illness or of acute mental attacks, or it may be due to fright and shock, or overexertion, mental or physical. The symptoms may be simply defective memory, incapacity for mental application, confusion of mind, and a proneness to self-indulgence. In severer cases these symptoms are greatly emphasized. *Permanent* dementia may be the result of acute mental attacks, or of severe injury to the brain, or it may be due to the encroachments of age—senile dementia. In many cases, as the dementia progresses, the patient is the subject of delusions and hallucinations of the kind described under delusional insanity. Finally he becomes bedridden.

In some cases the symptoms of dementia begin early in adult life; such cases are classified as *dementia præcox*—premature dementia. Most rfequently they occur in families tainted with epilepsy or some other nervous affection, or with actual insanity. In the majority of cases the onset takes place between the fifteenth and thirtieth years.

We need not enter into the question of treatment of the various forms of insanity, for it has, as a rule, to be carried out in special institutions.

INSOMNIA.—Of the changes which take place in the brain when the waking is exchanged for the sleeping state, little is known. One theory is that the processes which bring neighbouring brain-cells into contact with each other are retracted as the brain and the body generally become fatigued, and so the cells are for the time being disconnected, sleep being the result. Whether this is the true explanation or not, there can be no doubt that in those who suffer from insomnia there is often some measure of cerebral instability, which in many cases is inherited. In such persons, brain fatigue, instead of predisposing to sleep, leaves the brain irritated and restless. The same is true of worry: an amount of trouble or anxiety which would have no appreciable effect upon normally constituted persons may unfit for sleep those who are highly strung. It is sometimes supposed that sleeplessness is induced by great mental activity. This, however, is not so, unless the mental activity is associated with instability. Some men who have been famous as prodigious brain workers have been remarkable for being able to sleep almost, if not quite, at will.

Causes.—About the exciting causes of sleeplessness there is no mystery. Many cases are due to over-indulgence in tea, coffee, alcohol, and tobacco, which excite the heart and cause it to send too much blood to the brain. On the other hand a moderate dose of alcohol at bed-time may promote sleep, and when a person is "too tired to sleep," a cup of tea or coffee may act as a nervous restorative, and so induce sleep. Insomnia may also be caused by unhealthy states of the circulation. The brain may receive too much blood as in congestion of the brain, or too little as in anæmia. Or the temperature of the blood may be raised, and it may contain irritating poisons, as in gout, rheumatism, and malaria. Digestive disturbances, especially when they cause flatulent distension and palpitation, may be another cause of insomnia. Sleep, again, may be discouraged by mere discomfort, as from cold feet or from the bed being too warm.

Treatment.—If the digestion is at fault, the last substantial meal of the day must be taken not less than three or four hours before bed-time. If, however, sleep is difficult because of exhaustion from lack of food, a little light nourishment, such as malted milk, should be taken shortly before going to bed. If the trouble is due to constipation, this must be corrected. If the patient is plethoric the diet should be modified; if anæmic, a course of iron should be taken (*see* ANÆMIA). If the brain is overcharged with blood from severe mental application, mental work should cease at least an hour before bed-time, and a walk be taken, or the mind be diverted by light reading. If the bed is too warm, the remedy is obvious. If the feet are cold they should be well rubbed with a rough towel before getting into bed, and a hot-water bottle may be used. In some cases, especially where there is mental excitement, a hot bath is found to be serviceable. Many persons find that they are helped to go to sleep by having a warm drink the last thing. In all cases alike an effort should be made to control the thoughts. Too many people make the mistake of allowing themselves, when they get to bed, to muse over the events of the day. They should go to bed to sleep, and, hard as it may seem at first, it is possible to check the activity of the mind, either by conscious exercise of will or by counting certain numbers over and over again, or mentally repeating familiar words or lines of poetry without attending closely to their meaning.

A word of warning must be given with regard to sleep-inducing drugs (*see* NARCOTICS AND HYPNOTICS). If sleep is prevented by mental over-activity, bromide of potash or of soda, from 5 to 25 grains, in an ounce of chloroform water, may be taken, and a dose or two may also be taken during the day. In most cases belonging to this group nothing more will be necessary than this sedative. If it is ineffectual, a medical man should be consulted.

In cases where sleeplessness is due to severe pain as in neuralgia, bad headache, rheumatism, etc., hypnotics are of little avail, for they have no power to subdue pain. In such cases, a couple of 5-grain aspirin tablets may give the needed relief, and with the cessation of pain, sleep may come in due course. If, however, the pain is too great to yield to aspirin and the patient is suffering from the effects of prolonged sleeplessness, the medical attendant may feel it necessary to administer a narcotic, such as opium, in the form of laudanum, or of morphia, or of the preparation known as nepenthe. Narcotics, beneficial as they are in assuaging acute pain, must never be taken except in cases of necessity They leave behind them a train of disagreeable symptoms, such as constipation, indigestion, and headache, and there is danger of their setting up a craving for the drug which may lead to the formation of a habit worse even than the alcohol habit.

INSULIN (*see under* DIABETES MELLITUS).

INTERCOSTAL NEURALGIA (*see* NEURALGIA).

INTERNAL SECRETIONS (*see* DUCTLESS GLANDS).

INTERSTITIAL KERATITIS (*see* KERATITIS).

INTERTRIGO (*see* CHAFING).

INTESTINAL OBSTRUCTION (*see* BOWELS, OBSTRUCTION OF).

INTESTINES (*see* DIGESTION).

INTUSSUSCEPTION(*see*BOWELS, OBSTRUCTION OF).

INUNCTION (*see* OINTMENTS).

INVALID COOKERY(*see*COOKERY, INVALID).

IONIC MEDICATION (*see* ELECTRICAL TREATMENT).

IRITIS.—Inflammation of the iris, the coloured part of the eye, is in most cases due either to syphilis, rheumatism, or gonorrhœa, but it may also be the result of injury. The eye becomes bloodshot, and is usually very painful, and the bright spot in the centre of the eye—the pupil—becomes irregular in shape instead of circular, as well as small. The affection is too serious for domestic treatment. A mercurial ointment may be rubbed in, but reliance must be placed chiefly on dilating the pupil by instilling drops of atropine solution so as to draw the iris away from the lens and prevent it from adhering to that structure. If there is a tendency to rheumatism, salicylate of soda (10 grains) may be taken, or colchicum wine (10 minims) with iodide of potash (3 grains), thrice a day. The affected eye must be shaded and completely rested, and in cases in which light is very painful, both eyes should be protected.

IRRITANT POISONS (*see* Poisons and Poisoning).

ITCH.—The disagreeable affection known as "the itch," or scabies, is due to a minute animal parasite, *Acarus* (or *Sarcoptes*) *scabiei*, popularly termed the itch-mite. The mischief is entirely caused by the female acarus, which is just large enough to be visible to the naked eye as a whitish spot. Her plan of campaign, when she is ready to lay her eggs, is to bore her way into the skin, make a burrow from an eighth to half an inch long, and comfortably install herself at the end of it, remaining there a couple of months, and depositing about fifty eggs. As these are hatched they find their way out on to the surface. The male acarus does not enter the burrow, but remains on the skin and, being not more than half the size of the female, is only discoverable with the aid of a microscope. The parts specially attractive to the female are those where the skin is thin—the webs between the fingers and toes, the front of the wrist, the ankles, the elbows, various parts of the sexual organs, and the breasts in women.

Symptoms.—The itching which has given to this affection its name is often very troublesome, and is sometimes felt in places at a distance from the burrows made by the parasite. As a result of the scratching thus provoked, and of inflammation, pimples of various kinds appear, some of them filled with pus. In persistent cases, and in persons with an irritable skin, the trouble may not cease with the destruction of the parasite, but may be the starting-point of eczema or some other cutaneous affection, and if the itching is so severe and so constant as to prevent sleep, the general health may be seriously affected.

Treatment.—The patient should be stripped, and the affected parts soaked with hot water and scrubbed with soft soap to remove the superficial layers of the outer skin and lay open the burrows. Sulphur ointment, half a drachm to an ounce of vaselin, should then be well rubbed in at intervals of a few hours for two or three days, to destroy the parasite. For infants, and patients with delicate skins, either weak balsam of Peru ointment or stavesacre may be substituted. To soothe the skin, boric-acid ointment or carbolic-acid or menthol soap may be recommended. The itching may continue for some little time after the parasite has been destroyed. The clothing and bedclothes should be disinfected by boiling or by steam.

ITCHING.—This sensation, in the slighter degrees almost pleasurable, in its severer degrees almost maddening, is a feature of many skin diseases, including those due to attacks of parasites. But in some cases there are no lesions of the skin, and no indication of the presence of parasites, to account for the itching, and it is with these cases that we are concerned here. The *pruritus*—to use the medical name—may be either generalized or local. In *generalized* pruritus the itching may affect any part of the body. It is due to affections such as diabetes, Bright's disease, gout, rheumatism, jaundice, derangements of the liver and stomach. In one group of cases, peculiar to the winter months, the itching is usually limited to the limbs, is most felt when the patient is warm in bed, and is most often met with in the gouty and rheumatic. In another group (*senile* pruritus), degeneration of the skin as the result of age appears to be the cause, the affection seldom beginning until the age of sixty-five. *Local* pruritus specially affects the anus, the external female organs, the scrotum in men, the nostrils, the palms of the hands or the soles of the feet. In women it may be dependent upon some disorder of the internal sexual organs, and often occurs at the " change of life." When the anus is the part affected the irritation may be due to piles, to fissures or ulcers, or to the pressure of hard fæces in the lower bowel. Most of the cases of itching in the palms and soles are gouty.

Treatment.—If the itching is *generalized*, silk or linen-mesh underclothing should be substituted for flannel. If the external sexual organs are the seat of the irritation the urine should be examined for sugar, and if this is discovered the patient should be dieted as for diabetes. In all cases alike, if the itching is persistent, stimulants, including tea and coffee, should be avoided, as also should highly seasoned, salted and preserved foods. If gout is suspected, a Plummer's pill may be taken at bedtime. In many cases of pruritus, benefit is derived from carbolic acid ($\frac{1}{2}$ grain) and valerianate of zinc (3 grains) in a capsule, taken after meals. Other useful drugs are aspirin and antipyrin, which may be obtained in tablets. When the whole or a large part of the body is affected, Turkish baths, or a warm bath medicated with bicarbonate of soda, 2 ounces to 30 gallons of water, may give relief. In *local* pruritus the application of heat by means of a sponge squeezed out of hot water and firmly pressed on the affected part should be tried. Simple evaporating lotions, such as a mixture of ordinary vinegar with water in equal parts, or eau-de-Cologne and water in equal parts, will in many cases give relief for the time being. Another simple remedy is menthol ; the cone should be wetted with alcohol or water and the part rubbed with it. But itching is often a most intractable condition, and if the measures here recommended are ineffective and the patient's health is suffering from the persistent irritation, medical advice should be sought. In all cases alike care should be taken not to form a habit of scratching. The effect of much scratching is to roughen the skin and produce in its structure changes which themselves provoke further itching, a " vicious circle " being thus established.

J

JACKSONIAN EPILEPSY.—The form of epilepsy (q.v.) in which the convulsions are at first localized, named after Hughlings-Jackson, a famous English neurologist.

JAUNDICE.—This condition is due to obstruction to the flow of bile, which, remaining within the minute channels in the liver itself, or in the ducts which convey it to the intestine, is taken up by the blood, with the result that the structures of the various tissues of the body are stained yellow : hence the name, from *jaune*, the French for yellow. A common cause of the obstruction is the presence of gall-stones (*see* GALL-STONES). Another cause is a slight inflammation of the mucous membrane which lines the liver-ducts on the inner side, due to chill ; this form of the affection is known as catarrhal jaundice. Jaundice may be produced, again, by nervous disturbance, such as violent anger or intense fear, or by anxiety such as may be felt in sitting for an examination.. It may also be caused by poisons such as those of scarlet fever, typhoid fever, and other diseases ; by pressure of a tumour or of a pregnant womb ; or by disease of the liver. In addition to these kinds of jaundice there are epidemic and hereditary forms, some of them of a serious character.

Symptoms.—Discoloration of the skin and of the white of the eye is an unmistakable symptom of the condition. The urine is highly coloured and, indeed, may betray the presence of bile before the skin is affected ; the sweat takes on a yellow tinge, and even the saliva, the tears, and the milk may be discoloured. The motions, being unmixed with bile, which exerts an antiseptic effect, are particularly offensive, and are pale, drab, or clay-coloured. In most cases the patient is constipated—another consequence of the absence of bile, but in some cases, owing to the irritation caused by the decomposing fæces, there is diarrhœa with flatulence. The skin manifests the irritation caused by the presence of bile in the blood by itching and by eruptions. There is also a proneness to bleeding and to bruises.

The pulse slows down, and the patient is languid, drowsy, and depressed.

Treatment.—In cases where the cause of the obstruction can be dealt with, as when it is due to gall-stones, treatment will, of course, be directed to this. For the jaundice itself not much benefit is to be expected from drugs, except that tabloids of ox-gall —one twice a day immediately after food—may be taken to supply the digestive and antiseptic properties of the absent bile, while the constipation may be corrected by aperients, such as a grain or two of calomel at night, followed by a dose of Carlsbad salts in the morning. Relief may be found from itching by frequent warm baths and friction with towels, or by sponging with weak carbolic lotion. The patient, especially if the trouble originated in a chill, should take to bed and remain there until the attack subsides. Even then, however, he should avoid all exertion of body or of mind, for the effects of an attack of jaundice cannot immediately be neutralized. The pain and feeling of fullness in the liver region may be relieved by hot fomentations or linseed poultices. Until the bile resumes its normal flow, fatty foods must be avoided, and sweet and starchy foods used very sparingly. The patient should live chiefly upon milk which has been peptonized or diluted with soda water, beef tea, mutton, chicken and veal broths, with biscuits or a little toasted bread. As the attack passes off he may go on to bread-and-milk and light milk puddings, and return to his ordinary diet by way of fish, chicken, etc.

JOINTS (*see* BONES AND JOINTS).

K

KALA-AZAR.—This intractable and often fatal fever, occurring in certain warm climates, is due to a germ known as the Leishman-Donovan parasite. After a time the patient is either carried off by dysentery, which is much the most frequent termination of the disease, or begins to improve. The improvement may be spontaneous, or the result of treatment with tartar emetic or colloidal sulphide of antimony, supplemented by a nourishing diet and rest.

KERATITIS.—This is the technical name for inflammation of the cornea, the horny transparent structure in front of the coloured part of the eye. The affection, which is sometimes due to syphilis, is unsuitable for domestic treatment.

KIDNEY (*see* URINARY ORGANS).

KIDNEY, STONE IN (*see* STONE IN THE KIDNEY).

KIDNEYS, INFLAMMATION OF (*see* BRIGHT'S DISEASE).

KNOCK-KNEE.—Genu valgum, as this deformity is called in medical language, is sometimes a manifestation of rickets, but it may be simply a result of strain of the ligaments in the region of the knee while they are soft. The signs of it are most often noticed soon after the child begins to "run away," or during adolescence—which begins about the age of fourteen. When it is not a manifestation of rickets, it is brought about by faulty habits of standing or walking. Club-foot and flat-foot are frequently associated with it, sometimes as the result, but much more often as the cause.

Symptoms.—The patient is easily tired, and complains of an aching pain on the inner side of the knee. In attempting to run he often falls, from the knees knocking against each other. He walks cross-legged, and appears to be short and stumpy because of the bending of the legs. If he stands with the knees close together there is seen to be a space between the inner projections of the ankles, which in that attitude ought to meet.

Treatment.—If the defect is observed at the very beginning it can be prevented by insisting upon the child's standing and walking correctly, and, in cases where flatfoot is present, by providing boots of which the inner borders are raised, so that the strain upon the inner ligaments about the knee may be relieved. If the deformity has established itself, but is still in the early stages, it can be gradually corrected by bathing and rubbing the limbs in front of a fire daily, and by manipulations of the legs, which should be gently and steadily drawn straight for ten minutes every night and morning. If both knees are affected, a firm pillow should be placed between them, and the ankles tied together : if only one knee is affected, a well-padded splint should be strapped to the outside of the leg. In more advanced cases, a Thomas knee-brace, a steel bar running up beside the leg from the heel of the boot to the tip of the haunch-bone, should be used. The child must be put on a nourishing diet, and should take cod-liver oil and syrup of the iodide of iron. If treatment has been delayed, or the deformity does not yield to these palliative measures, operation will be necessary.

KYPHOSIS (*see* SPINAL CURVATURE, ANGULAR).

L

LABOUR.—To describe the preparations made for childbirth, the stages of the process, and the complications which may attend it would absorb more space than can be spared in a work such as this, and the reader must be referred to Chavasse's well known book, " Advice to a Wife " (Cassell & Co., Ltd.), where the subject is considered with all necessary detail.

LACTATION (*see* SUCKLING).

LARDACEOUS DISEASE.—This condition, known also as amyloid disease, is a degeneration of organs such as the liver, the kidneys, and the spleen, and is most frequently due to long-continued suppuration from a diseased bone, or in some deep-seated cavity which cannot easily be drained. It is also a result of late syphilis, both acquired and congenital, and is occasionally met with in some other diseases. It is termed *lardaceous* disease because the degenerated tissues, when cut, resemble raw bacon. It cannot be treated directly, but through the cause.

LARYNGISMUS STRIDULUS (*see* CHILD-CROWING).

LARYNGITIS.—Inflammation of the larynx, or voice-box, is predisposed to by breathing the vitiated air of hot, crowded or dust-laden rooms or conveyances, by fatigue, hunger, mental depression, or anxiety—by anything, in fact, which depresses the general condition. Among the exciting causes are excessive use of the voice, violent vomiting or retching, as on the sea or after an alcoholic debauch, and fits of passionate crying or sobbing. Laryngitis may also occur as a complication of an infectious fever. But in the great majority of cases the affection does not begin in the larynx, but spreads downwards from the nose or throat, although in a few cases it starts in the bronchial tubes and spreads upwards.

Symptoms.—The patient has a sense of discomfort in the throat, hoarseness sets in, the voice sinks in tone and may disappear, talking becomes painful, and there is a constant desire to clear the throat and swallow, both of which actions are painful. Coughing, however, is not a common symptom ; if present, it is of a hacking character. At first the expectoration is small in quantity and thin and watery. In average cases, at the end of twenty-four hours the symptoms begin to abate, and in from three to eight days from the onset of the affection the patient is quite well again. An ordinary attack of laryngitis, though requiring care, is not a serious affection, but in the aged or debilitated, and where it is a complication of one of the infectious fevers, it is of graver import.

Treatment.—The patient should have a hot bath and take 10 grains of Dover's powder to promote perspiration. He must be kept cosy in bed in a warm but well ventilated room, with a cold compress or a mustard-leaf applied to the front of the neck. At the same time ice may be sucked. The bowels should be cleared with whatever aperient the patient may be accustomed to. An inhalation of friar's balsam, a teaspoonful to a pint of hot water, will encourage the secretion of mucus and so relieve the cough, if present (*see* INHALATIONS). The diet at first should consist only of milk and milk puddings, with gruel or beef-tea ; to relieve thirst the patient may sip barley water and black-currant tea. If fever is a prominent symptom the following mixture may be taken :

Solution of acetate of
   ammonia .... 2 ounces
Salicylate of soda .... 60 grains
Bromide of potash .... 80 grains
Liquid extract of liquorice.. 1 ounce
Water to 8 ounces.
Two tablespoonfuls every three hours

If the condition does not quickly improve the doctor should be called in.

When the acute stage is past the following inhalation will be found useful :

Oil of Scotch pine.......... 1 drachm
Friar's balsam............. 1 ounce
Light carbonate of magnesia. 1 drachm
Rose water .... 1 ounce
Glycerin to 3 ounces.
One tablespoonful to a pint of water.

As soon as the symptoms have subsided the patient should go out of doors, but should be careful at first not to use the voice much. He must avoid dusty, crowded and over-heated rooms, should take alcohol, if at all, in strict moderation, and generally aim at keeping himself in good condition.

In *children* laryngitis is a rather more serious affection than in adults, and is apt to cause difficulty of breathing and spasm of the vocal cords. Unless the attack is obviously a slight one, a medical man should therefore at once be called in. Treatment is on the same lines as that for false croup (p. 97), a very similar affection, acute laryngitis in children being indeed sometimes called false croup.

LATERAL CURVATURE (*see* SPINAL CURVATURE, LATERAL).

LATERAL SCLEROSIS.—Lateral sclerosis means a degenerative hardening of a certain part of the spinal cord. The cause is not known. The disease comes on insidiously in early adult life or middle age, with a feeling of stiffness in the legs, which easily become tired. Presently the gait is obviously affected, the legs moving stiffly and awkwardly, and the steps growing shorter, and difficulty is experienced in raising the toes, so that there is a tendency to stumble in walking over uneven ground. Gradu-

ally walking becomes more and more difficult, and finally may be impossible. The upper limbs may be similarly affected. The tendency is for the disease slowly to progress, and in some cases the patient is ultimately bedridden. Little can be done except to massage the limbs in the hope of reducing the stiffness, and to prescribe periods of rest.

LAUGHING GAS (*see* ANÆS-THESIA).

LAXATIVES (*see* MEDICINES AND HOW THEY ARE MEASURED).

LEAD POISONING, ACUTE.—Lead is sometimes taken by accident or by design, in the form of sugar of lead, white lead, or Goulard's solution. An emetic should be given, and as soon as this has acted, follow it with a tablespoonful of Epsom salts in a tumblerful of hot water, then give milk, white of egg and water, and barley water. The pain in the abdomen may be relieved by pressure and the application of poultices.

LEAD POISONING, CHRONIC.—In spite of the precautions that are taken, chronic lead poisoning is still met with in industries in which lead is used. The disease is contracted chiefly by the inhalation or swallowing of lead dust, but it may also be conveyed by fumes containing lead, by eating with lead-contaminated hands, and in other ways. Cases of lead poisoning also arise through the contamination of drinking water by leaden pipes or cisterns, and this is especially likely to occur in water derived from peaty moorlands.

Symptoms.—The earliest symptoms are nausea, loss of appetite, and constipation. The breath is fetid, the patient is conscious of a sweet metallic taste in the mouth and of constant thirst, and is subject to paroxysms of

" lead-colic " caused by spasmodic contractions of the intestine. A blue or greyish line, due to the action of the tartar of the teeth upon the particles of lead, lines the edge of the gums. Dyspepsia and anæmia supervene, and the complexion takes on an earthy tint. Neuritis is set up, and in many cases certain of the muscles of the forearm are paralysed and " wrist-drop " occurs, the hand falling by its own weight when the arm is raised. The sensory nerves may also be affected, with resulting loss of sensation.

Treatment.—Exposure to the poison, whatever its source, must immediately cease. The colic may be somewhat relieved by pressure, but the medical attendant may find it necessary to administer morphia. To rid the system of the poison, the patient should be purged with Epsom salts and take a course of iodide of potash. The paralysed muscles should be treated with massage and electricity. *Prevention*, in the case of lead workers, consists in the wearing of respirators, in taking occasional doses of Epsom salts, in drinking lemonade containing sulphuric acid, and in the observance of rigid cleanliness; food should never be eaten in the workroom, or with unwashed hands, or in working clothes, nor should tobacco be used while at work. If the drinking water is contaminated, the lead pipes or cisterns should be changed for galvanized iron pipes, or for those lined with block tin, tar, bitumen, or glass. Failing this, the water should be treated chemically, by adding to it lime, powdered chalk, whiting, or carbonate of soda. If such measures as these are not practicable, or fail in their object, the water should be allowed to run off for a few minutes in the morning, and again before being drawn for use, and,

whether intended for drinking or for household purposes, should be filtered through animal charcoal.

LEADERS (*see under* MUSCLES AND TENDONS.)

LENS (*see* EYE).

LENTIGO (*see* FRECKLES).

LEPROSY.—This disease has claims to a high antiquity. By about the end of the fifteenth century, as the result, probably, of improved sanitary and social conditions, leprosy had almost disappeared from civilized Europe, but it lingered in isolated districts until about the end of the eighteenth century. Norway is the only European country where it is at all common, but there are a good many lepers also in Iceland. Leprosy is now considered to be a disease of tropical or subtropical climates, and within those limits it is widely distributed.

Cause.—In 1874 Hansen, of Bergen, discovered in cases of leprosy a germ which has been generally accepted as the cause of the disease, the *Bacillus lepræ*. How it enters the human body, whether in food, water, or air, or through the skin or some accidental abrasion, or by the bite of an insect, is not known. The late Sir Jonathan Hutchinson pointed out that the disease is associated with the eating of fish in a state of decomposition; he remarks that leprosy is more common on the sea-coast and in the neighbourhood of great lakes and rivers than elsewhere, and was especially rife in the Middle Ages, when there was a large consumption of salt fish, which formed the principal animal food throughout the winter, while to-day it is most prevalent among the Chinese, who with their rice habitually consume putrid fish as a condiment. This theory has not found wide acceptance ; but there can be no doubt that Hutchinson was right in regarding leprosy as a disease of semi-civilization —as distinct from civilization on the one hand and from savage life on the other hand, and the consumption of impure food may well be one, though only one, of the conditions which favour its propagation.

Types and symptoms of leprosy. —There are two distinct forms of leprosy, in one of which, the *nodular* or tubercular form, the brunt of the attack is borne by the skin, while in the other, the *anæsthetic* form, often styled nerve leprosy, the nerve-trunks are chiefly involved. In a third group of cases the symptoms of the first and second groups are combined—*mixed leprosy*. The disease is remarkable for the length of time that elapses between the act of infection and the appearance of the symptoms. This averages two to three years, but is occasionally very much longer. The first manifestations usually take the form of malaise, depression, itching and tingling, sweating, etc., which come and go perhaps for months, and are then succeeded by an eruption in the shape of spots and patches, from the size of a millet seed to several inches in diameter, of a reddish-brown colour, partly disappearing on pressure, roughly symmetrical, and situated on the outside of the arms and front of the legs and thighs, on the upper part of the face, and also on the trunk. After a time the skin under the eyes becomes swollen and puckered and the nose thickened, and in the *nodular* form flat, firm nodules or bosses appear, the size of split peas or beans, but often much larger, of a dirty-red colour, turning later on to brown or yellow, and with a smooth, greasy-looking surface. When these nodules are numerous and join together, the " leonine " expression so characteristic of the disease is produced. Later similar changes occur in other parts of the body, and the nodules soften and form ulcers, which exude sticky, offensive matter. The eyes and larynx also become affected in the same way and are ultimately destroyed, so that the sufferer becomes voiceless, blind, and most repulsive to look upon.

In *nerve* leprosy the eruption results in dark-red rings enclosing pale skin, in which sensation is lost ; or in large water-blisters, from the size of a pea to that of an egg. The eruption may get better or worse, but sooner or later neuralgic pains, tingling, and numbness occur, small nodules can be felt on the nerves, and mutilation of the fingers and toes may take place. Sensation is completely destroyed over a large part of the body, the limbs become twisted and deformed, the muscles waste and are partially paralysed, even bone is destroyed, and ulceration or gangrene (" mortification ") sets in.

The average duration of the *nodular* form is about nine years, of *nerve* leprosy about twice as long. In both cases the health becomes gradually more feeble and the vital powers exhausted, and after many years, it may be, the victim's sufferings are mercifully ended. by disease of the lungs or kidneys or by persistent diarrhœa.

Treatment.—The most important thing is to improve the patient's hygienic conditions by careful attention to cleanliness, by an abundance of fresh air and good food, and by the avoidance of fatigue and exposure. Under such a regimen the progress of the disease is for a time stayed, and in some cases has been permanently arrested. Europeans who have contracted leprosy in the tropics should return to the healthier modes of life of their native land. One favourite remedy is chaulmoogra oil, given in capsules, or it may be injected beneath the skin in the form of gynocardate of soda, or into a vein. Sodium morrhuate is sometimes combined with the gynocardate. Iodide of potassium, mercury, and salvarsan have also been tried, as well as various serums and vaccines, but none of these has stood the test of prolonged use.

LEUCOCYTES (*see* BLOOD AND LYMPH).

LEUCODERMIA.—In this affection, known also as *vitiligo*, white patches, with a coloured border, form on the skin, the result, probably, of some affection of the nerves. It is a rare condition in this country and in Europe generally, but is more common in the tropics, and especially in the dark races. To stay the progress of the disease, general tonic treatment is adopted.

LEUCORRHŒA.—This word, colloquially translated as "the whites," denotes an excessive discharge from the female genital passages—the vulva, the vagina and the womb. Sometimes it is the result of congestion, as in the leucorrhœa of pregnancy, in that just before and just after the periods, and in that due to misplacements of the womb. It may also be caused by inflammation (*see* WOMB, INFLAMMATION OF), by tumours, etc., but in many cases it appears to depend upon the general state of health. Thus, it is often met with in girls who are anæmic or have grown too fast. There may be a good deal of backache, and the patient may feel tired and out of sorts. If the trouble arises from the general state of health, the patient, if a girl, should not be hard pressed at

school, but spend as much time as possible in the open air, have a nutritious diet, and take cod-liver oil. If anæmic, she should have an iron tonic. If there is much pain or inflammation, injections should be used—boric acid, or subacetate of lead, or warm decoction of poppy heads, linseed or starch. When the inflammation has subsided, an astringent should be injected, such as alum (one or two teaspoonfuls to a pint of water), chloride of zinc (5 to 10 grains to a pint of water), or tannic acid (one to three teaspoonfuls to a pint of water). These astringent injections should also be given in cases in which inflammation is absent. The parts must, of course, be kept scrupulously clean, the bowels should be opened, if necessary, by aperients, and indigestion avoided by a careful diet. If such measures as these fail, a doctor must be consulted.

LEUKÆMIA.—A rare disease of the blood in which there is a great increase in the number of the white blood-cells. Its nature is not yet fully understood. The drug which had been most beneficial is arsenic.

LICE (*see* STINGS AND BITES).

LICHEN PLANUS.—This is a skin disease in which there is an eruption of groups of small tough pimples, usually flat-topped, many of them no larger than a pin's head. At first they are bluish-red or "lilac" in colour, but after a time the tint often becomes purple, and may be brown. The favourite sites for the eruption are the fronts of the wrists and the inner sides of the thighs near the knees, the forearms and shins, and the waist line. In most cases there is severe itching. The cause of the disease is not clearly understood, but nervous disturbance is known to have much to do with it; in some cases it has appeared suddenly after a mental shock, while other cases have been traced to prolonged worry. Children are seldom attacked; the favourite period is early adult life to middle age. Women are affected rather more often than men, and brain workers more often than hand workers. The disease is difficult to check, and may continue for as much as six months or even longer, while the large warty masses formed by the pimples around hair follicles may remain for years. For the ordinary type of eruption a good lotion is a drachm of liquor picis carbonis in 8 ounces of calamine or lead lotion. Internal treatment, however, is more important than external; the drugs most commonly employed are arsenic and mercury.

LIENTERIC DIARRHŒA (*see* Diarrhœa).

LIGAMENTS (*see* Bones and Joints).

LIGHT TREATMENT (*see* Electrical Treatment).

LINIMENTS.—Liniments or embrocations are applied to the skin by painting, anointing or rubbing; they contain either camphor, oil, soap, or glycerin. They are used to relieve pain, or to stimulate the nutrition of a part and remove the thickening and stiffness caused by past inflammation. For the latter purpose they are applied with more or less vigorous friction. The following will be found useful :

Sedative Liniment
Extract of belladonna ..... ½ ounce
Glycerin .... ½ ounce
To be smeared over the painful part.

A B C Sedative Liniment
Liniment of aconite .... ½ ounce
Liniment of belladonna .... ½ ounce
Liniment of chloroform .. ½ ounce
To be rubbed into the painful part.

Stimulating Liniment, "Hartshorn and Oil"
Solution of ammonia....... ½ ounce
Almond oil................1½ ounces
Shake together.

Another Stimulating Liniment
Liniment of turpentine .....1½ ounces
Solution of ammonia ......1½ ounces
Oil of cajuput .... ½ drachm
Olive oil to four ounces.

LINSEED POULTICES (*see* Poultices).

LIPOMAS (*see* Tumours).

LIPS, CHAPPED (*see* Chapped Hands and Lips).

LITHOTRITY (*see* Stone in the Bladder).

LIVE BLOOD (*see* Eyelid, Twitching of).

LIVER (*see* Digestion; Gall-Stones).

LIVER ABSCESS.—In warm countries there occurs a special type of liver abscess which is usually, if not always, associated with a certain form of dysentery—the amœbic form (*see* Dysentery). The treatment is to open the abscess and insert an indiarubber drainage tube, so that the discharge may escape. Liver abscess is attended by a heavy mortality.

LIVER, GIN-DRINKER'S (*see* Cirrhosis of Liver).

LIVER, INFLAMMATION OF (*see* Liver Abscess; Cirrhosis of Liver).

"LIVER SPOTS."—The irregular patches of fawn- or liver-coloured discoloration which are known as liver spots, or chloasma, may be caused by some external irritant; or may be due to dyspepsia, to consumption, or to uterine irritation during menstruation or pregnancy. The patches most often come on the forehead, cheeks, or nipples, but they may appear on any part of the face or of the body. Treatment is un-satisfactory.

LIVER, TROPICAL (*see* TROPICAL LIVER).

LOBAR PNEUMONIA (*see* PNEU-MONIA).

LOBULAR PNEUMONIA (*see* BRONCHO-PNEUMONIA).

LOCKJAW.—Tetanus, to give this disease its medical name, is due to a microbe, the *Bacillus tetani*, which flourishes in cultivated soil, and enters the body through a wound. The bacilli are believed not to pass into the blood-stream, but to remain at the point of entrance, where they create poisons which have a peculiar affinity for nervous tissues and find their way to the brain and spinal cord. In ordinary cases the incubation period varies between two or three days and as many weeks, but it may extend over several months. The sooner the symptoms appear the more acute they are. The earliest is usually a feeling of stiffness in the muscles of the neck, followed after a short interval by contractions of the muscles of the jaw and face, by which the jaws become "locked," and by spasms of the muscles of the trunk and limbs.

Treatment.—In cases in which the wound has not healed it should be cleansed and disinfected, and tetanus antitoxin injected with the least possible delay, in the hope that it may turn the scale in the patient's favour by neutralizing so much of the poison as has not yet been absorbed by the nervous system. Sedative drugs are also employed, and if the spasms are very severe the patient is allowed to inhale chloroform. He should lie in a dark room, and be protected as far as possible from any-thing that might provoke the spasms by which he is tortured. *Prevention*

is more important than remedial treatment. The microbe of tetanus being so commonly present in cul-tivated soil, antitoxin should be in-jected in all cases of crushed wounds, especially those contaminated by dirt or other foreign matter, without waiting to see whether symptoms of lockjaw appear. Its great value when it is thus employed preventively at this stage was demonstrated in the Great War.

LOCOMOTOR ATAXY.—The most dramatic symptom of *tabes dor-salis*, as this affection is also called, is a peculiarity of gait. The patient lifts the foot higher than is necessary, gives a kick forward, and then brings it down on the ground with a stamp. This and other symptoms are the result of a degeneration of the spinal cord, due, in the majority of cases, if not in all, to syphilis, supplemented in many instances by addiction to drink, by injury, worry, or other debilitating influences. The disease may appear during adolescence, and is then a result of congenital syphilis. In grown-up people the onset does not usually occur until ten or twelve years after the contraction of syphilis, and in extreme cases the interval may be as long as twenty-five years, or even more. Locomotor ataxy is much more prevalent in men than in women, the proportion being probably about two to one.

Symptoms.—The peculiar gait, which arises from the patent's in-ability to co-ordinate the action of the muscles used in walking, has already been mentioned. Among the earliest of the symptoms are pains which are known as "lightning" pains because of their darting or shooting character. They are usually attributed to rheumatism or neuralgia until their true nature is revealed by the supervention of other symptoms. There may also be pains in the bones or other organs which are known as " boring " pains, and the skin may be excessively sensitive in parts, so that the patient is unable to bear the slightest touch. Presently he becomes unsteady in walking or standing, especially if he is in the dark or has his eyes closed. Other symptoms take the form of what are called crises. Every few weeks, for example, there may be a very sharp attack of sickness and intense pain in the stomach, or there may be spasm of the muscles of the larynx, with a barking cough ; other organs, such as the kidneys, the bladder, and the lower bowel, may be similarly affected. The optic nerve may undergo atrophy, leading after some years to blindness. Various other symptoms may develop, but enough has been said to indicate the gravity of the disease.

Treatment.—Salvarsan, mercury, and iodide of potassium have been administered, but with results not at all corresponding with those produced in the earlier stages of syphilis. The best tonics are iron, arsenic, and quinine. Cod-liver oil should be given, and the diet must be nutritious. The difficulty in walking may be to some extent overcome by a course of special exercises known as Frenkel's exercises.

LONG SIGHT (*see* SIGHT, DEFECTS OF).

LOTIONS.—The chief differences between lotions and liniments is that the former are of a watery and the latter of an oily character, and that while lotions are applied on lint or rags, or are used for bathing the affected part, liniments are, as a rule, smeared over or rubbed into it. When cold water is used as a lotion the lint or rag should not be covered up, otherwise evaporation, which increases the effect of cold, will be checked. The evaporation may be increased by adding spirit to the water. The following medicated lotions may be recommended :

Evaporating Lotion
Solution of subacetate of lead 1 drachm
Rectified spirit .... 1 ounce.
Water to 8 ounces.

Carbolic-Acid Lotion
Pure carbolic acid liquefied
A tablespoonful to a pint of water makes a lotion 1 in 40 ; a dessertspoonful to a pint, 1 in 80.

Arnica Lotion, for Bruises
Add 20 drops of tincture of arnica to half a cupful of water.

Lead Lotion, to relieve Inflammation
Solution of subacetate of lead..40 minims
Water to 8 ounces.

Red Wash, to stimulate the Healing of Wounds
Sulphate of zinc .... 2 grains
Compound tincture of
   lavender ....12 minims
Water to 1 ounce.

Antiseptic Eye Lotion
Boric acid .... 8 grains
Distilled water to 1 ounce.
To be used in an eye-bath.

Astringent Eye Lotion
Boric acid .... 5 grains
Sulphate of zinc .... ½ grain
Distilled water to 1 ounce.
To be used in an eye-bath.

LUMBAGO.—This affection takes the form of a sharp pain in the muscles of the loins, which usually comes on quite suddenly. A person is stooping, it may be, to pick up something, and when he attempts to rise he feels a pain so acute that he may almost fancy he has been cut with a knife ; in some cases he is incapacitated from getting about, and may be unable even to turn over or raise himself in bed. Men are more liable to lumbago than women ; and it is rarely met with before middle age. Some regard it as a form of neuralgia, affecting the nerves of the loin muscles, but the present tendency is to interpret it as an affection of the muscles themselves, which is now called *myalgia*—that is, pain in the muscles. Lumbago is often brought on by cold and wet, especially after fatigue.

Treatment.—Except in slight cases the patient should take to his bed, where the affected muscles will have the benefit of rest and warmth. There is much virtue in the application of heat. A flannel may be wrung out of very hot water, laid over the back, and covered with oiled silk, or a dry flannel may be laid over the loins and a hot flat-iron passed over it. Another method is to apply a mustard leaf, or a very hot linseed poultice over which mustard has been sprinkled. In slight cases it may suffice to smear on equal parts of extract of belladonna and glycerin, or apply lint saturated with chloroform and belladonna liniments in equal parts, covering it with oil-silk, then with cotton-wool, and finally with a flannel bandage. In the later stages a course of Turkish baths will be serviceable. In obstinate cases electricity and massage may be tried. For internal treatment the patient, if not confined to bed, may take the following salicin mixture :

Salicin	2 drachms
Bicarbonate of potash	2 drachms
Tincture of orange	½ ounce.
Chloroform water to 8 ounces.	

Two tablespoonfuls every 2 or 3 hours.

If the patient is in bed, he may safely take the following mixture, which will promote perspiration :

Salicylate of soda ....1½ drachms
Bicarbonate of potash ..... 2 drachms
Bromide of potash ....80 grains
Compound tincture of car- damoms................. ½ ounce
Spirit of chloroform ....2½ drachms
Water to 8 ounces.

Two tablespoonfuls every 2 or 3 hours.

If the pain is not severe enough to require morphia, aspirin or phenacetin may be taken, two 5-grain tabloids of either for a dose. Anæmic and debilitated patients require tonics, such as quinine and iron, or arsenic.

LUNGS (*see* RESPIRATION).

LUNGS, CONGESTION OF (*see* CONGESTION OF THE LUNGS).

LUNGS, INFLAMMATION OF (*see* PNEUMONIA ; BRONCHO-PNEU-MONIA).

LUNGS, TUBERCULOSIS OF (*see* CONSUMPTION).

LUPUS ERYTHEMATOSUS.—This disease, an inflammatory affection of the skin and mucous membranes, received the name of lupus because the lesions bear resemblance to those of lupus vulgaris. There is no proof, however, that it is of tuberculous origin, as is lupus vulgaris, or that its occasional association with tuberculosis is anything more than accidental. The cause of the affection is obscure, but there is some ground for the view that it originates in some form of blood-poisoning which affects the nerves controlling the blood-vessels. It seldom appears before the age of twenty-five or after forty-five, and is much more common in women than in men. The part most frequently attacked is the face. The lesions start as red spots, either smooth, or covered with a scab or with greyish, paper-like scales. The disease spreads either by enlargement of the single spots or by the appearance of crop after crop of fresh spots, which run together into patches of considerable size. In many cases the lesions begin on both cheeks, and the red patches, with their covering of crusts or scales, spread inwards and meet in a narrow strip over the bridge of the nose, reminding the observer by their shape of a butterfly's or a bat's wings. After the face and neck, the hands and feet are most often attacked. The disease usually runs a slow course, which may spread over ten, fifteen, or twenty years, when it gradually disappears, leaving reminders, however, in the form of permanent scars and, in hairy parts, baldness.

Treatment.—Some cases are benefited by the Finsen light, electricity, or the X-rays. If the lesions are not much inflamed, the application of carbonic-acid snow may give good results in the earlier stages. In some stages cooling ointments and evaporating lotions are useful, as also is painting with tincture of iodine. Sea-air is not beneficial, but the patient should have plenty of fresh air and exercise, the food should be digestible and nutritious, and stimulants, including tea and coffee, should be avoided. Vaccine treatment is sometimes prescribed.

LUPUS VULGARIS.—This disease of the skin, called lupus (Latin for wolf) because of its destructive effects, is due to the same bacillus that causes consumption. Its progress, however, is much slower, and only with difficulty can the bacillus be found in the lesions. The disease begins, in most cases, in the nostril or on the nose, or elsewhere on the face, or on the neck, but no part is immune from attack. It is believed that the nostrils are infected in " picking " the nose, and that the bacillus also gains entrance through punctures, or through abrasions as from scratching, or is brought to the skin from tuberculous glands and other centres of infection in the body. Lupus usually begins during the first ten years of life, and is rare in middle age. Girls are much more liable to it than boys, and the poor than the

well-to-do. Cold is one predisposing cause ; measles appears to be another. The affection starts as a small swelling which is soft, brownish-red, and translucent, resembling apple-jelly, with which it is often compared. As this increases, other swellings, or nodules as they are called, appear in the same region, meeting each other as they spread, and so the circle of the disease is enlarged. Other parts of the body may be attacked independently until, in rare cases, the whole of the skin may be involved. In some cases the patch of disease, in course of time, heals up, but in most cases it goes on to ulceration which may not only extend through the skin, but may destroy cartilage, as in the nose and ear, though scarcely ever attacking bone. The patient suffers little pain, but lupus is a very obstinate affection, and even when the disease has disappeared it tends to recur.

Treatment.—Lupus differs so much in different cases that it calls for various methods of treatment. In the majority of cases the Finsen light yields the best results. In slight cases, in which there is no ulceration, the light alone is sufficient ; in others it may be desirable to give a preliminary course of X-ray treatment, or to resort to the X-rays after using the light. For mucous membranes, the X-rays are to be preferred. Another method which answers well in some cases is that of freezing, applied by carbonic-acid snow. If the patient is of scrofulous tendency, cod-liver oil and a nourishing diet are indicated, with sea air and general attention to hygiene. In some cases tuberculin is of service.

LYING-IN PERIOD, MANAGEMENT OF.—The great need of the mother after her child is born is *rest*.

Even her toilet must not be attended to until about an hour after labour is over ; then the vulva should be covered with a sterile pad, a binder applied, and a hot drink given. During the first twenty-four hours she should be kept as quiet as possible. After two or three days slight movement may be allowed. Towards the end of a week she may sit up for meals, being well propped up ; after this the semi-recumbent position may be encouraged, as it promotes drainage of the discharges. It is important that she should have at least six hours' unbroken sleep every night, and care must be taken that she is not disturbed by the infant during this period. As to how long she should remain in bed, opinions differ somewhat, but on the whole a rest of three weeks may be recommended. At the end of this time, she may be lifted on to a couch, and then to a chair ; she may now begin to walk, but great care should be taken to avoid fatigue.

Binders.—During the early lying-in period a binder is required ; a soft twill or linen band, at least 18 inches wide, may be fastened by safety pins or by straps and buckles, but not too tightly. If the breasts are full and pendulous, a breast-binder should be used, but care must be taken to apply it quite loosely. Troubles of lactation are described in the article SUCKLING.

Douching. — Vaginal douching should be avoided unless the discharge become offensive or hæmorrhage should occur. If douches have to be given, it should be by a trained nurse, and they should be hot. A good douche is one containing lysol 20 minims to the pint, brought to a temperature of 112° Fahr., rising to 115°. Douches may be given two or three times daily.

After-pains.—If there are troublesome after-pains, as sometimes happens in the case of women who have borne children before, it may be desirable to give a dose of antipyrin, 10 grains, repeated, if necessary, in two hours.

Diet.—During the first twenty-four hours the diet should be limited to milk, tea, oxo or bovril, cocoa, and custard. On the second day an egg and a little chicken or fish may be added. On the third day, after the bowels have been opened, ordinary diet may be returned to, except that it should be light ; meat and potatoes should not be taken more than once a day. Uncooked fruits and salads should be avoided for the sake of the child, but stewed fruits are permissible in moderation.

The bowels. — About thirty-six hours after the birth of the child, a dose of castor oil should be given so that the bowels may be opened. Afterwards the bowels should be opened at least once every day. In most cases a laxative is required ; liquid paraffin, half an ounce twice a day, may be used. If this is not sufficient, compound liquorice powder may be tried.

Micturition.—When six or eight hours have elapsed, the patient should be encouraged to pass water. In many cases she will be unable to do so while recumbent ; if so, she should be gently raised to a semi-recumbent or a sitting position. If further encouragement is needed, heat may be applied to the lower abdomen, or the vulva may be bathed with hot lotion. These measures failing, the nurse or doctor will have to pass a catheter.

Care of the infant.—As soon as the child is born, its eyelids are carefully wiped with pledgets of wool soaked in disinfectant, say weak boracic lotion, and the mouth and throat are cleared of mucus with a piece of wet cotton-wool ; the child is then wrapped in a towel or cloth so that it may not be able to rub its eyes. If the mother is believed to be suffering from gonorrhœa, further precautions must be taken, as described under Ophthalmia Neonatorum, in the article OPHTHALMIA. When the child has begun to breathe naturally and pulsation of the navel-string (umbilical cord) has become feeble, the cord should be tied. Two ligatures, consisting of three strands of thick thread which has been boiled, a foot long and knotted at each end, are tied securely round it, the first about 1½ in. from the child, the second an inch farther off, the ends are cut off, and the cord is divided with scissors between the two ligatures. When the third stage of labour—the expulsion of the afterbirth—is over and the baby has had its first bath, the stump, dried and passed through a hole cut

in the middle of a piece of clean sterile linen, is dusted with boric-acid powder, and folded up over the abdomen, and the binder applied. This dressing is carried out each day after the bath. The cord usually separates in about five to seven days. The feeding and care of the infant from this time onwards are described in the articles INFANTS AND YOUNG CHILDREN, FEEDING OF; and INFANTS, HYGIENE OF.

LYMPH (*see* BLOOD AND LYMPH).

LYMPH SCROTUM (*see* FILARIASIS).

LYMPH-GLANDS, INFLAMMATION OF (*see* ADENITIS).

LYMPHADENOMA (*see* HODGKIN'S DISEASE).

LYMPHATISM (*see* STATUS LYMPHATICUS).

M

MADNESS (*see* INSANITY).

MALARIA.—Ague, as this fever is popularly termed, was formerly quite common in England, but is now scarcely ever met with here except in patients who have contracted it abroad. Such cases became more numerous after the War, many of our men having been infected while serving in Macedonia and elsewhere.

History and causes.—The story of malaria takes us back at least to the fifth century B.C., when we find Hippocrates recognizing the existence of fevers which he divided into quotidian (recurring daily), tertian (recurring every third day), and quartan (recurring every fourth day). These fevers were undoubtedly the disease which we now term malaria, which divides up into just the same groups, according to the time at which the ague fits recur. (It should be

understood, by the way, with regard to the terms tertian and quartan, that in interpreting tertian as equivalent to *third*, and quartan as equivalent to *fourth*, the counting begins with the day on which the fever first occurs. The *third* day is therefore the next day but one to that on which the previous attack began, and the *fourth* day the next day but two). From classical times to the seventeenth century no advance had been made in our knowledge of malaria, but then (1640) it was discovered that cinchona bark (the source of quinine) is an antidote to malaria, and so this fever was definitely separated from others upon which cinchona bark exerts no influence. It had long been suspected that malaria was one of the diseases which are due to the action of parasites, but the ordinary view was that it was caused, as the word malaria (= bad air) suggests, by unwholesome exhalations from swamps. In 1880 Laveran, a French physician, pronounced that certain microscopic, dark-coloured cells present in the blood of malaria patients were not mere specks of pigment, but living parasites, and this view was speedily confirmed by other investigators.

How the parasite finds its way into the blood of malaria patients had still to be discovered. For centuries the peasants of Italy had believed that the fever was caused by the bite of a

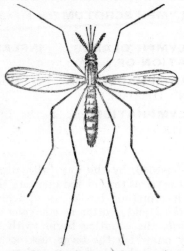

Fig. 31.—A malaria-carrying mosquito
(*Anopheles maculipennis*).

mosquito, and Koch, the German bacteriologist, found the same idea prevalent among the natives of German East Africa. It occurred to some medical authorities that by assuming the parasite of malaria to be derived from mosquitoes, the fact of the prevalence of malaria in marshy districts could be explained, for such districts are the breeding-grounds of mosquitoes. In 1894 the late Sir Patrick Manson propounded a definite theory on the subject, and Sir Ronald Ross, having put the theory to the test in India, proved that the malaria parasite spends one part of its life in

the mosquito, and is communicated to man in the act of biting. These observations were carried further by others, and it was shown that the guilty mosquitoes belong to a particular sub-family of wide distribution, the Anophelinæ (Fig. 31).

The mosquito is infected by the parasite when it bites a human being who is suffering from malaria. The parasite passes through certain stages of development in the mosquito's stomach, and then waits in its salivary glands until the next human being is bitten, when it escapes into a human host. Duly installed in the blood of its victim, it enters one of the red blood-cells and settles down here to raise a family. This it does by growing to as large a size as the red blood-cell will permit, and then breaking up into a number of tiny round bodies—its progeny. These burst out of the blood-cell and float free in the fluid of the blood, and then enter other blood-cells to develop into a new generation. Now, it is when the new generations burst out of the blood-cells that the ague fit occurs, possibly because they carry with them into the fluid of the blood poisonous substances. Some of the parasites take twenty-four, others forty-eight, yet others seventy-two hours to raise, so to speak, a new family; hence it is that we have quotidian, tertian, and quartan forms of malaria. After an attack, or a series of attacks, the symptoms may cease, either spontaneously or as the result of treatment, and if the blood is examined, no parasites will be found in it. But in some cases the attacks recur, after an interval of weeks or of months. What becomes of the parasites during the period of quiescence is not definitely known; but strain and depression of the vital forces appear to give them the opportunity of resuming their mischievous activity.

Symptoms.—The ague fit is often preceded by such symptoms as lassitude, bone-ache, headache, and loss of appetite. The fit itself divides into three stages. First the *cold* stage : the teeth chatter, the patient shivers from head to foot, his features become drawn and pinched, his skin looks blue and cold. All this while, cold as he feels, his temperature is rising, and at last, after lasting usually about an hour, the cold stage gives way to the *hot* stage. The shivering ceases, flushes of heat come on, the skin is very hot and dry, the face flushed, the eyes red, the pulse rapid and full, the respiration quick. There are severe headache and giddiness, with noises in the ears ; the back and the limbs ache, vomiting and diarrhœa are frequent, and the patient throws himself about in a state of intense restlessness and may wander in his mind. During this hot stage, which may last from three to four hours, the temperature rises, it may be to 105° Fahr. or higher. This phase passes into the *sweating* stage, and the patient's sufferings grow less, and he passes into a quiet sleep. During this stage also the fever disappears, the temperature falling in a few hours to the normal. Now comes an interval, which varies according to the time it takes for the parasite to produce a new generation, as explained above. During this interval the patient seems to be in no way the worse for his very unpleasant experience ; but if the case is not treated, after a time, as the fits follow one another, his health will be seriously affected, the spleen becoming enlarged and other serious symptoms developing.

We have described the more ordinary forms of malaria, but there are also other forms, including the serious forms which are styled *pernicious*.

Treatment.—Quinine may not always prevent the next succeeding fit, but it nearly always diminishes its severity. In 99 per cent. of cases no second attack develops. As long as the patient lives in a malarious district he should take occasional doses of quinine as a safeguard against recurrence. Great care should also be exercised—and this applies also to the non-infected—to avoid the bites of mosquitoes ; the risk is limited to the night. If it is necessary to be out of doors while mosquitoes are about, the face should be protected with a veil, the hands with gloves, and the ankles with high boots or leggings. The insects should be carefully excluded from the house by the use of gauze ; it is best to sleep in the upper storeys, as mosquitoes fly low, and the bed should be surrounded with mosquito netting.

MALFORMATIONS, CONGENITAL.—Children are sometimes born with one or more deformities as the result of imperfect development during ante-natal life. The most common of such deformities are club-foot and club-hand, webbed fingers, hare-lip, cleft palate, phimosis, imperforate anus, and spina bifida ; these are considered in separate articles.

MALIGNANT PUSTULE (*see* ANTHRAX).

MALIGNANT TUMOURS (*see* TUMOURS).

MALTA FEVER (*see* UNDULANT FEVER).

MANIA (*see* INSANITY).

MANY-TAILED BANDAGE (*see* BANDAGES).

MARASMUS (*see* WASTING IN CHILDREN).

MASSAGE.—This method of treatment, consisting in manipulations of the soft tissues of the body by the hand, has been used from time immemorial. It is referred to in Chinese manuscripts written some hundreds of years before the Christian era, it was practised by the Greeks and Romans, and, indeed, there are few lands, savage or civilized, in which it has not been employed. In modern times it has been much practised in France, whence we have borrowed the word, and also in Sweden, where it forms part of the gymnastic exercises for which that country is famous. In cases of neurasthenia, for which absolute rest is necessary, it is used as a substitute for physical exercise. In point of fact, it is in itself a form of exercise—exercise that is passive, as distinguished from active exercise. It accelerates the circulation, so causing an increased flow of blood to all the tissues, by which they are nourished and strengthened; it promotes the removal of waste products and the absorption of superfluous fluid, relieves congestion, breaks down adhesions, soothes or stimulates the nerves, according to the movement practised, and allays pain. It is particularly beneficial in obesity and in habitual constipation. It is also useful in stimulating the nutrition of paralysed muscles, in alleviating the pain of rheumatism, neuralgia, etc., and in the treatment of strains, sprains, and other injuries. Of late years it has been much employed in fractures, with the view of preventing fixation and pain. The chief movements in massage are stroking (effleurage), kneading (petrissage), percussion (tapotement), and vibrations—a form of percussion for which various mechanical devices are used.

MASTOID DISEASE.—In the mastoid process, the bone behind the ear, there are air-spaces, otherwise called air-cells, which are in communication with the middle ear, and when this part of the ear is inflamed, as not infrequently happens, the inflammation may extend to the mastoid air-spaces and an abscess may form. This is what is called mastoid disease, or mastoiditis. It is a serious condition, which may spread and involve the membranes of the brain and cause meningitis. The treatment is operative.

MEAD'S PLASTER (*see* DRESSINGS AND STRAPPING FOR WOUNDS).

MEASLES.—This highly infectious fever, known also as *rubeola* and as *morbilli*, is a malady of childhood, but it would no doubt be less uncommon among adults but that usually they are to some extent protected by having suffered from it in their early years. Even so, second attacks are by no means rare, for measles confers immunity in smaller measure than any other infective fever. The germ has not been clearly identified. The disease is infective at the very onset of the symptoms, three days before the rash appears to clear up the nature of the illness and demonstrate the necessity for isolation. Possibly, indeed, it is infective during the incubation stage —about twelve days—which precedes the first symptoms. Infection is given off by the breath and the mucus. The patient ceases to be infective two weeks after the appearance of the rash. The poison appears to be readily conveyed by the air, and for considerable distances. When a child has been exposed to infection, a quarantine of twenty-one days is usually enforced by school authorities. In Great Britain the mortality in epidemics seldom exceeds 5 per cent. of the patients, and frequently is not more than 1 or 2 per cent.

Symptoms.—The attack begins with a somewhat sudden rise of temperature. Reaching, it may be, nearly 104° Fahr. on the first day, the temperature then falls a degree or two, to rise once more on the fourth day. With the first rise of temperature there are aching pains in the limbs, headache and vomiting, but these may subside the next day, while those of a common cold develop. The glands of the neck may be enlarged; the throat may be red, and little bluish-white specks, known as Koplik's spots, make their appearance on the inside of the cheeks; earache also may be present. On the third day the symptoms become more pronounced, while the face becomes blotchy. About the end of the fourth day the rash appears on the face and neck, and during the next two days spreads all over the body. As soon as it is entirely out the temperature begins to fall, and becomes normal about two days later. On the face the rash has the appearance of dusky-red blotches of irregular shape; when these are viewed closely a number of fine red points are seen, which have a rough "feel" when touched with the finger. On the chest and the rest of the body the rash is more "spotty." On the sixth day the eruption is at its height, and then begins to fade, and is followed by a slight scurfiness. By the seventh or eighth day this will almost entirely have disappeared, leaving only a yellowish mottling or staining. The rash is attended by considerable irritation.

In children who enjoy good nursing, measles generally runs a quite mild course. Occasionally, however, *malignant* forms of the disease are met with, such as *hæmorrhagic* or *black* measles and *typhoid* measles.

Complications.—The most serious of the complications of measles, and the one which is the cause of death in most of the fatal cases, is broncho-pneumonia. Another complication is inflammation of the windpipe, which is sometimes so severe that tracheotomy has to be performed to save the patient from suffocation. Inflammation of the eyes, or ophthalmia, may occur in anæmic and unhealthy children, and ulcers may form on the eyes and permanently damage the sight. The swelling of the glands of the neck may increase and abscesses may form. The earache may develop into inflammation of the ear. Diarrhœa supervenes most often, though by no means exclusively, during hot weather. With its liability to such serious complications as we have enumerated, measles is clearly not to be regarded as a trifling complaint, mild as its symptoms frequently are in themselves. Moreover, even if complications are escaped, or survived, the patient often remains for months in a very low state of health, which predisposes him to bronchitis, pneumonia and tuberculosis. Another frequent sequel of measles is whooping-cough.

Treatment.—In ordinary cases little is required beyond rest, pure air, equable warmth, diluents and nourishment, but much may be done to promote the patient's comfort and ward off complications. As soon as the symptoms of catarrh above described give rise to a suspicion that they may be caused by measles, the patient must be confined to his room, and if feverish sent to bed. The temperature of the room should be maintained at 65° Fahr.; good ventilation must be secured. If cough is troublesome, the air may be moistened by the vapour from a steam kettle. The mouth should be cleansed by frequent irrigation with warm water or with an antiseptic. If the glands of the neck are swollen, hot fomentations sprinkled with belladonna liniment may be applied. The diet should consist of milk, broth, or meat jelly, while in quite mild cases custard, lightly boiled eggs, farinaceous puddings and bread and butter may be allowed. Such liquids as barley water, lemonade, black currant or tamarind drinks, cold water, and small pieces of ice, are useful in allaying the cough. Sponging parts of the body at a time with warm water to which a little sanitas has been added relieves the feeling of heat and itching and helps to bring out the rash. Irritation of the face may be soothed by the application of cold cream, and itching of the skin of the body by a daily warm bath and the use of carbolic soap, followed by inunction with the oily applications recommended in scarlet fever (p. 323). Where there is much fever, restlessness, and cough, solution of acetate of ammonia may be given in doses of half to two teaspoonfuls, according to age, in a wineglassful of water, every three or four hours ; to each dose a few drops of ipecacuanha wine may be added. The bowels should be gently regulated.

Further measures are called for in very severe cases. If the patient is a child, with a scanty rash, high fever, and signs of bronchitis or congestion of the lungs, the action of the skin must be stimulated so as to relieve the congested internal organs. To this end tepid sponging, hot packs, or mustard baths may be used. For a child under 2 years the mustard bath is the most satisfactory method. To water at a temperature of 100° Fahr., one tablespoonful of mustard to each gallon of water is added and the child is allowed to remain in the bath for three minutes and is then dried quickly and placed between blankets. If necessary the bath may be repeated in two hours. Linseed poultices on the chests of young children should be avoided, as they are heavy and may oppress the breathing ; hot fomentations and bran poultices are preferable. For older children the doctor may prescribe small doses of tartar emetic, in a teaspoonful of solution of citrate of ammonia, every three or four hours, provided it does not produce nausea. Alcohol, in the form of brandy, whisky, or wine should be administered if the pulse is weak and rapid or the tongue dry and brown.

When the crisis is passed, head symptoms may still threaten. To relieve them an ice-bag may be applied to the head, as advised in connexion with scarlet fever (p. 323). In severe cases of measles the eyes, nose and mouth should be bathed or mopped out with warm water. If ophthalmia supervenes, lead lotion is necessary, and the swollen eyelids should be raised to see that no injury to the eye occurs while attention is being directed to more urgent symptoms. Ulcers in the mouth should be touched with glycerin of borax or solution of boric acid. Earache may be relieved by a warm poultice, with a little laudanum dropped into the ear, and, if there is any discharge, by syringing with tepid water containing a little listerine.

The child should not be allowed to get up until the temperature has been down to normal for a week. In ordinary cases he may quit the room in three weeks from the appearance of the rash, and if he has been thoroughly disinfected it is not necessary to wait for the completion of scaling before allowing him to mix with other children. The greatest care must, however, be taken to prevent him from catching cold.

MEASLES,GERMAN(*see* GERMAN MEASLES).

MEDICINES, AND HOW THEY ARE MEASURED.

—Some persons profess to have no faith in the efficacy of medicine. In most cases this is obviously a mere pose. If such persons were to contract malaria, for example, they would be ready enough to resort to quinine. On the other hand, there are those who are much too fond of drugging themselves. It must be admitted that in the past medical men have been too much disposed to fall in with this weakness of their patients, but of late years the tendency in the profession has been not to administer drugs unless they are really required. The unwisdom of taking drugs needlessly is not yet, however, properly appreciated by the general public. In his clever and lively book on " Common Diseases," Dr. Woods Hutchinson records that in his student days in a London hospital a large vessel of an extremely nauseous but harmless mixture, known as the " dead-shot," was kept for the benefit of those who were too fond of medicine. It was composed of all the odds and ends of left-over drugs, with a handful each of crude quinine, aloes, and asafetida, and a pint of tincture of capsicum to strengthen the flavour and odour. Whenever a chronic medicine-taker complained that " his medicine didn't seem to have no strength in it " he was sent away with a bottle of the " dead-shot," which nearly always justified its name. Either the malingerer never returned, or he would come back to express his delight that the doctor had at last given him " something like a medicine," and to ask, " Why didn't you gimme that before, Doctor ? "

In the days when the apothecary was also the doctor, he was defined by Voltaire as " one who pours drugs of which he knows little into a body of which he knows less." The sarcasm has not yet lost all its point, for while a good deal of knowledge of drugs has been accumulated and many things about the human body that were mysterious are now understood, a medical man cannot know for certain, until he has actually administered it, what effect a drug will have upon a given patient. Thus, some patients are unable to take quinine, which at once gives them headache, buzzing in the ears, etc., and in other patients quite small doses of belladonna may set up very disagreeable symptoms. Such cases are, however, infrequent.

Classes of drugs.—Drugs are divided into groups according to their effects. Thus, those which soothe the nervous system are called *sedatives;* those which produce sleep, *hypnotics ;* those which produce both sleep and insensibility to pain, *narcotics ;* those which increase the action of the bowels, *laxatives* (weak aperients) and *purgatives* (strong aperients) ; those which cause perspiration, *diaphoretics ;* those which stimulate the action of the kidneys, *diuretics ;* and those which promote expectoration, *expectorants.*

Forms of drugs.—Instead of being given as pills (q.v.) and powders (q.v.), or as liquids, drugs are now frequently administered in the form of tablets and tabloids, capsules and cachets. *Tablets* and *tabloids* differ only in name ; they are usually devoid of unpleasant flavour, contain definite doses, occupy little space, and do not lose their efficacy, however long they may be kept, or in whatever climate. If crushed before being taken, they come into action more rapidly. *Capsules* are little cases of gelatin to contain drugs offensive to the taste ; they are swallowed, like pills, with a little water, and are rapidly dissolved in the stomach. *Cachets*, also used for unpleasant drugs, are little cases of wafer paper, and are made in various sizes according to the dose; they should be soaked in a tablespoonful of water, with which they may be washed down.

The time to take medicines.— For some classes of medicine there is a right and a wrong time to take them. Thus, acid medicines, hydrochloric acid, for instance, should, as a rule, be given from half an hour to two hours after the end of a meal, so that they may supplement the action of the gastric juice. Alkalis, such as bicarbonate of soda, often given to promote digestion by dissolving tenacious mucus in the stomach and to neutralize an excess of hydrochloric acid, should be taken about a quarter of an hour before a meal. Powerful drugs, such as arsenic and strychnine, are taken immediately after a meal, so that, mixing with the food, they may not injure the mucous membrane of the stomach and intestines.

Medicinal measures.—The *fluid* measures used in Medicine are these:

60 minims	=	1 fluid drachm
8 fluid drachms	=	1 fluid ounce
20 fluid ounces	=	1 pint
40 fluid ounces	=	1 quart
4 quarts	=	1 gallon

The popular equivalents of the fluid measures employed in Medicine are the following:

1 minim	=	1 drop
1 drachm	=	1 teaspoonful
2 drachms	=	1 dessertspoonful
½ ounce	=	1 tablespoonful
1 ounce	=	2 tablespoonfuls
2½ ounces	=	1 wineglassful
½ pint	=	1 tumblerful

Mixtures, unless they are put up in a graduated bottle, should be measured in a medicine-glass, for there are great differences in the sizes of spoons, wineglasses, and tumblers.

For *solid* drugs, apothecaries' weight is used. Here the equivalent of a drachm is 60 grains, but the ounce is not 480 grains, but $437\frac{1}{2}$ grains. A drachm, therefore, is a little more than the eighth part of an ounce.

MEDITERRANEAN FEVER (*see* UNDULANT FEVER).

MEDULLA OBLONGATA (*see* NERVOUS SYSTEM).

MEGRIM (*see under* HEADACHE).

MELANCHOLIA (*see* INSANITY).

MENIÈRE'S DISEASE.—Named after the French physician who first described it, this affection is sometimes a manifestation of disorder of the semicircular canals of the inner ear, so that they no longer enable the equilibrium of the body to be maintained. In other cases the trouble arises simply from blocking of the Eustachian tube, the canal which connects the throat with the middle ear, with consequent interference with the function of the semicircular canals.

Symptoms.—In most cases the patient, after hearing loud noises in the ears, suddenly becomes giddy; either he seems to himself to be reeling about, or the objects around him appear to be moving. In severe cases he may fall down, or may only save himself from doing so by clutching at the nearest object. In a few cases unconsciousness of slight duration supervenes. When the giddiness passes off it leaves the patient pale and perspiring; he feels sick, and may actually vomit; the vision may also be affected. The attacks occur at irregular intervals, sometimes following each other several times a day, at other times only once a week or once a month, but in bad cases they may increase in frequency until the patient is reduced to a state of permanent giddiness. The disease seldom begins before the age of forty, and is less common in women than in men. If the ear trouble progresses to complete deafness, the giddiness disappears with the sense of hearing.

Treatment.—The patient should lie down, and remain recumbent for some time, although even in that position he will not be free from a most disagreeable sense of giddiness during an attack. If the giddiness is caused by blocking of the Eustachian tube, the obstruction must be removed. The most useful drug in ordinary cases is bromide of potash, taken at first in 10-grain doses, gradually increased to 20 grains. In rheumatic cases salicylate of soda is indicated—in 10-grain doses ; in syphilitic cases, iodide of potash, in doses of 3 to 5 grains ; sulphate of quinine in 2-grain or 3-grain doses, in tablets, may also be recommended. All these drugs should be taken three times a day. In some cases the application of a blister just behind the ear gives relief. The general health must be carefully attended to.

MENINGES(*see*NERVOUS SYSTEM).

MENINGITIS, SUPPURATIVE. —Meningitis, the condition popularly known as " brain fever," consists in inflammation of the meninges, the membranes covering the brain, and in most cases the inflammation spreads to the substance of the brain and sets up encephalitis. Three forms of meningitis may be described : (1) suppurative meningitis, (2) tuberculous meningitis (*see* the next article), (3) infectious cerebro-spinal meningitis, known colloquially as " spotted fever " (*see* CEREBRO-SPINAL FEVER).

Causes.—Suppurative meningitis is in many cases the result of an extension of inflammation from the bones of the skull, originating in affections of the middle ear. It may also be caused by injury to the skull or brain, by exposure of the head to the direct rays of the sun, by erysipelas of the skull, or by infection conveyed from some other part of the body.

Symptoms.—In most cases the onset of the disease is sudden. There is severe and continuous headache, delirium, with pains in the neck and tenderness of the scalp, and vomiting. Usually there is a good deal of fever, the eyes are very sensitive to light, the ears to noise, the skin to touch. In many cases there are spasms or twitchings of the muscles, the head may be drawn backwards by retraction of the muscles of the neck, and there may be squinting or drooping of the upper eyelid from paralysis, etc. The duration of the disease varies in different cases ; the average may be taken as about a fortnight. Meningitis is attended by a high rate of mortality, and is, of course, unsuitable for domestic treatment.

Treatment.—The patient is put to bed in a darkened, airy room where he is out of the reach of noise, and the head should be raised. The bowels should be opened, and the aperient may be repeated from time to time. The head should be shaved, and cold lotions or ice applied to it to relieve the headache ; mustard plasters may be applied to the nape of the neck, and leeches behind the ears. Perspiration should be encouraged, and sedatives such as bromide of soda given. In cases in which the meningitis can be traced to some definite condition, such as middle-ear disease, a surgical operation is required, and a serum should be given.

MENINGITIS, TUBERCULOUS. —This serious disease is due to the germ that causes consumption of the lungs, the *Bacillus tuberculosis*. In some cases it follows tuberculosis in some other part of the body. It is usually children who are attacked, but adults also are liable.

Symptoms.—In some cases there may be premonitory symptoms; in others the attack begins with violent vomiting. Convulsions usually follow, and also headache, which may be so severe that the child screams continuously, or, putting its hand to its head utters a short sharp cry—the " hydrocephalic cry." There is fever, the temperature ranging between 101° and 103° Fahr. In many cases the little patient lies huddled up on his side, and if an attempt is made to straighten the limbs, the muscles offer automatic resistance. After a time the child loses consciousness, and although there may be intervals of apparent improvement, the hopes of recovery thus excited are usually fallacious.

Treatment.—This must proceed on the same lines as that of suppurative meningitis (*see* above).

MENOPAUSE (*see* MENSTRUATION AND THE MENOPAUSE).

MENORRHAGIA.—In the article MENSTRUATION AND THE MENOPAUSE it will be seen that the duration of the discharge in a menstrual period varies in different persons. In some quite healthy women the discharge may last only two days, in others it may extend over ten, and the quantity may vary from 2 to 6 ounces. When loss is excessive the subject will be anæmic and debilitated. The trouble may occur at any age, but is most frequent in early and later middle age, when fibroid tumours and the complications of pregnancy, both of them causes of excessive menstruation, are most common. In all cases of menorrhagia medical advice should be sought, for when the mucous membrane of the womb has once started

bleeding it is liable to continue, and in some cases the amount of blood lost in a few minutes is alarming. Very profuse bleeding is termed " flooding." If the excessive loss takes place during the monthly period, it is termed menorrhagia; if in the interval between one period and another, metrorrhagia; but the distinction is of no great importance, for in both cases the bleeding is from the womb.

Causes.—These are very diversified. Inflammation of the generative organs, displacements of the womb, abrasions and ulcers of its mucous membrane, threatened abortion, the conditions following confinement—these are among the local causes. To them must be added fibroid tumours and cancer, the latter most prone to occur when the child-bearing age is past. The general causes include inflammation of the kidney (Bright's disease), cirrhosis of the liver, the acute infectious fevers (in which the blood is abnormal, and clots with difficulty), hæmophilia and scurvy. Other general causes are emotional disturbance, excessive exercise, overwork at or near the time of the monthly period, chronic constipation, obesity, and high degrees of temperature.

Treatment.—The cause of the excessive bleeding in each case must be determined, and dealt with, if necessary, by surgical measures, such as dilating the neck of the womb and scraping away the diseased mucous membrane from the cavity (curetting). But the immediate requirement is to stop the bleeding. To this end the patient must take absolute rest in bed in the recumbent position, the hips being well raised. All exertion, whether of body or of mind, must be forbidden; even sitting up in bed would be harmful. The diet should be light and unstimulating; neither food nor drink should be taken hot, but at the most lukewarm, and alcohol must be withheld unless required to counteract faintness. If the bleeding still continues, cloths wrung out of ice-cold water may be applied to the lower part of the abdomen, and quite hot vaginal douches given (*see* DOUCHES). Resort may have to be had to drugs which will check the bleeding by causing contraction of the uterus, such as ergot and hydrastis ; these may be taken in the form of a compound hydrastin tabloid, or of a teaspoonful of the liquid extract of ergot in a tablespoonful of water, the dose being repeated in three or four hours if necessary. In bad cases the doctor may find it necessary to plug the vagina, first washing the passage clear of clots with a hot douche, and then, with due antiseptic precautions, inserting the plug.

MENSTRUATION AND THE MENOPAUSE.

—Menstruation is the periodical discharge of blood from the womb which marks the onset of puberty in the female sex. The name is derived from the Latin *mensis*, month. Alternative names are the menses, the catamenia, and, in common language, the courses or periods. All these terms have reference to the fact that the discharge, when normal as to time, occurs at regular intervals, i.e. intervals of twenty-eight days, reckoning from the beginning of one menstruation to the beginning of the next. The interval, however, is not seldom as short as three weeks, while it may be as long as five weeks or even longer. There is great variation also in the *duration* of the discharge, which averages five or six days, but may be only a single day, or as much as nine or ten days. Occasionally a day may be intermitted, the " loss " ceasing entirely and then beginning again.

Beginning of menstruation.— The average age at which the function begins is fourteen, but it may start two years earlier, or not until two or even four years later. It begins earlier in hot countries, and later in cold countries. Its onset may not be associated with indisposition, but more commonly it is preceded by some malaise. These symptoms return at the end of a month with greater severity, the girl may have sharp crampy pains in the stomach, the pulse may be quickened, and there may be slight feverishness and nausea. She then, with alarm if she has not been warned of what is pending, as girls ought to be, notices a blood-stained discharge from the vagina. As this becomes well established the disagreeable symptoms tend to abate, but she may feel weak and upset, and have dark circles round her eyes until the flow has ceased.

As time goes on, menstruation may entail no interference with usual habits and occupations, but the majority of women are not at their best during this part of the month. There is a sense of weakness and weariness, a feeling of fullness in the loins, with backache, headache, and pains in the lower part of the abdomen and in the thighs ; the breasts may swell and be tender to touch ; the mind is slack, and there may be a tendency to hysteria. In some cases the symptoms, both physical and mental, are more serious : the digestion is disturbed, the appetite capricious ; there may be diarrhœa and vomiting, the complexion loses its freshness, red spots and patches are to be seen on the face, and there may be distinct hysterical manifestations. As a rule, however, the only treatment required is rest in the recumbent position and quiet, the disagreeable symptoms passing off as soon as the discharge ceases. Even in cases in which the function is more normally performed, however, it is seldom wise for a woman to go about her duties as at ordinary times. She should take more rest than usual, avoid mental or bodily strain, restrict herself to gentle exercise, abstain from baths, shun exposure to cold and draughts, and wear clothing sufficiently warm.

Cessation of menstruation.—At the climacteric, or menopause, as this time is called, the capacity for child-bearing ends. The ovaries cease their activity, and the result is that the womb no longer becomes periodically congested with blood, menstruation is stayed, and the womb begins to shrink. When, after a time of more or less discomfort and stress, the periods finally cease, the woman seems to enter upon a new life, both looking and feeling distinctly younger, while her general vigour and energy are renewed. This change most often occurs between the ages of forty-five and fifty, the average age in this country being forty-seven. In a few cases, about one in seven, the change takes place quite suddenly, but as a rule it is gradual. One or more menstruations will be missed, then there will be the usual flow for a month or two, then another stoppage, with occasional returns at irregular intervals. This " dodging time," as it is called, usually spreads over two years and a quarter, but in rare cases lasts for ten or twelve years. The amount of the loss, as well as the time at which it occurs, becomes irregular, the discharge sometimes being scanty and at others profuse.

Symptoms of the menopause.— The cessation of menstruation is always accompanied by disagreeable and trying symptoms, such as heats and flushes, sensations of numbness, coldness, and tingling, digestive disturbances, constipation, headache, giddiness, failure of memory, wandering thoughts, and depression of spirits. In some cases these nervous symptoms may be so pronounced as to require special treatment.

Mode of life at the menopause. —At this trying time great care should be taken of the health. Indigestible food should be avoided, and less should, if possible, be eaten than before, so as to avoid the tendency to obesity which is characteristic of this stage of life. A special warning must be given against the temptation to resort to spirits to relieve the mental depression : in not a few cases this has been the beginning of the alcohol habit. Constipation may be corrected by cascara tablets or Carlsbad salts. To relieve the nervous symptoms warm baths may be taken. If there is difficulty in sleeping it should be met by healthy though not violent exercise, and the avoidance of excitement, rather than by hypnotic drugs. If necessary the following sedative mixture may be taken :

Bromide of potash ....80 grains
Sal volatile ....2½ drachms
Bicarbonate of potash ..... 2 drachms
Tincture of cardamoms .... 2 drachms
Chloroform water to 8 ounces.
Two tablespoonfuls three times a day.

MERCURY, POISONING BY, ACUTE.—Mercury is used as a disinfectant (corrosive sublimate, perchloride of mercury), and also in photography, etc. Give large quantities of white of egg beaten up with milk or water, or, failing this, flour and water, arrowroot, barley water, or gruel. The doctor when he comes will wash out the stomach. Stimulants to counteract the exhaustion, and laudanum to check the pain and purging, may be required.

MERCURY, POISONING BY, CHRONIC.—This condition may arise in those whose work brings them much into contact with mercury and its compounds. The mercury may be inhaled, or absorbed from food eaten with unwashed hands. A long course of mercury taken medicinally may give rise to similar symptoms, namely, an excessive flow of saliva (" salivation "), inflammation of the mouth and gums, offensive breath, nausea, and abdominal pain. These may be followed by symptoms of a graver character. To eliminate the poison, give iodide of potash in 3-grain or 5-grain doses three times a day. Antiseptic and astringent mouthwashes and gargles should be used, and tonics taken to improve the general health.

METRITIS (*see* Womb, Inflammation of).

MICROBES (*see* Germs).

MICTURITION, FREQUENT.—On an average the bladder is emptied five or six times a day in men, and three or four times a day in women. At night, when less urine is secreted by the kidneys, the function is usually in abeyance, though many persons, especially after middle age, find it necessary to rise at least once for this purpose during the night. In old age the bladder tends to become less sensitive, and water is passed less frequently. During hot weather less urine is secreted than normal, and micturition may be somewhat less frequent. It is sometimes found that on returning to this country from the tropics the call comes with embarrassing frequency, and in his work on Genito-Urinary Surgery, Sir John Thomson-Walker cites the case of an Indian civil servant and his wife who for two years after their return to England were unable, on this account, to dine away from home.

Frequency of micturition may be due to the secretion of an abnormally large amount of urine, as in diabetes and inflammation of the kidneys. In another group of cases it is the result of inflammation of the bladder, stone in the bladder, enlargement of the prostate gland, or inflammation of the urethra—the channel through which the urine finds its way from the bladder to the surface. In other cases the urine is at fault : it may be highly acid, may abound in oxalate-of-lime crystals, may be milky with phosphates, may swarm with bacilli or be mixed with blood. In yet other cases the trouble is referable to kidney disease, to irritation of the lower bowel by worms, or to pressure of the pregnant womb on the bladder ; or it may be purely nervous in origin, and be due simply to excitement or to fear. In many cases frequency of micturition is accompanied by pain, as when the urine is concentrated, or when the trouble arises from inflammation or ulcer of the bladder, or stone in that organ, or when, in women, the sexual organs are inflamed.

Treatment of frequent micturition will depend upon the cause. If, for example, acidity of the urine is present, Contrexéville or Evian waters should be taken, or bicarbonate of soda in doses of 15 to 20 grains. If there is excess of phosphates, acid phosphate of soda may be prescribed, or nitro-hydrochloric acid. If the urine is concentrated because too little fluid is drunk, the remedy is obvious.

MIDDLE-EAR DISEASE (*see* Ear, Middle, Inflammation of).

MIGRAINE (*see under* Headache).

MILK (*see under* Infants and Young Children, Feeding of).

MILK FEVER (*see* SUCKLING).

MILK TEETH (*see* TEETHING AND ITS TROUBLES).

MILIARIA PAPULOSA (*see* PRICKLY HEAT).

MINERAL WATERS.—In the article on Baths we have considered the medical and hygienic uses of ordinary baths; it remains to point out that there are also natural mineral waters, which may be applied either externally or internally, or both. They may be classified, according to their composition, as follows: (1) Saline (brine) waters, (2) Alkaline waters, (3) Bitter (sulphated) waters, (4) Sulphur waters, (5) Iron (chalybeate) waters, (6) Lime (calcareous) waters, (7) Indifferent thermal waters. There are also Bromide and Iodine waters and Arsenical waters.

1. The chief ingredient of **saline** waters is common salt, sometimes combined with carbonic acid. This group of wells includes hot springs as at Wiesbaden and cold springs as at Homburg; springs containing only 2 parts of common salt in 1,000, as at Baden-Baden, and others containing 300 parts in 1,000, as at Droitwich, which has the strongest brine springs in the world. They are chiefly employed in cases of gouty rheumatism, scrofula, and liver complaints. Taken internally, they improve the digestion, stimulate the kidneys, and encourage secretion generally. As baths they stimulate the skin. They occur at Ashby-de-la-Zouch, Builth, Cheltenham, Droitwich, Harrogate, Leamington, Nantwich, Woodhall Spa, and at many other watering places in this country. Among the best-known brine springs on the Continent are those at Bourbonne-les-Bains, Baden-Baden, Homburg, Kissingen, Kreuznach, Nauheim and Wiesbaden.

2. Of **alkaline** waters the chief mineral ingredient is bicarbonate of soda. They may be divided into two sub-groups—(1) the simple alkaline acidulous and (2) the alkaline saline. The former are impregnated with carbonic acid, and are useful in acidity, gout, gravel, gall-stones, indigestion, sluggish liver, and chronic catarrh of mucous membranes; there are springs at Clifton, Malvern, and Shap in this country, and at Bilin and Bachingen on the Continent. In the latter, common salt is present as well as bicarbonate of soda; these are less depressing than the others, and are beneficial in chronic mucous catarrh. They are found at Sandrock, Isle of Wight, at Ems, at Selters, and at Salzbrunn, etc.

3. **Bitter** waters contain sulphate of soda and magnesia, and sometimes, in addition, carbonate of soda and common salt; they are all aperients. They occur at Epsom (hence " Epsom salts "), Leamington, Scarborough, etc.; on the Continent at Apenta, Hunyadi Janos, Friedrichshall, Marienbad, Pullna, Seidlitz, and Carlsbad.

4. **Sulphur** waters are very disagreeable in flavour because of the presence in them of sulphuretted hydrogen or sulphides. They are prescribed in chronic gout and rheumatism, sluggish liver, chronic skin diseases, and chronic catarrh of the respiratory organs. They are met with at Builth, Harrogate (where the " old sulphur spring " contains 12·7 per 1,000 of common salt), Leamington, Llandrindod Wells, Moffat, and Strathpeffer. All these are cold springs. There are hot springs at Aix-les-Bains, Bagnères de Luchon, Cauterets, Barèges, Baden, and Aix-la-Chapelle.

5. In the best of the **iron** (or **chalybeate**) springs the iron is kept in solution by an abundance of free

carbonic acid, which makes the water at once more palatable and more digestible. This in part explains the great benefit produced in anæmia and in many female complaints by the very small proportion of iron present in the water. Among many other resorts in this country where iron waters can be drunk are Aberystwith, Bath, Builth, Cheltenham, Harrogate, Leamington, Llandrindod Wells, Scarborough, Tenby and Tunbridge Wells. Of Continental springs, those at Forges-les-Eaux, Pyrmont Spa, Schwalbach, St. Moritz, and Marienbad are among the best known.

6. Many of the **lime**, or earthy, waters differ little in composition from ordinary hard water, and it is not easy to understand the effects attributed to them, even when it is remembered that very large quantities are prescribed. They are said to correct over-acidity, and are therefore employed in some forms of dyspepsia and chronic diarrhœa. They are also used in chronic bronchial catarrh, and catarrh of the bladder and urinary passages, and are serviceable in rickets, as well as in some forms of eczema. They occur at Bath, Buxton, Cheltenham, Clifton and Matlock Bath, at Contrexéville, Vittel, Wildungen, and Loèche-les-Bains.

7. **Simple** or **indifferent thermal** waters are very feebly mineralized (hence the term " indifferent "), and are characterized by their softness and their temperature, which as a rule varies between 80° and 160° Fahr. They are taken internally for sluggish liver and dyspepsia, and are extensively employed as baths in chronic skin diseases, chronic rheumatism and gout, neuralgia, lumbago and sciatica, hysteria, general debility and the convalescent stage of illness. The waters of lower temperature occur at Buxton, Clifton, Malvern, Matlock; of higher, at Bath, Baden-Baden, Carlsbad, Gastein, Plombières, Vichy and Wiesbaden.

MINER'S ANÆMIA. — Technically, this disease was formerly styled *tropical anæmia*, but is now known as *ankylostomiasis*, after the ankylostome, a minute blood-sucking hookworm which in the egg stage of its life finds its way into the body through the medium of contaminated drinking-water, or food, and instals itself in the small intestine, where it fastens upon the mucous membrane lining that channel, drains it of blood, sets up a catarrh by the irritation it produces, and possibly crowns its evil deeds by manufacturing a poison for its involuntary host to absorb. In some cases the disease is caused by another hookworm, which bears the name of *Necator americanus*. Besides miner's anæmia, the complaint is sometimes called *tunnel disease* and *hookworm disease*. It is chiefly met with in those who work upon the soil, especially where they are massed together under conditions that make sanitation difficult, as in the case of miners, navvies, etc. The remedies most used are eucalyptus oil and beta-naphthol.

MINER'S ELBOW (*see* BURSÆ).

MINER'S NYSTAGMUS.—The word nystagmus denotes oscillation of the eyeball, and this is the chief feature of the disease known as miner's nystagmus. It is believed to be due mainly to the insufficient light in which miners work. In most cases the oscillations are accompanied by spasms of the eyelids, and the eyeballs and eyelids are red. There is dimness of vision, intolerance of light, and night-blindness, and it seems to the patient as though the lights in the pit, or on the surface at night, jump about or flicker. Miner's nystagmus is really a nervous disease, and the ocular symptoms are usually accompanied by headache, nausea, giddiness, sleeplessness, throbbing of the arteries and quickened pulse. For treatment the sight should be seen to, suitable glasses worn, and the general health improved. In severe cases the patient should have a long rest, and never return to work under ground.

MISCARRIAGE.—If a pregnancy terminates before a child is capable of independent life—i.e. before the eighth month, it is said to be a case of miscarriage or abortion (the latter term, however, is more often used for *early* miscarriage and for cases in which the pregnancy is terminated criminally). In miscarriages the child may no longer be living, while if living it will not survive birth. If the event does not occur until after the twenty-eighth week, then the case is said to be one of premature labour, and the child may possibly live.

Causes.—One of the most frequent causes of miscarriage is syphilis, which kills the child while in the womb. Other causes are injury, and a luxurious mode of life on the part of the mother, leading to a general want of tone. A pregnancy may be prematurely terminated also by a feverish illness. Slighter causes of miscarriage are indigestion, diarrhœa, the irritation set up by worms, the straining due to constipation, and a frequent use of strong purgatives. In highly-strung women, again, miscarriage may be brought on by violent emotions. It so frequently happens that one miscarriage is followed by others that it is not uncommon to speak of the "habit" of miscarriage. There is nothing remarkable about this when the miscarriage is due to such a cause as syphilis, which kills one child after another, expulsion from the womb

being then in the course of nature; but the habit is not so easily explained when the miscarriage is due to slighter causes not affecting the vitality of the child. Many miscarriages occur between the eighth and the twelfth week of pregnancy, but there can be no doubt that miscarriage occurs not infrequently at a much earlier period than this.

Symptoms.—In the first few weeks of pregnancy the symptoms of miscarriage resemble those of a painful monthly period; in the last three months they are like those of ordinary labour; in the intermediate stages they vary in severity according as they approximate to the one or the other of these extremes. In early cases the patient feels a sensation of weight and discomfort in the lower part of the abdomen, often accompanied by a feeling of coldness; she is also low-spirited and depressed. If the threatened miscarriage is not averted by such measures as those indicated below, these symptoms are followed by pains in the back, loins, and lower part of the stomach, gradually becoming severer, spreading into the groins and thighs, and assuming the character of mild labour pains accompanied by bearing-down sensations. There is often slight fever, manifested by shivering, a quick pulse, thirst, and digestive disturbances. A discharge of blood usually occurs quite early; at first slight, it becomes freer and more continuous. It may develop into "flooding," which is one of the chief dangers of miscarriage. In early and in late cases the hæmorrhage is not usually serious, but from the fourth to the sixth month, when the afterbirth comes away from the womb with difficulty, it is often alarming. Another symptom is a discharge of watery fluid, an indication that the membranes have burst, involving the death of the child.

Treatment.—Rest in the recumbent position is absolutely necessary. The patient should lie on a firm mattress, remain quiet both in mind and in body, put herself on a light diet, and avoid all hot foods or drinks. If the pains are severe the doctor may order 20 or 30 drops of laudanum to be given by the mouth, or stirred into a teacupful of thick starch and injected into the lower bowel, the dose being repeated until the symptoms have subsided or until a miscarriage is seen to be inevitable. If the treatment is successful in warding off the miscarriage, the patient should remain in bed for about eight days, and only very gradually return to her ordinary duties. If, on the other hand, miscarriage cannot be averted, it may be necessary to encourage the action of the womb by administering ergot, and by injecting an enema of soap and water into the bowel. In most cases, however, nature may be left to do her work unaided. If there is free bleeding, acid drinks are useful. Or the doctor may prescribe 2 or 3 grains of lead-and-opium pill. A drachm of liquid extract of ergot with water, repeated if necessary in three or four hours, will also help to check the bleeding, besides encouraging the pains. If these measures fail to check the bleeding it may be necessary to plug the vagina (*see* MENORRHAGIA). Until the afterbirth has all come away the bleeding is liable to recur ; it is necessary, therefore, that everything that is expelled from the womb should be preserved for the doctor's inspection. When everything has been expelled the patient should remain in bed from ten days to a fortnight, and must carefully avoid fatigue until she has returned to normal.

Among the precautions to be taken to prevent the formation of a *habit* of miscarriage is that of allowing an interval of some months to elapse before the beginning of another pregnancy, so that the womb may have time to recover its tone. When pregnancy again occurs the greatest care must be taken to avoid exertion and excitement, and to keep the general health up to par. As the time approaches at which the previous mishap occurred, these cares should be redoubled, the patient spending much of her time on the sofa, taking only the gentlest exercise, and of that, not more than enough to keep herself in health.

MOLES.—Moles consist of light brownish-yellow to black patches of skin which may be thickened and roughened, and are often the seat of an excessive growth of hair. They may be single, or may be present in great numbers, are usually small, though in some cases they occupy a large surface, and are most often met with on the face, neck, and trunk, but occasionally on the limbs. Either they are present at birth or develop soon afterwards. Of the cause of moles nothing is known. Unless for appearance sake, they should be left alone. If treated at all, they should never be irritated with caustics, but destroyed with carbonic-acid snow or removed by the surgeon's knife.

MONOMANIA (*see* INSANITY).

MORBILLI (*see* MEASLES).

MORNING DIARRHŒA (*see* DIARRHŒA).

MORNING SICKNESS (*see* VOMITING).

MORPHIA (*see* NARCOTICS AND HYPNOTICS).

MORTIFICATION (*see* GANGRENE).

MOSQUITO BITES (*see* STINGS AND BITES).

MOTHER'S MARKS (*see* BIRTHMARKS).

MOUTH, INFLAMMATION OF (STOMATITIS).—The form of this affection which is commonly called thrush is dealt with separately. In adults, inflammation of the mouth, in which the tongue may share, usually appears as painful little sores or ulcers, caused either by indigestion or by living under unhealthy conditions, such as breathing air polluted with sewer gas. Treatment aims at obviating the cause, whatever it may be, and using a mouth-wash consisting of boric acid 2 drachms, bicarbonate of soda 40 grains, tincture of eucalyptus leaves 6 drachms, glycerin ½ ounce, with water to 8 ounces. The mouthwash should be mixed with an equal quantity of warm water. In **children,** inflammation of the mouth is often associated with teething. It is important that it should receive attention, lest the surrounding glands should be implicated. The child should be allowed to suck a carefully cleansed finger-tip which has been dipped in boric acid and glycerin, and the mouth should be cleansed with wool soaked in a lotion made of borax ½ drachm, tincture of myrrh ½ drachm, glycerin 1 drachm, rose water to 1 ounce.

A more severe form of inflammation of the mouth in children, known as *ulcerative stomatitis*, is most frequent between the ages of six and twelve, when the permanent teeth are being cut. Rickety and tuberculous children are especially liable to it. At first the gums and the inside of the mouth are seen to be swollen and inflamed, and the breath becomes foul ; then the gums become spongy and bleed, the glands at the border of the jaw enlarge and are tender, there is an increased flow of saliva, and the inside of the cheeks and lips, and also the throat and tonsils, become ulcerated. For treatment, formalin tablets may be allowed to dissolve slowly in the mouth, and after food has been taken the gums should be mopped with glycerin of borax to which half as much tincture of myrrh has been added. For a time the diet should consist of finely pounded chicken, milk and barley water, cream, custards, and slops. Chlorate of potash in 5- to 10-grain doses may be given. A change of air is desirable, and it should be reinforced with cod-liver oil and with quinine and iron.

MOVABLE KIDNEY.—This condition, in which the kidney slips out of place, occurs much more often in women than in men, and in the great majority of cases it is the right kidney that is affected. A common cause is muscular strain, usually of a severe kind, but occasionally so slight as that set up by boisterous laughter. Among other causes are too early a return to ordinary life after confinement, constipation, and diseases of the kidney.

Symptoms.—Little, or much, pain may be felt in the loin of the affected side, and in the back and abdomen, accompanied by a sensation of dragging and weakness. The pain comes on when the patient is tired, or when the erect posture is assumed ; it is relieved by rest and aggravated by exertion. The digestive and menstrual functions may be deranged, various nervous and mental disorders set up, and the patient reduced to a state of invalidism, and, in cases where the stress falls upon the nervous system, she may develop melancholia and suicidal tendencies.

Treatment.—This may be either

palliative or operative. Palliative treatment may begin with the " rest cure " ; the patient keeps her bed, takes plenty of nourishment, the bowels are regulated, and massage is given to improve the muscular tone. She must then wear a special appliance, either Treves's truss or Suckling's belt. These appliances are most suitable when the kidney is movable in only a moderate degree and the patient is able to bear pressure. In other cases an operation may be necessary.

MULTIPLE NEURITIS (*see* Neuritis).

MUMPS.—This obscure disease is known among medical men as *parotitis*, because its chief symptom is inflammation of the salivary glands, among them the *parotid* glands at the sides of the face. It occurs in brief epidemics, and in any part of the world. It is favoured by cold and wet weather, and the seasons it prefers are winter and spring. The epidemics are often associated with outbreaks of measles, or of scarlet fever. Mumps usually attacks the young, especially those under 5 years, but the aged enjoy no immunity. Second attacks are rare. The breath is probably the chief vehicle of infection. The germ has not yet been discovered. A patient should be isolated for three weeks after the onset of the symptoms ; for the quarantine of a person who has been exposed to infection, four weeks is sufficient.

Incubation stage and symptoms. —The period between infection and the onset of the disease varies from eight to twenty-six days, and averages about nineteen days. The first symptom is usually fever ; the temperature may rise to 102° Fahr., with chilliness and headache. This is soon followed by stiffness, pain, and tenderness below

one of the ears. Swelling of the part follows, and gradually spreads. After a few days the other side of the face is liable to be similarly affected. The parts are so tender that it is difficult to speak or swallow, and in most cases biting is almost impossible. In a day or two the swelling begins to subside, and is quite gone in about ten or twelve days ; but if the spread from gland to gland is slow, that time may be exceeded. Sometimes the hearing is affected, and there may be earache. The general health is not much impaired, and recovery is complete and rapid. Serious complications may, however, arise : in boys the inflammation may attack the testicle, causing orchitis, with serious results ; in both sexes the brain or its membranes may be involved, with still graver results.

Treatment.—The chief requirement is the exercise of care to avoid chill, which might precipitate complications. The patient should therefore take to bed, remain there until the temperature has fallen to normal, and not leave the house until the swelling has entirely gone. The bowels must be regulated by a mild aperient. The swollen face should be smeared with belladonna liniment, or with equal parts of extract of belladonna and glycerin, or hot fomentations may be applied. If an abscess forms, the doctor will open it. The diet should consist of milk, strong soups, jellies, and beaten-up eggs. Thirst may be assuaged by lemonade to which a tabloid of bicarbonate of potash has been added. If there is much fever, the following mixture is suitable :

Solution of acetate of ammonium .... 1 ounce
Tincture of aconite .... 16 minims
Syrup of lemon .... ½ ounce
Water to 8 ounces.
Two tablespoonfuls every four hours (for a child of 10 years).

If the patient, when the symptoms have subsided, is anæmic and debilitated, cod-liver oil and a quinine and iron tonic may be given.

MUSCÆ VOLITANTES (*see* EYES, SPOTS BEFORE).

MUSCLES AND TENDONS.— (Plates XI, XII).—What we speak of as flesh is really muscle —the reddish part, with fat —the yellow or whitish part. Muscles are divided into two great groups, voluntary and involuntary.

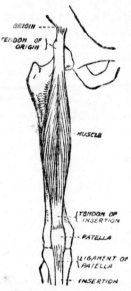

Voluntary muscles are under the control of the will; they are those by which the various joints are moved, and are connected with bones, cartilages,

Fig. 32.—Extensor muscle of the thigh, showing tendon of origin and tendon of insertion.

ligaments, etc., either directly or by means of fibrous prolongations called tendons and aponeuroses. The more fixed point to which a muscle is attached, and from which it acts, is termed its *origin;* its other end, attached to the structure upon which it acts, is called its *insertion.* Thus, the principal extensor muscle of the thigh (Fig. 32) has its origin on the pelvis, and its insertion on the patella, or knee-cap. **Involuntary muscles** are those not under the control of the will, but concerned in the automatic actions of the body; they are put into action by the sympa-

thetic nervous system (*see* NERVOUS SYSTEM). They are found in the blood-vessels, the different parts of the alimentary canal, the uterus, etc. Voluntary muscle is striated (Fig. 33), or striped—i.e. under the microscope a fine cross-shading can be detected in the fibres of which they are composed; involuntary muscle is non-striated. When a voluntary muscle contracts, the fibres swell out in the centre and its ends are brought nearer together. One may test this for oneself by bending the forearm upon the arm, when the biceps muscles can be seen to swell into a hard lump. The movements of the involuntary muscles are quite different; they are called vermicular movements, because they resemble the movements of a worm (*vermis*). It is by this vermicular action that food is passed downwards in its journey from the mouth to the end of the intestine. Heart muscle is striated, but the cells are somewhat different from those of voluntary muscle.

Tendons ("leaders") are white, glistening, fibrous cords. The tendon most generally known, perhaps, is the very powerful one called the Achilles tendon (Plate XII), which enables the muscle of the calf to raise the heel, into which it is inserted. The tendons of the hand and foot are of great length, for the muscles of which they are prolongations lie in the forearm and leg respectively (Plates XI, XII). These tendons run in sheaths, and, like joints, are lined with a membrane that secretes the glairy fluid called synovia, to enable them to move in their sheaths without friction. The tendons of broad and flat muscles, such as those of the abdominal walls, are flattened and ribbon-shaped, instead of cordlike; they are designated aponeuroses.

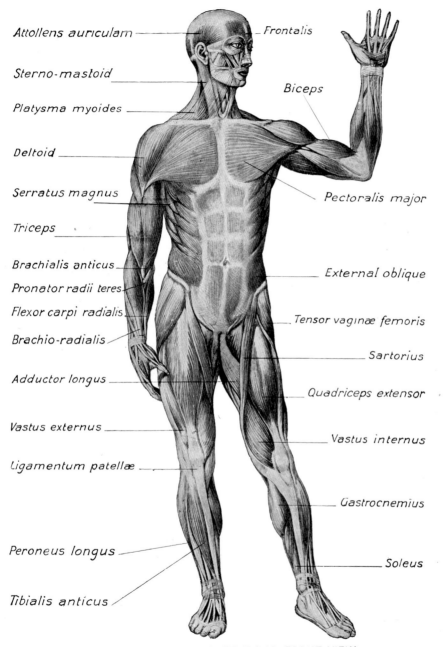

Attollens auriculam — Frontalis

Sterno-mastoid

Platysma myoides

Biceps

Deltoid

Serratus magnus

Pectoralis major

Triceps

Brachialis anticus

External oblique

Pronator radii teres

Flexor carpi radialis

Tensor vaginæ femoris

Brachio-radialis

Sartorius

Adductor longus

Quadriceps extensor

Vastus externus

Vastus internus

Ligamentum patellæ

Gastrocnemius

Peroneus longus

Soleus

Tibialis anticus

PLATE XI. MUSCLES AND TENDONS, FRONT VIEW.

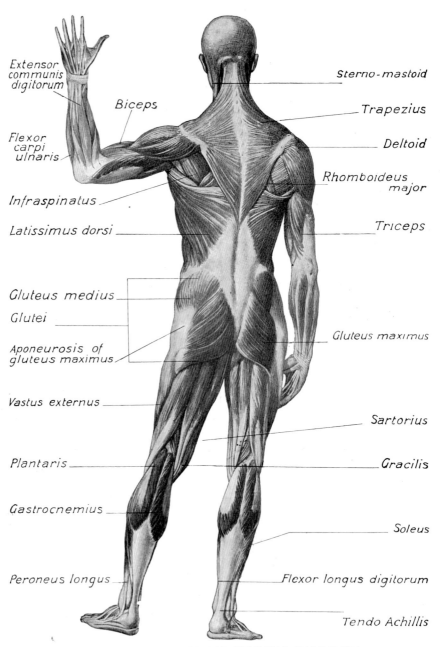

Extensor communis digitorum

Biceps

Flexor carpi ulnaris

Infraspinatus

Latissimus dorsi

Gluteus medius

Glutei

Aponeurosis of gluteus maximus

Vastus externus

Plantaris

Gastrocnemius

Peroneus longus

Sterno-mastoid

Trapezius

Deltoid

Rhomboideus major

Triceps

Gluteus maximus

Sartorius

Gracilis

Soleus

Flexor longus digitorum

Tendo Achillis

PLATE XII. MUSCLES AND TENDONS, BACK VIEW.

MUSCULAR RHEUMATISM
(*see* Rheumatism, Chronic).

MUSTARD PLASTER (*see* Plasters).

MYALGIA (*see* Rheumatism, Chronic).

MYELITIS (*see* Periosteo-myelitis, *under* Bone, Diseases of).

MYELOMAS (*see* Tumours).

MYOCARDITIS (*see* Heart Disease).

MYOMAS (*see* Tumours).

MYOPIA (*see* Sight, Defects of).

MYXŒDEMA. — This condition is remarkable because of the success with which it can be treated, so that, although it may persist for the rest of the patient's life, its effects can be entirely neutralized. It is allied to the cretinism of infants. In both diseases alike there is a partial or entire absence of the secretion of the thyroid gland, situated at the upper part of the windpipe. In myxœdema the gland wastes or undergoes degeneration, and may almost disappear, and although in some cases it may on the contrary become enlarged, the enlargement is only another form of degeneration.

Symptoms.—There is a great loss of muscular power; the patient's movements become feeble and slow, and the gait unsteady. The tongue swells, the speech is slow and often indistinct, the mind is inert. The face is swollen and expressionless, the complexion waxy, the nose flattened and broadened, the lips become thick and swollen, the eyelids are puffy. The hair of the scalp, with the eyelids and eyelashes, falls out, and in many cases the teeth are brittle and decayed. The circulation is languid, and the temperature of the body usually below normal. The body increases in size and weight, the abdomen protrudes, the hands are swollen, clumsy and spade-like, the fingers thick and defective in sensation. The œdema or dropsy thus present in many parts of the body is " solid "; if pressure is applied with the finger no depression is left when the finger is withdrawn. It is because of this solidity that the affection is termed *myxœdema*, the œdema consisting

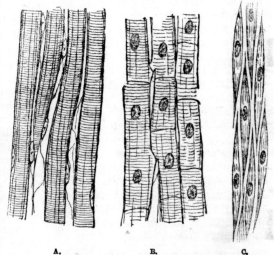

A.   B.   C.

Fig. 33.—Different kinds of muscle.
A, striped muscle; B, heart muscle; C, involuntary muscle.

not of the watery part of the blood, as in ordinary dropsy, but of a mucus-like substance.

Treatment.—This consists in administering extract of thyroid gland to compensate for the lack of the patient's own thyroid secretion. The medical attendant must ascertain the proper dose in each case. If the doses are too large the patient will complain of such symptoms as headache, or pains in the muscles. Most patients bear the treatment better if kept mainly on a suitable vegetable diet.

N

NÆVI (*see* BIRTH-MARKS).

NAILS, CARE OF.—The unsightliness of dirty finger-nails should be a sufficient reason for keeping them clean. There is, however, a further reason, viz. that in the handling of food it is possible to infect ourselves or others with disease. On both these grounds, therefore, it is one of the most important of the minor duties of life to brush the nails whenever the hands are washed. This is the proper way of keeping the nails clean; the improper way is to allow dirt to accumulate and then remove it with the point of a pen-knife, for the effect of this is to increase the space in which dirt can find lodgment. Keeping the nails clean is greatly facilitated by not allowing them to grow long; they should be trimmed at frequent intervals, at least once a week in winter and twice a week in summer. Finger-nails should be cut in a curved line, while toe-nails, especially the nail of the big toe, must be cut square—that is, straight across, otherwise the painful condition known as ingrowing toe-nail may arise.

NAILS, DISEASES OF.—Nails, like the hair and the teeth, are developed from a special layer of the skin, and are therefore regarded as appendages of the skin rather than as independent structures. The growth occurs at the root and at the bed (or under-surface); by the former the length of the nail is increased, by the latter its uniform thickness is maintained. It takes a finger-nail about four months to grow its own length; a toe-nail grows much more slowly. The nails are appreciably

Under this treatment the symptoms described will disappear, and will not return so long as it is continued.

affected by diseases which interfere with the nutrition of the body. Thus, in tuberculosis and other wasting diseases they are abnormally curved, as they are also in chronic heart disease owing to interference with the circulation at the tips of the fingers. In gout they may be deeply furrowed along their entire length, while in psoriasis and ringworm they tend to be furrowed from side to side, and to be dry, brittle and discoloured. The treatment of these nail troubles resolves itself into treatment of the conditions out of which they arise.

The independent diseases of the nails which must be considered here are—(1) Inflammation, (2) Ingrowing toe-nail.

1. Inflammation of the nail, technically known as onychia, and popularly as whitlow, is due to the presence of microbes, and is often the result of *injury*, as when a splinter is driven beneath the finger-nail. There is an accumulation of matter (pus) beneath the nail, which is loosened, and either lost permanently, or succeeded by an irregularly formed or an abnormally thin nail. In the milder forms of whitlow hot boric-acid compresses should be employed, and the finger soaked in hot water; the pain may be relieved by slinging the hand to the opposite shoulder. In the more severe forms the loose portions of the nail, or enough of it to allow the matter to escape, must be removed under an anæsthetic.

Inflammation of the nail may also be due to *syphilis*. The infection may be received in a crack beside the nail, in which case the inflammation forms the " primary sore " (*see*

SYPHILIS), or it may be one of the manifestations of the secondary stage of the disease.

In yet another group of cases inflammation of the nail (onychia maligna) is due to *tuberculosis*. It occurs in ill-nourished children after an injury to the nail, and several fingers may be affected. As the result the nail is shed, and an ulcer, which is slow to heal, is left. *Treatment* consists in giving an anæsthetic and removing the nail, if still adherent, scraping away the unhealthy tissue and applying iodoform gauze dressings. It is important that the child's general health should receive attention.

2. Ingrowing toe-nail.—In this condition, from causes such as the wearing of narrow-toed or ill-fitting boots, and cutting the toe-nail in a curve instead of square, the nail grows into the flesh and causes a troublesome sore. In almost all cases it is the outer side of the big toe that is affected. If the trouble is of recent origin, it may suffice to wear roomy, broad-toed shoes, and cut the nails square, packing a small piece of oiled cotton-wool or of gauze between the nail and the overhanging flesh with a clean probe, or the edge of a clean pen-knife, twice a day and gradually increasing the quantity of wool until it can be inserted under the edge of the nail. In addition, a notch may be cut in the centre of the top of the nail, for the nail will then grow in the centre instead of at the sides. If there is much pain and inflammation, a boric-acid compress may be applied. If ulceration is present these measures will be insufficient, and it will be necessary for the surgeon, under an anæsthetic, to remove the whole, or one half, of the nail, cutting out any unhealthy tissue that may be found, and applying an antiseptic dressing. The patient will be able to walk again in a few days.

NARCOTICS AND HYPNOTICS. —The chief narcotic is *opium*, which produces its effects by acting on the nervous centres. Whether as laudanum, the tincture, or as morphia (or morphine) or codeia, it is one of the most beneficent of drugs; it is the doctor's great stand-by when called upon to abolish intense pain, such as the agony caused by the passage of a stone, or the distress attending fractures, dislocations or other injuries. Opium also induces sleep in conditions in which mere hypnotics are insufficient, as in the insomnia of exhaustion, fever, or insanity; it is useful, too, in arresting diarrhœa and colic by checking the secretions and lessening the movements of the stomach and bowels, in staying hæmorrhage in the stomach or intestines, and in subduing cough. But when taken habitually, whether for the sake of the pleasurable sensations it produces, or to induce sleep, it is baneful beyond description. The first effect of a moderate dose is to stimulate the brain; the perceptions become clear and vivid, the tongue is loosened, and there is an enjoyable sense of exhilaration and mental freedom. All this, however, soon passes off, and gradually merges into drowsiness, and finally into deep sleep. If a larger dose is taken, the stage of stimulation is brief and is succeeded by insensibility so profound that it may be impossible to arouse the patient, and death may take place from paralysis of the respiratory organs. Some victims of the opium habit, or morphia habit as it is also called (morphia or morphine is the chief narcotic constituent of opium), take it for its stimulating as distinct from its narcotic effect, by drinking it, or by inhaling the vapour of the dried drug through a pipe. When the pleasurable sensations cease there is a corresponding reaction, and more of the drug is taken to escape the depression and recapture the vanished bliss. As the habit is continued the period of excitement becomes shorter and the depression deeper and more protracted, until at last the drug is taken more to purchase sleep than to procure pleasure. Its physical effects—dryness of the mouth, thirst, complete loss of appetite, nausea and vomiting, disagreeable as they are, are not so serious as its mental and moral effects—enfeeblement of the mind and perversion of the whole moral nature.

Chloral, an hypnotic, has little influence over pain, but is useful in nervous irritation and in checking delirium, and also in inducing sleep which is not followed, as is opium-induced sleep, by disagreeable after-effects. But this drug, again, should never be taken except under medical advice. It is very easy to form the "chloral habit," and its effects are as pernicious as those of the "opium habit." There is the same impairment of the mental powers, the skin is liable to serious eruptions, and abscesses may form. There is also the danger of an overdose, which may cause death by paralysing the nerve centre governing respiration.

Veronal, sulphonal, trional, etc., have no influence over pain, but are used simply as sleep-inducing drugs—hypnotics. The most powerful of the three is veronal, which, like trional, induces sleep in from half an hour to an hour. Sulphonal acts more slowly, and is also eliminated more slowly, so that there is often some drowsiness during the next day or two. Useful as these drugs are, they should only be resorted to when medically prescribed ; it is better to put up with occasional loss of sleep than to have recourse to hypnotics.

Cocaine, valuable as it is for its anæsthetic effects in slight operations (*see* ANÆSTHETICS) and in local irritation as in piles, and for subduing spasm as in asthma and hay-fever, is a most dangerous drug when used for its stimulating properties. Taken internally it spurs the mind into activity and imparts a sense of exhilaration, but these effects are followed by faintness, headache, breathlessness and other unpleasant symptoms. It has been used to enable people to overcome the craving for alcohol or for opium, but this is to invoke Beelzebub to cast out devils, for the cocaine habit, once formed, is said to be more difficult to break than the alcohol or even the morphia habit. Those who take it habitually lose flesh and suffer from impaired memory, sleeplessness and delirium. As one of the side-effects of the Great War there was a great increase in the number of cocaine and morphia "addicts," and vigorous measures have had to be taken to suppress the traffic in the drug.

Tobacco.—Nicotine, the active principle of tobacco, acts powerfully upon certain nerve-cells, and in this way slows the beating of the heart and increases the movement of muscles in the intestine and elsewhere. Smoking to excess causes the heart to beat rapidly and irregularly, setting up the condition known as "smoker's heart " ; the mucous membranes of the throat and bronchial tube are irritated, leading to frequent "hawking " and spitting, and the sight may be impaired (*see* Tobacco Blindness, *under* BLINDNESS). These are the effects of excessive smoking, and no inference is to be drawn from them adverse to moderate smoking. Moderation in smoking is difficult of precise definition, but everyone can discover for himself the point at which moderation passes into excess. There are a few persons who have an idiosyncrasy against smoking and should avoid it altogether, but smoking in strict moderation is ordinarily quite harmless, so long as the smoke is not inhaled or swallowed and the stomach is not empty ; it may, indeed, be distinctly beneficial, by soothing irritated nerves and inducing a sense of contentment. But it is known to have a deleterious effect upon the immature nervous system, and the habit should not, therefore, be formed until after the age of eighteen.

NASAL CATARRH (*see* CATARRH, NASAL).

NASAL POLYPUS (*see* POLYPUS, NASAL).

NEPHRITIS (*see* BRIGHT'S DISEASE).

NERVOUS SYSTEM. —The mechanism of the central nervous system is made up of the brain, the spinal cord, the nerves, and the groups of nerve-centres called ganglia.

The **brain,** enclosed in the skull, is enveloped by three membranes, the meninges—the *dura mater*, the outer one, the *arachnoid*, the intermediate one, and the *pia mater*, which is in contact with the brain. Between the intermediate and the inner membrane, and also filling a space at the base of the brain and the ventricles, small spaces in the centre of the brain, is the *cerebro-spinal fluid*, one object of which is to act as a water cushion, protecting the brain itself from jars and shocks. The brain consists of the cerebrum, or great brain, the cerebellum, or little brain, and the medulla oblongata— the bulb (Fig. 34). The *cerebrum* is

divided by a middle cleft, which passes from front to back, into two equal parts—the cerebral hemispheres, which are connected together underneath by crossing bands of fibres—the *pons Varolii*. The whole surface of the cerebrum is thrown into numerous ridges and furrows called convolutions and fissures. The outer layer, the *cortex*, consists of cells which are known as the " grey matter," being darker in colour than the " white matter " beneath, com-

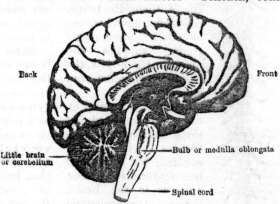

Back   Front

Little brain or cerebellum

Bulb or medulla oblongata

Spinal cord

Fig. 34.—Section of the brain.

posed of nerve-fibres which conduct impulses to and from the cortex. The cerebrum is the seat of the intellectual powers and of the will ; it receives all impressions from the external world, and originates muscular movements. The *cerebellum*, about the size of an orange, is situated behind and below the cerebral hemispheres, and is similarly composed of grey and white matter. Its functions are less clearly understood, but they are concerned in part with the co-ordination of movements on each side of the body. The *medulla oblongata* lies below the cerebrum, and connects both this part of the brain and the cerebellum with the spinal cord. It contains the nerve-cells which preside over circulation and respiration, so that any serious injury to this part of the brain is instantly fatal.

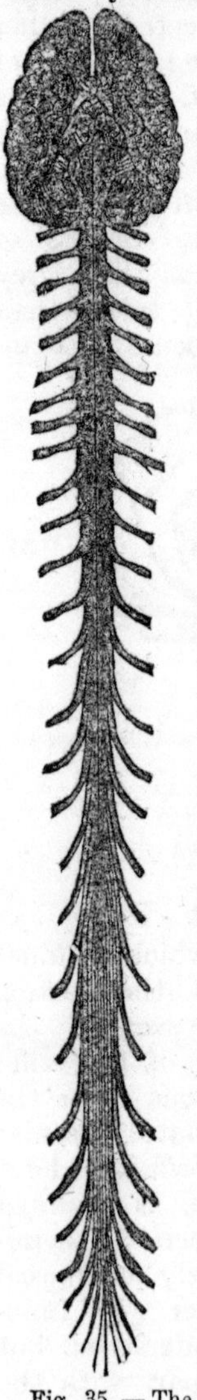

Twelve pairs of nerves, called the *cranial nerves*, are given off from the brain, and pass out through apertures (foramina) in the base of the skull to supply the organs of sight, hearing, smell, and taste, and the face generally, while one of them, the tenth, called the vagus because of its " wandering " course, supplies the pharynx, the larynx, the heart, lungs, gullet, and stomach.

The **spinal cord** (Fig. 35) is surrounded by three membranes continuous with those covering the brain, and bearing the same names, and, as in the brain, between the arachnoid and the pia mater is a quantity of cerebrospinal fluid, serving the same purpose of a pad or cushion. The spinal cord is a somewhat flattened cylinder of nerve substance, grey and white, but here the grey matter is within and the white matter without. It is enclosed in the *spinal column* (Fig. 36), which consists of seven cervical vertebræ at the top, twelve dorsal vertebræ, and five lumbar vertebræ, which are continued by the sacrum, the whole ending in the coccyx. The general office of the spinal cord is to transmit nervous

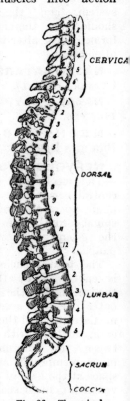

Fig. 35. — The brain and spinal cord.

impulses downwards from the brain to the body, and upwards from the body to the brain.

The *spinal nerves* arise from the spinal cord in pairs, thirty-one in number, and leave the spinal canal by small orifices between the vertebræ. The nerves which convey messages from the body to the brain, such as sensations of pain, cold, heat, touch, etc., are called sensory nerves ; those which convey messages from the brain that put the muscles into action are called motor nerves, or nerves of motion.

So far we have been describing the central nervous system. The **sympathetic,** or, as it is now sometimes called, the **vegetative** or **autonomic** system, has still to be mentioned. It consists of groups of nerves forming a chain that extends from the brain to the end of the spinal column. These nerves supply the lungs, heart, intestines, uterus, etc., and, in fact, all the involuntary muscles, including those of the blood-vessels.

Fig. 36.—The spinal column.

NERVOUS DEBILITY (*see* NEURASTHENIA).

NETTLE RASH (*see* URTICARIA).

NEURALGIA.—Literally the word neuralgia signifies pain in a nerve, but it usually denotes painful affections in which the structure of the nerve undergoes no visible degeneration. Among predisposing causes are debility, anæmia, and such diseases as diabetes, malaria, rheumatism, gout, and lead poisoning. In many cases the exciting cause of an attack is atmospheric—a draught of cold air, an east wind, exposure to cold and wet, etc. In other cases the trouble is set up by the abuse of alcohol, tobacco, tea or coffee, or by emotional disturbances. Yet other causes of neuralgia are decayed teeth, and a bruise or other injury to a nerve. The forms of neuralgia which will be dealt with here are (1) facial neuralgia, (2) neuralgic headache, and (3) intercostal neuralgia. Sciatica and neuritis are considered in separate articles.

1. Facial neuralgia. — Tic-doulereux, as this affection is also called, is the most severe of all the forms of neuralgia, and few affections are so refractory to treatment. The nerves affected are those supplying the side of the face and jaws, and they may all be affected at the same time, or the pain may shift from one to another. In some cases the eye is watery, painful, and bloodshot; in others the teeth are extremely tender, and the pain is greatly aggravated by eating or speaking. The neuralgia may extend to the neck and arm, and even over the trunk. The hair of the scalp may fall out, or a patch of hair may turn white. In some cases a breath of cold air or a loud noise may bring on an attack as suddenly as an electric shock. The patient may jump up in agony and rush about the room, or sit pressing his cheek, or rubbing it. These sudden attacks may occur, indeed, without any traceable cause.

2. Neuralgic headache.—In certain cases this form of neuralgia bears some resemblance to facial neuralgia. It is frequently started by a decayed tooth, an affection of the ear, or some defect of vision. If the eye is at fault an oculist should be consulted (*see* EYESTRAIN). Many of the nerves of the head have to pass through bony channels, and when inflamed, as the result of cold or injury, they press against the surrounding bone, and so pain is set up.

3. Intercostal neuralgia. — In this form of neuralgia the nerves in the spaces between the ribs are affected. The pain comes on in paroxysms, is sometimes very acute, and is greatly aggravated by any movement of the part. Frequently it is the first stage of an attack of shingles, the pain preceding the eruption by a few days, and continuing sometimes for months after the blisters have disappeared. It may be accompanied by palpitation of the heart, which may give rise to quite needless alarm.

Treatment of neuralgia.—In many cases neuralgia is singularly resistant to treatment, and it may be necessary to try a long succession of remedies. The first thing to attend to is to correct any trouble which may have set up the neuralgia, such as decayed teeth, imperfect sight, constipation, or the poison of rheumatism, gout, malaria, etc. The diet should be abundant and nourishing, and should contain a sufficiency of fatty substances, such as butter and cod-liver oil. The patient should take regular and systematic exercise, always stopping short of fatigue, which would aggravate the pain. The living and sleeping rooms should be well ventilated, and anxiety, worry, and every kind of strain should be avoided. Warm clothing should be worn, and the patient should, of course, be careful not to expose himself to cold or damp.

The drug which is most generally

used for neuralgia is quinine, in 5-grain doses twice a day in the form of pills or cachets. Some patients, however, cannot take quinine without getting headache; in these cases, and in others in which the drug has been used unsuccessfully, arsenic may be tried, 4 minims of the solution in water three times a day, after meals. A useful preparation is compound syrup of the hypophosphites. Other drugs are exalgin 1 grain, antipyrin 5 grains, aspirin 5 grains, antifebrin 3 grains, phenalgin 5 grains, phenacetin 5 grains.

In neuralgia of the face, butyl-chloral-hydrate, 5 grains taken as a pill every two or three hours, may be recommended, as also may gelsemium, 15 drops of the tincture every four or six hours, combined, if desired, with 15 grains of bromide of ammonium.

The pain of neuralgia is often mitigated by the use of local applications. One of them is menthol, which is made into cones, etc., to be rubbed on the site of the pain, or it may be combined with liquid drugs to form paints. Various liniments may be applied with a brush along the affected nerve, such as aconite, belladonna or chloroform liniment; or the A B C liniment, in which all three drugs are combined, may be used.

Counter-irritation, which sometimes gives relief, may take the form of hot poultices, mustard leaves, or blisters. In some obstinate cases electricity has been employed with good results. Where everything else fails, it may be necessary to resort to the surgeon.

NEURASTHENIA.—The meaning of this term, the medical equivalent of "nervous debility," is nerve exhaustion, and it is used to denote a state of the nervous system marked by great weakness and irritability, manifested in bodily as well as mental symptoms. The neurasthenic state is produced by over-fatigue, both mental and physical, worry, anxiety, and by many exhausting diseases, among them influenza. In most cases it may be regarded as the result of the wear and tear of life in a strenuous age. The most definite form of neurasthenia is that which is brought about by shock to the nervous system, either from direct injury to the nerves, with resulting pain and exhaustion, from fright, or from horror at the sight of accidents to others.

Symptoms.—The bodily symptoms include pains, crawling sensations, etc., in the head and various parts of the body. In some cases there is a sense of pressure at the top of the head; or the patient may complain of tenderness and weakness of the spine. Another symptom, especially in women, is flatulence, and there may also be dilatation of the stomach and constipation, together with " sinking " and " fainting " feelings. The heart-beat is in many cases quickened. The mental symptoms include a habit of magnifying small incidents, especially those connected with the patient's health. Generally, it may be said that the patient worries unnecessarily, and loses all self-confidence.

The simplest form of neurasthenia is that which is often met with towards the end of a year's work. The patient is mentally and physically overdone, work becomes an effort, there is lack of concentration, and mere trifles are magnified out of all proportion to their importance. Neurasthenia may thus be so slight an affection as to be cured by the usual annual holiday. On the other hand it may develop into a serious affection shading off into melancholia or hypochondriasis.

Treatment.—In serious cases nothing short of a rest-cure is efficacious.

It will probably have to be maintained for at least six weeks, and in some cases much longer. The patient should go to a nursing home, be isolated from friends and acquaintances, and protected from everything that would worry and disturb him. He must keep to his bed, and take exercise in the form of massage. He should live chiefly upon milk, so that the organs of digestion may be rested, and the bowels must be carefully regulated. In suitable cases electrical treatment is beneficial.

NEURITIS.—This affection may take either the localized or the multiple form, according to whether the inflammation is limited to a nerve, part of a nerve, or one group of nerves, or involves many nerves.

1. Localized neuritis may be due to injury to nerves, or to exposure to cold, or may be set up by poisons in the system, such as those of rheumatism, gout, or diabetes. The patient may feel an aching or boring pain along the course of the affected nerve and its branches; there may also be burning, pricking or tingling sensations, or numbness. In chronic cases, besides loss of sensation, there may be loss of power to move the muscles, which may waste. These symptoms may be present in a mild degree, or may cause intense suffering. The treatment of localized neuritis proceeds on the same lines as that for the multiple form (*see* below).

2. Multiple neuritis is usually due to poisons such as alcohol, arsenic, lead, and mercury; to those created by the germs of diphtheria, scarlet fever, influenza, syphilis, and other infectious diseases, and to those that accumulate in the system in jaundice, rheumatism, gout, diabetes, etc. The symptoms are very complex. They include tingling, numbness, pains, etc., in the feet and hands, loss of power over the hands and feet, loss of sensibility in the hands, feet, and legs, wasting of the affected muscles, etc. The *alcoholic* form, which is much the most common, occurs especially in women who are addicted to secret spirit-drinking. At first, in these cases, the patient may experience nothing but pains and tingling in the feet and hands, and tenderness of the muscles, but presently she feels that she is losing power over the feet and legs, and later over the hands and arms, and at last the hands and feet are " dropped "— i.e. the patient is unable to prevent them from hanging down from the wrist- and the ankle-joint respectively. These patients also suffer from loss of memory, and are subject to hallucinations. In *lead neuritis*, met with chiefly in painters, but also in workers in lead, there is usually wrist-drop but not foot-drop (*see* LEAD POISONING, CHRONIC). Of *arsenical neuritis*, which may be caused by the long-continued use of arsenic as a medicine, or by the consumption of food or drink which is contaminated with arsenic, the distinguishing feature is a deep-brown colour of the skin.

Treatment of neuritis.—In all cases of neuritis the same attention should be given to the general health as is described in connexion with neuralgia. If the attack is traceable to diseases such as rheumatism and gout, the treatment appropriate to those conditions will, of course, be followed. For the relief of the pain, similar remedies to those for neuralgia (q.v.) are suitable. In alcoholic cases the alcohol must, of course, be stopped. In most cases warm baths will be found helpful. As soon as the pains and tenderness have to a great extent subsided, gentle massage may be employed. Electricity is sometimes serviceable. It is important to apply passive movements to the affected limbs, so that contractions may be avoided.

NEUROMAS (*see* TUMOURS).

NIGHT BLINDNESS (*see* BLIND-NESS).

NIGHT TERRORS.—The proneness of some children to scream an hour or two after going to bed, and before they are quite asleep, is not so much a disease as evidence of nervous instability, and it demands wise management rather than medical treatment. The attack is frequently to be traced to nervous excitement during the day. Obviously, every care should be taken to save such children from all disturbing influences. Besides being excitable, they are often clever beyond their years, but their precocity should be checked rather than encouraged. Life should be for them a calm, quiet routine, and should be spent as much as possible in the open air. There should be an abundant supply of milk and cream. After an attack the child should be gently reasoned with, and encouraged to exert self-control, and each successful effort should be rewarded with praise. Unless the nervous instability is not checked by wise guidance and control, the danger is that the child may grow up to be flighty and hysterical.

NIPPLES, CRACKED (*see* SUCK-LING).

NITRIC-ACID POISONING.—Aqua-fortis, otherwise nitric acid, may be taken by accident. The lips, tongue, and gums are stained bright yellow, the clothes yellow, orange-red or brown. Lime-water or fluid magnesia may be given, in milk or gruel—a tablespoonful to a tumblerful. Or chalk, whiting, or carbonate of soda may be dissolved in a little water and administered in teaspoonful doses. Afterwards arrowroot or beaten-up eggs are suitable. No emetic should be given.

NITROUS-OXIDE GAS (*see* ANÆSTHESIA).

NOCTURNAL EMISSIONS (*see* SPERMATORRHŒA).

NOISES IN THE EAR (*see* EAR, NOISES IN).

NOSE-BLEEDING.—In nine cases out of ten of hæmorrhage from the nose the bleeding-point is situated in the front part of the cartilage which divides the nasal cavity into two parts, at a spot where the blood-vessels are very numerous. The bleeding, whatever the cause, usually ceases of its own accord. When it occurs spontaneously it may be salutary. In young people, for example, the flushing of the face, the buzzing in the ears, and the headache which may precede the attacks are all relieved by the bleeding. In elderly people the symptom may be of more serious import. *Treatment.* — The patient, having divested himself of any heavy clothing and loosened anything that is tight, should lie on his side and pinch the end of the nose with the thumb and forefinger for a quarter of an hour ; in most cases a bloodclot will be formed and the bleeding will cease. If this should fail, cotton-wool soaked in lemon juice or hazeline should be introduced into the bleeding nostril, which must then be compressed by the patient for fifteen minutes, the cotton pledget being left in for twenty-four hours. In some cases nothing more is necessary than to sluice ice-cold water freely over the face and neck, ice being at the same time sucked. In the last resort a medical man may have to plug the nostrils, both back and front, with lint. In some cases, having stopped the bleeding, he may advise the patient to have the bleeding-point cauterized in order to prevent recurrence of the trouble.

NOSTRIL, FOREIGN BODIES IN (*see* FOREIGN BODIES).

NOTIFICATION OF DISEASES. —The diseases which medical practitioners are under statutory obligation to notify to the Sanitary Authority are these : Smallpox, scarlet fever, typhus fever, typhoid (enteric) fever, relapsing fever, continued fever, puerperal fever, puerperal pyrexia, diphtheria, erysipelas, tuberculosis, acute primary and acute influenzal pneumonia, membranous croup, cerebrospinal fever ("spotted fever"), "sleepy sickness" (encephalitis lethargica), infantile paralysis, ophthalmia neonatorum, cholera, plague, malaria, dysentery, and trench fever. Yellow fever, measles, German measles, whooping-cough, chicken-pox and mumps may be made notifiable in the discretion of the various sanitary authorities. Certain industrial diseases, such as anthrax and lead-poisoning, are now notifiable.

NOVOCAIN (*see* ANÆSTHESIA).

NUMBNESS.—Those who are unduly concerned about their health are sometimes alarmed at a temporary loss of sensation in a limb, or part of a limb, which is commonly said to " go to sleep." The symptom, however, is devoid of serious significance. It means nothing more than that a nerve has been subjected to pressure long enough for its action to be slightly disordered. It most often occurs in the hand, from resting the elbow on the table, and in the leg, from pressure from the edge of a chair on the large nerve in the back of the thigh. In cases where pressure is long continued and frequently re-

peated it may lead to paralysis of the nerve affected (*see* PRESSURE PALSY).

NURSING, DOMESTIC.—In all cases of severe illness the services of a trained nurse or nurses are much to be desired, for the issue depends more upon good nursing than is generally understood. But trained nursing may not be available, and there are also less serious cases in which the wife or mother or other relative can undertake the duty. We will therefore, give some directions for the guidance of the amateur nurse.

Temperature of the sick-room. —A good average temperature for the sick-room is 60–65° Fahr., and it

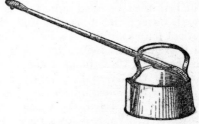

Fig. 37.—Bronchitis kettle.

should be kept at the same level day and night. The thermometer should be hung neither near the fire nor near the window. It is in the early hours of the morning that the room temperature needs most careful watching, for that is the coldest period of the twenty-four hours, and moreover the patient's temperature and vitality are then at their lowest. In most diseases of the respiratory organs, such as bronchitis and laryngitis, the air should be moistened by a steam kettle, either a special bronchitis kettle (Fig. 37), or an ordinary kettle with some contrivance for preventing the steam from passing directly up the chimney. In cases of pneumonia the room temperature should be about 60° Fahr., and plenty of air should be admitted, whilst in inflammation of the brain and some fevers it may be kept as low as 55°.

Water-bed.—If a water-bed is ordered, the bedstead must be strong to support the weight. A spring mattress must be made rigid by planks of wood laid across the springs ; on this a level hair mattress is placed,

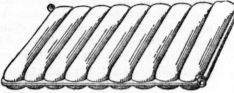

Fig. 38.—Air-and-water bed.

and the empty water-bed on the top. The bed must be filled quite full with tepid water ; if it is not full the patient may complain of a feeling akin to sea-sickness. Before he is placed on the bed a thick blanket should be stretched tightly and smoothly over it, then a long mackintosh sheet, and over this the linen sheet and the draw-sheet. Water-pillows may also have to be used to relieve various parts of the body from pressure and give support. For these pillows either water or air can be used, but a mixture of the two is generally to be preferred, and the same may be said of the bed (Fig. 38). Whether water or air is used, the pillows, unlike the bed, should be only half filled. A mixture of air and water may also be used for cushions (Fig. 39).

Draw-sheet.—This is very useful in cases in which the sheet is liable to frequent soiling. It consists of a large cotton sheet folded lengthwise into four, and so placed across the middle of the bed that it is under the patient's loins and thighs. When the part underneath him becomes soiled it is drawn away, and a fresh, clean portion used. If the bed is likely to be wetted, a piece of double-faced mackintosh may be laid between the under-sheet and the draw-sheet, or between the folds of the latter. It should be about 6 inches narrower than the draw-sheet, and fixed firmly to each side of the bed with safety pins.

Bedclothes, etc. — Whether a draw-sheet is used or not, the patient should be covered with an upper sheet, a blanket or two, and a light coverlet or eiderdown quilt—enough to keep him warm but not more ; if the covering is too heavy he will feel oppressed and exhausted. A bolster and several pillows will be required, and each bolster should have its separate cover, and not be wrapped round with the sheet. The patient's comfort depends not a little on the arrangement of the pillows. As a rule, the shoulders should be well supported. When he sits up in bed the bottom of the back should have the support of a pillow placed low down. If he sits up with a bed-rest, it is comforting to have the arms supported on small pillows, and sometimes a pillow placed under the knees is desirable. If this is rolled in a sheet, and the ends are tied to the top

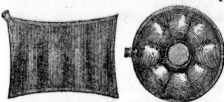

Fig. 39.—Air-and-water cushions.

of the bedstead, the tendency for the patient to slip down in the bed will be checked.

Changing the sheets.—The upper sheet should be changed from side to side by the following process : Remove all the upper bedclothes except the top sheet and one blanket ;

draw out the top sheet from one side while an assistant holds the blanket in place over the patient; then spread the clean sheet over the blanket, and while it is held in position by the assistant, draw out the blanket; finally, replace the remaining bedclothes over the sheet.

The changing of the under-sheet is by no means easy. If the patient is able to sit up he should move down to the foot of the bed; the sheet can then be removed from the upper portion of the bed, and the clean one arranged and tucked in; he then moves back on to the clean sheet and the lower part of the bed is made tidy. If the patient is incapable of moving, an assistant will be required.

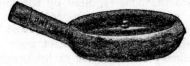

Fig. 40.—Bed-pan.

In this case the clean sheet, having been warmed, is rolled up from one side to half its width; the patient is turned well over on his side, preferably the right side, and retained in that position by the assistant while the nurse quickly removes the pillows and folds back all the upper clothes to half their width over him, taking care that he remains covered all the time. She then untucks the dirty sheet, rolls it up lengthwise to the middle of the bed against the patient's back, and lays the rolled-up clean sheet alongside and parallel with it. The clean sheet having been tucked in and laid smoothly over that half of the bed, the patient is turned first on his back and then on his left side, passing in the process on to and then over the two rolls of sheets, and while he is supported in this position by the nurse, the assistant removes

the dirty sheet and completes the rolling of the clean sheet.

In severe operations and fractures of the leg the patient cannot be moved about in this way, and it is then necessary for the sheets to be gradually drawn under him from the top to the bottom of the bed. First the dirty sheet is loosened from the top of the bed and rolled up as far as it is free, the clean one being rolled up with it and its upper end tucked in. Two persons, one on each side, by gradually raising first the shoulders, then the hips, and finally the feet, and rolling the sheet under each part in turn, can now remove the dirty

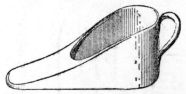

Fig. 41.—Earthenware "slipper" bed-pan.

sheet and put the clean one in its place without much disturbance to the patient.

The bed-pan.—There are several kinds of bed-pan, but the most convenient are the round (Fig. 40) and the slipper (Fig. 41) bed-pans, the latter with a thin end which makes its introduction under the patient easier. If the patient can move a little, the bed-pan can be easily brought into position, the nurse placing one hand under his back, and with the other slipping the receptacle into place. If he is quite helpless, she must have the help of another person. The bed-pan should never be dragged, otherwise the skin will be abraded and a bed-sore caused. Earthenware pans should be covered with flannel before use. When the pan, after use, is being removed from the room it should be covered. Unless the motion is to be kept for the doctor's inspection some disinfectant, such as carbolic acid, Condy's fluid, or Sanitas should be put into the pan before it is used. In some cases urinals have to be used; these can be obtained at the chemist's.

Cleaning the teeth.—When a patient is too weak to clean his teeth himself, the nurse should wrap a piece of lint or linen round the finger, dip it in water, and carefully go round the gums and teeth and roof of the mouth.

Washing the patient in bed.— Having got ready hot water, a bowl, soap and flannel, and towels, and put

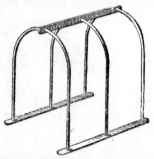

Fig. 42.—"Cradle" for supporting bedclothes.

a clean night-shirt warming in front of the fire, the nurse should close the window. The top bed-clothes, except the sheet, are removed, the patient's night-shirt is taken off, he is rolled in a thin blanket, the sides folded over the front of him, and the top sheet is removed. Only one part of the body should be washed at a time, and when finished should be wrapped up at once so that there may be no unnecessary exposure. When the washing is complete the clean night-shirt is put on, the top sheet replaced, the thin blanket removed and the bed made up in the usual way.

The prevention of bed-sores is dealt with in a separate article (*see* BED-SORES).

Lifting the patient.—By passing

her arms well beneath the patient, one under the hips, the other under the back below the shoulders, a strong nurse may be able to lift a patient single-handed. There is, however, some knack in this, and it is not wise for an inexperienced person to attempt it. When assistance is available the nurse stands on one side of the bed and the assistant on the other, and the patient is then raised or turned from side to side by means of a draw-sheet.

Sick-room appliances.—Among the appliances which are often useful, besides those already mentioned incidentally, is a *screen*, which may be used not only to ward off draughts but to protect the patient from the heat of the fire, or to guard his eyes from the light required by the nurse at night. If no proper screen is available, one may be improvised by fastening a shawl or sheet over an ordinary clothes-horse or by hanging one or the other from a clothes-line.

Bed-cradles are used to relieve the patient of the weight of the bed-clothes, and especially to keep them off a sensitive part (Fig. 42). One may be hired from a surgical-instrument maker's, or this appliance can easily be improvised, as by a three-legged stool or a band-box. In some cases it is comforting to the patient for his leg to be slung from the cradle by straps.

By use of the *bed-rest* or the *back-rest* (Fig. 43) the patient is enabled to assume any position, from the recumbent to the sitting, and to alter the angle of the body. With a bed-rest the pillows with which he is propped up can be used to much greater advantage, and prevented from slipping about in the bed, as they are apt otherwise to do. *Leg-rests* (Fig. 44) are particularly useful in cases of ankle sprain and gouty foot. Another useful appliance is the *bed-table:*

some are made to stand on the bed (Fig. 45), others to stand on the floor.

The best *hot-water bottles* are those made of india-rubber. Before being used they should be covered with

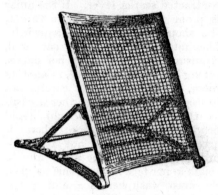

Fig. 43.—Back-rest.

flannel or other woollen material. This precaution is absolutely necessary in the case of young children or of paralysed and unconscious patients, otherwise serious burns may be inflicted.

A *feeding-cup* is useful to administer fluid nourishment and drinks when the patient is compelled to lie on his

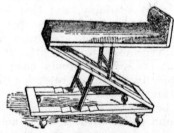

Fig. 44.—Leg-rest.

back. Feeding-cups with a spout should if possible be avoided, since it is difficult to keep the spout quite clean ; the cup shown in use in Fig. 46 is one of the best obtainable.

Taking the patient's temperature.—The doctor may expect the

amateur nurse to take and record the patient's temperature. The methods of doing this are described in the article TEMPERATURE, BODY.

The nursing of infectious cases.—In cases of infectious disease special precautions are necessary to guard against dissemination of the infection. A sheet should be suspended outside

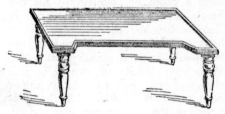

Fig. 45.—Table to stand on bed.

the door of the room or passage, the end of it resting in a bath containing carbolic solution, 1 in 40, with which solution it should be sprayed and kept wet. The chief use of this precaution is to serve as a danger signal, remind-

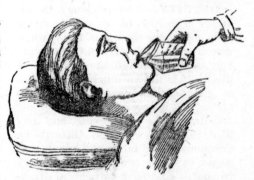

Fig. 46.—The "Ideal" feeding-cup in use.

ing members of the household that the room must not be entered. Discharge from the patient should stand for ten minutes in carbolic solution (1 in 40) before being emptied into the public drain. All books taken into the room must be burnt when the sickness is over, and the nurse will, of course, be careful not to do needlework in the sick-room, for this might afterwards convey the infection to others. All clothes for the laundry should be soaked for some hours in carbolic solution, and if possible should be boiled. Soiled sheets should be cleansed at once, before being put into disinfectant. The nurse should keep a basin of disinfectant for her hands, and dip them in it whenever she has touched the patient. When he is declared to be free from infection he should have a disinfectant bath. The head must be washed, and clothing put on that has never been in the sick-room. Before disinfecting the patient the nurse must change her dress, or put on a clean overall.

In all these infectious cases the nurse must be very careful to keep her own health up to par. A case is on record in which two medical students frequented the wards of a fever hospital for several weeks with impunity, but one day they entered a ward when tired out, and both contracted scarlet fever. If the nurse is prone to suffer from sore throat, she should use a gargle frequently. She must remember to eat well, cleansing and disinfecting her hands, taking her meals, of course, in another room, and being equally careful not to use the same cups or other utensils as the patient. She should avoid bending over him more than is necessary, and must not take his breath, nor should she allow him to cough in her face ; should this happen, she must wash her face and gargle her mouth with dilute Condy's fluid or boric-acid solution. If possible she should spend at least an hour out of doors every day.

O

OBESITY.—The tendency to an undue deposition of fat usually manifests itself after the age of forty, when men become less active in their habits and women undergo the " change of life." It is not so much a disease as a physiological process carried to excess, but it may have the discomfort and drawbacks of a disease, and may lead to heart weakness through an accumulation of fat in and round that organ, as well as promoting a tendency to gout. Excessive eating and drinking, the disproportionate use of fat-forming foods, such as fat, sugar, and starch, and indulgence in malt liquors and sweet wines, will account for most cases, but there are some in which obesity is found associated with rigid abstemiousness and careful avoidance of unsuitable food and beverages.

Treatment.—The only general principles that can be laid down are that no more food should be taken than is necessary to maintain the balance between intake and output, that sugar and starchy foods such as bread, potatoes, rice, etc., should be used most sparingly, and that little fat should be taken. The patient must rely chiefly on lean meat and green vegetables, with a little fruit, but as few persons would have the fortitude to be faithful to such a diet, stale bread, toast, rusks, and biscuits may be allowed in strict moderation. Tea and coffee without sugar and a little light dry wine are also allowable. The things to be specially tabooed are pork, duck, goose ; salmon, mackerel, herrings, and sardines in oil ; rice, tapioca, macaroni, oatmeal, and potatoes ; peas, beans, parsnips, carrot, and beetroot ; sugar and all kinds of sweets and pastry ; cocoa, milk (unless skimmed and diluted with water), cream, butter, malt liquors, and sweet wines.

The *Banting diet* once had a considerable vogue. It excludes starches and sugar, limits daily the quantity of fluid to 35 ounces—about a pint and three-quarters, and reduces the solids to about 25 ounces per day, of which about 14 ounces consist of animal food with 2 ounces of bread, the rest being made up of fresh vegetables. The details are as follows :

Breakfast at 8 to 9 o'clock : 5 or 6 oz. of meat or fish, or a couple of eggs, a little biscuit or dry toast (6 to 7 oz. of solids in all), and a breakfastcupful of tea or coffee, without either milk or sugar (9 oz. of liquid).

Dinner at 1 to 2 o'clock : 5 or 6 oz. of fish (not salmon, herrings, or eels), or meat (except pork), poultry or game ; vegetables (except potatoes, parsnips, beetroot, turnips, or carrots) ; a slice of dry toast, cooked fruit without sugar, dry sherry, 2 glasses ; or claret or madeira, 3 glasses.

Tea at 5 or 6 o'clock : 2 or 3 oz. of cooked fruit, a rusk or two, and a cup of tea without milk or sugar.

Supper at 9 o'clock : 3 or 4 oz. of meat or fish with a glass or two of claret or sherry and water (6 or 7 oz.).

This diet is not to be recommended indiscriminately, and should only be attempted under medical supervision. It may be too restricted for some persons, and may also, for the small quantity of fluid taken, lead to an accumulation in the body of deleterious waste products. These drawbacks are avoided in what is known as the *Salisbury diet*, introduced by Dr. Salisbury, of New York. Stated in the simplest terms, it at first limits food and drink to the lean of meat, preferably beef, and an abundance of quite hot water, a pint when dressing in the morning, a pint before lunch, a pint before dinner, and a pint before going to bed—not drunk, but slowly sipped. At meals only half or three-quarters of a tumblerful of water is allowed. The daily allowance of lean meat, 3 lb., is equally divided between the three meals. After a while, when the weight has been reduced, fats and farinaceous foods are gradually added in moderation. In many cases this diet has had good results, but no more than any other system should it be prescribed indiscriminately.

The taking of acids such as vinegar to reduce fat is a rather pernicious delusion, for it can only produce this effect by interfering with and perhaps seriously injuring the digestive organs. The patient should take as much exercise as he is capable of without fatigue ; if active exercise is impossible it should be replaced by massage. In some cases a daily cold bath is beneficial ; if there is no heart trouble a Turkish bath at regular, but not too frequent intervals may be advised ; and regular action of the bowels should be secured.

OBSESSIONS.—An obsession may take the form of a thought, an action, an impulse, or a fear. For example, a patient may be constantly imagining some dreadful thing, or may repeatedly perform some more or less irrational action, such as treading on every line in a pavement, or may feel impelled to commit suicide, or may have an intense fear of being in an open or a crowded space, as the case may be. These fears, by the way, are usually called phobias. The same patient may, of course, be the victim of two or more of these forms of obsession. They are all marked off from the illusion or the delusion of the insane by the fact that the patient knows perfectly well that they have no basis in fact. Obsessions are one of the manifestations of the psychasthenic state (*see* PSYCHASTHENIA).

OCCUPATION CRAMPS (*see* WRITER'S CRAMP).

ŒDEMA (*see* DROPSY).

ŒSOPHAGUS (*see* DIGESTION).

OFFENSIVE SWEAT (*see* SWEAT, OFFENSIVE).

OIL-OF-VITRIOL POISONING (*see* SULPHURIC-ACID POISONING).

OINTMENTS.—The substances most used as bases for ointments are lard, wax, lanolin, and paraffin. To one of these substances is added the active agent, the ingredients being thoroughly mixed or melted together. Ointments may be antiseptic, sedative, or stimulant ; they may be applied direct to the skin, or spread on the surface of a piece of lint. The one most often used is boric-acid ointment, which is mildly antiseptic, and promotes the healing of abrasions and other slight injuries to the skin. Zinc ointment, which is more stimulating, is also used for surface wounds. Mercury and iodide of potash ointments are employed to reduce inflammatory swellings and enlarged glands. Opium-and-gall ointment is serviceable in the treatment of piles. Drugs may be introduced into the system through the skin in the form of ointment by vigorous rubbing—" inunction."

OLD SIGHT (*see* SIGHT, DEFECTS OF).

ONYCHIA (*see* NAILS, DISEASES OF).

OPEN-AIR TREATMENT (*see under* CONSUMPTION).

OPHTHALMIA.—This term is applied to inflammation of the eye, and especially to the more serious forms of inflammation of the conjunctiva, the membrane lining the inside of the eyelid and the front of the eye-

ball. The simpler forms of inflammation of this membrane are dealt with under CONJUNCTIVITIS. Here we shall consider (1) purulent ophthalmia, with ophthalmia neonatorum, and (2) sympathetic ophthalmia.

1. **Purulent ophthalmia.** — This form of ophthalmia is very infective. It is transmitted from one person to another by the discharge from the eye, generally through the medium of a soiled towel, etc. ; it may also, it is believed, be conveyed by flies. Children are especially liable to it, and it sometimes runs as an epidemic through schools, barracks, etc. The eyelids are swollen and matted together, a severe burning pain is felt, the conjunctiva is puffy and bright scarlet in colour, and ulcers may form on the cornea, the transparent part of the eye, may seriously damage the sight, and may even cause blindness. The patient is feverish, and feels thoroughly out of sorts. The affection is, of course, too serious for domestic treatment. The inflamed membrane must be cleansed by the application of an antiseptic lotion, such as boric acid, a teaspoonful to a pint of warm water, or corrosive sublimate, 1 in 2,000 of warm water ; this should be used at hourly intervals during the day, and several times at night, the lids being gently separated with the finger and thumb, and the lotion introduced into the eye from a syringe or an undine (*see* p. 80). After the cleansing, a few drops of a 25-per-cent. solution of argyrol should be instilled into the eye, and the head so held that the solution runs well under the upper lid. The lids should then be smeared with lanolin or vaselin to prevent them from sticking together. Great care must be taken to keep the infection from spreading. The eyes should be wiped with clean rags or cotton-wool,

fallen on the clothes the stain will be brownish or reddish. Give no emetic, but draughts of dissolved chalk, whiting, lime, or whitewash off the wall or ceiling, and afterwards a dose of castor

P

PALPATION (*see* DIAGNOSIS).

PALPITATION OF THE HEART.—As a rule, a healthy person is unconscious of the beating of his heart, although in some cases the heart-beat may be felt when lying on the left side, a position in which the organ is brought more closely into contact with the wall of the chest. It may also be felt as the result of more or less violent physical exertion, such as running. But ordinarily the heart does its work without obtruding the fact upon our notice. If, however, there is organic disease, or the working of the heart is interfered with although its structure is undamaged, we may become disagreeably conscious of its activity.

Causes.—A common cause of palpitation is indigestion, and especially flatulence. Palpitation may arise, too, from pressure on the heart by tumours, from dropsy of the abdomen, or from tight clothing. Another cause is to be found in the condition of the blood. If this is " poor " as in severe anæmia, the heart is imperfectly nourished and its action interfered with ; as it is also when the blood contains large quantities of waste material. Hence it is that gouty people often complain of palpitation. Similarly the heart may be goaded into violent action by poisons which are introduced into the blood as the result of excessive indulgence in tobacco, or in tea or coffee ; in a few cases, even moderate indulgence in these luxuries is sufficient to produce palpitation. In another large group of cases the trouble is

oil. Drinks such as milk, lime water, barley water and gruel should be continued for several days.

OZÆNA (*see* CATARRH, NASAL).

brought about by the influence on the nerves of violent or distressing emotions. It is necessary, of course, to trace out the particular cause of the condition before instituting treatment, but the most important thing for the doctor to determine is whether the affection of the heart is organic or merely functional. The different characteristics of the two kinds of palpitation are clearly set out in the following table, compiled by Aitken :

Palpitation from organic heart disease
1. Usually comes on slowly and gradually.
2. Is constant, though worse at times.
3. Is accompanied by blueness of the lips and cheeks, congestion of the face, swelling of legs.
4. Heart action not necessarily quicker.
5. Palpitation often not much complained of by the patient, but occasionally attended with severe pain extending to the left shoulder and arm.
6. Palpitation increased by exercise, stimulants, and tonics, but relieved by rest.
7. Is more common in men than in women.
8. Beat stronger, heaving, and prolonged.

Palpitation from functional heart disease
1. Generally sets in suddenly.
2. Is not constant ; entirely absent between attacks.
3. Is not accompanied by blueness or swelling, face often pale.
4. Heart action usually quickened.
5. Palpitation much complained of by patient, often with pain in left side.
6. Palpitation increased by sedentary occupation, but relieved by moderate exercise, stimulants, and tonics.
7. Is more common in women than in men.
8. Beat abrupt, not heaving or prolonged ; fluttering sensation at pit of stomach.

Symptoms. — The sensations experienced during an attack of palpitation differ somewhat in different cases, but usually throbbing of the large arteries, as well as forcible or irregular action of the heart, is felt, and the pulse is irregular. Some difficulty is experienced in breathing, specks may be seen floating before the eyes and the eyeballs may feel disagreeably tense, noises may be heard in the ears, the patient may feel giddy, the face is flushed, the skin is moist with perspiration. In very bad attacks he may become partially unconscious, or may even faint. The attack may last only a few minutes, or several hours.

Treatment.—The late Sir William Broadbent found that in some cases an attack of palpitation might be cut short by taking " a dozen deliberate deep breaths." This simple remedy may be tried, though in many cases it will not be found to answer. If the attack is really troublesome the patient should lie down in a well ventilated room and keep quiet, anything tight about the neck and chest being loosened. A teaspoonful of sal-volatile and water may be taken as a stimulant. The discomfort caused by palpitation is relieved in some cases by the application of a belladonna plaster over the heart. If the attack is severe and protracted, and difficulty of breathing a prominent symptom, the inhalation of oxygen gas may be required. If the palpitation is associated with acidity of the stomach and flatulence, one or two soda-mint tablets may be taken in a little water, or dissolved slowly in the mouth, or hot water in which half a teaspoonful of bicarbonate of soda has been dissolved may be drunk. In all cases in which the condition depends upon digestive disturbances, whatever aperient the patient is accustomed to should be taken. If tobacco or tea or coffee appears to be the cause of the trouble it must, of course, be given

up for the time being and only returned to with caution. If the patient is full-blooded the diet should be reduced, and mineral or other aperients taken. Gouty and anæmic patients should be treated as described in the articles GOUT and ANÆMIA. Those who are debilitated should take a tonic such as arsenic. If the palpitation is nervous in origin, the remedy is to be found in avoidance of excitement, the exercise of self-control, and indulgence in moderate but not excessive exercise in the open air.

PALSY.—A synonym for paralysis (q.v.).

PANCREAS (*see* DIGESTION).

PANCREATITIS.— Inflammation of the pancreas is a grave but fortunately rare affection, of which the cause is not yet fully understood. Operative treatment is required.

PANDEMIC DISEASE (*see* DISEASE, CLASSIFICATION OF).

PAPILLOMAS (*see* WARTS).

PAPULAR URTICARIA (*see* URTICARIA).

PARAFFIN POISONING. — Paraffin (kerosine, petroleum) has occasionally been drunk in mistake for ginger beer. Treatment consists in giving an emetic (*see* EMETICS), following it with stimulants, and keeping the patient warm.

PARALYSIS.—This term covers loss of sensation and of power of movement, either partial or complete. It is due to disease or injury of the brain, the spinal cord, or the nerves. Bulbar paralysis, facial paralysis, general paralysis of the insane, locomotor ataxy, pressure palsy, and shaking palsy are dealt with in separate articles ; in this place we shall consider one-sided paralysis—hemiplegia, and paralysis of the lower part of the body—paraplegia.

Hemiplegia.—The most frequent cause of paralysis of one side of the body, i.e. one leg and one arm, is hæmorrhage on to the surface of the brain or into its substance (*see* APOPLEXY), but the condition may also be set up by arterial obstruction, so that the blood supply of the brain is cut off ; by meningitis—inflammation of the membranes covering the brain ; by encephalitis—inflammation of the brain itself ; by tumours ; by degeneration of the brain substance which takes the form of hardening, etc. The effects of hemiplegia which have, as far as possible, to be prevented are rigidity, contracture and wasting of muscles, and fixation of joints. *Treatment* consists largely in moving the paralysed limb for the patient—passive movements, and applying massage and electricity ; but the patient must be prompted to persevering endeavours to move the limb himself. If the power of voluntary movement is regained in some measure, it must be regularly exercised. Neither the arm nor the leg should be allowed to lie for long in one position, which would encourage rigidity. Fixation of the joints will not usually occur if movements, passive or active, are practised from the beginning of the illness. The wasting of muscles may be to some extent prevented by massage and the application of the faradic current.

Paraplegia.—In paraplegia there is partial or complete loss of power over the lower limbs, generally, but not always, accompanied by absence of sensation, by loss of control over the bladder and bowel, and by failure of nutrition, so that the muscles waste. It is most often the result of disease of the spinal cord, or of injury to it, as when the spine is fractured. In cases of disease of the spinal cord the treatment will vary with the particular

disease, but there are certain symptoms which are common to all forms, and demand the same treatment. Thus, the nutrition of the skin being impaired, there is special liability to bedsores (q.v.). The muscles will either have too much " tone " and become rigid, or will be toneless and limp. In the latter case massage, which in certain cases selected by the medical attendant may be supplemented by electricity, will be found beneficial. The former condition may be accompanied by involuntary spasms which it may be difficult to check. The clothes may have to be kept off the lower limbs by a cradle, and in some cases the attaching of weights to the ankles so as slightly to extend the lower limbs will avert or mitigate the spasms. If there is incontinence of urine, the patient will have to wear a urinal. If the contrary condition of retention of urine is present, the bladder must be emptied with a catheter. In cases where control over the motions is lost, it may be advisable to wash out the rectum daily with a large soap-and-water enema, so that the bed may be soiled as little as possible.

PARALYSIS AGITANS (*see* SHAKING PALSY).

PARALYSIS, FACIAL (*see* FACIAL PARALYSIS).

PARAPHIMOSIS (*see* PHIMOSIS).

PARAPLEGIA (*see* PARALYSIS).

PARAPSORIASIS (*see* PSORIASIS).

PARATYPHOID FEVER (*see* TYPHOID FEVER).

PAROTITIS (*see* MUMPS).

PASTEURIZATION OF MILK (*see* INFANTS AND YOUNG CHILDREN, FEEDING OF).

PEDICULOSIS (*see* STINGS AND BITES).

PELLAGRA.—This curious disease has a very wide range, occurring in parts of all the four continents, while it is not unknown in Australasia. Its history is comparatively recent. It was first described in Italy and in Spain about the middle of the eighteenth century, and it is still more common in those countries than in most others. Cases have of late years been met with in England and Scotland and in the United States. It is essentially a rural as distinct from a town disease, and most frequently attacks field labourers. In the northern hemisphere the disease always begins in the spring months, and the relapses which are one of its features take place year after year at the same season, although occasionally a relapse may occur in the autumn. There has been much speculation as to the cause. The present tendency is to include pellagra among the " deficiency diseases " (q.v.). According to this theory pellagra attacks those whose diet is poor in proteins and vitamins (*see* FOOD).

Symptoms.—The patient feels limp and lethargic, is very pale, has a peculiar stare, complains of headache, giddiness, and pains in the back and joints, becomes irritable, stupid and morose. The tongue, at first furred, becomes raw, the gums may be swollen and may bleed easily, red patches appear on the skin, especially in those parts of the body which are unclothed. As a rule the eruption lasts for about a fortnight, and is followed by scaling which leaves the skin rough, thickened, and permanently stained. This roughness of the skin it is which led to the disease being called " pellagra," the Italian for " rough skin." Besides the symptoms mentioned, there are others of a nervous character. After two or three months the symptoms subside, only

however, to recur in the following spring with greater severity, and so in succeeding years at the same season, and at last, unless he should succumb to some other disease, the patient is bedridden and completely demented.

Treatment.—There is not much hope of checking the progress of the disease except in the early stages. The drug which has given best results is arsenic, in the form of Fowler's solution, or of salvarsan. The diet should be rich in proteins and in vitamins, and the patient should migrate to an area where the disease is not endemic.

PEMPHIGUS, CONTAGIOUS. —The very contagious skin disease which bears this name, and is peculiar to warm climates, is allied to contagious impetigo (*see* IMPETIGO). It is undoubtedly due to a germ, which, however, has not yet been clearly identified. The lesions begin as tiny specks, which rapidly grow into watery pimples, and then into blisters : hence " pemphigus," from the Greek word for " blister." Treatment consists in the frequent application of bichloride-of-mercury lotion (1 in 1,000) and of a dusting powder of boric acid, starch, and zinc oxide in equal parts. Rigid cleanliness must be observed.

PEMPHIGUS VULGARIS.—This skin disease is qualified as *vulgaris* because it is less rare than some other and more serious varieties of pemphigus. The characteristic of all the varieties is an eruption of blisters (*see* PEMPHIGUS, CONTAGIOUS). The cause of pemphigus vulgaris is not known. It is a serious though fortunately not common affection, and is not suitable for domestic treatment. In a few cases it is hereditary. The blisters are usually preceded by a state of feverishness and accompanied by itching and burning sensations.

They attain their full size in the course of a few hours. Their contents are at first clear and transparent, but soon become opaque, the blisters then drying up and forming brownish-yellow scabs. There are successive crops of blisters, and thus the disease may be prolonged for several months. In weakly patients the discomfort the eruption causes and the consequent loss of sleep lead to great depression and exhaustion, and may even end in death. The first attack may be the last, but frequently, after some months or a year, the disease recurs, perhaps more than once. The drug which gives the best results internally is arsenic.

PEPTIC ULCER (*see* STOMACH, ULCER OF).

PEPTONIZATION (*see* Milk, Peptonized, and Beef Tea, Peptonized, *under* COOKERY, INVALID).

PERCUSSION (*see* DIAGNOSIS).

PERFORATION (*see* STOMACH, ULCER OF ; TYPHOID FEVER).

PERICARDITIS (*see* HEART DISEASE).

PERIOSTEUM (*see* BONES AND JOINTS).

PERIOSTITIS (*see* BONE, DISEASES OF).

PERITONITIS, ACUTE.—The peritoneum, the thin, smooth membrane which lines the wall of the abdomen and forms a covering for the organs of that cavity and of the pelvis, is very liable to become inflamed : this is peritonitis. In the acute form of the disease the immediate cause is to be found in a germ—most often the colon bacillus, which flourishes in the large bowel. Sometimes the germs find entrance to the peritoneum by a wound. In other cases the bowels, irritated by their contents, become inflamed, and

the germs, penetrating the walls of the intestine, reach the peritoneum. Peritonitis may also be due to disease of some other organ, such as the appendix (appendicitis), the stomach, the gall-bladder, the pancreas, or the womb. Other cases originate in a rupture which becomes nipped or strangulated, while in young women this serious affection may be due to so slight a cause as a chill contracted during the monthly periods. The infection may also be conveyed to the peritoneum by the blood-stream.

Symptoms. — The attack begins with violent pain which may be mistaken for colic, usually limited to a particular spot, but spreading rapidly over the whole abdomen, which is rigid and exceedingly tender. The patient shrinks from the slightest touch, and even the weight of the bedclothes is intolerable. He finds it least painful to breathe in quick, short gasps, and to lie on his back with the legs bent up to the trunk and the shoulders drawn forward. There is usually a high temperature, with violent sickness, and a rapid, feeble pulse. The appearance of the patient is highly characteristic : the face is pallid and drawn, and profoundly anxious in expression, and the sunken eyes are surrounded with dark rings. The abdomen is much distended with wind, and afterwards with fluid from the inflamed peritoneum.

Treatment.—In all cases in which the ordeal can be borne, an operation must be performed with the least possible delay, in order to remove the cause of the trouble. In some cases benefit is derived from the injection of large quantities of fluid. It is no longer considered desirable to administer opium to relieve the pain, except in hopeless cases. The patient must be fed by injections into the lower part of the bowel.

PERITONITIS, CHRONIC.— This form of peritonitis is in most cases due to tuberculosis, which may originate in the lungs or some other organ. In children the intestine is often attacked, and then the associated lymphatic glands.

Symptoms.—The peritonitis may come on suddenly, but more often it begins insidiously. There are shifting abdominal pains, the patient is emaciated, there may be diarrhœa and loss of appetite, the abdomen is tender under pressure, its surface may feel hot, as well as hard and resistant, and it may be either swollen or drawn in.

Treatment.—Abundance of sunshine and fresh air is one of the most important means of combating this disease. Sea air is very desirable, especially for children, and many of the patients are found to do well at Margate. The diet should be plentiful and nourishing, and should include a liberal supply of cow's milk. The abdomen may be painted with iodine daily, or every other day, and a layer of olive oil smeared over this to prevent evaporation; at the same time iodoform may be given internally. For diarrhœa, carbonate or subnitrate of bismuth may be given; for constipation, injections. When the fluid begins to absorb, cod-liver oil may be given to infants, and extract of malt, with iron or syrup of iodide of iron, to older patients. In very chronic cases it may be necessary to withdraw the accumulated fluid by puncture, or by aspiration (mechanical suction).

PERNICIOUS VOMITING OF PREGNANCY (*see* PREGNANCY, DISORDERS OF).

PERNIO (*see* CHILBLAIN).

PERSPIRATION, OFFENSIVE (*see* SWEAT, OFFENSIVE).

PERSPIRING FEET (*see* FEET, SWEATING).

PERTUSSIS (*see* WHOOPING-COUGH).

PES CAVUS (*see* CLUB-FOOT).

PETIT MAL (*see* EPILEPSY).

PHAGOCYTOSIS.—The process by which harmful germs and other injurious particles which invade the body are consumed by the white cells of the blood, etc. (*see* BLOOD AND LYMPH). The elements of the liquid part of the blood which prepare the germs for this fate are called *opsonins*.

PHARYNGITIS(*see* SORE THROAT).

PHIMOSIS.—In many male infants the orifice of the foreskin of the penis is contracted at birth, so that it is impossible to draw the skin back. In some cases the opening is absent altogether. Sometimes also the foreskin, besides being tight, is firmly adherent to the penis, and this also prevents it from being drawn back. In these various conditions water cannot be passed at all, or is passed with difficulty. In slight cases the trouble may be overcome by breaking the adhesions by the exercise of a little force, or by passing an instrument between the skin and the penis. But when the trouble is more pronounced the only remedy is the cutting off of the foreskin—circumcision, which is practised as a rite by Jews and Mohammedans and others. It is a quite simple operation, which no parent need hesitate to allow his child to undergo if it is advised by the medical attendant. In **paraphimosis** the foreskin, having been drawn back, cannot be drawn forward again, so that the penis begins to swell and become painful. Paraphimosis may be temporarily relieved by encircling the skin with the first and second finger of both hands and pressing it upwards while the thumbs press the end of the penis in the opposite direction, downwards. But circumcision is the only means of ensuring against recurrence.

PHLEBITIS.—This is the medical name for inflammation of veins, a condition usually, if not invariably, complicated by clotting of the blood. It sometimes occurs in the course of or as a sequel to infectious fevers, especially typhoid fever ; it may also arise when the tissues surrounding the vein are inflamed, or after surgical operations, or as a complication of varicose veins, or in states of anæmia and debility, or it may be a manifestation of gout (gouty phlebitis), or may occur after childbirth (*see* WHITE LEG).

Symptoms.—Aching or shooting pains are felt in the part affected, which is tender ; if the veins are on the surface they appear as bluish lines, and can be felt as hard cords. The circulation being interfered with, the parts from which the veins ought to drain the blood become swollen. When larger and deeper vessels are affected the patient will complain of cramps and of a sense of weight. If the phlebitis is due to the action of germs the clot of blood will become the seat of an abscess.

Phlebitis is not usually a very serious affection, except that there is danger of parts of the clot becoming detached and being carried by the blood-stream to some vital organ. To prevent this the patient must take to his bed and not leave it for any purpose whatever, and the affected limb must be kept completely at rest by being fixed to a splint or laid on a pillow. The pain may be relieved and the inflammation subdued by warm fomentations and the application of extract of belladonna and glycerin

in equal parts. If an abscess forms the doctor will incise it. The diet should be light and non-stimulating. When all the signs of inflammation have disappeared and the temperature has been normal for a week, light massage may be employed, but should never be instituted until three weeks after the onset of the symptoms. Such swelling as may remain should be treated by wearing a Martin elastic bandage. The patient may now be put upon a nutritious diet and may take a bark and ammonia tonic (p. 289).

PHLEGMASIA ALBA DOLENS (*see* WHITE LEG).

PHLYCTENULAR CONJUNC-TIVITIS (*see* CONJUNCTIVITIS).

PHOBIAS (*see* OBSESSIONS).

PHOSPHORUS POISONING.—In poisoning with phosphorus an emetic should be given (*see* EMETICS). Follow this with French (not American or German) oil of turpentine, 30 drops in an ounce of water every quarter of an hour for four doses, then three times a day. Half an ounce of Epsom salts dissolved in water may also be taken. Oils and fats must not be given, but milk and eggs are suitable. The pain and thirst may be relieved by barley water, and hot poultices applied over the pit of the stomach.

PHTHISIS (*see* CONSUMPTION).

PILES.—Hæmorrhoids, or piles, affect both sexes equally, and occur most frequently in middle age, though the trouble is not unknown in childhood. In many cases an hereditary predisposition can be traced. The most important cause is habitual constipation, aggravated by the use of strong aperients. The condition arises not infrequently in pregnancy owing to pressure of the pregnant womb on the affected part. Hæmorrhoids consist essentially in a varicose condition of the veins at the lower part of the rectum—the termination of the bowel—and the anus. They may take the form of external or of internal piles, according as to whether the swelling is outside or within the orifice of the anus.

External piles are composed of little flaps or folds covered with skin, and as a rule they give rise to discomfort rather than to pain—sensations of fullness, heat, pricking, etc. After an action of the bowels they may, however, become inflamed and irritated, when they cause a dull, aching, throbbing pain, increased by exercise and by standing.

Internal piles are distinctly painful. Burning, pricking, or smarting sensations are felt, especially after a motion. The patient feels as if the bowel were not emptied, and there is a bearing-down sensation, with a tendency to straining. Bleeding is a very common symptom, at first occurring only when the bowels move, but afterwards at other times, especially during active exercise. After a time the piles may protrude from the anus whenever a constipated motion is passed; later, as the muscle of the anus loses its tone, at other times also. Sometimes the protruding piles are nipped by the muscle of the anus, so that they cannot return, and they then become swollen, inflamed and painful; this is known as an " attack " of piles.

Treatment.—When an attack of piles occurs the patient should take an aperient such as Epsom salts, go to bed until the trouble has ceased, and put himself on a spare diet. The piles should be bathed with warm water or poppy fomentations, and smeared with ointment of gall and opium, or with hazeline cream. To check the bleeding, suppositories of cubebs may be used.

In the *local* treatment of piles generally, absolute cleanliness is an important factor. Every night and morning the parts should be washed with very hot or cold water, as well as after each motion. They should be smeared with pilewort, celandine, or gall-and-opium ointment, or with hazeline cream. In some cases astringent injections are found useful, such as 20 minims of tincture of steel, or 15 minims of tincture of hydrastis, each with 2 ounces of water. Suppositories of cubebs, belladonna and morphia, or suprarenal extract are often beneficial. Internal piles that are extruded should be washed, smeared with gall-and-opium or other ointment, and replaced by steady pressure applied with a piece of lint that has been smeared with ointment.

The *general* treatment of piles includes moderation in use of animal food, avoidance of stimulants, the securing of a regular daily action of the bowels—by the use of suitable food, if possible, supplemented if necessary by liquid paraffin and by general laxatives such as cascara sagrada, or sulphur in the form of lozenges—and the employment of tonics if the patient is debilitated.

The *operative* treatment of external piles is a simple matter; the doctor will snip off the redundant tags of skin with scissors after injecting novocain. The operative treatment of internal piles requires confinement to bed for two or three weeks. In cases associated with pregnancy, operation is unsuitable, and reliance must be placed upon such remedies as those described above. In these cases, when the child has been delivered and the patient has returned to normal habits the symptoms usually disappear

PILLS, HOW TO TAKE.—It is not everyone who can rely upon being able to swallow a pill at the first attempt by taking it into the mouth and gulping it down in a mouthful of water. Those who find this difficulty should try a method described by the late Sir James Cantlie in the British Red Cross Society's "Nursing Manual." The pill is placed on the floor of the mouth, underneath the tongue, and just behind the front teeth of the lower jaw. A large mouthful of water is then taken, and as in the act of swallowing the tongue is necessarily raised against the roof of the mouth, the water carries the pill to the back of the throat and washes it into the gullet. Tablets and tabloids can be taken in the same way, but unless they are nauseous it is better to crush them and treat them as powders (q.v.).

PITUITARY GLAND (*see* DUCTLESS GLANDS).

PITUITRIN(*see* ORGANOTHERAPY).

PITYRIASIS (*see* DANDRUFF).

PLAGUE.—This disease, the *pestis* of the ancients, can be traced back at least as far as the beginning of the second century before the Christian era. In the fourteenth century, starting probably from China, it spread over all Southern Europe in a specially malignant form which led to its being called the Black Death, and, finding its way to this country, it remained more or less prevalent here for several years. In the three following centuries various epidemics of plague occurred in Great Britain, culminating in the Great Plague of London in 1664–65, when upwards of 70,000 of the 460,000 inhabitants of the capital perished. The disease has long been suppressed in the West by improved hygienic conditions, and is now virtually a disease of warm climates—not so much because they are warm as because it is in such countries that sanitation is neglected and overcrowding most prevails. It is caused by the *Bacillus pestis*, a microbe discovered by Kitasato, the Japanese bacteriologist, and communicated to man by the fleas which infest rats. The rat flea becomes infected by biting a plague-stricken rat, and passes on the infection to other rats and to human beings by biting them.

Forms of plague.—The ordinary form of plague is that which is called *bubonic*, from the occurrence of a swelling or swellings (buboes) either in the groins or, less frequently, in the armpits, or, still less frequently, at the corners of the lower jaw. A much more deadly and more infectious form is known as *pneumonic* plague, because the lungs are specially affected. A third form, also very deadly, is termed *septicæmic* plague, or *pestis siderans*. Lastly there is the form called *abortive* plague, *pestis minor*, or *pestis ambulans*, in which the symptoms are so slight that the patient may be able to get about much as usual.

Incubation period and symptoms.—From the time of infection to the appearance of the symptoms the interval varies usually from two to eight days. The onset is generally somewhat sudden in the form of severe headache, giddiness, a staggering gait, and intense malaise. After a few hours or a day, rarely longer, fever develops, perhaps with shivering, the patient becoming either delirious or, more generally, unconscious. The buboes, due to inflammation of the lymphatic glands, may appear quite early, or as late as the fifth day. Other symptoms which may be present are profuse sweating, hæmorrhages under the skin, where they form the black patches known in the seventeenth century as "tokens" and thought to presage death; engorgement of the lungs, diarrhœa, and severe bilious vomiting. The mortality is greatest at the beginning of an epidemic, when as many as ninety cases out of a hundred may end fatally.

Treatment.—Little can be done in a case of plague except to combat the various symptoms as they arise. The buboes require local treatment. Where possible the patient, during treatment, should be kept in the open air. Haffkine's plague vaccine is chiefly of value as a preventive, but it also mitigates the severity of the disease if contracted, just as vaccination does in smallpox. The protection conferred is of no long duration, being measurable in months rather than in years. Other vaccines have been used for the same purpose, but none has yielded results comparable to those produced by Haffkine's.

PLASTER-OF-PARIS BANDAGE (*see* BANDAGES).

PLASTERS.—Plasters usually consist of an active ingredient, such as belladonna or mercury, with a basis of soap, oil, resin, etc. They are employed for their stimulating effect —mustard plasters, etc.; for their sedative qualities—belladonna, aconite, opium and menthol plasters, etc.; for reducing inflammatory thickening —mercury plasters, etc.; and for supporting, strengthening, or fixing a part—lead or diachylon plasters, etc. The old-fashioned mustard plaster has now been largely superseded by the mustard leaf. Neither mustard plasters nor mustard leaves should be kept on long enough to raise a blister; in old people and children special care is necessary to

avoid this effect. When they are removed a little olive oil should be smeared over the reddened surface, or a little zinc or boric-acid ointment applied and the surface then covered with cotton-wool. The belladonna plaster is much used to mitigate the pain of neuralgia or muscular strain, and is also applied to the breast to check the secretion of milk. The skin having been prepared by washing and drying, the plaster is warmed before the fire or by holding the back of it against a jug of hot water, and is then laid on the skin, and retained in position for a minute or two by pressure of the hand. It should be worn until it becomes loose, the edges being trimmed off with scissors as they come unstuck. After its removal the skin may be cleansed with olive oil.

PLEURISY.—The surface of the lungs is covered with a delicate, smooth, shining membrane, the pleura, which also lines the inner surface of the chest-walls; the space between the two layers is the pleural cavity. Pleurisy is inflammation of this membrane, and usually a result of the inflammation is that the watery part of the blood oozes out of the pleura into the cavity, so that the two layers, which normally are kept close together by the air-pressure within the lungs, become separated. The essential cause of pleurisy is invasion of the membrane by germs, which either first attack some adjacent organ or are carried to the pleura by the blood or the lymph. Most cases originate in tuberculosis of the lungs —consumption, a disease of which pleurisy is often one of the earliest manifestations. At one time or another, indeed, pleurisy occurs in every case of chronic consumption. It may also be set up by other diseases, or be an after-result of certain surgical operations, or may supervene upon a broken rib, or may follow injury due to a blow or fall on the chest. A frequent predisposing cause is exposure to cold and damp, or sitting in a draught. Pleurisy is too serious a disease for domestic treatment.

Symptoms.—Pain of a sharp stabbing character, the " stitch " of pleurisy, is felt in the side whenever a deep breath is taken or the patient moves. He feels chilly and may shiver, and the temperature rises, though usually only to a moderate extent, he has a dry cough, and the usual symptoms of feverishness. Soon the stitch in the side disappears, or becomes much less painful, but the breathing grows more difficult and more rapid, and if fluid continues to accumulate the affected lung may be put out of action. At the end of about a week the accumulation in most cases ceases, and the patient becomes convalescent. Other cases, however, do not follow this course, and if the fluid is allowed to remain a long time in the pleural cavity, the lung is unable to expand when it is withdrawn. In some cases, too, the fluid becomes mixed with pus, forming an empyema, or abscess of the chest, a serious complication which usually necessitates an operation.

Treatment.—The pain in the side may be relieved by hot linseed poultices, by a mustard leaf, by a belladonna plaster, or by painting with iodine. If it continues, the affected side must be firmly strapped up (Fig. 47). A large sheet of lead or other adhesive plaster about 18 inches square is cut into strips 3 or 4 inches wide.

One of the strips is warmed, and when quite moist, at a moment when the patient has emptied his

chest of air as completely as possible, is applied to the lower part of the chest, beginning at the spine, passing downwards and forwards towards the ribs, and ending about the middle line in front. The second strip begins just below the first, and crosses it on the way to the middle line in front. The third strip runs parallel

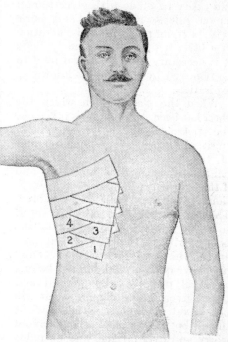

Fig. 47.—Strapping in pleurisy.

to the first, which it overlaps by about an inch, the fourth runs parallel with and similarly overlaps the second, and so on until the painful part of the chest is quite covered. Before each strip is applied the patient must empty the chest of air, as at the beginning.

To relieve the pain, three aspirin tablets of 5 grains each may be given, followed, if necessary, at intervals of three or four hours, by 10-grain doses until three or four doses have been taken. Or the following mixture may be taken :

> Dover's powder.............. 30 grains
> Citrate of potash ....120 grains
> Ammonium acetate solution   12 drachms
> Water of camphor to 8 ounces.
>
> Two tablespoonfuls every 3 or 4 hours until the pain is relieved.

The diet should be nutritious but quite light. A useful mouth wash can easily be made with glycerin and lemon juice, or glycerin and boric acid, in equal parts, with the addition of a little hot water. In many cases it is necessary for the pleural fluid to be removed by the process known as aspiration.

When the plaster with which the chest has been strapped up is taken off, the stickiness may be removed with spirit of turpentine. The lower half of the affected chest may then be painted with tincture of iodine, and if the skin is kept a little sore, absorption of the fluid will be promoted. The regular use of a mineral water, so as to cause a free action of the bowels, will also tend to the disappearance of the fluid. When the fever and pain have quite ceased, but not before, a liberal diet may be allowed and tonics given, and a change of air will be found beneficial. The patient should be warmly clad, should avoid worry and over-fatigue, and no pains should be spared to secure a complete return of health. Until then he should remain under medical supervision, lest the case should prove to be one of consumption.

In *children* pleurisy sometimes develops after exposure to cold, but is usually a complication of consumption, pneumonia, scarlet fever, or rheumatism. It may appear as an acute illness with high fever, or in mild chronic form. When it complicates some other disease it may easily be overlooked. If the pleurisy is " dry " or the quantity of the fluid not excessive, the child in most cases recovers, and is restored to health within a reasonable time. In cases where this disorder is associated with scarlet fever or consumption, the outlook is less favourable. Treatment proceeds on the same general lines as in adults. To reduce the fever and inflammation, salicylate of soda, 5 to 10 grains, or antipyrin, 2 to 6 grains, is useful. To assuage the pain, hot poultices or fomentations may be applied, or, if it is very severe, one or two leeches. As an anodyne, 1 to 3 drops of compound tincture of camphor may be given to babies, and half to one grain of Dover's powder to older children. To promote the absorption of fluid, the chest may be painted with tincture of iodine diluted with glycerin, and this may be followed by giving syrup of iodide of iron with maltine, and a sufficiency of nutritious food and fresh air. As in adults, it may be necessary to remove the fluid from the pleural cavity by aspiration, or, if the fluid has become purulent and continues to accumulate, a drainage tube may have to be inserted.

PLEURODYNIA (*see* SIDE-ACHE).

PNEUMONIA.—Inflammation of the lungs may be either lobar or lobular. In the lobar form it affects the whole of one lobe of a lung ; in the lobular it affects a lung in patches. In the latter form, disease begins in the bronchial tubes (bronchitis) and spreads to the tissues of the lung— i.e. the air-cells ; a better designation for this form is broncho-pneumonia, under which it is treated in this work. In this article we are concerned with *lobar* pneumonia.

As a result of the inflamed state of the lung tissue, a thick fluid exudes into the air-cells so that this part of the lung becomes solid and is no longer available for breathing. In most cases only one lung is involved. If both are affected the case is said to be one of " double pneumonia." In most cases, again, the inflammation, beginning in the tissues of the lung, extends to the pleura and sets up pleurisy. These cases can be distinguished from those in which pleurisy is not present by an acute pain that is felt in breathing. Pneumonia often occurs in the course of infectious fevers and in the final stage of many chronic diseases. This secondary pneumonia, however, is not quite the same as primary pneumonia.

Causes.—The disease is due to a germ, though not necessarily the same kind of germ in every case. It sometimes occurs in epidemics, nearly always in winter or in spring, and some of them are attended by a high mortality. Some persons, quite apart from their surroundings and general state of health, have a special liability to this disease. Thus an eminent London surgeon, who lived to be well over fourscore, had pneumonia six times, and cases have been reported in which the disease has recurred up to twenty-eight times.

Symptoms.—After an incubation period varying from two to seven days the patient begins to feel slightly out of sorts. He is then seized with a violent shivering fit, and in a few hours his temperature mounts to 104° Fahr. or higher; he feels very ill, and his expression becomes anxious. The urine is scanty and high-coloured. Both the pulse-rate and the breathing are quickened, the latter much more than the former. From twelve to twenty-four hours after the shivering fit the pain of pleurisy may be felt in the side. The sputum (phlegm) is small in quantity, but extremely sticky, and is usually of a " rusty "

or reddish or tawny hue from mixture with blood. When the fever is at its height the patient may become delirious, especially in the evening or during the night. In most cases in which the disease ends in recovery the fever terminates " by crisis "—i.e. suddenly; this usually occurs between the fifth and eighth days. In from six to twenty-four hours the temperature falls to normal or even below. At once the pulse and the breathing become less rapid, and the patient's general condition shows an astonishing improvement. In a minority of cases the fever terminates " by lysis "—i.e. the temperature falls gradually.

Treatment.—The disease is, of course, much too serious for domestic treatment. The patient must be put to bed; light woollen underclothing, not heavy enough to cause perspiration, should be worn. It used to be the fashion to apply a " jacket " poultice; but this is better dispensed with. The room should be airy, and well lighted; this is important because pneumonia is infectious, though not in a high degree. The expectoration should be disinfected by placing a strong solution of caustic soda in the sputum cup. Dry sweeping or dusting should be avoided, and if possible the patient should be isolated. The nurse should not handle or remain in close proximity to the patient more than is necessary, should carefully cleanse her hands, and should use an antiseptic mouth-wash at frequent intervals. The room should be kept at a temperature of about 60° Fahr.; 65° should be regarded as the maximum. The window should be open and the patient protected from draughts by a screen. Some authorities believe that a modified form of open-air treatment is beneficial in pneumonia, and recommend that the patient should be placed on a roof or a verandah, or at any rate in a large sunny room with open windows. If this treatment is adopted the patient, in cold weather, must be kept warm by extra clothing and by use of hot-water bottles, etc.

The fever may be reduced by doses of phenacetin with hydrobromide of quinine, one grain of each, given at frequent intervals. Aspirin is also valuable, for it tends not only to check the fever but to allay the pain. A more generally useful method of combating the fever is cold sponging. If the patient becomes delirious, as is very likely to happen, an ice-cap may be applied to the head. In cases in which the delirium depends upon a special nervous excitability, or is a result of exhaustion at a late stage of the disease, chloral and bromide of potash may be given, 15 grains of the former and 25 grains of the latter, dissolved in an ounce of camphor water, the dose to be repeated when necessary. Great *difficulty of breathing* is usually an indication of commencing heart-failure. To meet this respiratory difficulty the doctor may withdraw blood from a vein in the arm or may institute dry cupping. The patient must also be allowed to inhale oxygen at frequent intervals. No attempt should be made to check the cough so long as it is attended by expectoration. If expectoration is absent it is because the sputum is too tenacious to be discharged, or because the cough is due to some irritation of the larynx. Should the former condition appear to be present the following spray may be used by means of a spray producer :

Bicarbonate of soda . . . . 10 grains
Chloride of soda . . . . 5 grains
Glycerin of carbolic acid. . . . ½ drachm
Cherry-laurel water . . . . 2 drachms
Water to one ounce.
To be used as a spray, warm.

The patient should also have an occasional drink of Vichy water, mixed with a little hot milk and a teaspoonful or two of brandy or whisky. If the cough is due to laryngeal catarrh, 2 or 4 grains of Dover's powder mixed with a little chloroform water may be given occasionally. The pain in the side may be relieved by applying from 3 to 6 leeches and afterwards a hot compress sprinkled with laudanum. It may be necessary to strap up the chest, as described under PLEURISY. In ordinary cases the use of alcohol is better avoided, at any rate until the stage of convalescence is reached, but in drunkards, and in the aged, it can hardly be dispensed with, and it may have to be given in large doses. Digitalis is often prescribed to stimulate the heart.

When the temperature is reduced to normal, the lower part of the chest on the affected side should be painted once a day with tincture of iodine in order to promote the absorption of the material which has accumulated in the lungs. Careful nursing and suitable diet are at least as important as medical treatment. The patient must be disturbed as little as possible. The diet must at first be fluid, and light ; the best staple food, so to speak, is milk diluted with water, or, if there is any tendency to sickness, with soda water ; but the diet may also include light clear soups and broths. To assuage thirst, iced lemonade may be sipped, or, if the patient prefers it, toast-water or barley-water or the juice of an orange. An occasional cup of tea or coffee may also be allowed, and the coffee may be made strong, for it acts as a tonic to the heart. When the time comes for more nourishing diet, strong beef tea or meat juice and arrowroot may be given with a little brandy or whisky, also eggs beaten up with boiling water and laced with a little alcohol. A draught of cold water may be given every hour or two to promote the flow of urine ; it may be flavoured with a little syrup of lemon and a few grains of salt.

When the patient seems well enough to get out of bed he must be carefully watched, for the exertion is likely to bring on a fainting fit. At first he should only remain out long enough for the bed to be made comfortable, the time being increased as strength returns. A suitable tonic is half a teaspoonful of compound syrup of the hypophosphites in a tablespoonful of water, three times a day. Or a bark and ammonia mixture may be taken, as follows :

Compound tincture of bark .   ½ ounce
Carbonate of ammonia ..... 24 grains
Syrup of orange ....   ½ ounce
Water to 8 ounces.
Two tablespoonfuls 3 times a day before meals.

The return to health and strength may be a long process, and the doctor may find it necessary to give other tonics, for example Easton's syrup, to allow a moderate amount of good wine such as port or burgundy, and to send the patient to the seaside, or to a mountain resort.

The treatment of pneumonia which is secondary to some other diseases, such as an infectious fever, will vary with the treatment required by the original disease. It may be said generally, however, that as soon as the pneumonia is detected, warm mustard and linseed poultices, or hot flannel sprinkled with turpentine, may be applied. In these cases there is usually a tendency to heart-failure, and stimulants are indicated.

In *children*, pneumonia, while following the same general course as in adults, presents some special features. Thus, breathing is accompanied by a short grunting noise. Infants lie quiet because of the pain felt at any movement of the chest, older children will complain of pain and refer it to the stomach. In extreme cases the pulse may rise as high as 160 beats per minute, the breathing to 60. In healthy children, in most cases the temperature begins to fall between the sixth and ninth days, and, as in adults, is in a few hours reduced to normal, the patient then falling into a quiet sleep and perspiring profusely. When he awakes the breathing has become easier, a large quantity of urine, which before had been scanty, is passed, appetite returns, and there seems to be little the matter except that the little patient is thin and anæmic. In some cases the disease is " aborted," and comes to an end in about three days from the onset. In others, vomiting and diarrhœa are excessive. In yet others the cerebral symptoms are pronounced —headache, delirium, convulsions, or drowsiness; these cases may easily be mistaken for meningitis. Pneumonia in children may have serious complications : the kidneys, or the membrane covering the heart, may become inflamed, or jaundice may set in.

A temperature of not more than 103° Fahr. may be dealt with simply by sponging with tepid water, and by giving tincture of aconite in 1-minim doses every three or four hours. A temperature of 104° or 105° Fahr. calls for a wet pack (q.v.) at 60° or 70° Fahr. ; if there is delirium or convulsions the child may be put into a warm bath and the temperature of the water gradually reduced to 60° Fahr. In these cases also aconite is the medicine of choice, but if it should induce

11   289

indigestion it may be replaced by the following mixture :

Citrate of potash .... 1 drachm
Solution of acetate of am-
monia .... 3 drachms
Ipecacuanha wine.......... 1 drachm
Syrup of tolu.............. 3 drachms
Water to 1½ ounces.

A teaspoonful every 3 hours.

If there are signs of heart-failure, the doctor may add two or three minims of tincture of digitalis to each dose. If the patient is very restless or in great pain, ½ to 2 grains of Dover's powder may be given at night.

PNEUMONIC PLAGUE (*see* PLAGUE).

PNEUMONOCONIOSES. — This rather formidable word denotes diseases of the lungs that have their origin in irritation from the inhalation of dust. In this category are silicosis (q.v.), dust-bronchitis, dust-pneumonia, dust-phthisis and dust-asthma. Except in the case of asthma, the dust does its mischievous work by so irritating the bronchial tubes, or the air-cells of the lungs, as to render them specially liable to the attacks of germs. Among the dusts which so act are those of quartz, flint, sandstone, emery, glass, basic slag, certain hard woods, and the husk of cotton, flax, jute, and hemp. The treatment of the different diseases is much the same as when they are induced by more ordinary causes.

POISONS AND POISONING.— The symptoms and treatment of poisoning are described in separate articles under the name of each poison. Here we may (1) show how poisons are classified, and (2) give some general indication of first-aid treatment.

1. Classification.—Poisons have been divided, according to their effects, into (*a*) irritants, (*b*) corrosives, (*c*) narcotics, (*d*) deliriants.

(*a*) *Irritants* are so called because they irritate the mucous membranes with which they come in contact. The most familiar irritant poisons are metallic, such as arsenic, antimony, lead, mercury, phosphorus and zinc. The symptoms are a burning pain in the throat and stomach, a metallic taste in the mouth, with retching and vomiting, followed by cramps in the muscles, cold sweats, exhaustion, collapse, and finally, in severe cases, either convulsions or the state of profound insensibility that is termed coma. In some cases there is violent diarrhœa.

(*b*) *Corrosives.*—These poisons are similar in their action to irritants, but instead of merely irritating the tissues they destroy them. They may be either acids, alkalis, or salts. The corrosive acids include sulphuric acid (oil of vitriol), hydrochloric acid (spirit of salts), nitric acid (aquafortis), oxalic acid (salt of lemon or sorrel), carbolic acid, and acetic acid (aromatic vinegar and glacial acetic acid) ; among the alkalis are caustic potash and soda, strong ammonia and quicklime ; the salts may be represented by corrosive sublimate, a powerful disinfectant.

Among the symptoms of poisoning by *acids* are burning and discoloration of the lips, mouth, throat and stomach ; there may also be signs of suffocation, from blocking of the air-passages by swellings of the contiguous mucous membranes. The symptoms of poisoning by *alkalis* are similar, but the tongue, instead of being covered with a black, yellow, or white coating, as in acid poisoning, is denuded of its covering and looks like raw meat. In *corrosive-sublimate* poisoning the lips and mouth are white and shrivelled, the throat feels as though it were closed up, and there is a metallic taste in the mouth.

(c) *Narcotics.*—This group of poisons consists mainly of opium and its many derivatives and preparations, such as morphia, codeia, laudanum, paregoric, syrup of poppies, and Dover's powder. Opium is also contained in chlorodyne and nepenthe (*see* OPIUM-POISONING). Among the narcotics is alcohol; poisoning by this drug is considered separately in the article on ALCOHOLISM.

At first narcotics cause exhilaration, which quickly subsides into a drowsiness that passes into deep sleep and finally into coma. The face is pale, the pulse-rate and breathing are slow, the latter being also stertorous (snoring), and the pupils of the eyes are contracted to mere points—" pinpoint pupils."

(d) *Deliriants.*—Among the deliriants are belladonna, henbane, strychnine and aconite. Besides delirium, which is their chief effect, they dilate the pupil of the eye. They also produce dryness of the mouth and throat and flushing of the face.

2. First aid in poisoning.—(1) Send for the doctor. (2) Decide whether an emetic is required. *An emetic should be given in every case unless the lips and mouth are charred or burnt, or unless the patient is unconscious* (*see* EMETICS). If the lips and mouth are burnt the case is one of corrosive poisoning ; the stomach will be much burnt, and the strain of vomiting might cause its wall at some point to give way, probably with a fatal result. In these cases, instead of an emetic, something should be given which will neutralize the poison. Thus, in poisoning by a corrosive *acid*, chalk, whiting, lime, or whitewash off the wall or ceiling, should be dissolved in water and given freely. In poisoning by an *alkali*, a well-diluted acid should be given, such as vinegar, or lemon or orange juice. If the patient is *unconscious*, the emetic, or the vomited fluid, might get into the airpassages and choke him.

(3) In all cases in which the patient is able to swallow, milk, raw eggs, olive or linseed oil, strong tea or coffee may be given after the emetic (if an emetic is suitable). The only exception to this rule is in phosphorus poisoning, in which oils, by dissolving the phosphorus, would promote its assimilation. Milk forms curds in the stomach which will envelop the poison and help to carry it out when vomiting takes place. The white of eggs acts similarly. Oils soothe the stomach and form a protective coating over its surface. Either olive or linseed oil is suitable, but not, of course, mineral oils. Tea and coffee are not only stimulants, but are actual antidotes to many poisons.

(4) Keep the patient warm and give him stimulants to sustain him under the shock.

(5) Endeavour by all means to prevent him from going to sleep. If he is already unconscious, try to arouse him by flicking him with a wet towel, pouring cold water over his head, shaking him, and shouting into his ear.

(6) If his breath is failing, employ cold affusion as just described. Should breathing cease, apply artificial respiration (*see* RESPIRATION, ARTIFICIAL).

(7) If the poisoning is due to bad food, hot applications to the abdomen may be employed while the doctor is coming.

POLIOMYELITIS, ACUTE (*see* INFANTILE PARALYSIS).

POLYPUS, NASAL.—The growths known as polypi are sometimes the result of disease of the nasal bones, but the causes are not well understood. They occur most frequently between the ages of twenty and thirty, and men are said to be more liable to them than women. They may come singly or in large numbers, and on one or both sides of the nose. There is a watery discharge which is constant; the patient feels out of sorts, in many cases the mind is dulled, and there is liability to such complications as disease of the middle ear, deafness, noises in the ear, and laryngitis. Treatment consists in removal of the polyps. In many cases there is recurrence; the patient, therefore, should go to his doctor for examination at regular intervals.

POLYURIA.—When the quantity of urine passed during the twenty-four hours is greatly in excess of the normal 2½ pints (50 ounces), the condition is termed polyuria. It may be a symptom of serious disease such as diabetes, or inflammation of the kidney, or stone in the kidney, or it may be transient, as after a fever or an epileptic fit. Another group of cases is classified as hysterical; the patients are nervous and excitable young adults of either sex who for a few hours, or even weeks, from no traceable cause, are troubled with frequent and excessive micturition; there are no attendant symptoms, except that scalding is felt as the urine is passed, and also some abdominal pain. In these cases no treatment is called for. When polyuria is a symptom of serious organic disease, treatment must, of course, be directed to the antecedent disease.

PORT-WINE STAINS (*see* BIRTHMARKS).

POTT'S DISEASE (*see* SPINAL CURVATURE, ANGULAR).

POTT'S FRACTURE (*see* FRACTURES).

POULTICES.—Poultices are not so much used as they were formerly, for they have obvious drawbacks. They are heavy, they become hard, they crumble into the bed if badly made, and finally they are not antiseptic; they should therefore never be applied to broken skin or to any form of wound; for such lesions a boric-acid compress is far preferable (*see* COMPRESSES). Poultices, however, still have a useful place in medical treatment. As a general rule, it may be said that large poultices should be changed once at least every four hours, and small poultices every two hours. The fresh poultice should be ready before the old poultice is removed. When, finally, poultices are discontinued the skin should be gently washed with warm water and covered with a warm piece of gamgee tissue or cotton-wool.

Bread poultices.—These are used to relieve inflammation and assuage pain. Prepare a sufficient quantity of bread-crumbs, stir them rapidly in boiling water, well beat the mixture, cover it with a saucer, then place the vessel over a saucepan of hot water so that the bread may swell. Having thoroughly drained off the water, spread the poultice evenly with a heated knife on the calico or other material, turn the edges neatly in, spread some olive oil or cold cream on the top to prevent sticking, and apply, placing one edge of the poultice against the part, and laying on the rest as soon as the heat can be borne, then covering it with wool and bandaging it on. A hot bread poultice must be changed very frequently, as the heat is soon lost. In some cases cold instead of hot poultices are used.

Linseed poultices.—These are used for much the same purpose as bread poultices, and also in inflammation of internal organs, attacks of colic, etc. They act as mild counter-irritants by drawing the blood to the surface. They are usually made not of the linseed meal of commerce, but of crushed linseed. If the former kind of linseed is used, olive oil should be smeared over the poultice as soon as it is made, to prevent adhesion. Place the linseed before the fire, and heat the basin, spoon and knife with boiling water. Pour some of this into the basin, half a pint for every 4 ounces of meal, and gradually sprinkle in the meal with the left hand, while stirring it with the spoon in the other hand until it is just thick enough and is free from lumps. Then turn it out on to a piece of calico, spread it evenly, fold it up, place it on the palm of the hand or a hot plate, and apply like a bread poultice. If the patient is a child or the skin is delicate, the surface of the poultice should be smeared lightly with vaselin, or it should be covered with muslin. Ordinary linseed poultices should be about half an inch thick.

Mustard poultices have been to a great extent succeeded by the mustard leaf, but we may here explain how a linseed-and-mustard poultice can be made when required in painful muscular affections, such as lumbago. The strength will, of course, depend upon the proportion of mustard to the linseed. In a moderately strong one two tablespoonfuls of mustard are used for the amount of linseed required for a poultice of average size. The mustard is put in a basin and mixed smoothly with boiling water that is poured in gradually, the linseed being then added. The poultice should be kept on long enough to cause redness, but not blistering ; the only guide as to time is that furnished by the patient's feelings.

Bran poultices.—Put the bran in a flannel bag and saturate it with boiling water. The water can be squeezed out of the poultice with help of two boards, or by passing over it a rolling-pin.

Yeast poultices.—These are employed to mitigate the pain of boils and carbuncles. Mix 6 parts of beer yeast, 14 parts of flour, and 6 parts of water at 100° Fahr., and place near a fire until the mixture rises, but do not allow it to boil.

Poppy head and camomile poultices.—This kind of poultice is useful in neuralgia and toothache. Having boiled the camomile flowers, boil the poppy heads until soft, remove the seeds, crush up the heads, and then mix with the camomile flowers.

Hemlock poultices.—In cancer and other very painful diseases hemlock poultices are of service for their anodyne effects. Mix together 1 ounce of hemlock seeds and 3 ounces of linseed meal, and then gradually stir in a tumblerful of boiling water.

POWDERS, HOW TO TAKE.—If allowed to remain in water for a few hours, say in a wine- or liqueur-glass, most powders will sink and be suspended in the water, instead of floating on the surface. They can then, in the water, be transferred to a tablespoon and swallowed without difficulty. The cachets in which very nauseous drugs may be enclosed can be soaked in a tablespoonful of water, which is then poured into the mouth and swallowed. If a dry cachet is put on the tongue and an attempt is made to wash it down, it may burst.

PREGNANCY, DISORDERS OF.—Most of the minor troubles of pregnancy are sufficiently considered in the articles HEARTBURN, WATERBRASH, CONSTIPATION, DIARRHŒA and VOMITING. Another minor trouble in a few cases is *excessive production of saliva*, chiefly present in the early months. This may be relieved by clearing the bowels with a dose of Carlsbad salts and the frequent use of a mouth-wash, say chlorate of potash, 10 grains in two tablespoonfuls of water. In some cases there is *loss of appetite*, which may pass into an actual loathing for food. This is best treated by exercise, plenty of fresh air, the correction of constipation, and a digestive tonic, such as those specified in the article INDIGESTION. In other cases the patient is troubled with *excessive appetite*. Here the only remedy is the exercise of self-control. In certain cases there is *perversion of appetite :* the patient may long for things that are not merely indigestible but actually inedible or repulsive. The cravings of a pregnant woman should be gratified so long as the things desired are not harmful : it may be the expression of some obscure physiological need, and even if it is not, there is no need to impose upon her needless limitations. Where, however, the things she wants are repulsive or would be injurious she must, of course, be encouraged to deny herself.

Among the more serious troubles of pregnancy are *varicose veins in the legs* and *piles*. These are sufficiently considered in the articles VARICOSE VEINS and PILES, but in consulting them the reader should understand that in pregnancy operative treatment is unsuitable.

Swollen legs and feet may be due to varicose veins or may be an indication of anæmia. In the former case a bandage should be applied. In the latter, it is not desirable to take iron without having a doctor's opinion, for there is some ground for believing that Nature has provided a somewhat anæmic state in pregnancy as a safeguard against more serious troubles during confinement. In some cases the swelling is an indication that the kidneys are affected (*see* later). Another trouble of pregnancy is the presence of *cramps in the legs*, caused by pressure of the womb on the nerves of the legs as they pass through the pelvis. The patient may try the effect of getting out of bed and walking about the room, or may tie a bandage rightly round the limb. If the muscles affected are knotted and very painful, they should be gently rubbed with warm oil or belladonna liniment and fomented with hot water. During the day a firm elastic bandage or stocking should be worn.

In some cases, especially in first pregnancies, discomfort may be caused by *distension of the abdomen;* relief may be found by applying hot fomentations or poultices. If the skin of the abdomen should become sore, or crack, warm olive oil or lanolin ointment should be rubbed in. In other cases, especially in women who have borne children in rapid succession and have not been careful to use a firm binder in convalescence, there is trouble from *pendulous abdomen*. The patient should take plenty of rest on the sofa, and when up and about should wear a carefully fitted abdominal belt, the lower edge fixed round the hips and the upper extended above the most prominent part of the swelling; it should be fastened with a lace, or with straps and buckles, so that it may be accommodated to the size of the gradually enlarging abdomen.

The patient may complain of *painful breasts* if they should increase in size very rapidly. Fomentations should be applied, and warm olive oil rubbed in night and morning; if the rubbing proceeds from the circumference towards the nipple, a thin fluid may be expressed. If the breasts are very heavy, they should be supported with a bandage arranged as a sling. The bowels may be relieved by a dose of saline aperient, such as Apenta water. With this trouble may be coupled *itching of the external reproductive organs*. Warm lead lotion or Goulard water may be frequently applied, or equal quantities of vinegar and water. Warm sitz baths, continued for about ten minutes, are also useful, especially if a small quantity of washing soda or table salt is dissolved in the water. If the parts are red and swollen and painful, hot poppy lotion, made by crushing poppy-heads in water, should be applied for a few minutes.

Another group of troubles is associated with the bladder and the kidneys. In pregnancy there is always some amount of irritability of the bladder, and the result may be *frequency of micturition*. As a rule, this annoyance ceases by the time quickening occurs—that is, when the pregnancy has run about eighteen weeks. While it lasts, the diet must be carefully regulated, and only light, unstimulating articles of food taken ; alcohol in every form must be avoided ; the bowels must be kept active, and water or linseed tea drunk freely. A teaspoonful of sweet spirit of nitre may be taken at bedtime in water, and a belladonna pessary, containing 2 grains of extract of belladonna, may be placed in the vagina at bedtime to allay the irritability.

In the later months of pregnancy the pressure of the much enlarged womb on the bladder may cause *incontinence of urine*, the water escaping constantly, and putting the patient to much inconvenience. She should rest as much as possible in the recumbent position, and during the day should wear a well-fitting abdominal belt ; it should be put on while she is lying down, and tightened first at the lowest part, so as to lift up the womb and keep it from pressing on the bladder. In other cases, the patient has to complain of a *sluggish bladder :* the urine is retained and the bladder becomes distended. If so, she must be careful to pass water every four or six hours, even though she receives no call to do so. In some cases there is positive *inability to pass water*, either because the womb is pressed against the neck of the bladder (*see* Retroversion, under WOMB, DISPLACEMENTS OF), or, in the last weeks of pregnancy, because the bladder is compressed between the child's head and the bone of the pelvis. In the former case the doctor must restore the womb to its natural position ; in the latter, the patient should place herself on her elbows and knees, when the womb will probably fall away from the bladder by its own weight. A firmly applied abdominal belt should be worn.

The presence of *albumin in the urine* is a not infrequent complication of pregnancy. It is an occurrence that must not be disregarded, for in some cases, fortunately not many, it leads to the serious condition called *eclampsia*, in which the patient falls into convulsions. This is a manifestation of what is called *toxæmia*—that is, blood-poisoning. Other toxæmias of pregnancy are *acute yellow atrophy of the liver* and *pernicious vomiting*. Fortunately these toxæmic states are so rare that they need not further be considered in this work.

PREGNANCY, DURATION OF.
—The duration of pregnancy varies in different cases. The laws of England and America do not presume to fix the maximum limit, but leave the question to be decided in each individual case. The French law, more daring, specifies 300 days as the extreme limit, but Nature has not chosen to recognize this ordinance, and there are cases on record in which pregnancy extended to 317 days, and even longer, and important questions in connexion with the inheritance of property or title and the chastity of the wife have depended upon this point. On the other hand, there are examples of fully grown, perfectly developed children being born well within the traditional period of nine calendar months. Conception can only occur in the interval which separates two monthly flows, and the most likely time is during the seven days following the cessation of a flow. The common custom is to count from the last day of the last menstrual flow, to reckon nine calendar months forward, and then to add seven days. Another method is to count 273 days from the last day of the last menstrual flow, and to expect the confinement during the following week ; thus the date of labour will fall in the interval

between nine calendar months (273 days) and ten four-weeks months (280 days). In these calculations the four-weeks month is usually called the "lunar" month, but this is a misnomer, for a lunar month—the time from one new moon to another or from one full moon to another—is not 28 days, but 29½ days.

In these calculations two sources of error must be noted. (1) A woman may have one, two, or even three monthly flows after conception; if this should occur, labour will, of course, take place considerably before the time calculated. (2) In not a few cases fertilization takes place immediately before a period, instead of during the seven days after a period; if so, the calculation will, of course, be out by any number of days up to fourteen. It is desirable, therefore, that the calculation, whichever method is adopted, should be checked by the date of " quickening " (see the next article). This most often falls about twenty-two weeks before labour is due, or about a fortnight before the middle of pregnancy. A skilled midwife or a doctor will be able further to check the calculation by the apparent size of the child and by the " falling " of the womb. This latter sign is an indication that labour is imminent. When this occurs in a multipara, a woman who has borne a child or children before, labour may be expected in a day or two; in a primipara, a woman who is bearing for the first time, labour may be somewhat delayed, in some cases as much as a fortnight.

PREGNANCY, SIGNS AND SYMPTOMS OF.—The first indication of pregnancy is the *cessation of menstruation*. This, however, may occur as the result of anæmia or of some other abnormal condition of mind or body; in itself, therefore, it is only a probable indication of pregnancy. The probability is strengthened if two, and still more if three periods are missed. The second indication of pregnancy, in order of time, is *morning sickness*, which generally comes on about six weeks after conception, and continues for about the same time. It may, however, begin earlier or later than the time stated, and may continue much longer than six weeks. The third sign, *changes in the breasts*, is usually observed about the same time as the morning sickness. The breasts grow larger and firmer, the veins can be seen as blue lines coursing under the skin, and the coloured part round each nipple—the areola—becomes deeper in colour, a more vivid pink in the blonde and a deeper shade of brown in the brunette. Later, a milky fluid may be squeezed out of the nipple by pressure. This is more significant of pregnancy in a primipara than in a multipara (for these terms *see* the preceding article), but even in the former, too much importance must not be attached to it, for the breasts may be stimulated to produce such a fluid by disorders of the womb. Pains in the breast also are felt. The fourth sign, *enlarged abdomen*, is not usually perceived by the woman herself until about the end of the third month. By the end of the fourth month it is fairly obvious. By the end of the fifth month the rounded upper border of the womb is midway between the pubic bone and the navel; it reaches the lower margin of the navel by the sixth month, and a month later is half-way between the navel and the ribs. By the end of the seventh month it lies immediately below the margin of the ribs. The fifth indication of pregnancy occurs about the eighteenth week; it is commonly known as "*quickening*," and is often compared by those who experience it to the fluttering of a bird. It means, of course, that the movements of the child have become sufficiently vigorous to be felt by the mother. The sixth sign is *alteration in the navel*. In the early days of pregnancy the depth of this depression may appear to be increased, but gradually the hollow fills up, until somewhere about the sixth month it becomes level with the skin. All these signs and symptoms are felt or can be observed by the patient. There are others, more unequivocal in their significance than those described, which can only be perceived by the midwife or doctor.

PRESBYOPIA (*see* SIGHT, DEFECTS OF).

PRESSURE PALSY.—This is a designation given to loss of sensation and power in nerves which have been subjected to pressure. The nerves most often affected in this way are the musculo-spiral nerve and its branches, in the arm. They may be compressed by the new growth that surrounds the ends of a fractured bone, by leaning on crutches (crutch paralysis), or by the arm hanging for a long time over a chair, etc., as when a person is under the influence of alcohol or of an anæsthetic. In these ways such symptoms as loss of sensation and wrist-drop may be set up. The lost functions are generally recovered in the course of a few days, but the interval may be longer, especially in the case of elderly people.

PRESSURE - POINTS   OF ARTERIES (*see* HÆMORRHAGE).

PREVENTIVE MEDICINE.—The Public Health Service of the country is sometimes called State Medicine, because it is organized by the State. It is also known as Preventive Medicine, because its ultimate aim is the prevention of disease, technically styled prophylaxis; in so far as it compasses the cure of disease it does so as a means to that end—prevention —rather than as an end in itself. It acts partly by measures for checking the dissemination of infectious diseases, and partly by the enforcement of sanitary regulations. The system has grown up gradually, and few realize the extent of its ramifications or how much the individual citizen owes to it. It is carried out mainly by medical officers of health, who work under the local authorities; but these authorities, in turn, are supervised by the Ministry of Health, the chief organ of the Public Health Service, although the Home Office also plays an important part in the system by its supervision of factories, workshops, prisons, etc. The Health Ministry controls sewerage and drainage, ensures a pure water supply, guards against the adulteration of food, sees to the sanitary condition of dwelling-houses, schools, public institutions, etc., secures isolation and disinfection in cases of communicable disease, and imposes quarantine regulations where necessary. Its care for the future citizen begins before he is born, and continues until after he is dead, only ceasing when he has been buried or cremated. Of late years it has made an important departure by undertaking the medical inspection of school children. Formerly it attended to the sanitary condition and suitability of the school buildings, but took no thought for the children except to guard them from exposure to infectious diseases. Now, every child who attends school undergoes medical inspection, and a large proportion of them are found to be suffering from defects of vision, adenoids and enlarged tonsils, decay of teeth, etc. Such of the defects as are remediable are cured, and the children thus have a reasonable chance of profiting from the education they receive. For those who are blind or deaf, or labour under other serious infirmities, physical or mental, special schools are provided.

A more recent development of Preventive Medicine is in connexion with venereal diseases (*see* VENEREAL DISEASES).

PRICKLY HEAT.—The medical name for this affection is *miliaria papulosa*, because it manifests itself in an eruption of papules (hard pimples) which are as tiny as millet seeds. It consists in inflammation of the sweat-glands, with the result that the ducts which bring the sweat to the surface become blocked. Most common in the tropics, it is not infrequent in this country. One attack appears to predispose to others. The little pimples, bright red in colour, come out suddenly in thick clusters, after profuse perspiration, and give rise to a pricking and tingling so acute as to be painful. The treatment required is to apply boric-acid ointment or dusting powder to relieve the irritation, and to take a dose of magnesia or fruit salts as a cooling aperient. An alkaline or bran bath will also be found beneficial. Only light food should be taken for a few days, and no alcohol.

PROCTITIS (*see* BOWELS, INFLAMMATION OF).

PROGRESSIVE MUSCULAR ATROPHY.—In some forms of muscular wasting the seat of the disease is the muscles themselves, but what is called progressive muscular atrophy is the result of a degeneration of certain parts of the spinal cord and brain. Why they undergo this degeneration is not fully understood, but there can be little doubt that for some of the cases syphilis is responsible. The disease more often assails men than women, and it usually begins in the thirties or forties. As a rule, the arms are first attacked; an aching pain is followed by wasting of the muscles. Later, the muscles of the trunk are attacked. Death may be caused by respiratory difficulty from wasting of the muscles used in breathing. This is but one type of progressive muscular atrophy. It is not necessary to describe the others, but in all alike the disease tends steadily to progress, though in some cases its course is arrested. Treatment consists in massage and remedial exercises and in maintaining the general health by cod-liver oil and tonics such as iron, arsenic, and strychnine.

PROLAPSE OF THE BOWEL (*see* BOWEL, FALLING OF).

PROLAPSE OF THE WOMB (*see* WOMB, DISPLACEMENTS OF).

PROPHYLAXIS (*see* PREVENTIVE MEDICINE).

PROSTATE GLAND, ENLARGED.—The prostate gland (Fig. 48), which surrounds the male urethra near the neck of the bladder, is peculiarly liable to undergo enlargement after the age of 50. The late Sir Henry Thompson made observations which led him to conclude that after the age of 55 one out of every three men is thus affected. There are various theories as to the cause of the enlargement, but none of them commands general assent. Fortunately the condition is not in itself serious, though it becomes so if it interferes with the passing of water. The bladder in cases of enlarged prostate is never entirely emptied, and as a result it is irritated, and water has to be passed more frequently, especially at night. The irritation may pass into inflammation, and finally the bladder may be so distended that the urine, no longer under the patient's control, constantly dribbles away.

Treatment.—Whatever the degree of enlargement, the patient should avoid bicycling and horse exercise, which cause pressure on the prostate, and for the same reason should avoid constipation. He must not indulge in highly spiced food, which tends to render the urine irritating, should abstain from alcohol while drinking freely of other fluids, and should take as much exercise as possible. In many cases "catheter life" becomes necessary—i.e. a tube is passed along the urethra to draw off the water from the bladder. The catheter may have to be used regularly or only occasionally, but the tendency is for the frequency to increase. The patient can easily be taught to use the catheter himself, but he must be brought to see the absolute necessity for keeping the instrument surgically clean by disinfecting it with an antiseptic, such as carbolic-acid lotion, 1 in 20, every time it is used. If this is not done with unfailing regularity a severe form of inflammation of the bladder may be set up. If he avoids this danger the patient may go on to the end of his life without being seriously troubled. In some cases, however, it is necessary for the gland to be removed, either entirely or in part.

PROTEINS (*see* Food).

PROTOZOA (*see* Germs).

PRURIGO.—The term prurigo is derived from the Latin *prurire*, to itch, and is applied to this affection

because it is characterized by the most intense itching. The cause of prurigo is not understood, but it is believed to be of nervous origin, and to be predisposed to by alcoholism, affections of the womb, and other conditions that depress the general health. Although it may develop in childhood, it most often begins between the twentieth and thirtieth years. After two or three weeks the affection may disappear, or it may persist for several months, but in either case it is apt to recur, and the recurrence may take place at the same season each year. The itching must be dealt with on the

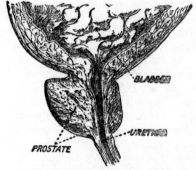

Fig. 48.—The prostate gland.

lines described in the article on that subject. In some cases benefit has been derived from radium, the X-rays, or electricity.

PRURITUS (*see* Itching).

PRUSSIC-ACID POISONING.—Prussic acid, otherwise hydrocyanic acid, received its common name from the fact that it was first made from prussian blue. As soon as the acid is swallowed, or immediately afterwards, the patient, whose breath smells of bitter almonds, becomes giddy, loses all power, and rapidly lapses into insensibility, with dilated pupils and staring, glistening eyes. The first thing to do is to give an emetic, if he is able to swallow (*see* Emetics).

Then remove the patient to the open air, dash cold water over him, or pour it from a height on to his head and spine. If he can still swallow, give him brandy or any other spirit which is at hand. Meanwhile artificial respiration should be carried out.

PSORIASIS.—The characteristic feature of this affection of the skin is the formation, in patches, of dry scales which are whitish or silver-grey on the surface, and bright as frosted silver beneath. The cause of the affection, in spite of the most elaborate researches, is not understood. It occurs more frequently in youth than in later adult life, is uncommon in early infancy, and seldom begins after the age of fifty. Though not more frequent at one time of year than another, it is apt to become worse in the spring and the autumn. In many cases it follows childbirth, suckling, nervous shock, emotional disturbance, or depressing influences such as insufficient nourishment. In some cases it is apparently hereditary.

Symptoms.—The eruption begins as papules (hard pimples) of the size of a pin's head, at first red but afterwards becoming white and scaly. The pimples spread outwards from the centre and form patches. After extending for a time the patches may remain stationary for a long while and then gradually disappear, or, continuing to spread, they may run into each other and cover large areas of skin. The patches of psoriasis are especially likely to occur in parts where the skin is thick and frequently stretched, and is exposed to friction with clothes, etc. Almost always the disease starts at the point of the elbows (Plate XIII) or the front of the knees. Other favourite sites are the scalp and the loins. The face is seldom attacked, and the palms and the soles still more

rarely. The appearance of the patches varies somewhat with the part affected. In some cases the nails are attacked, with the result that they may be split and pushed out of their bed, or may be thickened. Severe itching is seldom a feature of this affection, and in most cases itching is absent. If not treated, the disease may last for months or even years, with periods of intermission during which it may entirely disappear. It is liable also to sudden exacerbations, due to such influences as change of climate, mental shock, or some particular food. When it has disappeared it is extremely likely sooner or later to recur.

Treatment.—The first thing to do is to remove the scales, which should be softened and loosened by being well washed with hot water and soft soap, or kept immersed in tepid water, or treated with oil or vaselin. If the patch is in an early stage, and has a zone of redness, it should be covered with olive oil or cold cream. In chronic cases a stimulating ointment is needed, such as pyrogallic acid (10 grains), or resorcin (10 grains), mixed with an ounce of prepared lard or lanolin. These ointments must be used with caution. Under the X-rays, or radium, or the high-frequency electric current the patches frequently disappear, but the proneness to recurrence continues as with other forms of treatment. In chronic cases, sulphur baths, such as those of Harrogate and Strathpeffer, are often beneficial, and arsenic is of service in many cases. A dose of 3 minims of Fowler's solution, freely diluted, may be taken thrice a day, after meals, and gradually increased to 5 minims, but the medicine should not be continued for more than two or three weeks without a break.

Somewhat allied to psoriasis, but

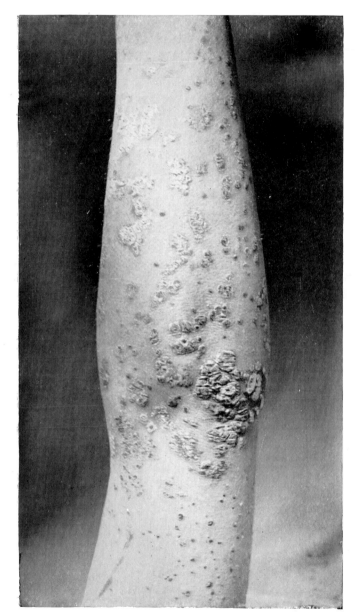

PLATE XIII. PSORIASIS IN A COMMON SITUATION, OVER THE ELBOW

with important differences, is the eruptive affection known as **para-psoriasis.** The lesions are round, oval, or irregular in shape, may be either smooth or covered with a fine scale, and vary in colour from fawn to pale red. The favourite sites for the eruption are the trunk, arms, and legs, and sometimes the back of the hands and feet; the scalp and face are avoided. It takes a long time to develop, is very persistent, and is curiously resistant to treatment, making little or no response to remedies which effectually remove the lesions of psoriasis. The cause is not known.

PSYCHASTHENIA.—The psychasthenic is unable to regulate his ideas and actions in a rational manner, finds it difficult to concentrate his mind upon any subject, and in severe cases develops obsessions (q.v.), and is subject to the emotional crises popularly called hysterics. In many cases there is nervous instability to start with, and the psychasthenia develops under exposure to some emotional strain. One of the worst effects of psychasthenia is difficulty in sleeping. When at last the patient falls asleep, the thoughts which he has been able, more or less, to repress while awake reappear as nightmares, so that he wakes in terror, although often he may have no recollection of his dream. Treatment is entirely mental (*see* PSYCHOTHERAPY).

PSYCHOTHERAPY.—This term means treatment not by material or physical means, but by psychical (mental) influence. Obviously, psychotherapy is mainly applicable to disorders arising chiefly from psychical or mental causes. It is of some service even in certain forms of actual insanity; but it is in the group of cases coming between ordinary physical diseases and insanity—i.e.

functional nervous disorders, in which there is no traceable organic disease of the nervous system—that psychotherapy finds its chief sphere of usefulness (*see* PSYCHASTHENIA, NEURASTHENIA, OBSESSIONS). The chief methods of psychotherapy are suggestion (including hypnotism), persuasion, and analysis. By *suggestion* the patient is brought to believe that the affection from which he suffers, say the paralysis of a limb in hysteria, no longer exists, and as the paralysis has no physical basis it now disappears. Suggestion may avail itself of physical aids, and this is the explanation of the benefit derived from electricity and even from drugs in these cases. When suggestion takes the form of hypnosis, it is still more potent (*see* HYPNOTISM). The difference between suggestion and *persuasion* is that the former may be quite independent of reason, whereas persuasion consists mainly in explanation and argument, though here also the personality of the medical man counts for a good deal. In *psycho-analysis* the physician sets himself to discover the precise mental causes of the disorder. Often they lie in the depths of the patient's mind, and much skill is required to bring them to the surface and appreciate their significance. This method is not without its dangers: it is possible to harm sensitive, ill-balanced minds by suggesting or stressing obnoxious ideas, and the most delicate discretion is required.

PTOMAINES (*see* FOOD-POISONING).

PTOSIS.—This word means a falling, and it is used in connexion with various organs of the body, such as those in the abdomen, but when it is employed alone it usually signifies a drooping of the upper eyelid (*see* EYELID, UPPER, DROOPING OF).

PUBLIC HEALTH (*see* PREVENTIVE MEDICINE).

PUERPERAL FEVER.—Child-bed fever, to give this affection its popular name, is a form of blood-poisoning, the result of infection of the mother with germs after the birth of the child. The germs may be conveyed by the nurse or midwife, or may be derived from the patient herself; they enter the blood through one of the raw surfaces caused by the delivery of the child. The affection is a serious one, but fortunately, owing to the antiseptic precautions now taken, it is much less frequent than it used to be. The pioneer of the movement which has brought about this improvement was an Austrian physician of the name of Semmelweiss, who in 1846 joined the staff of the General Hospital at Vienna. At that time the death-rate from puerperal fever in the hospital had reached alarming proportions. As the result of prolonged research, Semmelweiss came to the conclusion that the disease was due to infection, conveyed from the dissecting room by the hands of medical students, and he therefore insisted that before a midwifery patient was examined, the hands should be thoroughly washed with liquid chlorine or chlorinated lime water. The result was that in a few months the death-rate fell from over 12 per cent. to a trifle over 3 per cent., and the next year it fell as low as $1\frac{1}{4}$ per cent. At first, however, the new method aroused hostility, which became so bitter that in 1850 Semmelweiss left Vienna. He continued to defend his method, but with little success, and in 1865 lost his reason, and was consigned to an asylum, where within a few months, by the irony of fate, he died of blood-poisoning. Up to this time no scientific basis had been found for the use of antiseptics, for the germs to which blood-poisoning is due had not been discovered. It was in this very year, indeed—1865—that Lister entered upon the patient researches that led to the establishment of antiseptic principles on a rational basis. To few diseases have these principles been applied more successfully than to puerperal fever. As a general rule, to which there are but few exceptions, it may be said that this disease would never arise if proper antiseptic precautions were taken. Treatment will, of course, be directed by the medical attendant.

PUERPERAL INSANITY.—The causes of insanity after labour, either within a few days, or later when the patient has become exhausted from suckling her child, are much the same in all cases, and are of the same order as those which produce insanity during pregnancy. The patient is the victim of nervous instability to start with, and her brain fails under the strain of the emotion, hæmorrhage, physical exhaustion, and pain which are associated with pregnancy, childbirth, and lactation. These causes may be powerfully reinforced by worry and grief, and, if the woman is unmarried, especially by shame. In the insanity of pregnancy the patient becomes depressed and anxious, is often suspicious of her husband, and develops delusions which may continue after the birth of the child. In such cases removal to a mental hospital is necessary, unless she can be kept under constant supervision at home. If this is possible, it is much to be preferred, so that the child may not bear the stigma of having been born in a mental hospital. In the insanity of lactation the baby should be weaned and taken away from the mother. In simple cases **recovery**

usually takes place as the patient's bodily health improves, but there are cases in which she passes into a condition of chronic or recurrent insanity. Whether insanity occurs in pregnancy, in childbirth, or later, the patient must have plenty of fresh air and nourishing food, and usually tonics will be found necessary. Often the doctor will have to give drugs to procure sleep.

PULMONARY TUBERCULOSIS
(*see* CONSUMPTION).

PULSE, THE.—With each contraction of the left ventricle of the heart an impulse is communicated to all the arteries which causes them to expand, and wherever an artery comes close to the surface of the body this impulse can be felt by the finger. This is what is known as the pulse. In ordinary circumstances it is most conveniently taken at the wrist, but when, for example, the wrists are covered with wrappings, or the patient is in a wet pack, it is necessary that it should be taken elsewhere. Among other places at which it can be felt are the front and inner side of the ankle, the groin, at the bend of the elbow and inner side of the arm, the front of the neck but away from the middle line, in front of the lappet of the ear (the tragus), and at the edge of the hair between the temple and the brow.

To take the pulse.—The pulse may be felt in either wrist, standing or sitting (according to the position of the patient) on the outer side of the arm. The fore-, middle and ring fingers of the right hand are placed about half an inch from the outer side of the forearm, which is supported by the thumb. In the unoccupied hand is held a watch with a second hand, and the pulse-beats are counted for a minute.

The frequency of the beats will vary with the age and position of the patient, and other circumstances. In the new-born infant the rate is 130 to 140 beats a minute ; at the age of 6 it is about 100 ; in men the average is about 72, and in women about 80. The rate varies also with position, being some eight beats more frequent in the standing, and about the same number of beats less frequent in the recumbent position, than in the sitting posture. It is quickened by exercise, and by taking food, especially if alcohol is drunk, and as the movements of the heart are controlled by the nervous system, it is affected by excitement in a marked degree.

Variations from the normal.—In endeavouring to understand the meaning of departures from the normal pulse, it must be borne in mind that in some persons the rate is exceptionally slow or exceptionally quick. Thus, men of gouty tendencies may have a slow pulse, and it is usually slow also in those who have had a protracted attack of jaundice. Allowances must be made for individual peculiarities, and if the patient is aware of any such peculiarity he should inform the doctor of it.

A *frequent* pulse occurs in fevers, in heart-failure, and in hysteria and other nervous affections. A *slow* pulse is often met with in convalescence from acute fevers, in some forms of heart disease, and in compression of the brain. In the *irregular* pulse some of the beats are more distinct than others. This is one of the indications of failure of the heart. It is common in digestive troubles, when it is only a temporary feature, and it may occur in tuberculous meningitis. In the *intermittent* pulse one or two beats are absent at intervals. This condition, like irregularity of the pulse, may be present in heart disease, but it may also be due to indigestion, constipation, flatulence, acidity, gout, nervous excitement, overwork, excessive indulgence in tea, coffee, or tobacco. A feeble beat— the *low-tension* pulse—may be a sign of heart-failure, and is often met with in fevers when the heart is weak and the blood-vessels are dilated. A strong beat—the pulse of *high-tension* —which resists the pressure of the finger, indicates high blood-pressure and may be symptomatic of disease of the kidney, but is not necessarily associated with any organic disease.

PUPIL (*see* EYE).

PURPURA.—As the result of bleeding into the skin, red or purple spots, or lines, or large or small patches are seen, which will not disappear under pressure of the finger. This may be a symptom of other diseases, such as the infectious fevers, blood-poisoning, etc., or may be due to the taking of drugs. When there is no other condition to account for it, it is regarded as a separate disease—" simple purpura," though probably it is still only a symptom of some other condition which cannot be traced. The treatment of simple purpura, which is all that need be described here, is to rest in bed, take plenty of nourishing food, and a quinine and iron tonic. The patient should keep to his bed for some time after the eruption has gone, so as to lessen the chances of recurrence.

PURULENT OPHTHALMIA (*see* OPHTHALMIA).

PUS IN URINE (*see* URINE, NORMAL AND ABNORMAL).

PYÆMIA (*see* BLOOD-POISONING).

PYONEPHROSIS (*see* HYDRONEPHROSIS).

PYORRHŒA ALVEOLARIS.—Of late years this disease of the tooth sockets, known also as *Riggs' disease*, has been recognized as one of great importance on account of the grave results which accrue to the patient's health from swallowing the poisons discharged into the mouth from the gums. It seldom comes on before middle age. Often the patient is not aware that anything is seriously wrong with the mouth until the doctor whom he consults because he is feeling altogether out of sorts, or has indigestion, or rheumatic pains, examines the gums and finds that they have an angry appearance; then, perhaps, gentle pressure is followed by the oozing of pus. The cause of the condition is not fully understood, but it is of microbic origin. It attacks sound teeth as often as those that are decayed. Insufficient care of the teeth, so that particles of food collect beneath the border of the gums and there decompose, may have something to do with its onset. If the disease is in an early stage, nothing more may be needed to arrest it than for the dentist to remove all deposits and flush the space between gums and teeth with a solution of hydrogen peroxide or a 2-per-cent. carbolic-acid lotion. If the disease still advances, the doctor may advise vaccine treatment. If this also fails, the affected teeth should be extracted, but this should be regarded as the last resort, not the first.

PYREXIA (*see* FEVER).

PYROSIS (*see* HEARTBURN).

Q

QUARANTINE.—In the old sense of the term, denoting the detention of crew and passengers on board a ship where cases of infectious disease had occurred, quarantine no longer exists in Great Britain. What happens now is that the Customs Officer, who is the first to board an incoming ship, obtains a written declaration that there has been, or has not been, during the voyage, a case of cholera, yellow fever, or plague. If such a case has occurred, every person on board is medically examined, and all who are found to be infected are removed to a hospital or, if that is impossible, kept on board until free from the disease. Before others on board are allowed to leave they must give their names and the addresses to which they are going, and in each case the name and address are forwarded to the sanitary authority of the district, so that the " contact " may be kept under observation until the incubation period has expired. Before leaving its moorings the ship is thoroughly disinfected.

Certain measures of domestic quarantine are carried out in cases of the infectious fevers, and are found to be extremely useful in checking the spread of infection. If the patient is removed to an isolation hospital and the house thoroughly disinfected, it is only necessary that the household should remain under observation for the maximum incubation period of the disease (for the *average* incubation periods, *see* Incubation Periods). If the case is treated at home the household must remain under observation until disinfection has been carried out. In both cases, during the quarantine period, no child from the house should be allowed to attend school (except in typhoid fever), nor should any member of the household engage in milk traffic, in nursing, in washing, or in trades in which food is handled. Such forms of homework as tailoring and dressmaking are forbidden for the time being. Injunctions are given against admitting persons, especially children, into the infected house, but

at present there is no power to inflict punishment if this precaution is disregarded. It is especially necessary that the most rigid precautions be taken in all cases of smallpox. In some towns, in connexion with the isolation hospitals, quarantine stations are provided where, in cases of smallpox, the other members of the household can be accommodated during the quarantine period and while the house is being disinfected.

QUICKENING (*see* Pregnancy, Signs and Symptoms of).

QUINSY.—This term is often applied to acute inflammation of the tonsils, but it is really a distinct affection, in which, although the tonsils are inflamed, an abscess forms not in them but in adjoining tissues. Quinsy is most frequent in autumn and spring, rarely attacks children under fifteen or persons who are over thirty-five, and is due to infection with germs derived from unhealthy conditions of the mouth and teeth, the nose, or the middle ear. It may follow in the wake of an attack of tonsillitis, or may occur independently of that affection.

Symptoms.—The patient feels generally out of sorts, is feverish, and possibly has a violent shivering fit. Soon he complains of acute pain behind the angle of the jaw, extending up to the ear and down the neck on the same side. He can neither swallow nor expectorate except with great pain, and allows the thickened saliva to dribble from his mouth. The breath is offensive, the tongue coated with fur, the head held stiffly forward and inclined on the affected side. The skin is hot and moist, and the temperature in the early stages may rise to 102° or even 105° Fahr. There is rapid loss of weight, and the patient sinks into a condition of prostration. As the " gathering " matures the symptoms may somewhat abate. Apart from treatment the disease may run its course in from five to ten days. In most cases only one side of the throat is involved, but occasionally the other side is affected as soon as the first attack has subsided. Although a painful and prostrating affection, quinsy is scarcely ever fatal, and Trousseau, the eminent French physician, said that during his long career he had never known a case to end in death.

Treatment.—The patient should take to his bed and will require careful nursing. At the outset a thorough evacuation of the bowels must be secured by a purge such as Epsom salts. The doctor may consider that the most suitable medicine for children is aconite, and for adults salicylate of soda. It is useless to give gargles or sprays or paints, for the patient in most cases would be unable to use them, and if he could use them they would do him no good. The mouth and throat may be cleansed by syringing the back of the throat with copious tepid lotions, such as one composed of sodium benzoate 2 drachms, resorcin 1½ drachms, antipyrin 1 drachm, with glycerin to 8 ounces ; a teaspoonful to half a tumbler of tepid water. A hot poultice of linseed meal may be placed across the throat from ear to ear. The patient will have no appe-

tite, but he should take soft foods such as bread and milk, light milk puddings, blancmanges and jellies, and may drink as freely as he can of milk and water, barley water, beef tea, etc. In many cases it is easier to swallow soft solid foods than liquids.

It is much better not to wait until the abscess bursts, but to allow the doctor, having painted it with cocaine, to open it, so that it may discharge. Some of the pus will escape into the stomach, and the purgative should therefore be continued. As the symptoms subside and the temperature falls, the salicylate of soda, or the aconite in the case of children, must be given less frequently, and discontinued altogether when the temperature becomes normal. The throat may now be covered with cotton-wool or flannel, and the affected part painted with glycerin of tannic acid. Or a gargle may now be used —say 40 grains of alum to 8 ounces of water.

The patient will need a nutritious diet for a few days, and also a tonic —bark and ammonia (*see* p. 289), or if he is anæmic, quinine and iron (*see* p. 42). If there is a tendency for the quinsy to recur, the throat and back of the neck should be sponged daily with cold water and the throat gargled every morning with 2 grains of borax and a few drops of tincture of myrrh in two tablespoonfuls of water.

R

RABIES (*see* HYDROPHOBIA).

RACHITIS (*see* RICKETS).

RADIANT HEAT (*see* ELECTRICAL TREATMENT).

R A D I U M   TREATMENT.— Radium is a chemical element which was discovered a few years ago by two eminent French workers in

chemistry, Mme. Curie and her husband. It is perpetually emitting four different kinds of rays with a velocity almost equal to that of light, but in spite of this a fragment of radium undergoes no appreciable loss of weight, and it would take hundreds of years to exhaust the energy of a single grain of this marvellous substance. It is used with success in many affections of the skin, such as rodent ulcer, sarcoma, port-wine stains, lupus vulgaris, and scars. It is also inserted into the body so as to act upon deep-seated cancers, and though it cannot be considered curative for such conditions it has decided palliative virtue, and is also a valuable adjunct to operation. Radium gives off a gas which discharges the same rays as the salt and produces similar effects.

RAT-FLEA (*see* PLAGUE).

RAYNAUD'S DISEASE.—This affection, named after a French physician, is allied to chill and frostbite. It is known also as symmetrical (i.e. double-sided) gangrene of the extremities, "extremities" including not merely the fingers, toes, and heels, but also the ears and the tip of the nose. It is not always, however, symmetrical, though usually so. Persons with weak circulation, and especially those who are subject to "dead" fingers or to chilblains, are particularly liable to attack. It is usually associated with a sluggish circulation and nervous instability, and it may follow an attack of such diseases as scarlet fever, measles, and diphtheria. In bad cases suppuration of the affected part takes place; in slighter cases, after the superficial tissues have been more or less damaged, healing takes place, the part, however, remaining thinned. Galvanism and hot-water baths are the treatment indicated. The diet should be nourishing, and should contain foods rich in starch and sugar, and a sufficiency of outdoor exercise should be taken. Tonics, especially quinine and arsenic, are useful.

RECURRENT MANIA AND MELANCHOLIA (*see* INSANITY).

RED CORPUSCLES (*see* BLOOD AND LYMPH).

REDNESS OF THE SKIN (*see* ERYTHEMA).

RED-GUM.—This affection manifests itself in an eruption of small red pimples scattered over the body, accompanied by acute itching. In most cases it is the result of some disturbance of the digestive organs, due to vaccination, or teething, or unsuitable food; it may also be set up by profuse perspiration, caused by the child being too warmly wrapped up. The first attack is liable to be followed by others, and thus the affection may continue off and on for years. The treatment is simple. For the irritation of the skin, soothing lotions such as lead lotion may be used. The bowels should be occasionally cleared with a mild aperient such as a one-grain powder of mercury and chalk, and to remove acidity a few doses of chalk mixture, which the chemist will supply, may be given. Irritating clothing must be avoided. The child must be kept scrupulously clean, must have plenty of fresh air, and any food that disagrees should be discontinued.

REEF-KNOT (*see* BANDAGES).

REFRACTION AND ACCOMMODATION, ERRORS OF.—The chief defects of sight that come under this designation are long sight, short sight, and astigmatism, which are errors of refraction, and old sight, which is an error of accommodation. They are all described under SIGHT, DEFECTS OF.

REFRIGERATION, TREATMENT BY (*see* CARBONIC-ACID SNOW, TREATMENT BY).

RELAPSING FEVER.—In many countries, especially in the tropics, a curious form of fever is prevalent which comes on suddenly, lasts for a period varying from one to seven days, subsides, and after an interval, also varying between one and seven days, recurs, and may do so an indefinite number of times. It is met with in tropical Africa and Asia, and in Norway, Denmark, Germany, Russia, and Turkey, and in Russia sometimes appears as an epidemic, as when it attacked the Grand Army in the retreat from Moscow, the Allied Armies in the Crimea, and the armies of both sides in the Russo-Turkish

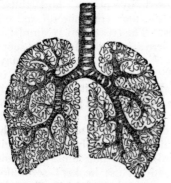

Fig. 49.—The bronchial tubes and air-sacs.

War. It has also visited the United States in epidemic form, and is widely distributed throughout Central and South America. Formerly it was not uncommon in the British Isles, especially Ireland, but is now rare. It is due to a germ belonging to the group of spirochætes. It is transmitted by body vermin, and in Africa by tiny insects known as ticks—hence the name tick fever, which, however, should be discarded, for this is not the only fever in which the tick plays the rôle of communicator. The disease is only infectious in a low degree. Neo-salvarsan, which is so inimical to the germ of syphilis, is not less so to that of relapsing fever.

Prevention consists in rigid personal and domestic cleanliness, and the use, where necessary, of insect powders.

RELAXED SORE THROAT (*see* SORE THROAT).

RENAL COLIC (*see* STONE IN THE KIDNEY).

RESPIRATION.—Respiration, or breathing, is made up of two acts—inspiration and expiration. *Inspiration* is brought about by the action of muscles which, by raising the ribs, increase the size of the chest cavity; at the same time the diaphragm, the great muscle which separates the chest from the abdomen, is flattened out and enlarges the size of the chest downwards by pushing down the organs beneath it. The increased space in the chest thus produced can only be filled by air rushing in through the air-passages (*see* below) and distending the lungs. In *expiration* the ribs fall, the diaphragm relaxes, the distended lungs contract, and the air is driven out until the pressure within and without is equalized.

The *air-passages* are the nose, the pharynx or back of the mouth, the larynx, the windpipe (trachea), and the bronchial tubes (Plate XIV). These bronchial tubes become smaller and smaller as they penetrate the lungs until they terminate in air-sacs (Fig. 49). The air-sacs are covered with little cells called alveoli which on one surface of their walls have a network of tiny blood-vessels known as capillaries, whilst on the inner surface they are in contact with the air which has been inspired. Thus the air from without and the blood brought to the lungs come so close together that the blood can take oxygen from the air and give up to the air the carbonic acid gas it has brought from the tissues.

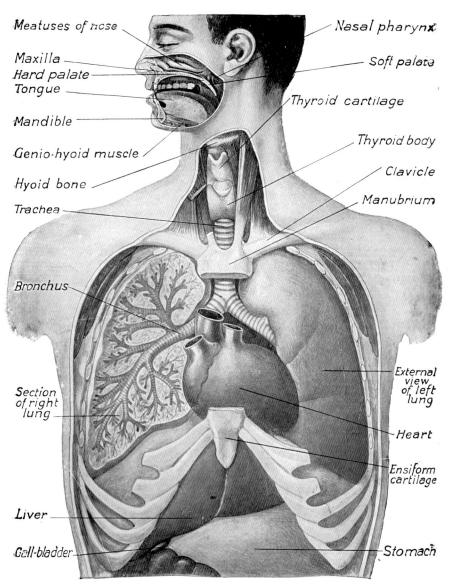

Meatuses of nose

Maxilla

Hard palate

Tongue

Mandible

Genio-hyoid muscle

Hyoid bone

Trachea

Bronchus

Section
of right
lung

Liver

Gall-bladder

Nasal pharynx

Soft palate

Thyroid cartilage

Thyroid body

Clavicle

Manubrium

External
view
of left
lung

Heart

Ensiform
cartilage

Stomach

PLATE XIV. THE RESPIRATORY TRACT.

Essentially, therefore, and in brief, respiration consists in supplying oxygen to the blood and removing from it carbonic acid gas.

The *lungs* are composed of the air-sacs and the connective tissue which

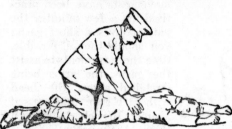

Fig. 50.—Schafer's method of artificial respiration: first movement.
(*British Red Cross Society's First-Aid Manual.*)

supports this multitude of tiny cells. The right lung consists of three and the left of two lobes; they are enveloped by the *pleura*, a membrane which is reflected back upon the inner surface of the chest. The pleura is moistened with a fluid which prevents friction between its two layers (the one lining the lungs, the other the chest cavity) as the lungs contract and expand.

RESPIRATION, ARTIFICIAL.— Special measures to restore respiration may be required not only for persons who have been immersed in water until breathing has stopped, but also in cases where poisonous fumes or gases have been inhaled, or where there is choking from particles of food or foreign bodies in the air-passages, or where strangulation has been effected. Of the various methods of artificial respiration in use we shall describe Schafer's, Sylvester's and Howard's.

In all alike the clothing round the neck, chest and abdomen must be loosened and the air-passages freed from obstruction so that air may enter the lungs without

difficulty. Foreign bodies and food particles must be removed with the finger; the mouth must be cleared of water, dirt and froth with a cloth, and the water allowed to escape by laying the patient face downwards. In Sylvester's and Howard's methods the tongue must be held out of the mouth so that it may not obstruct the windpipe. If an assistant is at hand he may hold the tongue between his finger and thumb with the corner of a handkerchief; if not, a piece of string or torn handkerchief having been attached to it, it should be drawn forward and the string or torn handkerchief tied firmly under the jaw. In cases of drowning, resuscitation should be attempted even if a person has been submerged for ten minutes or longer. Cases have occurred in which patients have been restored after several hours of unconsciousness, and the attempt should not cease until the body temperature has fallen fifteen degrees below the normal 98·4° Fahr.

1. **Schafer's method.—**Put the patient on the ground with his face downwards, his head turned to one side, and the arms stretched out forwards; a rolled-up coat may be

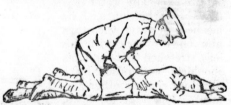

Fig. 51.—Schafer's method of artificial respiration: second movement.
(*British Red Cross Society's First-Aid Manual.*)

put under the lower part of the chest. Kneel astride the patient, facing his head, and lay the hands on each side (Fig. 50). Then gradually bend forward your body, throwing your weight on his chest (Fig. 51). In this way the air is forced out of the patient's chest by compressing the lower ribs. Next raise yourself slowly into the kneeling position, removing all pressure from the chest. The chest will now expand by virtue of its natural elasticity, and

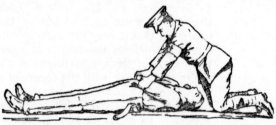

Fig. 52.—Sylvester's method of artificial respiration : first movement.
(*British Red Cross Society's First-Aid Manual.*)

will draw air into the lungs. Repeat these two movements every four or five seconds regularly until natural movements of breathing are re-established.

The advantages of this method are that it is less fatiguing than Sylvester's, that there is no need to hold the tongue forward, and that no changes of position are required.

2. Sylvester's method.—Put the patient face downwards or on his side and squeeze the lower part of his chest hard with a hand on each side, to expel any water that may be in his lungs, if he has been in water, then turn him on his back with his legs stretched out and his shoulders well raised by a rolled-up coat or other garment. Kneel at his head, and take hold of both his arms just above the elbows. Press the arms into the sides of the chest (Fig. 52) so as to expel any air in the chest, and get an assistant to press on the pit of the stomach. Draw the arms away from the sides outwards and carry them upwards and backwards until they

rest on the ground as illustrated in Fig. 53. Pause in this position for two seconds, to allow air to get into the lungs, and repeat the process again and again at the rate of 15 times a minute. In many cases, after these movements have been practised for a few minutes the patient gives a short gasp ; you should then, if possible, time the movements to assist the gasps, the arms being stretched above the head with each gasp, and pressed against the chest between them. As the natural breaths become deeper, the movements should gradually be discontinued, but they must be recommenced if breathing begins to fail again. While these movements are being carried out, assistants may dry and warm the feet, may rub the legs towards the body to encourage the flow of blood, and may put on warm dry clothing. Care, however, must be taken to avoid interference with the movements, which are the essential part of the treatment.

This method has the merit of simplicity. The disadvantage of it is that it is very fatiguing, and can only

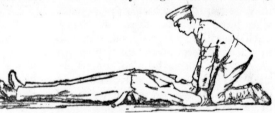

Fig. 53.—Sylvester's method of artificial respiration. second movement.
(*British Red Cross Society's First-Aid Manual.*)

be carried on by the same person for a few minutes at a time.

3. Howard's method.—Lay the patient on his back with a folded coat under, and slightly below, the shoulder-blades so that the abdomen projects forwards and the head hangs well back. Place the hands above the head. Kneel astride the patient's thighs, bend up your arms, and fix your elbows firmly against your sides. Place your hands spread out over the lower part of his chest on each side of the pit of the stomach ; now lean forward until your mouth is nearly over the patient's, squeezing his two sides together by bringing all your weight to bear on him, as if you wished to force everything in the chest upwards towards the mouth. Remain in this position for about three seconds, and repeat the movements again and again with great regularity. In this way the air is forced out of the chest by the pressure, and is drawn into it by the elastic recoil of the chest-walls. The movements should be repeated ten times a minute.

This method can be employed when the patient's arm is broken. It can be carried out by one person and, as it is less exhausting than Sylvester's, can be continued much longer.

" REST CURE."—This method of treatment, especially successful in cases of nervous exhaustion, is described under NEURASTHENIA. In suitable cases it is undoubtedly beneficial, but it has sometimes been prescribed where less expensive treatment would have sufficed, nor, except in extreme cases, is it necessary that it should be carried out in its entirety. It was devised by Dr. Weir-Mitchell, a very able American physician who was also eminent as a man of letters, and it is often called by his name.

RETENTION OF URINE (*see* URINE, RETENTION OF).

RETINA (*see* EYE).

RETROFLEXION (*see* WOMB, DISPLACEMENTS OF).

RETROVERSION (*see* WOMB, DISPLACEMENTS OF).

RHEUMATIC FEVER (*see* RHEUMATISM, ACUTE).

RHEUMATIC GOUT (*see* ARTHRITIS DEFORMANS).

RHEUMATIC HEADACHE (*see* HEADACHE).

RHEUMATISM, ACUTE.—This disease is known popularly as rheumatic fever, a high temperature being one of its constant features, and the common view is that it is caused by exposure to cold and wet, associated, it may be, with over-exertion and fatigue. In some cases, undoubtedly, these factors play their part, though only a subordinate part, in causing the disease ; but in many cases they are absent. In about one-fourth of the cases, too, there is a history of rheumatism in one or both parents. But this again is only a predisposing cause. The actual or exciting cause is undoubtedly a germ, for the whole course and character of " rheumatic fever " are those of an acute germ disease. The great majority of cases occur between the ages of ten and twenty.

Symptoms.—For two or three days the patient feels chilly and generally out of sorts, has sore throat and headache, and restless nights ; he then wakes up in the morning with a temperature. He complains of severe pain in one or more of the joints, and the affected joint or joints rapidly swell. The disease may not confine itself to one joint or set of joints, but may, and usually does, shift from one to another. In some cases, termed sub-acute, the affection of the joints may be slight and the pain not severe, but more often the pain is so great that the patient cannot bear to move or to be moved. As far as his restlessness will allow, he lies motionless in bed on the flat of his back, his legs stretched out and his arms folded across, anxiously watching every movement of those in attendance lest they should move the bed and shake him. The whole body is soaked with sour-smelling sweat. The face is flushed, the tongue furred, the pulse quick and full, the urine high-coloured and scanty. Appetite is lost, but there is a raging thirst. So the patient remains day after day, and the pain may not begin to subside until all the joints liable to attack have had their turn.

Complications.—The worst feature of acute rheumatism is the serious complications which frequently arise. It is important, therefore, that from the beginning of the attack the nursing should be of the most careful kind, and that every possible precaution should be taken to safeguard the patient against cold, undue exertion, or any kind of indiscretion. The most common complications are those affecting the heart. Besides palpitation and rapid pulse, there may be inflammation of the inner membrane—*endocarditis ;* of the outer membrane—*pericarditis ;* or of the heart-muscle—*myocarditis.* These complications occur more often in women than in men, in children than in adults. Acute rheumatism may also be complicated by inflammatory affections of the breathing organs, such as pneumonia, bronchitis, and pleurisy. Skin eruptions often occur, or little lumps (nodules) may be seen and felt underneath the skin, especially in severe cases. The sore throat which has been mentioned as one of the early symptoms sometimes takes the form of tonsillitis, and some authorities believe that the germ finds its way into the blood through the tonsils, as it does in some other diseases.

Treatment.—The helplessness of the patient makes it important to secure the services of a skilled nurse. The sheets should be removed, so that the patient may lie between the blankets. He should wear woollen nightshirts, split from top to bottom along the front, and from neck to cuff along the seam of the sleeve, so that any part of the body may easily be uncovered for washing or to apply treatment ; tapes should be stitched on to the garment to fasten it up. The copious, sour-smelling perspiration will necessitate frequent changing of the nightshirt and occasional changing of blankets.

In some cases the sweating ceases and the pains vanish but the temperature rises with alarming rapidity, and may mount to 110° Fahr., or even higher, and delirium or violent convulsions may follow. In such cases the measures recommended against hyperpyrexia must at once be adopted (*see* FEVER).

The best drugs in the treatment of this disease, as of other rheumatic affections, are salicylate of soda and salicin. A simple salicylate mixture is the following :

Salicylate of soda .... 3 drachms
Syrup of ginger............ 1 ounce
Water to 8 ounces.
One tablespoonful every 3 hours.

Aspirin, a derivative of salicylic acid, is also useful, 10 to 15 grains for an adult, 3 to 5 grains for a child, dissolved in lemon water or in cold milk, one dose every three or four hours.

The patient should be supplied freely with effervescing potash or soda water mixed with milk or lemon juice. If there is great exhaustion, alcohol is needed. Nourishment must be given in fluid form (*see* FEVER), and at short and regular intervals, both night and day. When the fever has subsided, light clear soups and broths may be given, and a little pounded beef or chicken may be mixed with them. Bread and milk, and milk puddings, are also suitable.

Local treatment will be needed. Each painful joint should be covered with a thick layer of cotton-wool kept in position by a firm but not tight bandage, and changed when it becomes soaked with sweat, the joint being sponged with warm water in which carbonate of soda has been dissolved. Hot fomentations often give relief ; they must be applied very gently, and as hot as can be borne. In most cases nothing more will be necessary, but if the joints are very painful the doctor may order a laudanum and bicarbonate-of-soda lotion—1 part of laudanum to 6 parts of hot water, with 20 grains of bicarbonate of soda to the ounce, or a belladonna-and-glycerin liniment may be used.

The patient must still be carefully watched during convalescence. He should remain in bed for a week or two after all fever and pain have disappeared ; if the heart has been implicated, the period of absolute rest should be prolonged for some weeks. When he gets about he should wear warm woollen clothing, take special care of the throat, and avoid fatigue, for acute rheumatism, so far from giving immunity, as many germ fevers do, predisposes to further attacks.

In *children* the high fever and soaking perspirations are absent, the temperature seldom rising above 102° Fahr. ; often, too, the joint-pains are insignificant, and the joints but little swollen. The pains, in fact, are what is usually called " growing pains "—a misleading designation which may lead to the illness being regarded as trivial. Trivial it certainly is not, because of the frequent occurrence of heart complications. Treatment proceeds on the same general lines as in adults, but the salicylate of soda should be replaced by salicin, as in the following prescription :

Salicin .... 60 grains
Carbonate of potash........ 60 grains
Tincture of orange .... 2 drachms
Syrup .... ½ ounce
Water to 3 ounces.
A dessertspoonful every 4 to 6 hours for a child of 5 years ; dose to be modified according to age.

Complete rest in bed, however slight the symptoms, is of the first importance as the most promising means of averting heart and other complications, and it should be continued for at least a fortnight after all the symptoms have disappeared. During convalescence cod-liver oil is of great service.

RHEUMATISM, CHRONIC.— This designation was formerly used in Medicine to denote a chronic affection of the muscles, when it was called chronic *muscular* rheumatism, and a chronic affection of the joints, when it was called chronic *articular* rheumatism. It is now, however, being abandoned, the muscular affections which it covered being grouped under the general heading of myalgia (i.e. pain in muscles) and divided up into lumbago, side-ache, etc. (*see* LUMBAGO, SIDE-ACHE, WRY-NECK), and the joint affections into osteo-arthritis and rheumatoid arthritis, both of which are described in the article on ARTHRITIS DEFORMANS.

RHEUMATISM, MUSCULAR (*see* RHEUMATISM, CHRONIC).

RHEUMATOID ARTHRITIS (*see* ARTHRITIS DEFORMANS).

RHINOPHYMA (*see* ACNE ROSACEA).

RICKETS.—Rachitis, to give this affection its technical name, is said to be the most common of all infantile diseases. In the vast majority of cases it begins between the ages of 3 months and 3 years, but occasionally it appears later, though usually as a recurrence of early rickets. In a few cases on the other hand, symptoms are present at birth.

Causes.—The cause of rickets is not fully understood. Some authorities hold that the disease is due to a germ, others that it is a deficiency disease, due to the lack of a vitamin (*see under* FOOD) or of lime salts, others that it is caused by lack of sunlight, and yet others that it is due to bad hygiene in the widest sense of the term, including unsuitable food, lack of fresh air and sunshine, and the other disadvantages of slum life.

Symptoms.—Rickets manifests itself gradually. The child becomes irritable and fretful, and loses his appetite; the bowels act irregularly. The complexion grows sallow and pale, sleep is disturbed, and perspiration is profuse. There may be slight fever, especially towards night. Often there is what has been called a "diffuse soreness of body," so that the child cannot bear to be moved, and cries on being touched. Convulsions are set up by very slight nervous irritation, and vary in severity in different cases from passing spasms to fatal attacks. When the child is excited he may have what are called "breath-holding spasms"; the face flushes and the breathing ceases for some seconds, and then he seems as well as before. On the slightest exposure to cold there is great liability to catarrh. There is protrusion of the abdomen, partly because of the great tendency to excessive distension of the bowels with wind. Owing to imperfect development and softness

the bones bend with great readiness and become distorted and thickened; the thickening of the ends of the ribs at the points where they join the gristle that fixes them to the breast-bone produces a row of knobs or "beads," the so-called "rickety rosary," passing downwards and outwards on each side of the chest, while the breast-bone is pushed forward and is more projecting than natural—"pigeon breast." These and a great variety of other deformities do not all appear in any one case, and in slight cases there may be nothing worse than an enlargement of the wrists, and of the ribs on each side of the breast-bone.

While a serious disease, rickets is in itself seldom fatal, though it much increases the dangerousness of other infantile maladies. It may be years before the symptoms subside, but in most cases, sooner or later, they disappear, and no trace of the disease is left but the deformities, slight or gross according to the severity of the attack.

Treatment.—This consists mainly in attention to hygiene and diet. If the child is living in an overcrowded dwelling in a city, removal to the country or the seaside is necessary. The bedroom and living room must be well ventilated, and as much time as possible spent in the open air and sunlight. The greatest care must, however, be taken to avoid chills; warm woollen clothes should be worn, and the face and chest protected. If the child is being nursed, the mother must have plenty of animal fats—butter, cream, etc. —and meat. If her milk is still defective in quality or in amount, it should be supplemented with appropriately modified cow's milk (*see* p. 207). In the case of hand-fed children, if cow's milk has to be diluted, cream must always be added to make up for the deficiency of fat. The bowels must be kept regular by enemata or suppositories or simple aperients (*see* p. 83). Cod-liver oil is beneficial in most cases; it may be given as an emulsion with maltine.

After the ninth month, rusk and milk, the yolk of an egg, and meat gravies may be added to the diet. After twelve months, rusk and butter, bread and butter, stewed apple and prunes, and milk puddings may be given, and the yolk of an egg at least once daily.

Exercise and massage are both useful, but must always be followed by sufficient rest. In a mild case complete rest is not called for, but in more severe cases in which the bones are bent as a result of sitting or walking, etc., splinting by long external splints is desirable, the splints to be worn both day and night, but taken off morning and evening so that the limbs may be bathed in salt water (1 oz. of rock salt to two gallons of water) and well rubbed with a towel or massaged. For the correction of deformities the child should be taken to an orthopædic hospital. At a later stage operation may have to be performed.

A rare form of rickets, known as **late** or **adolescent rickets** does not begin, as a rule, until between the sixth and the twelfth years. It usually occurs in children who have suffered from rickets at an earlier period, and is commoner in girls than in boys. It resembles ordinary rickets, and, in the main, treatment is on the same lines.

RIGGS' DISEASE (*see* Pyorrhœa Alveolaris).

RIGOR.—A rigor is a shivering fit which indicates the onset of an attack of malaria or other fever, or of inflammation of some internal organ or structure, as pneumonia and peritonitis, or the formation of an abscess. A rigor may also be caused by the passage of a catheter or by the pain set up by the movement of calculi (" stones "). The shiverings are followed by a hot stage, the temperature rising rapidly until the patient is bathed in perspiration. He should be made as comfortable as possible. During the cold or shivering stage he should be wrapped up in warm blankets, foot-warmers should be applied, and a hot drink, which may contain alcohol, given. The hot stage may be mitigated by tepid or cold sponging, with barley water to drink.

RIGOR MORTIS.—Rigor mortis is the stiffening of the muscles which follows death. The immediate effect of death is a relaxation of the muscles, but from three or four to ten hours afterwards the relaxed muscles of the lower jaw, and then those of the rest of the body, become rigid. The stiffness usually lasts from twenty-four to forty-eight hours, but the muscles may become flaccid again within an hour or so, or not until a week has elapsed. The time at which rigor mortis comes on and passes away depends largely upon the vitality of the muscles at death. If their vitality is low, as after an exhausting illness, the rigidity appears early, and, as a rule, is quick to pass away, and vice versa. In some cases of death from violence, rigor mortis sets in spasmodically at the moment of death. This explains how it is that, when a suicide shoots himself with a revolver, the weapon is often found tightly clutched in his hand.

RINGWORM. — This contagious disease is caused by fungi belonging to two different families, the smallspored and the large-spored parasites. It may affect the scalp or other hairy parts, or the hairless skin. The disease may be " caught " not only from human beings, but also from cats, dogs, and horses. It may be transmitted directly, by contact with a patient, and also indirectly, by caps, hair-brushes, towels, clothes, etc.

Ringworm of the *scalp* (tinea tonsurans) is seldom met with except in children. The affection begins as a tiny scaly spot or a small red pimple round a hair ; the pimple spreads, becomes scaly, and soon grows into a round or an oval patch, slightly raised above the level of the surrounding skin, and covered with a layer of fungus and scurf, forming a dirty, greyish-white powder. Smaller patches form elsewhere, and run together. The skin becomes inflamed, and little watery spots appear, which may become " mattery " and break, leaving dirty-looking scabs. The affected hairs are shrivelled and twisted, and break off close to the skin. By joining each other, the patches may lay bare large areas of the scalp. The patches may itch, but in uncomplicated cases they give rise to no other symptom, and even in ill-nourished children the general health is unaffected. Only in very bad cases is ringworm followed by permanent baldness.

Ringworm of the *hairless skin* (tinea circinata) begins as a small, red, slightly-raised spot, which slowly spreads into a ring, and becomes more or less scaly. The circle gradually enlarges, and may expand so as to cover a considerable area. There may be only one of these areas, or several. The surface is covered with dirty scurf, and at the edge little blisters may form and become pustular (" mattery "). If so, the patient may complain of pain, but usually the only symptom is itching. In this, as in ringworm of the scalp, if the spots become inflamed and discharge, the lymphatic glands may be infected, and abscesses may form.

Treatment. — Ringworm of the scalp, beard, etc., should be treated with the X-rays. By this treatment cases that would take many months to cure by the older methods can be cured in a few weeks. It cures by removing the diseased hairs and with them the parasites. If the X-rays are not available, treatment must begin by pulling out, one by one, as many as possible of the diseased hairs, and also a ring of healthy hairs around them, with forceps. If done carefully, this causes little pain. The hair that is left should be clipped to a length of not more than half an inch, so that the scalp may be easily inspected. Among many useful remedies that may now be applied—and the same remedies are appropriate in ringworm of the hairless skin— are equal parts of white precipitate ointment and vaselin, or of sulphur and carbolic-acid ointment, rubbed into the spots with a stall-covered finger twice a day for ten minutes. For simple cases, painting on tincture of iodine until the skin becomes sore is sufficient. Stronger remedies may have to be resorted to, but they should only be used under medical direction.

RISUS SARDONICUS (*see* STRYCHNINE POISONING).

RODENT ULCER.—Rodent ulcer is regarded as a form of cancer, but it has features which mark it off sharply from all other kinds of malignant tumour. It advances with extraordinary slowness, it causes comparatively little suffering, even when there is great destruction of tissue, it does not injure the neighbouring tissues, as do cancer and sarcoma, and, again unlike them, it is never carried to other parts of the body, there to reproduce itself. Another curious feature of rodent ulcer is that, though it may occur on almost any part of the body, in the great majority of cases it has its seat in the face, most often at the inner corners of the eyelids, and on or close to the nose, less often on the lips and chin. It occurs more frequently on the right side of the face than on the left, and it has been suggested by Dr. Sequeira, of the London Hospital, that this may be explained by the fact that as the great majority of people are right-handed, the right side of the face is more often scratched to relieve slight itching than the left, the irritation thus caused probably acting as a predisposing cause. Men are subject to rodent ulcer rather more than women, and the middle-aged and elderly than the young. As a rule the ulcer is single, but there is at least one case on record in which there were as many as twenty. The disease usually begins as a small red pimple, which may remain stationary for a long period, or may enlarge very slightly, and then become covered with crust, on removal of which it is seen that the pimple is ulcerating. Gradually it is entirely converted into an ulcer, which slowly becomes larger and deeper. Even when it has destroyed a great deal of tissue, there may be little pain, unless nerves are involved, and no appreciable effect on the general health.

Treatment.—If possible, the ulcer should be removed by excision. But in parts where this cannot be done, as between the nose and eye, radium should be employed. Both with radium and with X-rays better results have been obtained in rodent ulcer than in any other form of cancer. Several other modern methods of treatment, such as freezing with carbon dioxide snow, and the introduction of solutions of drugs into the tissues by means of an electric current (ionization), have also been used with success.

ROLLER BANDAGE (*see* BANDAGES).

RÖNTGEN RAYS.—A synonym for X-rays (*see* ELECTRICAL TREATMENT).

" ROSE," THE (*see* ERYSIPELAS).

ROSE RASH.—Any rose-coloured eruption is a rose rash, but the name is used especially for a rash of slightly raised patches which often occurs during hot weather and is usually caused by errors of diet, though in young children it may be due to teething. The spots appear on all parts of the body, and usually have no regular shape. They are accompanied by a slight rise of temperature, and the patient complains of dryness of the throat. The affection is not at all serious, and generally disappears in the course of a few days, but it receives a good deal of attention because of its liability to be confused with scarlet fever and measles. The rise of temperature, however, is usually considerably less than in most cases of scarlet fever; while from measles the disorder may be distinguished by the absence of any signs of cold in the head. No treatment is required beyond keeping the patient quiet and warm, putting him on a light diet and giving a mild aperient.

ROSEOLA, EPIDEMIC (*see* GERMAN MEASLES).

RÖTHELN (*see* GERMAN MEASLES).

ROUNDWORM (*see* WORMS).

RUBELLA (*see* GERMAN MEASLES).

RUBEOLA (*see* MEASLES).

" RUNNING FROM THE EAR " (*see* EAR, DISCHARGE FROM).

RUPTURE.—A hernia, to use the technical term for rupture, is the escape of a portion of intestine through a weakened spot in the wall of the abdomen, so that a lump appears above the level of the surface. The points at which ruptures most often occur are the navel (umbilical hernia) and the groin (inguinal hernia). The immediate cause may be an increase of the pressure within the abdomen, very heavy manual labour, the blowing of wind instruments, coughing or screaming, repeated pregnancies, the strain to pass water in cases of stricture of the urethra, or to pass motions in constipation. Sometimes a rupture occurs at the site of an operation, the tissue left by the healing of the operation wound not having the elasticity of true muscular tissue. When a rupture occurs a bulging is noticed at the site on any exertion or strain, gradually increasing to a distinct lump, which, however, is not constant, but disappears when the patient lies down or applies slight pressure. Under pressure the lump slips back suddenly, often with a gurgling sound. *Treatment* consists in operation, or in the wearing of a truss. The circular spring truss is the one most in use ; it must be made to fit well, and must be strong enough to restrain the rupture without causing discomfort. It must be worn whenever the patient is not lying down, and should be adjusted to its proper position before he leaves the recumbent posture. An extra appliance should be kept in reserve in case anything should go wrong with the one in use, and a special waterproof-covered truss should be worn in the bath. If the rupture is allowed to remain protruding, there is always the danger of the bowel being nipped by the parts surrounding it at its point of escape. The symptoms of *strangulation*, as this condition is called, are acute pain, violent vomiting, and intestinal obstruction. The rupture cannot now be returned by pressure or by lying down. The patient should be put into a hot bath, and the doctor sent for, no attempt meanwhile being made to return the rupture, or to induce movement of the bowels by aperient drugs. If the doctor is unable to reduce the rupture by manipulations, an operation will have to be performed.

In **children** rupture may either be present at birth, as the result of imperfect development, or may occur later. In some cases *umbilical* rupture arises during the first few months of life from the yielding of the scar of the navel. As a rule, the bulging is slight, and even if untreated will usually undergo spontaneous cure. Treatment consists in gently pushing back the swelling with the finger while the child is quiet, and applying a simple pad of lint or linen wrapped round a piece of cork or lead not smaller than a threepenny bit, keeping the pad in place by strapping. It should not be taken off, except to apply a fresh one, until the weakened spot has become quite strong again.

The most frequent cause of *inguinal* rupture in children is straining in the passing of water owing to a tight foreskin (*see* PHIMOSIS). Other causes are coughing during attacks of bronchitis or whooping-cough, violent crying, and straining in the passing of motions. Boys are more liable to this form of rupture than girls, and it is sometimes associated with a testicle that has not descended into its bag, the scrotum. Most of the little subjects of inguinal rupture are delicate children who suffer from indigestion and constipation. As a rule, the rupture can be returned by gentle pressure; this can be more easily done if the child is laid on his back with the hips supported on a pillow.

A rupture becomes strangulated much less frequently in children than in adults. If the rupture is due to some definite, ascertained cause, such as phimosis, this must, of course, receive attention. In many cases nothing more is necessary. If, however, the protrusion remains, a truss must be obtained, and worn both day and night; a rubber truss should be substituted when the child is being bathed. The truss should be changed when the child is on his back, and is not crying or straining. The skin underneath the pad of the truss must be kept dry, and should be dusted with a powder containing oxide of zinc and boric acid. If the child is less than a year old, a rupture that can be prevented from coming down for three months is usually cured. Older children must wear the truss longer, and until the doctor advises that it can be left off. If the rupture remains after the truss has had a fair trial, the question of an operation should be considered.

RUSSIAN BATH (*see* BATHS).

S

ST. ANTHONY'S FIRE (*see* ERYSIPELAS).

ST. VITUS'S DANCE. — This affection is known in medical literature as *chorea*, from a Greek word that signifies " dancing." It derives its popular name from the fact that dancing pilgrimages were at one time made to the shrine of St. Vitus. A disease of children between the ages of five and fifteen, it attacks girls more often than boys, and ill-nourished and neglected children more than those of the well-to-do classes. It is mainly a manifestation of injury done to the nerves by rheumatism, for in most cases the nervous symptoms are preceded by a rheumatic attack. Often the symptoms are brought on by a sudden fright or some other shock to the nervous system, the involuntary movements which characterize the affection beginning the next day or a few days afterwards. In other cases eyestrain or over-study in delicate children who are outgrowing their strength appears to be the exciting cause. Some children seem, to superficial observation, to succumb to the affection from mimicking others, but the act of imitation is not in itself sufficient to account for the affection.

Symptoms. — St. Vitus's dance often begins as an exaggeration of the fidgetiness common in children, or it may begin with failure of attention and the dropping of things. The hands, the knees, the facial muscles are in constant and spasmodic action. The movements may be general, or may be confined to one limb or one side of the body. Their intensity varies much in different cases : in one case they are hardly perceptible, in another it may be impossible to keep the patient in an ordinary bed. The movements are very irregular, and are never repeated time after time, as in tics (*see* TICS). They are aggravated by excitement, or by reproof and correction. The hands are especially affected, so that the child can only shake hands awkwardly and with difficulty, while if the tongue is put out, it is suddenly withdrawn to avoid being bitten. The child makes peculiar grimaces, and the effect of these, combined with spasms of the tongue and jaw, is to make talking and eating difficult. The breathing may be jerky, and queer noises may be made in the throat. Movements which are made voluntarily are lacking in precision; thus, if the patient is asked to pick up a small object from the floor, the fingers move irregularly round it before it is grasped. During sleep the involuntary movements cease, but often sleep is difficult to obtain. Before long the muscles of one or more of the limbs lose their power and, sooner or later, mental symptoms, such as dullness, inattention, defective memory, appear, and hysteria may develop. As a result of the preceding rheumatism, the valves of the heart may be damaged. While it lasts, St. Vitus's dance is a troublesome and exhausting affection, but the tendency, fortunately, is to recovery, and from four to twelve weeks may be given as the average duration. There may, however, be a relapse just when the symptoms appear to be subsiding, and after recovery there may be recrudescence, but in the majority of cases the affection disappears entirely.

Treatment.—Rest, both of body and of mind, must be ensured, and in all but slight cases the child should remain in bed for a week or two. Throughout the illness the diet must be nutritious but light, should include an abundance of milk and cream, and be supplemented by cod-liver oil and steel wine, a teaspoonful of each three times a day after meals. It is better that the patient should see as little as possible of other children, and excitement should be avoided, but care should be taken to provide quiet amusement and occupation. If the movements are violent and the child cannot sleep, bromide of potash and chloral hydrate, 10 grains of each, may be given at bedtime and repeated every three or four hours until sleep comes. Rheumatic symptoms are seldom present during an attack, for usually they precede it, but if the two conditions coincide, 5 grains of salicylate of soda or of aspirin may be given every three or four hours. In some cases arsenic is useful—2 or 3 drops of the solution, well diluted with water, three times a day after food. Convalescence may be aided by a stay at the seaside and by tonics containing iron.

SAL VOLATILE (*see* STIMULANTS).

SALISBURY DIET (*see* OBESITY).

SALIVA (*see* DIGESTION).

SALVARSAN (*see* SYPHILIS).

SARCOMA.—The sarcomas form one of the chief groups into which malignant tumours are divided, the other main group being constituted by the carcinomas (*see* TUMOURS). Sarcoma is much less prone than cancer to follow chronic irritation; on the other hand, it is more frequently the sequel of injury, as from a blow, a fracture of a bone, etc. Another difference between the two kinds of tumour is that sarcoma is much more common in early life, while cancer is a disease of middle and later life. Like cancer, sarcoma may attack almost any part of the body, and, like cancer again, parts of the growth may be carried, chiefly by the blood, to other organs, especially the lungs, and there start growing again. What is said under CANCER about cause and treatment applies generally to sarcoma. It may be added, however, that in some cases of sarcoma in which operation is impracticable, a measure of success has been obtained with the antitoxin known as Coley's fluid.

SCABIES (*see* ITCH).

SCALDS (*see* BURNS AND SCALDS).

SCAR.—A scar, or cicatrix, consists of new tissue which has formed after the destruction of tissue by inflammation or by a burn or other injury. In many conditions it is coloured, as often in shingles and in carbuncle, but frequently it is white. If the scar is composed of very fibrous tissue it is sometimes called cheloid ; scars of this kind are usually tender, and the patient may complain of itching or burning. Ordinary scars require no treatment, but when they take the cheloid form it is sometimes desirable to treat them with radium or with X-rays.

SCARLATINA (*see* SCARLET FEVER).

SCARLET FEVER.—This infectious disease is known alternatively as scarlatina, a term which is sometimes used popularly, but without justification, to denote a mild attack. The germ to which it is due is now believed to be the *Streptococcus hæmolyticus*, which attacks the throat. In England the disease is least prevalent in March and April, and most prevalent in October. It is chiefly a disease of childhood. In their first year children are seldom attacked ; from the first to the fifth year they become increasingly susceptible ; after the fifth year susceptibility gradually declines. The mortality is greatest in infancy, or in the second year of life ; then it gradually diminishes. The few cases, however, which occur after the fifteenth or twentieth year are apt to be severe. The death-rate from this disease in England and Wales is declining, owing not to lessened prevalence but to diminished severity.

Infection.—The disease is infective from the beginning of the attack, before the eruption appears. It is disseminated by contact with or proximity to a patient, or by means of infected articles or contaminated milk. Infection is given off by the breath and the secretions from the nose, mouth and throat—most freely in the earlier and acute stages. The degree to which the scales of the skin are infective is not certainly known, but probably in the later stages of the "peeling," contrary to the ordinary belief, they are innocuous, unless contaminated by the secretions. The patient remains infective for at least five weeks, and not seldom for more than two months. If there is no discharge from the ear or nose, he may, as a rule, be safely discharged from hospital after six weeks' detention. The poison clings to clothes, and to household articles that have been in contact with the patient, with great tenacity, and may retain its virulence for many months. One attack generally confers immunity for the rest of the patient's life. If there has been exposure to infection a ten days' quarantine should be enforced. It is now possible by means of what is known as the *Dick test* to ascertain whether a person is susceptible to the disease. A filtrate of a culture of the germs is injected into the skin ; if no redness appears around the spot in from four to six hours, the subject is not susceptible. If susceptibility is present, some degree of immunity may be conferred by inoculation.

Incubation period and symptoms.—The incubation stage may be as long as seven days, or less than twenty-four hours : the average is from two to three days. The patient is suddenly attacked with sore throat, headache, vomiting, and occasionally diarrhœa, accompanied by chilliness, aching pains, furred tongue, hot, dry skin and raised temperature. The more severe the onset, the worse the attack is likely to be. The pulse is quicker than in any other fever. Within twenty-four hours the eruption—minute red spots, which soon unite and form a general bright scarlet blush—shows itself, first on the chest, neck and arms, then rapidly spreading over the whole body during the next twenty-four hours. It fades away in the same order, leaving the neck and chest first, and by the end of the week has usually quite gone. With the rash there is often a good deal of swelling of the skin, and sometimes there are crops of blisters surrounded by rings of red. As the redness subsides the skin of the part "peels," the peeling beginning on the parts first attacked by the rash. In four weeks the peeling is usually completed on the body generally, but it may be some three weeks longer before the palms and soles are clear.

A frequent though not an invariable symptom of scarlet fever is the "*strawberry tongue*." If the patient's tongue is examined it is seen to be red and raw-looking at its tip and edges, and dirty, with a thick coating of fur along its centre; through this white fur little red spots show themselves. At the end of three or four days the fur has disappeared, the back of it clearing last, and the tongue is left red, raw, and rough like a ripe strawberry. Such a strawberry tongue occurring with sore throat is almost sufficient to prove the case to be one of scarlet fever. The throat is more or less inflamed and painful, the glands below the jaw are enlarged and tender, cause much pain in swallowing, and may give rise to troublesome abscesses. The temperature goes up suddenly with the onset of the disease to perhaps 102° Fahr., and on the third or fourth day, when the rash is fully out, it may be as high as 104°. It then begins to abate, and disappears with

the eruption. In the height of the illness delirium is common at night.

Such are the symptoms of an ordinary case of scarlet fever. But the attack may be much slighter, so slight as almost to escape notice, or may be so severe as to be termed *malignant*. In one group of cases the brunt of the attack falls upon the throat; the tonsils become deeply ulcerated and covered with a membrane much like that of diphtheria; the glands of the neck swell greatly and may break down into abscesses; and a state of blood-poisoning ensues.

Complications.—Although there is nothing alarming in an ordinary case of scarlet fever, it is necessary to keep a careful watch, even in quite mild cases, for the onset of complications. One of the most serious of them is *inflammation of the kidneys*. Another serious, and more frequent, complication is *inflammation of the middle ear* —otitis media, set up by spread of inflammation from the throat along the Eustachian tubes (*see* EAR). It is most likely to occur in severe cases, at the end of the first week, and in young children.

Treatment.—This consists in careful management, good nursing, and dealing with the symptoms, rather than in attempting to influence the disease itself. The patient must at once be put to bed in a room suited for isolation, and in charge of a skilful nurse or nurses. The room should be kept at a temperature of not less than 60° Fahr., and should be well ventilated, draught being prevented by the use of a screen. During the feverish stage the food should consist of milk, but when the temperature falls, bread-and-butter puddings and milk puddings may be allowed, and in a few days a return may be made to ordinary diet. Ripe, fresh fruit, such as oranges and grapes, will be grateful to the patient, and he may drink water freely. Every evening the body should be sponged all over with warm water, with due care against chills; the effect of this is to soothe the skin and promote sleep. If the skin is very irritable, it may be anointed, after the bath, with eucalyptus and olive oil— 2 drachms of eucalyptus oil and 1 drachm of carbolic acid, with olive oil to 8 ounces. The anointing, however, must be discontinued as soon as the irritability is subdued, so that the skin may be left free to do its work of excretion. After the temperature has reached the normal, a daily warm bath should replace the sponging. The bowels must be regulated by simple aperients, say compound liquorice powder for adults and syrup of senna or figs for children. The patient should remain in bed for three weeks, and should not leave the sick room until " peeling " has ceased. He should be dressed warmly, and be careful to avoid chills, for there is still liability to inflammation of the kidneys, and the urine should still be tested for albumin every few days.

In cases marked by high temperature the application of cold to the head and neck is often beneficial. It may take the form of an ice-bag applied to the head, or of pieces of lint or linen soaked in ice-cold water to which a little vinegar or eau-de-Cologne has been added. A broad strip of lint, or soft linen, soaked in the same water should be wrapped round the neck and throat and frequently renewed, and the throat should be treated with antiseptics. A good disinfectant is a " free chlorine gargle," which can be obtained from the chemist; others are Condy's fluid with warm water, of a pale purple colour.

If after the patient has left his bed there should be much albumin in the urine, he should at once return to bed,

wear a flannel nightdress and lie between blankets, the sheets being removed. A good purge should be taken, either a teaspoonful of Epsom salts, or 30 grains of compound jalap powder, for an adult, which should be repeated, so as to keep the bowels loose. A hot poultice should be applied to the loins and a hot-air bath given if that can be managed; and the doctor will probably prescribe a mixture to act upon the skin. Large enemata are sometimes useful. The food must be fluid—milk with soda or barley water, or peptonized milk, and it should be taken in small quantities frequently. Solid food should only be returned to very gradually as the urine becomes normal.

If there are swollen glands, fomentations should be applied. Earache and inflammation of the middle ear may be treated as advised in the articles on those affections. In rheumatic cases the affected joints should be wrapped in cotton-wool and aceto-salicylic acid given.

To assist the peeling of the thick skin of the soles of the feet, they may be soaked for five or ten minutes, once a day, in a solution of washing soda, and then in hot soapsuds for a further ten minutes, and dried by friction with a rough towel.

SCHICK TEST (*see* DIPHTHERIA).

SCHISTOSOMIASIS (*see* BILHARZIASIS).

SCIATICA.—This painful affection is the result of an inflammation of the sciatic nerve—the large nerve which passes down the back of the thigh. Often the inflammation is set up by poisons such as those of rheumatism or gout or diabetes, but in many cases it is a simple neuralgia, caused by exposure to wet and cold or by strain or injury. The pain may extend from the thigh downwards into the leg. The patient finds that he is most comfortable when he bends the leg at the knee and hip. If he extends the limb, the pain is worse. In severe cases he should remain in bed, and take a purge such as a blue pill at night and a black draught in the morning. Aspirin or phenacetin, whichever is found to suit better, should be given, and counter-irritation applied in the form of hot poultices, mustard leaves or plasters. Ionization (*see under* ELECTRICAL TREATMENT) is useful in some cases. When the pain has been subdued, massage and electricity will be found beneficial if the muscles have wasted. In very intractable cases it may be necessary for the surgeon to operate.

SCLERODERMIA.—In this little-understood and very peculiar cutaneous affection, affecting chiefly young adults, and women more often than men, the skin becomes hard and rigid, either generally or in patches. Mild cases of generalized sclerodermia sometimes undergo spontaneous cure; the severer often end fatally. Cod-liver oil and massage are useful, and warm clothing should be worn, the patient being specially susceptible to cold. In the local form of the disease, in which the skin is affected only in patches, the drug known as thiosinamin sometimes has a beneficial effect.

SCLEROTIC (*see* EYE).

SCOLIOSIS (*see* SPINAL CURVATURE, LATERAL).

SCROFULA.—This term used to cover a number of affections that are now definitely known to be forms of tuberculosis, such as enlarged and inflamed glands (*see* ADENITIS; CONSUMPTION OF THE BOWELS). It is still serviceable, however, as denoting a constitutional condition which prepares the way for tuberculosis and other diseases, and also renders the patient vulnerable to slight injuries. Thus, in a scrofulous subject injuries are prone to undergo chronic inflammation, with a pronounced tendency to suppuration and the formation of unhealthy sores; mucous membranes are easily irritated, lymphatic glands readily become enlarged and the eyes inflamed and sore. The scrofulous constitution offers less resistance than the normal constitution to attacks of measles and scarlet fever, and there appears to be more than the average liability to inflammatory and other affections of the bones. Children born with the scrofulous taint fall into two greatly contrasted groups. In one they are tall, slight, graceful, with fine silky hair, clear complexions and quick intelligence; in the other they are short and thick-set, with coarse skin and features and dull, apathetic minds. Scrofula is of historical interest as the "king's evil," which was held to be cured by a touch of the monarch's hand, and among those to whom this cure was applied was Dr. Johnson. In these days there is less faith in the virtue of royalty's touch, and trust is reposed rather in nourishing food, cod-liver oil, syrup of the iodide of iron, and fresh air, especially at the seaside. Such treatment must be carried out patiently and perseveringly, and care must be taken to secure the healing of slight injuries of the skin, patches of eczema, etc., lest they become the seat of chronic inflammation.

SOURFINESS (*see* DANDRUFF).

SCURVY.—Until recently it was believed that the lack of certain salts, owing to the absence of fresh vegetables from the diet, was the explanation of the scurvy which used to be rampant among our sailors, and also among soldiers in camp. Now, however, the theory which finds most acceptance is that the disease is due to the absence of a substance the exact nature of which is not known, but which is called a vitamin (*see* Vitamins, under Food). It is present in green vegetables and fresh fruits, including lemons and oranges. It is present also, in small amounts, in milk and fresh meat. In an untreated case of scurvy the patient loses energy, both physical and mental, has pain in the back and limbs, the complexion is sallow and unhealthy, the gums are puffy and spongy and liable to bleed, the teeth loosen, the tongue is coated and swollen, the bowels are confined, the breath is fetid. The skin is dry and rough, and hæmorrhages may occur, the patient becomes profoundly anæmic and sinks into a condition of extreme weakness. He must remain in bed and be put upon a diet into which vegetables and fruit, milk, eggs, scraped raw meat, and raw-meat juice enter largely, and these foods should be supplemented by lemon juice.

Scurvy sometimes appears in infants. In all but a few cases those attacked have been fed on proprietary foods. The only treatment required is to add a little steamed potato to the milk in the bottle, and give three or four teaspoonfuls of orange juice each day.

SEA-BATHING (*see* Baths).

SEA-SICKNESS.—This condition, although it reduces the sufferer to the depths of misery and despair, is usually regarded as a subject for merriment. Although nearly always its effects soon pass away, in exceptional cases it leads to great prostration and has even ended in death. Many drugs have been tried as preventives, but there is none which answers in all cases. Among them are chloretone, bromide of soda and of potash, phenacetin, caffeine, and chloral hydrate.

Perhaps the best of them is chloretone, of which 5 grains may be taken in a cachet, the dose being repeated, if necessary, after an interval of two hours. If this does not suit, $1\frac{1}{2}$ drachms of syrup of chloral and 30 grains of bromide of potash in 4 tablespoonfuls of water may be taken in teaspoonful doses at intervals of five minutes until relief is obtained or the patient falls asleep. It is well to have a sufficient but not heavy meal from two to three hours before going on board, and those who are especially liable to sea-sickness might take a mild aperient the day before.

SEBACEOUS CYSTS (*see* Cysts).

SEBORRHŒIC DERMATITIS.— The chief manifestation of this disease is the formation of scales on the scalp, which is described in the article Dandruff. The eyebrow, moustache and beard may also be attacked, and the disease may spread over the scalp to the face, the trunk, and the muscles. The scales may be removed by applying an ointment consisting of three parts each of sulphur and salicylic acid to 94 parts of soft paraffin.

SEBORRHŒIC WARTS (*see* Warts).

SEDATIVES (*see* Medicines, and how they are Measured).

SEIZURE, APOPLECTIC (*see* Apoplexy).

SEMICIRCULAR CANALS (*see* Ear).

SENILE PRURITUS (*see* Itching).

SEPTICÆMIA (*see* Blood-Poisoning).

SERUM TREATMENT (*see* Vaccine and Serum Treatment).

SHAKING PALSY. — Paralysis agitans, to give this affection its medical name, is a form of trembling paralysis which usually sets in between the ages of forty-five and sixty. The cause is not known, but injury, shock, worry, and other such influences may be the apparent starting-point of the disease. The tremors are generally first noticed in one hand, later they may affect the arm also. From one hand or arm they often spread to the leg on the same side, and thence to the hand on the other side. As the disease progresses, the head, face and jaws may all be affected. It is a curious fact that the patient is able to control the movements for a few seconds by an effort of the will, but in severe cases any attempt to check them in one limb generally leads to increased movements in another. It is also found that they cease entirely during sleep. Another feature is rigidity of the muscles, manifesting itself in various ways. Thus the patient may be bowed like an old man with the head inclined forward and the body bent, the features fixed and expressionless, the voice dull and monotonous, the gait peculiar : he takes short rapid steps and has difficulty in stopping when he has once started ; it has been wittily said that he looks as though he is trying to catch his centre of gravity. The rigidity may develop until the whole body is more or less affected, so that any kind of voluntary movement is almost impossible and at last the patient becomes bedridden. In the way of treatment, little can be done except to endeavour, by both active and passive movements, to check the rigidity. Hot baths with light massage are also useful in this direction. The general nutrition must be maintained, and the patient should spend as much time as possible in the open air, and must aim at living a passive life, the tremors being always aggravated by excitement.

SHINGLES.—Medically, this affection of the skin, often preceded by a chill, is known as *herpes zoster*, or as *zona*, because in rare cases the eruption forms a complete girdle or zone round the body. The vesicles (little blisters) appear in clusters on patches of reddened skin. Their favourite site is the trunk, but they may appear on almost any part of the body. The attack usually begins with neuralgic tenderness in the affected area, and there may also be slight feverishness. As a rule the neuralgic pain ceases when the eruption appears, but the lesions themselves cause a good deal of tingling and smarting, and the affected nerve may become inflamed. In children pain is usually slight, but in the elderly it may be severe, and very persistent. The vesicles come out in crops, and it takes about a week for the eruption to reach its full development, and from two to three weeks for the attack to subside, the yellowish or brownish crusts which form on the burst vesicles then falling off. In some cases bleeding into the vesicles occurs, and leads to the formation of little ulcers which may leave permanent scars behind them, white or coloured. There is seldom a second attack, but some persons are liable to little crops of painful blisters whenever they are out of health or are subject to nervous strain. The best-known cause of shingles is chill, which probably acts by setting up neuritis ; but not seldom shingles is associated with infection, as from tuberculosis, pleurisy, pneumonia, etc. Some medical men believe that shingles is allied to chickenpox, for it has been noticed that shingles sometimes occurs in persons who have been exposed to chickenpox infection, and vice versa. This question deserves further investigation.

Treatment.—As a rule the affection

will disappear spontaneously in from two to three weeks, and the object of treatment is not so much to speed the parting guest as to mitigate the pain. The vesicles should be protected from friction and kept warm by applying zinc ointment, or by powdering flour over the part and then covering with a thick layer of cotton-wool. A good dusting powder is one consisting of oxide of zinc and bismuth in equal parts ; or a layer of flexile collodion may be painted over it with a soft brush ; the collodion will evaporate, leaving behind a protecting film. If the pain is severe, menthol ointment should be applied. Middle-aged and elderly persons should keep their beds for a few days. Internally, aspirin or antipyrin in 5-grain doses may be taken for its sedative properties ; tonics, too, such as the compound syrup of hypophosphites, are often beneficial in combination with a nutritious diet.

SHOCK.—After severe burns or other injuries, or an operation, or as a result of terror or mental distress, the condition known as shock may supervene. The breath becomes rapid, the pulse can hardly be felt, the face becomes white, the skin is bathed in a cold perspiration, the patient is only semi-conscious. Great loss of blood alone is sufficient to produce shock, but the condition may arise in the absence of hæmorrhage. If the shock is due to mental causes, the patient may be treated as for a fainting fit ; if the result of physical injury, besides being kept flat with the head low he should be put to bed between blankets and warmed with hot-water bottles, and hot tea, coffee, milk or soup administered. A little alcohol may be given, unless the condition is caused by loss of blood ; in this case the stimulant would re-

start the hæmorrhage. In bad cases artificial respiration (q.v.) must be resorted to. If the patient is unable to swallow, stimulants may be given by enema. The stimulant treatment must be stopped as soon as the patient begins to feel better. (*See also* TRANSFUSION OF BLOOD).

SHORTNESS OF BREATH (*see* BREATHING, DIFFICULTY OF).

SHORT SIGHT (*see* SIGHT, DEFECTS OF).

SICK HEADACHE (*see under* HEADACHE).

SICKNESS (*see* VOMITING).

SICK-ROOM (*see* NURSING, DOMESTIC).

SIDE-ACHE.—Pleurodynia, or side-ache, is one variety of " stitch in the side," the other being due to pleurisy. A sharp pain is felt in the muscles of the side of the chest whenever the patient coughs or makes a sudden movement. It may be slight, but is sometimes severe ; it feels as though the muscles were being cut with a knife. As a rule, the only treatment required is to keep the ribs from moving by fixing the affected side with strips of plaster 3 or 4 inches wide and overlapping each other for about an inch (*see under* PLEURISY). The strips must, of course, cover the site of the pain, and should extend from the middle line in front to the middle line at the back. Belladonna plaster may be recommended, for besides controlling the movements of the ribs it soothes the pain. Pain may also be relieved by a mustard plaster, or a turpentine stupe (*see* FOMENTATIONS).

SIGHT, DEFECTS OF. — The common defects of sight are (1) long sight, (2) short sight, (3) old sight, and (4) astigmatism. Fortunately, they all admit of easy correction by the use of appropriate glasses. These should be prescribed not by an optician, but by an oculist, who will not only order just the glasses that are needed, but will examine the eye to make sure that no more serious eye trouble is present.

1. Long sight (hypermetropia).

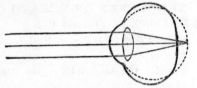

Fig. 54.—Long sight.

—To make this condition intelligible, we must first direct attention to the normal eye, of which the outlines are roughly indicated by the dotted line in Fig. 54. It will be seen that the rays of light coming from the left-hand side and passing through the lens are brought to a focus at the dotted line, indicating the retina. In long sight the eyeball is shorter than normal, and the rays therefore meet the retina (here represented by the thick curved line) before they have come to a focus, so that every object looked at appears blurred and indistinct. In advanced cases this is true of distant as well as of near objects; in earlier or slighter cases the ocular muscles are able to accommodate the eye to distant objects so that they are seen clearly. Long sight is present at birth, but may not be recognized in early childhood. When, however, the child has to read and write or sew, trouble begins, and symptoms such as mistiness of vision, watery and painful eyes, headache and sleepiness are complained of. These symptoms are particularly pronounced at the end of the day, or of the school week, when the eye-muscles are fatigued by use. In many cases a squint develops, the two eyes looking toward each other (convergent squint) until the defect settles in one eye, which then ceases

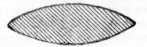

Fig. 55.—Double convex lens.

to be used. The remedy is to wear convex lenses (Fig. 55)—lenses that are curved *towards* the rays of light so as to bring them to a focus before they travel so far as they would in the absence of the lenses. Children should wear the glasses always, but adults, in whom the defect occurs in but slight degree, need wear them only when reading.

2. Short sight (myopia).

—In short sight the eyeball, instead of being shorter from back to front than normal, is longer, so that the rays of light come to a focus before they reach the retina (Fig. 56). Although short sight is sometimes congenital, it is more often acquired by misuse of sight, as by excessive reading, especially of very small print, or by doing very fine work in a bad light. The eyes become congested and inflamed at the back, and the affected parts bulge backwards and so increase the length of the eyeball. As a rule, short-sighted eyes are large and prominent, and the pupils are often much dilated. The patient complains that he cannot see distant

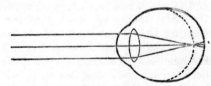

Fig. 56.—Short sight.

objects and has to hold near objects, such as a book, inconveniently close. After a while spots may be seen before the eyes, a squint outwards may develop, and ultimately the retina may be seriously damaged. For short sight the lenses must be concave on both sides (Fig. 57). They act by making the rays of light more divergent, so that the image is formed farther back in the eye. They will

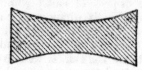

Fig. 57.—Double concave lens.

have to be worn out of doors, and in bad cases reading glasses may also be necessary. The reading and work of short-sighted children should be carefully regulated, so that they may never work or read except in a good light, may not attempt to read small print, and may avoid bending down the head. In some cases it is necessary to forbid all work for some months, until the eyes have been thoroughly rested. If the eyes are intolerant of light, smoked glasses should be worn. The trouble may disappear suddenly when the time for growth has ceased, except when the patient is run down, and in later life the sight may so improve that it is possible to do without the glasses which formerly were indispensable.

3. **Old sight (presbyopia).**—This defect of vision arises simply from failure of the power to accommodate the eyes to objects according to their distance. The trouble is with the lens of the eye, which loses its elasticity, so that the ocular muscles can less readily alter its shape than they were able to do earlier in life. A book, for example, has to be held farther and farther away before it can be read, and a better light is required. After the age of forty-five the onset of old

sight is natural, but those with long sight suffer from it earlier than those with short sight, and very short-sighted persons may never experience it at all. The glasses suitable for old sight are convex, as in the case of long sight. As age advances it will usually be necessary to change them occasionally for stronger ones.

4. **Astigmatism.**—In some cases the curvature of the cornea, the transparent structure in the front part of the eyeball, is so irregular that the image of an object lacks distinctness; this is astigmatism. In this condition it is especially important that the glasses be prescribed by an oculist.

For other affections of the eye *see* AMBLYOPIA; BLINDNESS; CATARACT; COLOUR BLINDNESS; CONJUNCTIVITIS; EYESTRAIN; GLAUCOMA; OPHTHALMIA.

SILICOSIS.—This is the name of a fibrous degeneration of the lungs which is caused by the inhalation of silica dust, i.e. the dust of flint, sandstone, granite, rock crystal, etc., so rendering them specially liable to the attacks of the tubercle bacillus. In the case of some industries, the existence of silicosis entitles the sufferer to compensation under the Workmen's Compensation (Silicosis) Act, 1918.

SKIN.—The skin (Fig. 58) consists of two chief layers—the outer or scarf skin, called the cuticle or epidermis, and the inner or true skin, the dermis or corium, and each is made up of several different strata. The **epidermis** is in some parts only $\frac{1}{240}$ in. in thickness, but in regions exposed to wear and tear, such as the palms of the hands and the soles of the feet, it is some ten times as thick. The deepest part of the epidermis, resting upon the true skin, contains a quantity of dark pigment, and it is this pigment that modifies the colour of the skin. Thus, there is comparatively little pigment in the skin of white races, and less in blondes than in brunettes ; in yellow races there is more than in white, and in negroes most of all. The epidermis has neither nerves nor blood-vessels. An injury to it, therefore, causes neither pain nor

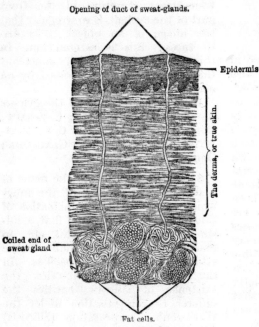

Opening of duct of sweat-glands.

Epidermis

The dermis, or true skin.

Coiled end of sweat gland

Fat cells.

Fig. 58. —The skin.

bleeding. The **dermis**, the true skin, on the other hand, is richly supplied with both nerves and blood-vessels. In the deeper layers of the dermis are sweat-glands (*see* Fig. 58), coiled tubes of which the ducts pass up through the epidermis and open on the surface. These glands secrete the perspiration, which contains a little solid matter. Even when one is not conscious of perspiring, the process is constantly going on, and about $2\frac{1}{2}$ lb. of fluid are thus daily discharged from the body. Hair and nails are appendages of the skin. Everywhere, except in the palms and soles, hairs grow from little depressions called follicles ; the portion within the follicle is called the bulb or root, and that outside it, the shaft. On the inner walls of the hair-follicles are the orifices of small glands, the sebaceous glands, which secrete an oily fluid needed by the skin for lubrication.

By its toughness and elasticity the skin is well fitted to defend the parts lying beneath it from injury. Besides being, as we have seen, an important excretory organ, it is the principal organ of the sense of touch, and is also supplied with nerves which enable it to appreciate sensations of heat and cold. And it is through the skin that the nervous system regulates the temperature of the body, as explained in TEMPERATURE, BODY.

SKIN, TUBERCULOSIS OF (*see* LUPUS VULGARIS ; SCROFULA).

SLEEP, DISTURBED.—Inability to sleep is considered under the head of INSOMNIA. In this place we have to deal with the disturbed sleep from which young children often suffer. It is important that the cause of it should be discovered, for while it may be due simply to the child being in an uncomfortable position, or to its being cold, or to some passing digestive disturbance, or to teething, it may also be an indication of illness. The child's temperature should therefore be taken. If there is feverishness, medical advice should be sought. The child may have adenoids, or enlarged tonsils, or both —for the two conditions often go together; he cannot breathe comfortably through the nose, and when, on his falling asleep, the mouth closes there is a constant waking up with a sensation of suffocation. A child with enlarged tonsils or adenoids tends to lie with the head thrown back and the mouth open. If there is heart or lung trouble with consequent difficulty of breathing, he will be apt to lie with the head and shoulders raised high on the pillow. If he lies on his face, the probable cause is that something is wrong with the eyes, so that he cannot bear the light. If he suddenly starts up from sleep with a scream, joint disease, especially disease of the hip-joint, is to be suspected. In all these different cases, treatment must, of course, be directed to the condition responsible for the disturbed sleep. Sedatives should never be given to children unless prescribed by a doctor. If the trouble is not due to illness, but to mere restlessness, the child should have a warm bath; this, in many cases, will have a soothing effect, and enable him to get quiet and refreshing sleep (*see also* NIGHT TERRORS).

SLEEPING SICKNESS (*see* TRYPANOSOMIASIS).

SLEEPLESSNESS (*see* INSOMNIA).

"SLEEPY SICKNESS" (*see* ENCEPHALITIS LETHARGICA).

SLEEP-WALKING.—This strange condition, in which, while consciousness is suspended, the brain generally may be in a state of heightened activity, must be regarded as an indication of some nervous instability. There is often a distinct exciting cause, such as the imperfect digestion of a heavy meal taken too near bedtime, grief, fright, physical or mental exhaustion, or the disordered action of

organs such as the ovaries or the liver. There are strange cases on record which suggest that in somnambulism the senses are preternaturally acute, or that the patient is able to exercise a kind of clairvoyance. For example, one patient was accustomed to rise from her bed and write in complete darkness. Darkness, indeed, seemed to be a necessary condition of the performance, for if the least light, as from the moon, entered the room she was unable to write. In another case the patient, while fast asleep, was seen by her husband to go to a dark boxroom adjoining their bedroom, open a trunk and assort, without making a single mistake, various articles of clothing which had been bundled in indiscriminately. Yet another case was that of a student who translated a passage from Italian into French in complete darkness, looking up difficult words in a dictionary. Somnambulism is not an alarming or a serious condition in itself, but it is a very undesirable one, for the common notion that a sleep-walker may get into very perilous positions with impunity has no foundation in fact. Moreover, it is possible for a somnambulist, like an epileptic, to do deeds of violence of which he has no recollection when he wakes, or which recur to his memory only as a horrid dream.

Treatment. — It is very undesirable to waken a sleep-walker roughly or suddenly. He should be addressed with quiet authoritativeness, and directed to return to bed, or should be gently led there. If the condition recurs at a regular hour, he should set an alarum to awaken him at that time. In other cases he should be awakened after the first hour of sleep, which is usually the deepest—for in most cases the trouble occurs during deep sleep rather than in the lighter sleep that comes as daybreak approaches. A sleep-walker should avoid lying on the back, the head should be as high upon the pillow as is consistent with comfort, the bedclothes should not be heavier than is necessary to keep the sleeper warm, and the bedroom should be well ventilated. If the trouble is brought on by emotional disturbance, a dose of bromide of potassium (10 grains for an adult) may be taken three hours before bedtime, and another on retiring.

SLUGGISH LIVER (*see* BILIOUSNESS; TROPICAL LIVER).

SMALLPOX.—This loathsome disease, also called *variola*, is due to a germ which has not yet been definitely identified. When the patient has been successfully vaccinated (*see* VACCINATION) the disease usually takes the form of " modified " smallpox (*see* below). Since the beginning of the twentieth century two different types of smallpox have occurred simultaneously in Great Britain, one being the European or African type and the other the American type. The former has a mortality of 16·8 to 24·7 per cent., the latter of 0·45 to 0·5 per cent. The American type is sometimes called *alastrim*, a name derived from a Spanish word indicating the scattered distribution of the eruption, but most of the authorities regard it as a mild form of smallpox, and not a separate disease.

It is believed that the breath of a smallpox patient is infective from the beginning of the disease. The exhalations of the body and the pocks are also highly infectious. The virus finds lodgment in clothing, and retains its vitality with great tenacity. Under favourable conditions infection can be conveyed through the air, and

for considerable distances. After exposure to infection a person should be regarded as suspect for seventeen days. Successful vaccination within a day or two of exposure is an almost certain preventive. Second attacks are rare, except after an interval of several years.

Symptoms.—After an incubation stage of about twelve days the patient is seized with a shivering fit, and has headache, backache and feverishness, sometimes with vomiting and profuse perspiration, while there may also be a faint rose-coloured rash resembling that of scarlet fever, and diffused more or less over the whole body. The eruption proper usually appears on the third day, on the same day of the week that the infection was acquired; it is accompanied by a decrease of the fever. Beginning as a mere fleck, the size of a pin's head, the spots swell into smooth, round, hard, red pimples; after two days a small blister forms on each, and they gradually increase in size, the tops becoming flattened or hollowed out. Spots may also be seen on the inside of the mouth and in the throat. The eruption is fully out by the eighth day of the disease, and some of the spots now fill with yellowish matter and become larger and rounder, and at the same time the temperature again rises, and the patient feels worse. In *discrete* cases each spot or " pock " remains distinctly separated from the others, and dries up rapidly or bursts, leaving a scab; the temperature reaches normal by about the tenth day, and the patient soon becomes convalescent, though it is some time longer before the scabs fall off. Another mild variety of the disease is called *modified* smallpox or *varioloid*. It runs a shorter course, and the lesions fall short of full development.

After three days of feverishness, a few pimples come out which rapidly dry up and disappear, or the pimples turn into blisters but dry up without becoming "mattery," and without any more feverishness. It must not be forgotten, however, that in some cases of modified smallpox the feverishness and illness before the spots come out may be as severe as in ordinary smallpox. A special form of modified smallpox is that in which all the initial symptoms, including the early rash, are present but there is no eruption proper. Such cases are sometimes mistaken for influenza. They are apt to occur in persons who have recently been vaccinated.

Of the severer types of the disease, one is the *confluent*, so called because the pocks run together, instead of remaining separate and distinct. In these cases there is a high mortality. The severest form, *hæmorrhagic, malignant, black* or *toxic* smallpox, as it is variously called, is nearly always fatal.

Treatment.—If not removed to a smallpox hospital, as should be done whenever possible, the patient must be isolated in a large, well-ventilated room. Only those who have had smallpox, or have recently been vaccinated, are suitable as nurses. The room, preferably a room on the top floor, should be divested of all carpets and hangings and unnecessary articles of furniture, and across the doorway should be suspended a sheet wrung out in a strong solution of carbolic acid. To neutralize the disagreeable odour emitted by the patient, the bed-clothes should be frequently sprayed with some deodorant, such as ozonized water ; or pieces of blotting-paper soaked in eucalyptus oil may be placed about the room, or it may be sprinkled with powdered camphor, or spirit of tur-

pentine. The patient must be fed at frequent and regular intervals with easily-digested liquid nourishment ; his thirst may be assuaged with water or bland drinks. Lanolin or vaselin may be applied to the skin to relieve itching and help to loosen the scabs, and cold compresses to the swollen eyelids, and it is better to cut the hair short. The mouth should be kept clean. Stimulants are generally needed when there is much " mattery " discharge. Delirium calls for extra nursing, and inflammation of the windpipe or larynx must be carefully watched for, lest necessity should arise for the operation of tracheotomy to prevent suffocation. The patient must not be considered free from infection until all the scabs are removed from the body. This process may be hastened by the application of glycerin and rose-water to the skin and the daily use of warm baths.

SMELL, PERVERSIONS OF.— Disturbances of smell, usually of an unpleasant character, are most often caused by functional nervous disorder—disorder in which there is no organic disease of the nervous system. Nothing can be done in the way of treatment, but, like perversions of taste, they are usually fleeting, and will disappear spontaneously.

SMOKING (*see* NARCOTICS AND HYPNOTICS).

SNAKE-BITES (*see* STINGS AND BITES).

SNOW-BLINDNESS (*see* BLINDNESS).

SOFT CORNS (*see* CORNS).

SOFT SORE.—Soft chancre, or soft sore, or ulcus molle, the third and much the least serious of the venereal diseases (*see* VENEREAL DISEASES), is named by way of distinction from the *hard chancre* of syphilis, with which it is sometimes confused. In many cases the two infections are conveyed together, when the lesion is termed a *mixed sore*. The disease is attributed to what is known as Ducrey's bacillus. As a rule, there is more than one sore, and yet others may appear afterwards, as a result of self-inoculation. The sores appear a few hours or from two to three days after sexual intercourse with an infected person; they are always on or in the immediate neighbourhood of the sexual organs. They soon develop into pustules, which presently burst. The nearest lymph-glands enlarge and become very painful, but instead of hardening, as in syphilis, they tend to suppurate. Soft sore never passes into a constitutional stage. Usually the sores heal up in from three to six weeks, but they require treatment in the form of applications, say, of carbolic acid, followed by powdering with iodoform, or boric acid, or subgallate of bismuth. Hot baths should be taken and scrupulous cleanliness observed. In dirty and debilitated patients the ulceration may spread and cause extensive destruction of tissue.

SOMNAMBULISM (*see* SLEEP-WALKING).

SORE NIPPLES (*see* SUCKLING).

SORE THROAT.—This is a popular expression which covers any inflammation or painful affection of the pharynx (the back part of the mouth) or of the surrounding parts—the soft palate, tonsils, uvula, larynx (voice-box), and upper part of the trachea (windpipe). The most common forms of sore throat are acute and chronic pharyngitis, and these will be dealt with here, together with hospital sore throat.

1. *Acute pharyngitis.*—When one speaks of having a sore throat, this is the condition most often intended. In most cases it occurs as an extension of inflammation of the nasal mucous membrane—a common cold, or the inflammation may arise not in front of the pharynx in the nose, but below it, in the larynx, and extend upwards. Predisposing causes are previous attacks and a low state of health. Rheumatism, gout, digestive disorders, and excessive indulgence in alcohol or tobacco also act as predisposing causes.

Symptoms.—Dryness and discomfort in the throat, with slight hoarseness and a cough, are often preceded by chill and feverishness, headache and a feeling of general malaise. The sensation in the throat may be just a slight irritation, leading to hemming and hawking, or it may be a pain so intense as to make the swallowing even of saliva an agony. The voice is thick and woolly from accumulation of mucus, the breath is offensive, the tongue coated, the patient is thirsty, and usually there is constipation.

Treatment.—If the symptoms are at all severe, the patient should remain in bed, and take an aperient (say 3 grains of calomel at night with a hot glass of mineral water such as Friedrichshall in the morning), should talk little, abstain from smoking and from alcohol, and take nothing but soft, bland food. A warm compress may be applied externally or, if the patient prefers it, a hot fomentation. If he is feverish, a tablet of 5 grains of aspirin may be taken three times a day. The inflamed parts of the throat may be painted several times a day with glycerin of boric acid, and ice may be sucked, or lozenges of menthol, krameria, or red gum. Thirst may be assuaged with plain water, barley water, or Vichy water. When the inflammation has subsided, an abundance of nutritious food should be taken, and a dose of quinine and iron three times a day after meals.

2. *Chronic pharyngitis.*—This form of sore throat is known also as relaxed sore throat or, because it is often met with in preachers and others who have to use the voice much, as " clergyman's sore throat." It is often a sequel of attacks of acute pharyngitis, or of measles or scarlet fever, or it may be due to exposure to dust or dirt, or irritating vapours, as in certain industries ; dram-drinking and the excessive use of tobacco must be held accountable for a proportion of cases ; and, like acute pharyngitis, it is predisposed to by ill-health and bad hygiene.

Symptoms.—The symptoms exhibit great variety. Perhaps the one most often present is a sense of discomfort in the throat, very slight in some cases, amounting to pain in others. The patient feels that the throat needs clearing, and hawks, but often there is very little mucus so show for the exertion. In some cases there is a frequent desire to swallow, and the act is attended with some pain. The cough is of a rasping or scraping character, or it may be a " stomach cough," hollow and alarming, or abortive and give rise to spasm of the larynx. The voice is often weak and lacking in resonance, is apt to crack or to drop suddenly to a whisper, and may be entirely lost for a time. If the throat is examined, the uvula, which hangs down like a curtain from the soft palate, is seen to be long, flabby, and relaxed ; the hinder part of the pharynx is roughened and covered with small elevations, and there may be a coating of thick mucus, or the surface may be dry and shiny, with red patches.

Treatment.—In many cases this is tedious. Where the voice particu-larly is affected, the chief indication is complete rest, not for the body generally—for the patient will be benefited by exercise and fresh air —but for the throat and voice. Smoking should cease entirely, and if alcohol is taken, it should be in the strictest moderation. The diet must be nutritious. The food should be neither too hot nor too highly spiced. Glycerin of tannic acid may be painted on the affected part two or three times a day, or tincture of iodine, at first diluted with an equal quantity of water, afterwards without dilution, may be applied in the same way. Compound benzoic acid, chlorate of potash and borax, or chloride of ammonium lozenges may be recommended. Externally, a cold compress may be applied when going to bed and worn during the night, and in the morning the throat should be thoroughly sponged with cold water. It may also be sprayed thrice a day with a lotion consisting of two tablespoonfuls of water with 5 to 20 grains of alum, or 5 to 15 grains of tannin, or 5 to 10 grains of sulphate of zinc.

3. *Hospital sore throat.*—This, the popular name of what is more technically known as acute septic inflammation of the throat, has reference to the fact that the condition is sometimes met with in nurses and others employed in hospital wards if they are overworked and take too little fresh air and out-door exercise. But it most often occurs in alcoholic subjects and in persons who are broken down in health from privation. It varies greatly in severity ; it may be quite mild and run a course of several days, or death may ensue in a few hours, it may be from heart-failure, or from swelling of the larynx so that the patient is suffocated.

Treatment.—If the patient's surroundings are unhealthy, he must be removed from them. In any case, he must keep his bed and, after a brisk aperient has been administered, be put upon a diet of beef tea, raw eggs and milk. The graver type of cases may require brandy and strychnine, and operative measures, including tracheotomy, may be called for. In milder cases an antiseptic gargle, such as the following, with formamint tablets to suck, may suffice :

Glycerin of carbolic acid ... 3 drachms
Water to 8 ounces.
To be warmed and used as a gargle.

The nutritious diet may be reinforced with an iron and quinine tonic. During convalescence a change of air is desirable, and the holiday may have to be prolonged, recovery in these cases being often a slow process.

SOUR MILK.—This is the name by which milk artificially soured and curdled by introducing into it lactic acid bacilli is known. It would be more correctly termed " soured milk." It undoubtedly has antiseptic properties, and a few years ago it was advocated as a cure for rheumatism and other conditions, but less is heard of it now. Metchnikoff was of opinion that by drinking sour milk the advent of old age might be postponed. The theory has found few adherents.

SPAS (*see* Mineral Waters).

SPASMS (*see* Cramp).

SPEECH, DISTURBANCES OF (*see* Voice, Loss of ; Aphasia).

SPERMATORRHŒA. — In this condition there is a discharge of seminal fluid independently of voluntary sexual excitement. It may take place during sleep (nocturnal emission) or as a result of straining at stool, or of irritation of the sexual organs during walking or riding, or of such local conditions as a long foreskin, varicose veins, intestinal worms, and constipation, or the fluid may be discharged with the urine. In many cases the fluid discharged is that secreted by the prostate gland, not by the testicles. The patient is apt to form an exaggerated estimate of his condition and to get into a depressed and altogether morbid state of mind, in which he easily becomes the prey of quacks. He should lose no time in putting himself into the hands of a medical man, who will set right any local cause of the trouble, and will see to his general health. Cold hip-baths are usually beneficial. The patient should sleep on a hard bed, take ample but not excessive exercise, and seek cheerful companions instead of indulging in solitary brooding. A bromide of potash mixture is useful in many cases—for example :

Bromide of potash .... 2½ drachms
Syrup of orange .... ½ ounce
Water to 8 ounces.
Two or three tablespoonfuls at bed-time.

SPHAGNUM MOSS (*see* Dressings and Strapping for Wounds).

SPICA BANDAGE (*see* Bandages).

SPINA BIFIDA.—As a result of imperfect development in ante-natal life there may be a gap in the bones of the spinal column, so that a part of the spinal cord, or of its membranes, escapes in the form of a round soft protrusion which becomes tense when the child cries. The malformation is a serious one. In a few cases there is spontaneous recovery. In some other cases an operation should be performed.

SPINAL ANALGESIA (*see* Anæsthesia).

SPINAL CARIES (*see* Spinal Curvature, Angular).

SPINAL COLUMN (*see* Nervous System).

SPINAL CORD (*see* NERVOUS SYSTEM).

SPINAL CURVATURE, ANGULAR.—This form of curvature is called also *kyphosis* and *spinal caries*, as well as *Pott's disease*, after a famous surgeon. It is an inflammatory disease of the bones of the spinal cord, and is nearly always tuberculous. The immediate cause may be exposure to cold or external injury, such as a fall, blow, strain, severe jerk, or a sudden twist, but there is usually also a predisposing cause at work, such as anæmia or a constitutional tendency to tuberculosis. The tubercle bacillus finds its way to the spinal column through the blood-stream, coming in many cases from the tonsil or the lung. The disease usually begins between the third and the tenth year, but sometimes adults are attacked. At first the symptoms may be ill-defined, but presently the destruction of bone and the consequent collapse of the spinal column lead to deformity. If the disease is in the neck the deformity is slight ; if in the back, the chest is distorted, the ribs are brought too close together, and the shoulders are raised so that the head looks sunken between them. When the neck is affected, the child supports his head with his hands, and stoops or turns round slowly and carefully ; when the lower parts of the spine are involved the child, in an instinctive effort to keep the spine from moving, bends the knees and hips to pick up an object from the floor, instead of bending the back. In many cases the destruction of bone is followed by a process of repair (ankylosis), new bone being created. In other cases an abscess forms, and the " matter " (pus) may make its way to the surface in the loin or elsewhere. The bladder may become inflamed or paralysed as a result of pressure on, or inflammation of, the spinal cord ; the lower limbs, too, may be paralysed in various degrees, and the damage to the spinal cord may predispose to the formation of bedsores. In these bad cases the end may come in two or three months, or may be delayed for as many years.

Treatment.—If resident in a big town, the patient should be removed to the country, and spend as much time as possible in the sunshine and open air. Absolute rest must be enforced so that the diseased bone may be immobilized. The doctor may administer tuberculin, which is sometimes beneficial. When pain and tenderness and any complications of the disease have disappeared, a mechanical appliance such as a plaster-of-Paris jacket should be worn so that the patient may move about while the spine is protected from any sudden or excessive movement. This should be worn for a year, and be succeeded by a light support, such as a celluloid jacket. An abundance of nutritious food should be supplemented by cod-liver oil and syrup of iodide of iron. Abscesses may be punctured and the contents withdrawn by aspiration, or an open operation may have to be performed. In paralytic cases extension may be applied to the lower limbs by weight and pulley.

SPINAL CURVATURE, LATERAL.—In lateral curvature, known technically as *scoliosis*, there is no destruction of bone ; the disease consists in weakness of the spine, leading to twisting of the column sideways. It generally comes on between the ages of ten and eighteen, and is more frequent in girls than in boys. It may be regarded as a form of rickets, but environment and habit play their part in its production, contributory causes being insufficient food, lack of pure air and sunshine, over-rapid growth, sitting in cramped attitudes, standing with one knee bent, and carrying heavy weights on one arm or on one shoulder. If the case is neglected, the curvature becomes permanent ; the spinal bones are bent on one side and twisted on each other, so that the ribs become more or less flattened and straightened out, while the shoulder-blade rests unevenly against the wall of the chest (hence the disease is sometimes called "growing out of the shoulder.") There may also be undue prominence of the hip on one side. The patient may be attacked by severe pains, cramps, or numbness, and may become emaciated. The deformity of the chest may embarrass the action of the heart and lungs, with consequent palpitations, irregular pulse and difficulty of breathing. The disease may proceed slowly or rapidly ; in some cases it reaches a certain point and then makes no further progress ; in other cases the deformity may to a great extent be corrected, but unless treatment is begun while the deformity is slight, correction will be only partial.

Treatment.—The remedy for this form of curvature consists in attending carefully to the general health, correcting anæmia and dyspepsia if present, and strengthening the muscles by appropriate exercises. Standing should be avoided, but the patient should do plenty of walking or should practise with a skipping-rope, dumb-bells, horizontal bars and trapeze. A reclining-board fitted with extension apparatus for the head and arms should be used for the systematic training of the spinal and other muscles. Breathing exercises with the hands holding some fixed object will also tend to strengthen the enfeebled muscles.

A celluloid or plaster-of-Paris jacket, with metal reinforcement, may be used to support the chest and to promote one-sided breathing so as to develop the side of the chest which is compressed. If there is extreme muscular weakness, friction and douching with a strong solution of bay-salt may be useful. The patient must have plenty of nourishing food and fresh air, should lie recumbent for two hours after the mid-day meal, and should take a tonic containing iron.

SPINAL NERVES (*see* NERVOUS SYSTEM).

SPIRAL BANDAGE (*see* BANDAGES).

SPIROCHÆTES (*see* GERMS).

SPLEEN, ENLARGED.—An enlarged spleen (*splenomegaly*) is a feature of quite a number of infectious and other diseases, including malaria, several forms of anæmia and jaundice, and tumours. In some of these diseases the treatment is operative.

SPLENOMEGALY (*see* SPLEEN, ENLARGED).

SPLINTS.—In rendering first aid in cases of fracture, the injured bone must be rendered immobile by means of splints, extending beyond the joint above and below the fracture, before the patient is moved. They may be improvised from all sorts of articles. Anything that is sufficiently stiff to prevent " giving " under strain, as when the limb is bent, will answer the purpose—for a broken leg, a walking stick, an umbrella, a broom-handle, a rifle, or a couple of billiard cues ; for a broken arm, a ruler, a hammer, straw bottle-covers, cigar-boxes, a thick piece of folded card-board, or newspapers folded into a thick roll. Splints, especially those to be applied to bony prominences, should be padded with some soft material to prevent them from causing pain and injuring the skin. For this purpose, towels, cotton-wool, tow, oakum, hemp, dry ferns, rushes, or even pieces of paper may be used. The bandages for applying the splints may be improvised out of handkerchiefs, neckties, braces, belts, bootlaces, thick cord, straps, strips of linen, etc.

SPONDYLITIS DEFORMANS.—This term denotes inflammation of the joints of the spine, due to the affections described under Arthritis Deformans.

SPONGIOPILINE (*see* Fomentations).

SPONGY GUMS (*see under* Breath, Offensive).

SPORADIC DISEASE (*see* Disease, Classification of).

SPOTS BEFORE THE EYES (*see* Eyes, Spots before).

SPOTTED FEVER (*see* Cerebrospinal Fever).

SPRAINS AND STRAINS.—A sprain is the wrenching of a joint ; a strain the wrenching of muscles or of tendons (" leaders ").

Sprains.—In a sprain, one or more of the ligaments of a joint are stretched or torn completely through, so that there is displacement of the bones of the joint ; bleeding occurs into the joint and the surrounding tissues, as can be seen from the part turning " black and blue " ; the membrane of the joint becomes inflamed and pours out its lubricating fluid (synovia) in abundance, so that the joint swells. Much pain is felt, and the joint becomes powerless. However careful the treatment, the inflammation is slow to subside, and even when it has disappeared the joint may be stiff and weak for a long time ; while if there is any tendency to rheumatism or gout the poison is apt to settle in the injured joint. A sprain, therefore, is an injury to be taken seriously, and treated with the utmost care. The first thing to do, if the patient is out of doors, is to apply firm pressure in the form of a bandage to the joint, so as to check any bleeding from the torn ligaments and keep down the swelling. The joint that is most frequently sprained is the *ankle*, and this accident most often occurs out of doors. It will be well to describe with some detail how the patient is to be got home. As Sir James Cantlie writes in the " First-Aid Manual " of the British Red Cross Society, the shoe ought not to be removed, but laced up more tightly. Then a strap, belt, or two handkerchiefs knotted together should be applied below the waist of the shoe, the ends crossed over the instep and carried round and round the ankle and lower part of the leg and secured quite firmly. If alone, the patient may do this himself. Cold water, if obtainable, may then be poured over the bandaged foot, or the foot dipped in a pool or bucket of water, the bandage thus being tightened, while the cold water tends to relieve the pain. It is much better that a patient with a sprained ankle should not attempt to walk, even with help, but if no conveyance is available, he can be assisted to shelter, as Sir James points out, in this way :—" Supposing it is the left ankle that is sprained, the helper stands on the left side of the patient (that is, on the same side as the injury), brings the patient's left arm over his (the helper's) left shoulder, tucking his right shoulder beneath the patient's left axilla. The helper now grasps the patient's left wrist with his (the helper's) left hand ; passes his right arm round the patient's waist so that the hand appears well forward on the patient's right side on a level with the haunch-bone. In this position, if the patient raises his left foot from the ground, he can, with the assistance of the helper, hop along on the right foot quite quickly, even at a running pace. The helper, by bringing the patient's weight on his right side, can carry the patient over obstacles, or for a considerable distance if the patient is faint." As soon as the patient has been got home, he should lie down on a bed or couch. The bandages having been removed, the shoe-laces should be cut, and also the shoe if necessary: then the sock is cut from the top to the toe, and the foot raised upon a pillow or cushion and wrapped in a large towel wrung out of cold water (ice-cold water, if possible), and the cold maintained by squeezing water from a wet sponge over the towel from time to time. Or a rag wrung out of evaporating lotion made of spirit and water may be laid over the joint. After a time heat in the form of fomentations or of linseed, bran, or oatmeal poultices will give more relief than cold. Recovery may be expedited by massage and passive movements of the part.

This treatment of a sprained ankle-joint applies generally to sprains of other joints, and it need only be added that special care should be taken when the knee-joint is thus affected, for it is the largest and most complicated joint in the body.

Strains.—In a slight strain a muscle or tendon is stretched; in a more severe strain there may be not only stretching but tearing. The most common situations of strains are about the shoulders, hips and back. Acute local pain is felt, the part becomes swollen and tender, and afterwards stiffness may set in, which may be persistent in persons prone to rheumatism. In the case of a limb, it may be necessary to apply a splint to keep the joints immediately above and below the injured muscle at rest. In all strains the pain may be mitigated by a hot fomentation or a bran poultice. If the bran poultice is to be applied to the loins, it should be enclosed in a muslin bag. Strains in the back require rest in bed until the pain has been subdued. A course of massage and passive movements will be found beneficial, followed by electricity and hot douches.

SPRUE.—Other names for this affection are *tropical diarrhœa, Ceylon sore mouth,* and *psilosis.* It consists in severe chronic catarrh of some part or the whole of the alimentary tract, which stretches from the mouth to the anus. It is probably of microbic origin, although no germ has yet been clearly identified. It is met with in most parts of the tropics and in many sub-tropical regions. The treatment is predominantly dietary.

SQUINT.—Strabismus, to give this affection its technical name, is due to defective action of the muscles that regulate the movements of the eye. Most babies squint at first, not from any defect in the ocular muscles, but because those muscles are not properly controlled until they have been exercised for some time. Squint, as a disorder, is usually first noticed between the ages of five and ten. It should be understood that there is no such thing as squinting with both eyes; a squint exists only when one eye is looking straight ahead and fixing an object, while the other assumes an abnormal position, either inwards, outwards, upwards, or downwards. The commonest deflection in childhood is inwards, towards the nose.

This is the *convergent* squint, the squint outwards being called *divergent*. For a time the child sees double, but to avoid this double vision he learns to look with one eye only, and the squinting eye is practically disused. Squint may be due to the irritation set up by unsuitable food, or by worms; in such slight cases it will disappear with the removal of the cause. When it is of a more permanent character it is, in most cases, the result either of long or of short sight. It may, however, be a sequel of inflammation of the eye, a patch of opacity on the cornea being formed in the centre of the line of vision, and the eye being turned to one side so as to avoid the patch. It may also be a symptom of hydrocephalus, of cerebral tumour, or of meningitis. When due to defect of vision it may usually be corrected by the use of glasses, if these are adopted in time. If the case is neglected, the defective muscles may have to be operated upon.

STAMMERING.—This affection is not uncommon in children belonging to families in which there is some nervous trouble. It may be induced by severe illness, or a child—more often a boy than a girl—may have been underfed or overworked. Though often an expression of nervous instability in one of the child's parents, it is seldom noticed before the age of six. In many cases it appears to be the result of unconscious mimicry, but the probability is that the child would be able to avoid the involuntary imitation if the predisposition were not present. The letters over which stammerers most often stumble are the labials, such as *p* and *b*. Much may be done by patient and judicious treatment to enable the child to overcome the difficulty.

The most important thing is to gain his confidence. He should be made to feel that there is nothing in stammering that he need be ashamed of. He should be induced to take his time in speaking, and not to haggle over a word, but to begin again at the beginning. He should be encouraged to sing and to learn poetry for recitation, for stammerers can both sing and recite without difficulty, and when they feel sure of this, they will be able to hope that presently the trouble will disappear from their ordinary speech. The general health must be watched, for it is a matter of universal experience that stammering is always worse when the patient is run down.

STAPHYLOCOCCI (*see* GERMS).

STARTING-PAINS (*see* HIP DISEASE).

STATUS EPILEPTICUS (*see* EPILEPSY).

STATUS LYMPHATICUS.—When a patient dies under an anæsthetic the medical evidence sometimes assigns status lymphaticus, or lymphatism, as the cause. In this condition there is overgrowth of the lymphatic tissue in the body—the lymph-glands, the tonsils, the adenoid tissue in the upper part of the throat, the spleen, the thymus gland, etc. Of the cause of lymphatism nothing is known; and unfortunately the condition, while readily recognized in a post-mortem examination, is exceedingly difficult to detect during life. It may lead to death not only while the patient is under an anæsthetic, but after any trivial injury or shock, such as a slight burn, or a warm bath, or mental excitement.

STERILITY.—Formerly it was thought that if a marriage was childless the defect was in the wife. Now it is known that the defect is often in the husband, and while statistics vary greatly, the fact appears to be that the sexes are about equally responsible for sterile marriages. In women the trouble may arise from defects of development, or from fibroid tumours, but in a large group of cases the cause is to be found in inflammation of the internal sexual organs, often a late result of gonorrhœa. In men also gonorrhœa is one of the most frequent causes of sterility, others being syphilis, tuberculosis, affections of the prostate gland, and congenital malformations. Sexual exhaustion may also be named, but the effect of this is usually only temporary. Both in men and in women the treatment will, of course, depend upon the cause.

STERILIZATION OF MILK (*see under* INFANTS AND YOUNG CHILDREN, FEEDING OF).

STIFFNECK (*see* WRY-NECK).

STILL'S DISEASE (*see* ARTHRITIS DEFORMANS).

STIMULANTS.—*Alcohol* is commonly regarded as a stimulant, though it is much more appropriately classified as a narcotic, its depressant being more important than its stimulating properties. *Methylated spirit* is a form of alcohol which is sometimes consumed as a beverage by persons of depraved taste. *Ether*, a liquid from which the alcohol and some of the water have been extracted, is also sometimes used as a beverage, especially in large manufacturing towns. It resembles alcohol in its effects, but acts more rapidly, and its results pass off more quickly. *Absinthe* (wormwood) is a very powerful and extremely pernicious stimulant. It does not act as a depressant, but sets up convulsions resembling those

of epilepsy. *Ammonia*, a general stimulant, of great value as a medicine, is usually taken in the form of salvolatile, which is the carbonate of ammonium. As it readily causes nausea and vomiting, it is seldom taken except for medicinal purposes.

STINGS AND BITES.—Of the larger parasites which infest the human skin, perhaps the most persistent and the most objectionable is the **louse.** Its attacks and their effects are dignified with the name *pediculosis*. The *head-louse* frequents the hair of the scalp, especially in neglected children, and on occasion will make a home in the eyelashes and the beard. The *body-louse* infests adults and elderly persons more than children, dwells in the underclothing, but does not disdain the outer garments, and is particularly partial to the inner surface of the collar. The *crab-louse* is most at home in the hairs round the genitals (hence " pubic pediculosis "), but may wander to other parts. The body-louse deposits its eggs on clothing ; the head- and crab-louse lay theirs on hairs, only one egg (nit) being, as a rule, fixed to a hair, to which it is bound so firmly by a glutinous substance as to be difficult of detachment. The headlouse and the body-louse vary in colour with the colour of the hair or skin of the different races to which they pay their attentions ; thus the body-louse is black in the negro, yellowish-brown in the Chinaman, and dirty grey in the European. All the species alike feed by driving into the orifice of a sweat-duct a membranous sucker, at the same time injecting an irritant fluid to encourage the flow of blood. When the creature has had its fill it withdraws the sucker, leaving at the point of penetration a tiny red speck due to the blood which wells up the duct as the sucker is extracted. Any other lesions which the skin of a lice-infested person may present are caused by scratching provoked by the intense itching. In children inflammation may thus be set up, and there may be a mattery discharge which binds the hairs together and may lead in extreme cases to abscesses in the glands of the neck. Usually it is people who are not scrupulously clean who are the victims of pediculosis, but old age may also act as a predisposing cause so far as the body-louse is concerned.

Treatment.—In *pediculosis of the head* in children the hair may be cut short and the scalp treated with white precipitate ointment; in adults the nits may be run down the individual hairs nearly to the end and the hairs then cut just above, or the hairs may be wetted with acetic acid so as to dissolve the glutinous material which binds the eggs to them, and then well combed with a small-toothed comb, the process being repeated until the eggs have all disappeared; the scalp should also be well smeared with white precipitate ointment. If the scratching has produced crusts, these should be detached by softening them with carbolized oil or carbolic-acid lotion. White precipitate ointment is not less useful in *pubic pediculosis* than in pediculosis of the scalp; it may be followed by an application of calamine lotion. In *body pediculosis* all the clothes must be baked in an oven at a temperature of at least 212° Fahr., and the patient should take hot baths and make free use of carbolic soap. During the Great War it was found that what is known as N.C.I. powder (naphthalene 96 per cent., creosote 2 per cent., and iodoform 2 per cent), dusted on the underclothing, and vermijelli rubbed into the seams of the coat and trousers, formed an efficient preventive against lice. It is all the more important that infection with body-lice should be avoided because they are known to be carriers of typhus and relapsing fever.

Bug-bites cause a wheal with a whitish centre round a dark point. Like lice, these insects inject an irritant to increase the flow of blood. Linen soaked in eau-de-Cologne, toilet vinegar, lead lotion or strong ammonia or weak solution of tar should be applied to the bites. If they are extensive, a hot solution of boric acid or soda, as strong as it can be made, may be applied. A useful preventive is oil of lavender smeared on the exposed parts, or oil of eucalyptus, or peppermint.

The bites of the **harvest-bug** are often a source of irritation to those who have to work in the fields in July and August. Bright-red wheals and hard pimples appear, most often on the ankles and legs, and there is a good deal of itching. The little creature must be picked out of the bite, and naphthol or weak mercurial ointment then applied. Anointing with tincture of benzoin is recommended as a deterrent.

The **flea** leaves its mark in the form of a small red spot with a darker point in the centre. The irritation is less pronounced than that caused by bug-bites, but if the skin is specially sensitive, a little lead lotion may be applied on linen.

The bites of **gnats** and **mosquitoes** raise wheals, which in some persons may be of considerable size. The remedies recommended for bug-bites will be found suitable. Or a piece of washing soda may be rubbed on the affected part. If the insect has left its " sting " in the puncture, it should be picked out with a needle. A good preventive is oil of lavender or of eucalyptus or of citronella, smeared on the exposed part.

The stings of **wasps** and **bees** are painful but not dangerous, unless the tongue or the throat is stung, when there may be so much swelling as to threaten suffocation. If the sting has been left in the wound, it should be removed with tweezers, and the smarting allayed with a little moistened bicarbonate of soda or ammonia, or some sal-volatile and oil may be rubbed in. Should there be much swelling, a hot bicarbonate-of-soda fomentation may be resorted to.

Snake-bites.—The only venomous snake indigenous to Great Britain is the adder or viper, the bite of which, though setting up serious symptoms, is seldom fatal. The wound rapidly reddens and swells and becomes painful, and the patient falls into a state of prostration and may collapse. Treatment consists in tying a tight band round the limb between the wound and the heart, to prevent the poison from being disseminated, and then swabbing the wound with a strong solution of permanganate of potash or rubbing in permanganate of potash crystals. Brandy or some other stimulant should be given to counteract the shock to the system, and the area round the wound may be gently rubbed with warm oil to assuage the pain.

" STINK NOSE " (*see* Ozæna, *under* NASAL CATARRH).

STITCH IN THE SIDE (*see* SIDE-ACHE ; PLEURISY).

STOMACH (*see* DIGESTION).

STOMACH, DILATATION OF. —The stomach may be overfilled with food or stretched to its utmost capacity with gas, but if, when relieved of its contents, it returns to its normal size, it has been simply distended. Dilatation is the condition which supervenes when from prolonged distension the walls of the stomach lose their elasticity and fail to contract. It may be the result of the defective muscular tone which follows in the wake of anæmia, or it may be set up by nervous exhaustion, by excessive indulgence in alcohol or tobacco, or by other causes of a general character. In another group of cases it is caused by obstruction at the pylorus—the narrow end of the stomach, through which its contents pass to the intestine. Dilatation arises gradually. Vomiting is a constant symptom ; it may occur some hours after taking food, or at intervals, and many pints, it may be, of sour, frothy fluid, of a dirty-brown colour, are brought up. As the nourishment taken is not assimilated, there is a craving for food, and, if the dilatation persists, the body wastes. If the trouble is due to a tumour, or to obstruction of a permanent character, an operation will be necessary. In other cases medical measures should be tried. Only food that is easily digested should be taken, and that in strictly moderate quantities. If necessary, pre-digested food may be used. Very little drink should be taken with solid food, but half a pint of hot water may be sipped an hour or more before the meal. Vegetables that leave an unabsorbable residue, as cabbage does, should be avoided.

STOMACH, ULCER OF.—Gastric (also called peptic) ulcer usually occurs between the ages of twenty and forty-five. A round or oval ulcer, which may be as small as a threepenny bit or as large as a half-crown, forms on the mucous membrane— the inner surface—of the stomach. It may heal spontaneously or under medical treatment, or may eat its way through the walls of the stomach until " perforation " takes place, with the result that the contents of the stomach escape into the peritoneal cavity and set up peritonitis. The cause of gastric ulcer is not fully understood. It is not improbable that dental abscesses and septic gums account for some cases; it is believed that germs from burns or from a septic appendix are responsible for others. It is possible, too, that abstention from food for long periods is another factor. Heredity seems to be yet another. Thus Sir William Willcox records that he has met with gastric ulcer in three generations— grandfather, father and son. This, however, may be only coincidence.

Symptoms.—In almost all cases there is a good deal of burning or stabbing or cramping pain, usually coming on within an hour of a meal, and persisting until the stomach is emptied, either by the food passing into the intestine or by vomiting. A curious feature of the pain is that there may be long periods in which it is absent. In some cases lying down gives relief; in others, stooping forward or lying on one side. Vomiting, usually preceded by nausea and a flow of saliva, is a frequent, though not an invariable, symptom. Bleeding may also occur. If the hæmorrhage is profuse, the blood will be vomited; smaller quantities may pass into the intestine and make the motions black. In addition to the pain, there is often a feeling of weight in the pit of the stomach, with flatulence and the bringing up of extremely acid fluid. The most serious complication of gastric ulcer is perforation. Sudden and agonizing pain is felt in the abdomen, the patient collapses, and the only hope of saving his life lies in prompt operation.

Treatment.—At first medical, as distinct from surgical, treatment should be employed. The mouth should be carefully examined and any source of oral sepsis removed. The patient must go to bed, and not only the body in general but the stomach in particular should be rested. In severe cases, especially if there has been vomiting of blood, the gastric rest should be complete, nourishment being given in the form of enemata. In less severe cases, and in bad cases when they begin to improve, nothing but milk, either alone or mixed with lime-water or soda-water, or peptonized, should be given by mouth, so that the ulcer may be spared all irritation and may have a chance to heal. Some patients find it impossible to retain milk; in such cases buttermilk may be tried as a temporary expedient, or albumen water, or small quantities of chicken or veal broth, or water arrowroot sweetened to taste. Whatever its nature, the food must be given in very small quantities— a tablespoonful every hour gradually increased to a teacupful every two or three hours. After a time meat extracts and, later still, beaten-up eggs may be given. Unless there is hæmorrhage, the food should be warm. When there is reason to believe that healing of the ulcer has taken place, the medical attendant will permit a very gradual return to ordinary diet, but the greatest care must be taken to avoid all indigestible food for several months.

If after prolonged trial medical treatment is unavailing, operation will no doubt be advised. In a large percentage of cases this effects a cure.

Ulcer of the *duodenum* sets up symptoms similar to those of gastric ulcer, and requires similar treatment.

STOMACH-ACHE (*see* Colic; Flatulence).

STOMATITIS (*see* MOUTH, INFLAMMATION OF).

STONE IN THE BLADDER.— We may begin the present article by considering the causes of urinary calculi generally. A urinary calculus is an agglomeration of crystals formed by the solid constituents of the urine which are normally held in solution, and the mass is held together by substances in the nature of cement, which can also be detected in normal urine. Whether stones are formed in the kidneys, the bladder, or the other parts of the urinary tract, the causes are much the same. Food and drinking-water play an important part. For example, an excess of nitrogenous food (*see* FOOD) or of alcohol tends to the undue formation of uric acid, especially if too little exercise is taken; digestive disorders lead to the deposit in the urine of crystals of oxalate of lime; and hard water furnishes an excessive amount of lime salts. Heredity, too, has to be taken into account.

In the article URINE, NORMAL AND ABNORMAL, it is pointed out that this secretion contains solid constituents such as uric acid, oxalate of lime, and phosphates, which sometimes form deposits after the fluid has been standing for some time. These solid constituents may be deposited before the urine is passed, being present in urine as tiny granules —commonly spoken of as " gravel " —while it is still in the urinary passages, but in some cases they combine into stones (calculi). These may be formed in the kidneys, the ureters (the tubes leading from the kidneys to the bladder), the bladder, or the urethra (the tube leading from the bladder to the surface of the body). In this article we shall consider those formed in or carried to the bladder

from the kidney—vesical calculi, as they are called.

Stone in the bladder is very much more frequent in men than in women, and less frequent in children than in adults. The stones are composed almost wholly of uric acid, phosphates, or oxalate of lime, in that order of frequency. They seldom, however, consist of a single ingredient, and when one speaks, for instance, of a uric-acid calculus one only means that uric acid is the chief constituent. In many cases the centre or nucleus consists of uric acid; around this layer after layer is deposited until the stone is formed, weighing on an average from half to three-quarters of an ounce. Oxalate-of-lime stones form very slowly, and years elapse before they attain a moderate size. Uric-acid stones form more rapidly, and a large phosphatic stone may form in a few weeks.

Cause.—The causes of calculi in general have already been touched upon, but it may be added that in some cases bladder-stones result from changes in the urine due to the action of bacteria.

Symptoms.—The earliest and most common symptom is a frequent and urgent desire to pass water, caused by irritation of the neck of the bladder from contact with the stone. When the patient lies on his back the stone falls away from the bladder-neck and the urgency ceases. The passing of water leaves a sense of discomfort, and the patient feels that the bladder has not been emptied; a dull, aching pain is felt in the bladder, aggravated when he moves about, and especially if he rides on horseback or on a bicycle, or is subjected to the jarring of a bus. At the end of micturition a few drops of light blood are often passed, and a sharp cutting pain is felt in the bladder and at the end of the penis. When children scream on passing water, it is usually because of calculus, and small boys will pull at the penis in a vain endeavour to relieve the pain. The urine contains crystals ; if the bladder becomes inflamed, mucus and pus are present, and the water is offensive to the smell. Severe pain is experienced in the bladder in the middle of the act, and the stream suddenly ceases, the stone having blocked the orifice through which the urine passes out of the bladder. If the patient lies down, the stone rolls away, and the act can be continued.

Fortunately, stone in the bladder is not difficult to diagnose. When symptoms are present which suggest it, a metal instrument called a sound is passed into the bladder, and a click is heard when it comes into contact with a stone. Or the X-rays can be employed, or by means of a cysto-scope the surgeon can actually see the stones in the bladder and determine their number and position.

Treatment.—The best method of removing a stone in the bladder, unless it is very large, is that known as lithotrity or litholapaxy, which is not a cutting operation : the stone is crushed by an instrument called a lithotrite, which is passed along the urethra into the bladder. The fragments are washed out by injecting fluid into the bladder and withdrawing it by suction, and finally the bladder is flushed with an antiseptic. In cases in which this procedure is not suitable, as for instance if the stone is too large to be grasped by the litho-trite, or is fixed, the old operation of lithotomy is performed, the bladder being opened by an incision and the stones removed by forceps. In women the urethra is much shorter than in men, and in many cases it can be stretched sufficiently to enable the stones to be removed. In a small proportion of cases of stone the con-dition recurs ; if so, the operation, whether lithotrity or lithotomy, can be repeated. How the formation of stones may be prevented is described in the article STONE IN THE KIDNEY.

STONE IN THE GALL-BLADDER (*see* GALL-STONES).

STONE IN THE KIDNEY.—Renal calculus most often occurs in middle age, but the beginning of the trouble may date back to a much earlier period, and in some cases can be traced to infancy or childhood. The disease is more common in East Anglia and the east of Scotland than in other parts of Great Britain, possibly owing to the presence of a larger proportion of lime salts in the drinking-water. In most cases there is but one stone in the kidney, but there may be many. The kidney is always more or less damaged by stone. Inflammation is set up, and the organ may either enlarge or waste away. The outflow of urine into the ureters, the tubes which conduct it to the bladder, may be obstructed, and so the kidney may be dilated and its secreting powers destroyed, and abscesses may form. In about 50 per cent. of the cases, sooner or later the other kidney is attacked.

Symptoms.—In rare cases the stone in the kidney may give no clear sign of its presence for years, but usually a distressing train of symptoms arises before very long. A dull aching pain, aggravated by movement, or jarring, as in walking over rough ground, or in horseback or bicycle exercise, or in driving, is felt in the loin on the affected side, and may also be felt in the front of the abdomen. If the patient takes complete rest the pain disappears for the time being. In some cases pain is felt, too, in the sole of the foot or the heel, in the thigh or leg, in the testicle, in the bladder, or in the unaffected kidney ; these are " referred " pains. In about half the cases blood appears in the urine. Pus may also be detected there, and the urine may be excessive in quantity.

The most striking of the symptoms of stone in the kidney is that known as *renal colic*, caused by the passage of the stone down one of the ureters into the bladder. If the stone is quite small, it may pass along the ureter without attracting attention, but if large it causes agonizing pain, which begins in the loin and shoots downwards to the thigh or groin, or even as far as the leg. The patient becomes faint, breaks out into profuse perspiration, may roll about in his agony, may be violently sick, and soon becomes exhausted. There is a constant and very urgent desire to pass water, which is seen to be stained with blood, and may contain blood-clots. If the stone catches in the ureter, so that its progress is for the time being arrested, the acute pain sinks into a dull aching, but is raised to its former intensity when the stone resumes its journey. As soon as it has entered the bladder the pain ceases. An attack of colic may last for an hour or two or for two or three days. In a few hours, or days, the stone may be passed with the urine, or it may remain in the bladder until removed by the surgeon.

Treatment.—If both kidneys are seriously affected, operation is not desirable. If small stones are frequently passed, and the X-rays reveal the presence of no large stones, operation is useless, for it would not stop the formation of further small calculi ; in this group of cases, medical and spa treatment is indicated. In other cases the patient should consent to operation if this is advised by the doctor.

Treatment of *renal colic* should begin with a hot bath, or the patient should be got to bed, and hot linseed poultices or fomentations, sprinkled with laudanum, applied to the painful part. The medical attendant may administer opium, or omnopon ; the pain usually subsides within half an hour of the injection, but the injection may have to be repeated more than once. In very bad cases chloroform may have to be given and the patient kept lightly under its influence for an hour or more. The bowels should be cleared out with copious enemata of hot water.

If the urine passed is always very acid and contains large quantities of solids that form visible deposits, *preventive treatment* is called for so that the formation of stone may be avoided. Meat should be taken only sparingly, and veal and pork, kidney, liver, brain and sweetbreads, duck and goose, and high game not at all, and the food generally should be quite moderate in amount, especially as to sugar and fats. The digestive organs must be maintained in good working order and the bowels in regular action, and a sufficiency of out-door exercise must be taken. Heavy wines must be tabooed, and tea and coffee, if taken at all, should be very weak. Plenty of water which is known to be free from a large proportion of salts must be taken, not with meals, but at other times. Bicarbonate of soda and tartrate of potash are to be recommended for their effect in neutralizing acidity. Carbonate of lime or prepared chalk, 20 or 30 grains in mucilage of gum, with some peppermint water, may be taken with advantage three or four times a day. Natural mineral waters such as those of Contrexéville or Evian are beneficial. Turkish baths, massage, and radiant-heat baths are valuable adjuncts to treatment.

STRABISMUS (*see* SQUINT).

STRAINS (*see* SPRAINS AND STRAINS).

STRAPPING (*see* DRESSINGS AND STRAPPING FOR WOUNDS).

STRAWBERRY MARKS (*see* BIRTH-MARKS).

STRAWBERRY TONGUE (*see* SCARLET FEVER).

STREPTOCOCCI (*see* GERMS).

STRICTURE OF URETHRA (*see* URETHRA, STRICTURE OF).

STRIDOR (*see* BREATHING, DIFFICULTY OF).

"STROKE" (*see* APOPLEXY).

STRYCHNINE POISONING.— Strychnine is the basis of many vermin-killers, and is also much used in medicine. In strychnine poisoning breathing becomes difficult, the body is convulsed and becomes stiff and arched, and the limbs rigid ; the muscles of the face are drawn into what is called *risus sardonicus* (the sardonic grin), the eyes protrude and the pupils dilate. The patient should be taken into a darkened room and kept quiet, and an emetic given without delay, and continued unless the spasms make swallowing impossible. As a sedative, bromide of potash in 2-drachm or 3-drachm doses may be given, and chloroform inhaled. If death threatens, artificial respiration should be performed (*see* RESPIRATION, ARTIFICIAL).

STUPES (*see* FOMENTATIONS).

STUPOR (*see* INSANITY).

STUTTERING (*see* STAMMERING.)

STY.—A small abscess round the root of an eyelash, though sometimes met with in children who are not delicate, and even in adults, is most common in children who are weakly or run down. First, at the edge of the lid, there is a little redness and swelling (Frontispiece, Fig. 1), which increases until the whole lid may be involved. Pus (" matter ") forms, and in due course is discharged, when the discomfort quickly subsides. If sties grow in rapid succession, it is an indication that the general health needs attention. Accordingly, the bowels should be regulated, the child should be encouraged to take plenty of nourishing but easily digested food, and cod-liver oil with steel wine should be given. It is seldom necessary to puncture the " gathering "; it is sufficient to bathe it with hot water or to apply warm compresses.

SUCKLING.—In this article the troubles of mothers who nurse their children are dealt with. One of them, known as *milk-fever*, is much less common than it was in the days when it was considered that a woman exhausted by the pain and strain and hæmorrhage of labour required to be half-starved on a diet of weak gruel. But even now milk-fever sometimes occurs, it may be from distension of the breasts through the child not being allowed to suck sufficiently early, or because the mother's diet is not nutritious enough. The symptoms are a rise of temperature and some constitutional disturbance. Treatment consists in carefully emptying the breasts at regular intervals, clearing the bowels by simple aperients, and taking plenty of nourishing food.

If there is *deficient secretion of milk*, warm fomentations should be applied to the breast. The bowels should be kept freely open by gentle aperients and abundance of nourishing but not rich food taken. Highly seasoned dishes, pickles, acid drinks, pastry, raw vegetables and fruit should be avoided, as likely to upset the baby by affecting the milk.

Instead of deficient there may be *excessive secretion of milk*, so that it runs away, causing much discomfort by wetting the night-dress and bed-clothes. This is an indication for reducing the proportion of liquid food. Some of the milk should be drawn off with a pump, or squeezed out with the fingers, before putting the child to the breast.

The commonest trouble of suckling is *cracked nipples*. This is one of those conditions which, although simple and free from danger, cause great pain. Putting the child to the breast, which ought to be a delight, becomes a dread. The nervous system may be so upset as to disturb the secretion of milk, and not infrequently nursing has to be suspended, if not terminated. The nipples should be carefully prepared for some two months before the child is born by being bathed night and morning with an astringent lotion, such as glycerin and eau-de-Cologne (or brandy) in equal parts, or 10 grains of tannin in an ounce of glycerin. During nursing the nipples should be gently but thoroughly washed and dried as soon as the child is taken from the breast, and if there is any tendency to soreness the astringent lotion should be used. If a crack appears the nipple may be protected by a nipple shield and dressed with strong tea, but if this is ineffectual the lotion must be resumed. To keep the nipple dry it may be powdered with equal parts of oxide of zinc and starch. If the pain is acute the crack may have to be touched with a stick of lunar caustic.

Abscesses of the breast begin as hard lumps, and are often slow to heal. As soon as lumps appear, treatment must be instituted, in the hope of preventing inflammation. The child must be put to the breast at regular intervals, so that no large quantity of milk may accumulate. The swelling should be gently rubbed in the direction of the nipple with clean fingers moistened with oil or with belladonna liniment. If this is not done, or if the breast is exposed to cold, or inflammation spreads to it from a cracked nipple, the lumps may become inflamed. Even if they do, suppuration may be prevented by smearing a liniment of equal parts of belladonna and glycerin over the painful part and covering it with hot fomentations or poultices frequently renewed. Nursing should be suspended, and the breast supported by a handkerchief tied round the neck. It is better that the abscess should be opened by the surgeon's knife than that it should be left to burst through the skin, for this intervention will shorten the patient's sufferings and less scarring will be left.

SUFFOCATION (*see* Respiration, Artificial; Foreign Bodies in the Larynx and Windpipe, *under* Foreign Bodies).

" SUGGESTION " (*see* Hypnotism; Psychotherapy).

SULPHONAL (*see* Narcotics and Hypnotics).

SULPHURIC ACID POISONING.—Oil of vitriol, which is a form of sulphuric acid, is sometimes taken in mistake for olive oil, or with suicidal intent. The tongue, cheek and gums are white to brown or black, and if there are any spots on the clothes they will be dirty brown, with red edges. No emetic must be given. Instead, give large draughts of soap and water. Washing soda, chalk (from the wall or ceiling, if no other is available), or whiting may be dissolved or broken up in a little water, and given in teaspoonful doses, frequently repeated. Later, lime-water or fluid magnesia may be given in milk or gruel, in the proportion of a tablespoonful to a tumblerful, or olive oil, a quarter of a pint in a pint of water. Such drinks may be continued for several days.

SUMMER DIARRHŒA (*see* EPIDEMIC DIARRHŒA).

SUNLIGHT TREATMENT.— Exposure to the rays of the sun, technically called heliotherapy, is a special form of the open-air treatment, that is briefly described under CONSUMPTION. It has come into prominence of late years in the treatment of various forms of tuberculosis, especially tuberculosis of bones, joints and glands, but not excluding tuberculosis of the lungs, and also in the treatment of rickets. The effects are due partly to general stimulation and exhilaration, but the rays also have a direct action on the skin and on the blood and other tissues of the body. The treatment has to be administered with great care so that the patient may not be burnt or over-stimulated. He has to be acclimatized by gradual and progressive exposure, and the head has always to be protected ; and it is found that those whose skin bronzes readily best tolerate the treatment and derive from it most benefit. In *artificial sunlight treatment* the short ultraviolet rays of light (invisible in the sun's spectrum) are administered by means of carbon-arc and other electric lamps. This treatment has been found beneficial in varying degrees in ulcers and wounds, tuberculosis of bones and joints, etc., some cases of tuberculosis of the lungs, rickets, and many skin diseases such as eczema, acne, barber's itch and loss of hair. High blood-pressure is slightly lowered. Mental fatigue is relieved and vitality stimulated, but these effects may be largely psychological—i.e. due to suggestion. This method of treatment has recently attracted a good deal of popular notice, but its precise value has yet to be determined.

SUNSTROKE (*see* HEATSTROKE AND SUNSTROKE).

SUPERFLUOUS HAIRS (*see* HAIRINESS).

SUPPOSITORIES.—Suppositories are conical preparations, an inch or two in length and about a quarter of an inch in breadth at the base, consisting of drugs mixed with wax or cacao butter, which melts at a temperature a little lower than that of the body. The finger and the suppository are smeared with vaselin, and the suppository is then pushed as far into the bowel as the finger can reach. Suppositories may be employed for their astringent, their sedative, or their aperient effects. If the astringent effect is desired, as when it is desired to check hæmorrhage or mucous discharge from the bowel, tannic acid, hazeline, or compound lead is used ; if a sedative effect, morphia ; if an aperient effect, glycerin. A home-made suppository, useful in the constipation of infants and young children, consists of a piece of ordinary yellow soap of the size of a small thimble. Nutrient suppositories are also employed.

SUPPRESSED GOUT (*see* GOUT).

SUPPRESSION OF URINE (*see* URINE, SUPPRESSION OF).

SUPPURATION (*see* INFLAMMATION).

SUPPURATIVE MENINGITIS (*see* MENINGITIS, SUPPURATIVE).

SUPRARENAL GLANDS (*see* DUCTLESS GLANDS).

SWALLOWING, DIFFICULTY OF (*see* GULLET, STRICTURE OF).

SWEAT, OFFENSIVE.—Bromidrosis, to give this condition its technical name, may be the symptom of some serious disease, such as rheumatic fever or scurvy, or may occur independently, either with or without excessive perspiration. It may be general, but is more often confined to a part such as the armpits or, most frequently of all, the feet. The sweat is not foul-smelling when first secreted, but becomes so afterwards owing to the action of germs. A contributory cause is lack of cleanliness, but the condition may be present in those who are guiltless of such neglect. If the armpits are the seat of the trouble, they may be shaved and frequently powdered with boric acid. For treatment of sweating feet, *see* FEET, SWEATING.

SYCOSIS, COCCOGENIC (*see* BARBER'S ITCH).

SYMMETRICAL GANGRENE OF THE EXTREMITIES (*see* RAYNAUD'S DISEASE).

SYMPATHETIC OPHTHALMIA (*see* OPHTHALMIA).

SYNCOPE (*see* FAINTING).

SYNOVITIS.—Inflammation of the synovial membrane, which forms the lining of joints, may be acute or chronic.

Acute synovitis may be set up by injury, such as a strain, or by germs or their poisons, such as those of gonorrhœa, syphilis, tuberculosis, dysentery, blood-poisoning. The joint—in many cases the knee—becomes hot and painful, and swells from the excessive synovial fluid which is poured out by the membrane. There is also some general feverishness. If the inflammation is due to blood-poisoning, the fluid accumulated in the joint may become purulent ("mattery"), the patient may have high fever and become seriously ill, and permanent stiffness may be left behind. In cases due to rheumatism there may be a good deal of stiffness, but usually there is no formation of pus and no high fever. If injury is the cause, the symptoms gradually subside with rest and suitable treatment, and there are no after-effects. The first requisite of treatment is rest: the limb must be immobilized with a splint and rested in the position most comfortable to the patient. An ice-pack should be applied to relieve the inflammation. If the fluid becomes purulent the joint must be opened by a surgeon and the cavity washed out with an antiseptic solution. In other cases the joint may be painted with strong tincture of iodine. In rheumatic and gouty cases the rheumatism or gout must be treated by drugs given internally, as advised in the articles on those subjects.

Chronic synovitis is a sequel of the acute form. The pain is much less severe than in acute synovitis, and the swelling is due less to the accumulation of fluid in the joint than to thickening of the synovial membrane. As in the acute form, the joint must be immobilized. Blistering should be resorted to, and after the blisters have healed, compound mercury ointment should be applied on strips of linen 2 inches wide and sufficiently long to go round the joint and overlap ; eight or more of these straps may be used, beginning from below and reaching to well above the joint. Strips of diachylon adhesive strapping of the same size, spread on "moleskin," should be applied over the others, so as to form a case for the whole joint and make firm pressure upon it. This case may be worn for some weeks. Chronic synovitis is very intractable.

SYPHILIS.—The most serious of the three venereal diseases (*see*

VENEREAL DISEASES) was brought to Europe from America in the fifteenth century : how it originated in the Western Continent is not known. The germ to which it is due usually, perhaps always, finds its way into the human system through a breach in the skin or the mucous membrane, but the breach may be so slight that the patient is unaware of it. Contagion is usually *direct*—that is, by contact with the discharge from a syphilitic sore or with one of the secretions of a patient, but it may be *indirect*—that is, the germ may be received from a contaminated object, such as a razor, a drinking vessel or a glass-blowing implement. In direct contagion the disease is usually contracted in sexual intercourse, but it may be communicated by kissing, and it has often been " caught " by wet nurses who suckle syphilitic infants, and by medical men, midwives and others who have handled syphilitic patients.

Symptoms.—The slight breach in the surface of the skin or mucous membrane through which the germ enters heals up, and for a period which averages from three to six weeks (the incubation period) the disease gives no signs of its presence. Then a sore appears on the spot where infection was received. This is the " primary sore " called also the *hard chancre*, to distinguish it from soft sore (*see* SOFT SORE). It is hard at the base, and the nearest lymph-glands also become hard. As a rule, the primary sore heals, even if not treated, in a few days or weeks, but occasionally it ulcerates in spite of treatment and causes much destruction of tissue. Even before the primary sore has disappeared the disease has begun to affect the constitution, the germs, constantly multiplying, being carried along in the blood- and lymph-

vessels, and forming colonies in various organs. Evidence of this diffusion of the germs is seen within a few weeks of the appearance of the primary sore by the breaking out of a rash which may imitate almost every known skin disease. The lymph-glands enlarge, ulcers may form on the mucous membranes, and the bones, joints, arteries, the nervous system and the eye may be the seat of painful inflammations. These symptoms form what is called the *secondary stage* of syphilis. The *third* (tertiary) stage usually begins in the third year after infection, but may be delayed much longer. It consists in a process of slow inflammation, leading to the formation of swellings (gummata) on the skin and mucous membranes, the bones, nerves, and organs generally. The swellings near the surface give rise to ulcers ; the less superficial ones may do irreparable damage to the structures they attack. There is still another stage of the disease, the *fourth stage*, which may be delayed for many years. In this stage the optic nerve may atrophy, causing intense pain and ending in blindness, or the patient may suffer from the serious nervous affection called locomotor ataxy (q.v.) (otherwise tabes dorsalis), or, worse still, he may become the victim of general paralysis of the insane (q.v.).

So far we have been considering syphilis as an acquired disease. But it is also a congenital disease, which is usually communicated to the unborn child by an infected mother, and possibly in some cases is communicated by the father to the unborn child without the mother being infected. As a rule, no sign of the disease is present at birth, but a few weeks afterwards the child suffers from " snuffles." The larynx (voice-box) becomes inflamed, a rash appears on the skin, the face grows wrinkled

12a

and wizened and looks more like that of an aged person than of an infant. Left untreated, the disease follows the same general course in the child as in the adult.

Syphilis, then, is one of the most serious of all diseases. Fortunately, however, its progress can almost always be arrested if treatment is begun in the first stage. Fortunately, also, methods of diagnosis are now available which make it easy of detection.

Treatment.—The historical remedy for syphilis is mercury, which undoubtedly has great efficacy, though it is not an absolute antidote. A few years ago a more potent remedy was devised—salvarsan, an arsenical compound. Even salvarsan, however, is not an absolute remedy, for in some cases in which it is used the disease, after lying dormant for months or years, once more becomes active. This being so, the custom now is to combine the two remedies ; salvarsan is injected and is followed by a course of mercury, and this sequence is repeated time after time ; iodide of potash being also given if tertiary symptoms appear.

SYSTEMIC CIRCULATION (*see* BLOOD, CIRCULATION OF).

T

TABES DORSALIS (*see* LOCOMOTOR ATAXY).

TABES MESENTERICA (*see* CONSUMPTION OF THE BOWELS).

TALIPES (*see* CLUB-FOOT).

TAPEWORMS (*see* WORMS).

TARTAR EMETIC POISONING (*see* ANTIMONY POISONING).

TASTE, PERVERSIONS OF.— Imaginary sensations of taste, usually disagreeable, may be due to an affection of the brain, but they may also be the expression simply of a functional nervous disorder, i.e. a nervous disorder in which there is no traceable disease or injury of the organs constituting the nervous system. Taste disturbances of this latter group are usually fleeting, and disappear as the nervous disorder is subdued.

T-BANDAGE (*see* BANDAGES).

TEARS, OVERFLOW OF (*see* EPIPHORA).

TEETH, CARE OF.—There is hardly any structure of the body which calls for the exercise of so much care as the teeth, for they are constantly surrounded by dangerous enemies in the form of microbes that dwell in the mouth. Although they are made of hard substances, dentine (ivory) and enamel—the latter the hardest substance in the body—they are so constantly exposed to attack that it is rare for adults to preserve them all in their integrity. After a meal, food is apt to lodge between the teeth, where, especially if it is of a starchy nature, it undergoes fermentation which exposes it to invasion by microbes, with the result that injurious acids are formed. The necessity for carefully cleansing the teeth at frequent intervals is therefore evident. There appears to be ground for believing that the process of fermentation is more active during the night than in the day. The cleansing ought, therefore, to be done not merely in the morning but also at night, and if it can be repeated after meals during the day, so much the better. The teeth should be brushed in the up-and-down direction, as well as across, and where teeth have been lost and the tooth-brush can be introduced into the vacant space, the sides of the teeth should receive attention. The cleansing of the teeth will be aided by the use of a simple tooth-powder, such as carbolic powder, or camphorated chalk, or magnesia. A visit should be paid to the dentist at regular intervals, say once in six months, so that the teeth may be kept free from tartar, and decay stopped in an early stage. With such precautions as these a person in sound health may hope to carry a fairly good set of teeth into late middle or even old age. If so few of us have this good fortune, it is mainly because we awake too late to the importance of taking care of these precious but precarious organs.

TEETH, DECAY OF.—The influence of lack of care of the teeth in favouring dental decay, known technically as *dental caries*, has been touched upon in the preceding article. There can be no doubt that the almost exclusive use of foods that have been rendered soft by cooking contributes to the same end. The mastication of hard foods tends to cleanse them and keep them in good condition, and largely explains why the lower animals and the lower races of mankind usually have sound, bright teeth, although they are never consciously cleansed. In the first stage of dental decay no pain is felt, but as the layer that covers the sensitive pulp in the interior of the tooth grows thin, a pang is experienced when anything hot or very cold is taken into the mouth. When the pulp is actually exposed, inflammation is set up, and the pain, as everyone knows, may be intense. The inflammation may spread along the root of the teeth and cause a gumboil, which is accompanied by a throbbing pain. (*See* GUMBOIL.)

In many cases the pain of toothache spreads to other branches of the nerve which supplies the tooth, or to the nerve of a different tooth, and neu-ralgia is felt in the side of the head, or the eye, or the ear. This neuralgic pain is sometimes relieved by a good dose of quinine, or by aspirin (10 grains), or by tincture of gelsemium (15 drops in water). Occasionally, however, the pain associated with a decayed tooth is due to rheumatism, and is relieved by iodide of potash in doses of 3 to 5 grains, or by aspirin. In cases of toothache generally, the gums may be painted with mild tincture of iodine. Sometimes the pain is subdued by placing bicarbonate of soda in the cavity after well cleansing the mouth with an antispetic wash. Or a little piece of cotton-wool soaked in pure carbolic acid may be inserted in the cavity, care being taken not to touch it with the fingers, nor to allow it to come into contact with any part of the mouth except the tooth, since carbolic acid is a strong caustic; it should then be covered with a small piece of wool soaked in friar's balsam. Other remedies are (1) oil of cloves, with the addition of 5 per cent. of cocaine, and (2) flowers of camphor 1 drachm, chloral hydrate 1 drachm, cocaine 5 grains. As these remedies contain cocaine, a prescription must be obtained from a dentist or a doctor.

TEETHING AND ITS TROUBLES.—Although dentition is a physiological process, not a disease, it may give rise not only to a great deal of local irritation, but even to constitutional disturbance, and often an infant may need careful watching and attention as each tooth is cut. The temporary or milk teeth number twenty, and usually begin to appear at the sixth or seventh month. In rare instances teething begins at the age of three months, and there are cases on record in which children have been born with teeth already cut. According to Shakespeare, Richard III.

was one of these abnormal children, for he could " gnaw a crust at two hours old." The first teeth to appear are the lower central incisors —the two teeth in the centre of the lower jaw : these are usually cut by the eighth month. Then, after three to six weeks, the four central teeth of the upper jaw—the central and lateral incisors—begin to come, following each other at intervals of a week or two. Two or three months later the two lower lateral incisors are cut, followed by the upper and lower

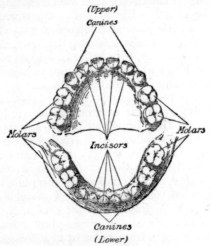

(Upper)
Canines

Molars   Molars

Incisors

Canines
(Lower)

Fig. 59.—The temporary teeth.

front molars or first double teeth, which usually have all come through by the end of the fourteenth month. The upper canines or eye-teeth come next, within three or four months ; the lower eye-teeth are through by the twentieth month, and the posterior or second molars complete the set at the age of two to two and a half years. (Fig. 59.) This is the usual sequence, but variations are quite common. Thus, the upper central incisors may come through before the lower, and in some instances the set is never completed. If the child is affected with

rickets, teething may be considerably delayed.

One of the troubles of teething is the dribbling of saliva, so that it is necessary frequently to change the bibs. The child may be feverish at night, although during the day he may seem to be quite comfortable. If on examination of the gum it is evident that a tooth is about to be cut, the process may be expedited by gently rubbing the gum with the point of the finger. In these circumstances a little bromide of potash will be useful in doses of from 1 to 5 grains dissolved in water and syrup, and the gums may be rubbed also with the medicine. If the mouth becomes sore, so that sucking is painful, the finger should be dipped in boric acid and glycerin and the child allowed to suck it, and the mouth should be cleaned out with wool soaked in weak solution of borax and tincture of myrrh—half a drachm of each with a drachm of glycerin and rosewater to the ounce. In these cases of sore mouth the glands under the jaw or at the side of the face may be tender and enlarged ; if so, they should be fomented. Skin eruptions are another frequent complication of teething ; they may be eczematous, or may take the form of nettle-rash or red gum. The treatment of these eruptions is described in the articles on those subjects, but in addition the bowels should be cleared out by a powder, as follows :

Grey powder .... ½ grain
Bicarbonate of soda .... 2 grains
Bromide of ammonium .... 2 grains
Cinnamon .... ½ grain
Send six powders. One to be given twice a day.

These powders are also useful in checking the diarrhœa, vomiting, and stomach-ache which are sometimes caused by teething, etc. During dentition it is particularly desirable that food should not be given in excess or at irregular hours. If digestive troubles occur, the milk, if the child is bottle-fed, should be further diluted with water, or peptonized (p. 91) or a third of its volume of lime-water added. Occasionally teething is accompanied by convulsions, the treatment of which is described in the article on that subject. In cases where the child's health is seriously disturbed, the gums may have to be lanced, but this is seldom necessary, and should be avoided whenever possible.

When the milk teeth have been cut, they should receive more care and attention than is often bestowed upon them, for the permanent teeth are greatly influenced by their predecessors. They ought to be cleansed regularly with warm water, and any fragments of food removed from their interstices, and if possible they should be inspected at regular intervals by the dentist. Whatever care is taken of them, however, they will begin to disappear about the age of six to make way for the *permanent teeth*, thirty-two in number (Fig. 60). The first to come through are the front molars ; then, about the age of seven, appear the central incisors, and next, at eight, the lateral incisors. At nine the front bicuspids replace the first

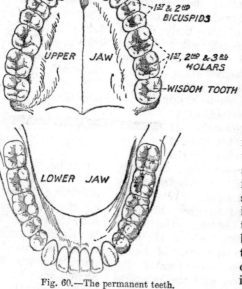

Fig. 60.—The permanent teeth.

temporary molars, and at ten the back bicuspids replace the posterior molars. The canines are cut at eleven or twelve, the second molars from twelve to thirteen, and the third molars or wisdom teeth may appear from seventeen to twenty-five, or even later, or they may never come through at all. In many cases they are so decayed or ill formed that it is necessary to extract them before they come through. It is conjectured that wisdom teeth are so irregular in their behaviour because the human mouth is smaller than it was in primitive man, whose plentiful use of raw meat provided more ample exercise for the jaw. The second dentition is a much less troublesome business than the first, but in delicate children it may give rise to gastric and intestinal disturbance, and there is extra liability to bronchitis, as well as to nasal catarrh. In children whose nervous system is delicately poised, epilepsy or St. Vitus's dance may develop. Teething, however, is only the occasion, not the cause, of these affections, which would probably declare themselves under some other stress, if not under this.

TEMPERATURE, BODY.—The temperature of cold-blooded animals, such as snakes and fishes, varies with that of the surrounding medium, be it air or water ; that of warm-blooded animals, including man, remains fairly constant, whatever the temperature of the air. The normal temperature of the human body averages 98·4° Fahr. ; it fluctuates about 2° during the twenty-four hours, being lowest in the early hours of the morning, between 3 and 6 a.m., reaching the normal towards midday, being slightly higher than normal in the evening, between 5 and 8 p.m., and returning to the normal about midnight. It might be supposed, from the uncomfortable sense of heat at the surface of the body during hot weather, especially after physical exertion, that the body temperature is considerably higher than at other times. In point of fact, the temperature under such conditions is seldom more than about 1° higher than normal. It varies so little because of the automatic action of the heat-regulating mechanism, operating through the skin and controlled by the nervous system. When the body is exposed to great heat the nervous system expands the superficial blood-vessels, which therefore contain a larger quantity of blood, the sweat-glands consequently become more active, and the perspiration they pour out on the surface undergoes evaporation, by which the body is cooled. When, on the other hand, the body is exposed to cold, the blood-vessels of the skin contract, there is therefore more blood in the internal organs, and so loss of heat is prevented, while, as a result of the extra amount of blood in the interior of the body, the production of heat is stimulated—for body-heat is generated not only by muscular contractions and the movements of joints, but by the combustion of food, and the functional activity of all the

organs of secretion, absorption and excretion, as well as by chemical changes that go on within the body. Heat is lost to the body not only by radiation from the skin, but in the air expelled from the lungs in breathing, and in the excretions from the kidneys and intestines. But much the greater part of it escapes through the skin, and this is the only one of the eliminating channels which can be controlled—by the use of suitable clothing.

How to take the temperature.— The temperature is most often taken in the mouth. The bulb of the clinical thermometer (Fig. 61) should be placed not between the cheek and the teeth, but beneath one or other side of the tongue, as far back as possible, and obliquely. The mouth

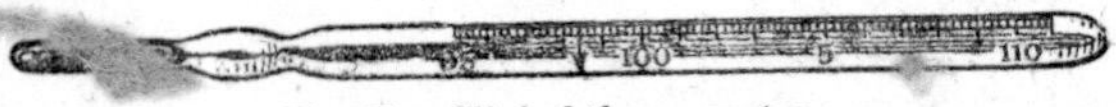

Fig. 61.—Clinical thermometer.

must be tightly closed, so that no cold air may enter, the patient breathing through the nose and holding the instrument with the lips, not with the teeth. This precaution must be rigidly carried out if accuracy is to be ensured, and the patient must, of course, be careful not to talk. Sometimes the temperature cannot be conveniently or correctly taken in the mouth ; if so, the thermometer may be placed in the armpit and the arm held against the side of the chest. This method requires a longer time than the other. Sometimes, especially in children, the thermometer is inserted in the bowel, being pushed up for a distance of about two inches. It should be remembered that the temperature is usually about half a degree less under the armpit, and nearly one degree more in the bowel, than in the mouth. After the temperature has been read, the mercury should be shaken down, and the instrument washed, not in hot water, which might break the glass, but in cold.

TENO-SYNOVITIS.—This is the technical name for inflammation of the sheaths of the tendons or "leaders" about the wrist or the ankle-joint. It may be the result of a sudden severe strain, as after a jump from a height, or in taking a stroke at golf, or it may be due to a poison, such as that of the gonococcus, the germ of gonorrhœa. The pain comes on abruptly, and rapidly becomes worse, but is only felt when the tendons are moved. Its most common site is the wrist, which feels stiff and weak. If the hand is placed on the affected part while the joint is in movement a creaking sensation can be felt, caused by friction between the tendon and its sheath. In treatment the most important thing is rest; to this may be added rubbing with camphor or some other stimulating liniment. As soon as the joint can be moved without much pain, gentle movements should be performed once or twice daily, to prevent adhesions. This may be followed by massage. When the patient returns to his ordinary employment he will do well, if the trouble has been in the wrist, to wear a wristlet for a time.

TETANUS (*see* LOCKJAW).

TETANY.—This disease must not be confused with tetanus (lockjaw), although the muscular spasms which are the principal symptoms somewhat resemble those of the more serious disease. It most often attacks rickety children, but is sometimes met with in adults, and occasionally occurs in epidemics. The cause is probably a deficiency of calcium salt. The spasms are often preceded by sensations of tingling and numbness, and it is usually the hands and feet that are most affected by them. They may cause a good deal of pain and tenderness. In some cases they pass off in a few months; in others, they may last for years. They are more alarming than dangerous. Warm baths during the attack sometimes have a beneficial effect. In children the bowels should be moved by a dose of castor oil or, if necessary, by enemata, and the general health must be carefully supervised. Sedatives are required, and the doctor may prescribe chloral or one of the bromides.

THERMOMETER, CLINICAL (*see* TEMPERATURE, BODY).

THREADWORMS (*see* WORMS).

THROAT, FOREIGN BODIES IN (*see* FOREIGN BODIES).

THROAT, SORE (*see* SORE THROAT).

THROMBOSIS (*see* ARTERIES, DISEASES OF).

THRUSH.—Other forms of inflammation of the mouth have been considered in the article MOUTH, INFLAMMATION OF; here we have to deal with the form which is due to the growth, in the mucous membrane of the mouth, of a fungus known as *Oïdium albicans*. It is most common during the first few weeks of life, and is generally the result of lack of cleanliness and unsuitable food. In older children, in adults, and in the elderly, it sometimes appears in the wasting stages of exhausting diseases. It is contagious, and is sometimes communicated from child to child by the feeding-bottle. The notion that everyone must have an attack of thrush, and that it occurs either in the first or the last month of life, is, of course, a mere superstition, which has no other foundation than the fact that the affection most often occurs in infants and that if it occurs in the aged it is usually in the final stages of a fatal disease.

Symptoms.—First the inside of the mouth is hot, dry and tender. Then round, milk-white spots appear which join each other, forming flakes with a white, curd-like covering. The upper surface of the tongue, the inside of the lips and cheeks, are the parts affected, and the fungus may spread backwards to the throat, and into the gullet, and thus into the stomach and intestine. The mouth becomes very tender, and the child can only suck with pain and difficulty.

Treatment.—The child's mouth should be brushed after each feed with a solution of sulphite of soda, one drachm to the ounce, followed by the application of glycerin of borax. If this proves unavailing, a solution of carbolic acid, 2 grains to the ounce, may be tried. The bowels should be regulated with magnesia, and the child should be as much as possible in the open air. If the mouth is so sore than he cannot suck, the medical attendant will have to feed him artificially by passing a tube through the nose into the throat. The most rigid cleanliness must be practised in feeding. *Prevention* consists in carefully cleansing the teat and feeding-bottles. If breast-feeding is not available, the milk should be sterilized and mixed with a little lime water or a little bicarbonate of soda.

THYMUS GLAND (*see* DUCTLESS GLANDS).

THYROID EXTRACT (*see* ORGANOTHERAPY).

THYROID GLAND (*see* DUCTLESS GLANDS).

TIC-DOULOUREUX (*see* NEURALGIA).

TICS.—A tic is a convulsive movement, gentle or violent, which may at the outset have been instigated by some external cause, but has become habitual and purposeless. For example, a grain of dust blown into the eye will cause blinking. The blinking may be repeated when the irritation has subsided, until it becomes habitual; it is then a tic. The variety of tics is endless. One of the most common of them is blinking; others are licking, sucking, biting, pouting, nibbling, mumbling, head-nodding, head-tossing, scratching, rubbing, scraping, stroking, tapping, etc. They occur in both sexes and at any age, except in very young children. They are associated with nervous instability, though in some cases it may be very slight, and they are predisposed to by fatigue, anxiety, worry, mental or physical strain. They disappear in sleep, and seldom occur when the attention is engaged or the mind is concentrated. In some cases the impulse to the act is almost irresistible, and its suppression is attended with a feeling of malaise; in others it is a mere habit, acquired imitatively or from a wish to attract attention. In treatment, attention to the general health is important. The patient should endeavour to avoid the movement for a longer and longer time each day, and should exercise the muscles involved in it. Bromide of potash, 5-grain doses in half a wineglassful of water thrice a day, continued for many weeks, may be beneficial.

TINEA CIRCINATA (*see* RINGWORM).

TINEA CRURIS (*see* DHOBIE'S ITCH).

TINEA TONSURANS (*see* RINGWORM).

TINNITUS (*see* EAR, NOISES IN).

TOBACCO (*see* NARCOTICS AND HYPNOTICS).

TOBACCO BLINDNESS (*see* BLINDNESS).

TOENAIL, INGROWING (*see* NAILS, DISEASES OF).

TONGUE, APPEARANCE OF, IN DISEASE.—Fur on the tongue is the result of a thickening of the surface layer, caused in many cases by the accumulation of food particles, germs, etc., mixed with saliva and mucus. The colour ranges from white to dark brown or black, but a dark colour in itself means little, for it may be due to smoking or chewing tobacco, or to taking medicines of which iron is one of the ingredients. A furred tongue is not an infallible indication that something is wrong with the health. Some persons normally have what is called a " dirty " tongue, which in their case is no indication of digestive disorder. Those who sleep with the mouth open, again, may have fur on the tongue in the morning, but it will disappear after breakfast. On the other hand, there are disorders in which the tongue remains clean, and this is even so in some cases of indigestion. Generally, however, the furred tongue is a sign of disordered health. It may be a sick headache, catarrh of the stomach and intestines, inflammation of the mouth or tonsils, kidney disease, or fever. In gout the tongue is coated with a brownish fur. In rheumatic fever a very thick white fur is seen. In other fevers the fur may be brownish. In scarlet fever one of the most unmistakable signs is the " strawberry tongue " (*see* SCARLET FEVER). Fur may cover the whole tongue, or may be limited to the middle and back of it. If present on one side only, it may be due to neuralgia of one side of the face, or to irritation from the teeth on one side, or to inflammation of one tonsil. In anæmia, general debility, and long-continued indigestion, the tongue may be large and flabby, and at its edges may be seen dents caused by pressure against the teeth. In acute peritonitis it is small and contracted. In diabetes it may be red and cracked, and may look like raw beef. Sore spots or ulcers at the sides or back of the tongue suggest indigestion, but they may be, on the other hand, an indication of syphilis. In thrush the throat, as well as other parts of the mouth, may be inflamed from the growth of the fungus of that disease. In alcoholics and the subjects of general paralysis of the insane the tongue, when put out, is tremulous. In one-sided paralysis and other diseases in which the muscles of the tongue are paralysed, it is protruded to one side instead of keeping the middle line. In St. Vitus's dance it is put out and drawn back with a jerk.

TONGUE, INFLAMMATION OF.—Glossitis, to give this affection its technical name, may be set up by biting, cutting, pricking, or scalding the tongue, or by exposure to wet and cold, but it is often difficult to trace the cause. The tongue swells, and there is severe throbbing or burning pain, increased by swallowing or speaking or by mastication. Generally, after three or four days the inflammation and swelling begin to subside, and disappear in about a week or ten days from the onset. *Treatment.*—Give a good dose of whatever aperient the patient is accustomed to take, and let him wash out the mouth with hot water, or suck ice, whichever is found to give the greater relief. Chlorate of potash (10 grains to the ounce) may be added to the mouth-wash. The outside of the throat should be fomented. If an abscess can be found, the surgeon should incise it. He may consider it advisable to draw blood by making small pricks in the tongue with a sharp-pointed instrument, or a long cut on either side of the middle line, or by applying leeches externally. Every endeavour should be made to induce the patient, in spite of the pain, to take warm fluid food, such as milk and water, in small quantities at a time.

TONGUE-TIE.—The frænum, or " rein," of the tongue, the band near the tip of its lower surface which prevents it from being drawn back into the throat, is in some infants too tight, so that they are unable to suck properly. The defect is usually cured by putting the band on the stretch, snipping the edge with a blunt-pointed pair of scissors, and then tearing through the rest of it sufficiently to give the requisite freedom of movement. Simple as this operation is, it must not be attempted by an unskilled person.

TONSILLITIS, ACUTE.—This affection is sometimes regarded as identical with quinsy, but in the latter an abscess forms in the tissues adjoining, but outside, the tonsils (*see* Quinsy), while in the former it is the tonsils themselves that are inflamed, and usually without the formation of an abscess. In some cases, however, the two conditions occur together. The disease, which is common between the ages of ten and thirty, may be " caught " from contaminated water or milk, and is sometimes infectious as between one case and another. It is more common in spring and autumn than in the other seasons. Sewer gas, overwork in a vitiated atmosphere, and anxiety are believed to act as predisposing causes. Enlarged tonsils are more liable to attack than normal tonsils. In some cases a rheumatic or gouty element appears to be present.

Symptoms.—Acute tonsillitis may begin with malaise, prostration, thirst, loss of appetite, and feverishness. In other cases, besides symptoms such as these, with headache and backache, there is a sense of fullness in the throat, amounting to sharp pain which radiates up to the ear, and makes swallowing difficult. In both cases alike the voice soon becomes muffled. The senses of smell and taste, and sometimes that of hearing, are lost. Both tonsils are usually affected together. The glands in the corner of the lower jaw swell and become extremely tender, so that the head is held stiffly; the temperature may rise as high as 105° Fahr. In many instances the breath is foul, the tongue is coated, and in acute cases can only be protruded with difficulty. In mild cases the trouble may last only three or four days; more often it is not until the fifth day that the symptoms begin to abate.

Treatment. — The doctor will probably begin by ordering a purge, such as 2 to 4 grains of calomel with 3 grains of bicarbonate of soda, placed on the tongue and washed down with a sip of milk, and followed in about eight hours by a black draught or a few teaspoonfuls of Rochelle salts. In many cases salicylate of soda is beneficial—10 grains, repeated in an hour, then in two hours, and afterwards at three-hourly intervals, or as required. If there is headache or neuralgia, antipyrin may also be given, 3 to 5 grains being added to each dose of the salicylate. In cases where salicylate of soda is not considered suitable, aspirin or a dose of salol (3 to 5 grains) may be given. Some paint the tonsils with 5 per cent. menthol and guaiacol in almond oil, or, in milder cases, with 25-per-cent. argyrol. The neck should be covered with a hot fomentation. As in quinsy, it may be easier to swallow some semi-solid food, such as custard puddings, or beef tea thickened with arrowroot, than liquids. It is less painful to suck fluids through a straw than to attempt to drink them. Lemon squash in which the whites of eggs have been broken up can be taken in this way. When the symptoms have subsided the patient should be put upon a nourishing diet, and tonics such as quinine and iron, or in children syrup of iodide of iron, given ; and restoration to normal health will be promoted by a change of air.

TONSILLITIS, CHRONIC (*see* TONSILS, ENLARGED).

TONSILS, ENLARGED. — As childhood advances, the tonsils tend to shrink, but in many children they begin to enlarge about the age of three or four, sometimes following an attack of scarlet fever, measles, diphtheria, or whooping-cough, or repeated attacks of acute tonsillitis. The condition appears to " run in families," and is often associated with adenoids. Occasionally it is met with in adults. It is sometimes called chronic tonsillitis, but " tonsillitis " means inflammation of the tonsils, and as inflammation may be absent the term is better avoided.

Symptoms.—The tone of the voice becomes thick and " woolly," speech may be indistinct, and there may be slight deafness. Swallowing is somewhat difficult, and a lump may be constantly felt in the throat. In many cases there is indigestion, and the patient is very likely to retch if the mouth is widely opened, as for inspection. In some cases complaint is made of a " rotten " taste in the mouth, and offensive " cheesy " matter may be spat out. From the absorption of such matter the general health is affected, as evidenced by anæmia, languor, and general feebleness. In many cases the glands of the neck are enlarged. The patient breathes through the mouth instead of through the nose, snores, and suffers from shortness of breath, but it is not always possible to determine how far these symptoms are set up by overgrown tonsils and how far by adenoids. In bad cases the tonsils may be so large as to meet each other. In exceptional instances the enlarged tonsils may cause no great inconvenience, and may persist through life, and only be discovered by accident. If not so bad as to necessitate removal, they usually disappear at puberty.

Treatment.—In slight and early cases the enlargement may be arrested by gargling with a solution of resorcin (1 in 200), by brushing the tonsils daily with a paint of carbolic acid (15 grains) and glycerin of tannin (1 ounce), by giving a course of Parrish's food or cod-liver oil with syrup of iodide of iron, and by taking the child to the seaside. In most cases, however, it is better that the tonsils should be removed. For the first twenty-four hours after this little operation the diet should be limited to iced milk, and for the next day or two to milk and soft foods.

TOOTHACHE (*see* TEETH, DECAY OF).

TOPHI (*see* GOUT).

TORTICOLLIS (*see* WRY-NECK).

TOURNIQUET (*see* HÆMORRHAGE).

TRACHEOTOMY (*see* DIPH-THERIA).

TRACHOMA (*see* CONJUNCTI-VITIS).

TRANSFUSION OF BLOOD.— As a remedy for shock to the system (*see* SHOCK) which is associated with serious hæmorrhage, blood is some-times transfused from an artery or vein of the person who consents to act as " donor " into one of the patient's veins. The method has of late years been coming into more frequent use, and some large hospitals now have a regular service of donors.

TREMORS.—Trembling is seen in an extreme form in certain organic nervous diseases, such as paralysis agitans, popularly called " shaking palsy," which forms the subject of a separate article. It is often present in old age, and when due to senility is not amenable to remedy. In younger persons it may occur as a result of the excessive use of alcohol, tea or tobacco, or from taking large doses of certain medicines. In such cases it ceases with the correction of the faulty habit or the discontinuance of the drug. It may also be a symp-tom of debility, in which case the remedy consists in bringing the health up to par by tonics, plenty of nourish-ing food, and avoidance of worry and excitement.

TRENCH FEVER.—This fever was first recognized among troops during the War, but cases sometimes occur among civilians. It is caused by a microbe which has not been definitely identified, but which is undoubtedly conveyed by lice—not by their bites, but by their crushed bodies or their excreta being rubbed into the abraded skin. It is charac-terized by intermittent " burning " or " tearing " pains in the shins, knees, ankles, elbows, forearms and shoulder-

blades, associated with great tender-ness. The disease may become chronic and persist for months. In the acute stage benefit may be derived from phenacetin and caffeine, or aspirin, or compound powder of ipecacuanha. In the later stages, to relieve the pains, a mixture contain-ing colchicum wine (10 minims) and iodide of potash (2 grains) may be given three times a day for one week, or for two ; useful local applications are hot or cold compresses or evapora-ting lead lotion or menthol ointment.

TRIANGULAR BANDAGES (*see* BANDAGES).

TRICHIASIS (*see* EYELASHES, INGROWING).

TRICHINOSIS. — This disease, sometimes called *trichinelliasis*, is rare in this country, and much more frequent in Germany, where uncooked or imperfectly-cooked pork is freely eaten. It is named after a tiny worm, *Trichina* (or *Trichinella*) *spiralis*, which is the cause of it. This parasite is communicated to man by eating the uncooked or insufficiently-cooked flesh of infected pigs, rabbits, oxen and other animals. When such meat is eaten, the worms are set free in the human intestine, and the embryos penetrate the intes-tinal wall, enter the muscles, and there remain, setting up severe local pain as well as general symptoms. Death may occur in the third or fourth week or later, from suffocation, ex-haustion or bronchitis. In less severe cases the symptoms gradually subside as the parasites settle down in the muscles. If the worms are to be prevented from invading the muscles they must be removed from the stomach by an emetic, taken as soon as the patient begins to feel ill, and from the intestine by brisk purges. A dose of mustard-and-water is a suitable emetic ; for the purge, a black draught, followed by another a few hours later, and this by periodic doses of calomel during the first five or six weeks. When once the parasites have worked their way through the walls of the intestine, it is too late to effect a cure, and nothing can be done beyond supporting the patient's strength with good food and stimulants, and treating the symptoms—the pain with hot baths and aspirin, and if necessary with morphia, the profuse sweats with atropine.

TRIONAL (*see* NARCOTICS AND HYPNOTICS).

TROPICAL ANÆMIA (*see* MINER'S ANAEMIA).

TROPICAL LIVER.—This rather loose term covers all those irregularities of the liver that are frequent in hot climates, from mere occasional " sluggishness " to inflammation. As the result of too luxurious a life with too little exercise, the liver becomes congested. One step further and the congestion passes into actual inflammation, with sharp pain in the liver and with fever. The patient grows thin, feeble, anæmic and sallow, and at last sinks into chronic invalidism. *Treatment.*—If inflammation of the liver is present the patient must keep to his bed and go upon a milk diet ; free purges must be given at night, and 20-grain doses of chloride of ammonium, well diluted with water, three or four times a day ; and large hot poultices should be applied all over the liver region. In dysenteric cases emetine (*see* DYSENTERY) must be administered ; in malarial cases, quinine. Cases that have not passed the congestive stage may be treated less drastically. Here the remedy consists chiefly in simple living and ample though not excessive exercise ; but the bowels should be regulated by saline aperients, such as Carlsbad salts.

TRUE CROUP (*see* CROUP).

TRYPANOSOMIASIS.—This disease, which prevails extensively in Central Africa, is due to infection with parasites belonging to the genus of trypanosomes, communicated by the bite of the tse-tse fly. It is virtually confined to narrow belts along the banks of rivers and the shores of lakes, for it is in such belts that the tse-tse fly dwells. In South America a similar disease, caused by another species of trypanosome, is disseminated by the bite of a bug. The patient has successive feverish attacks, he becomes anæmic, and enfeebled both in mind and in body. The glands in the neck and elsewhere swell, and cramps, neuralgic pains and inflammatory swellings may supervene. In most cases the spleen is enlarged, and there may also be enlargement of the liver. In a few cases the disease now begins to subside ; in others, cerebral symptoms appear, and the patient either succumbs, or gradually passes into the *sleeping-sickness stage*, and, unless carried off by some complicating disease, finally dies in a state of coma, or life flickers out from sheer weakness. It is only in the earlier stages that treatment can do more than delay the fatal termination. It consists in injecting the drug known as " Bayer 205," or preparations of arsenic and antimony.

TUBERCULIN (*see under* TUBERCULOSIS).

TUBERCULOSIS.—The most common form of tuberculosis is that popularly called consumption (q.v.), that is, tuberculosis of the lungs. But tuberculosis may attack many other organs than the lungs. All forms of tuberculosis alike are due to the activities of the tubercle bacillus, a thin, rod-shaped germ which in a dry condition may remain alive and capable of mischief for some six to nine months, if not longer. It may enter the body through the air-passages, as when infected dust is inhaled in the street or in the house in which a consumptive person dwells, or through the digestive organs, as when the imperfectly cooked flesh of tuberculous animals is eaten or the milk of tuberculous cows is drunk. It may also gain entrance through a wound or slight abrasion of the skin.

Perhaps the most frequent source of tuberculous infection is air-borne dust. A patient carelessly expectorates in the street, the sputum containing the bacilli dries, and the bacilli are carried with the dust into the air-passages of wayfarers. Or the disease may be inhaled indoors, if a tuberculous patient dwells in the house, and even when the sputum is received into a closed vessel, for the germ is contained not only in the expectoration but in the tiny particles of moisture which are expelled from the mouth in coughing. If the bacillus is so widely diffused, and may so easily be inhaled or taken into the body with meat and milk, it may seem strange at first that so many of us appear to escape its attacks. The fact is that most of us *are* attacked, and the germs even find lodgment in the body. From examination of the bodies of persons who during life have been free from tuberculous symptoms, it has been found that over 60 per cent. of the whole population bear scars of early tuberculous infection of the lungs, and if the other forms of tuberculosis are included the percentage is very much larger. The reason why, in so many cases, the germ fails to establish itself in its human host is

that the tissues of the body, unless their vitality is lowered by vitiated air, lack of light, or other unhygienic conditions, by dust, alcoholism, or, it may be, an hereditary predisposition —although this factor is doubtful— are able to offer to it a successful resistance, so that it is only when the germs attack in great force (" massive infection "), or a person is repeatedly exposed to infection, that they are able to work mischief. Fortunately, they rapidly succumb to light. Direct sunlight kills them in three minutes, and daylight in a few days. Probably, therefore, most of the germs we inhale in dust are either dead or inert.

One of the commonest forms of tuberculosis is that in which the lymphatic glands, especially the glands of the neck, are infected (*see* ADENITIS). When the skin is affected the disease is termed lupus vulgaris (q.v.). The stomach is seldom the seat of tuberculosis because the gastric juice exercises a restraining effect upon the germs, without, however, destroying them. Passing into the intestine, they may set up tuberculosis there and in the intestinal glands (*see* CONSUMPTION OF THE BOWELS). If the peritoneum is invaded, we have a form of peritonitis (*see* PERITONITIS, CHRONIC) ; if the membranes covering the brain, meningitis is set up (*see* MENINGITIS, TUBERCULOUS). Tuberculosis of the bones and joints is considered in the articles BONE, DISEASES OF, and HIP-DISEASE ; tuberculosis of the suprarenal glands, the glands above the kidneys, is noted under ADDISON'S DISEASE.

We have now mentioned all the chief forms of tuberculosis, but sometimes, in children who are debilitated by measles or some other illness, or by lack of nourishment, the disease is not confined to a single organ but is generalized. In such cases it runs a very rapid course, and ends in death in from one or two to five or six weeks in acute cases, while in other cases the child gradually wastes to a skeleton, and at last dies from exhaustion or some complication such as pneumonia or meningitis.

The best treatment for tuberculosis is hygienic—fresh air and sunlight, carefully regulated exercise, abundant nourishment. Drugs are of little avail, but *tuberculin*, which consists of the dead bodies or the products of tubercle bacilli, is gradually finding its true place as the most serviceable of all the adjuncts of hygienic treatment. It was introduced by Koch in 1881, but the claims made for it were put far too high, and it was used with such little discrimination that the results were disappointing, and in many cases disastrous, and before long it fell into disfavour. The reaction has now spent itself, and the best authorities hold that tuberculin is not only of the greatest value in diagnosis, but in carefully selected cases is extremely valuable as a supplement to general treatment.

TUBERCULOSIS OF BONE
(*see* BONE, DISEASES OF).

TUBERCULOSIS OF THE HIP-JOINT (*see* HIP-DISEASE).

TUBERCULOUS MENINGITIS
(*see* MENINGITIS, TUBERCULOUS).

TUMOURS.—In medical literature the word tumour may denote a swelling due to any cause, or a new growth. It is in the latter sense that the term is used here. So used, it indicates, as one authority expresses it, " a new formation of tissue which . . . serves no useful purpose in the economy." Tumours are divided into two great classes—(1) benign, innocent or simple tumours, and (2) malig-

nant tumours. The *benign* tumour is generally enclosed in a capsule or covering which separates it from the surrounding parts. It does not invade and destroy the tissues around it, except that if it attains a very large size it may by mere pressure absorb them. It can only, speaking generally, endanger life by its position, as for instance when it grows on the larynx (voice-box) and obstructs breathing, or by becoming so large as to interfere with the functions of some vital organ. A *malignant* tumour, on the other hand, gradually encroaches upon and destroys the surrounding tissues, and, moreover, it undergoes dissemination —that is, by means of the lymph or the blood it is carried to other parts of the body, such as the lungs or the liver, and there begins to grow again. Both innocent and malignant tumours are divided into groups according to the tissues of which they are composed. The two great groups of malignant tumours are dealt with separately under CANCER and SARCOMA. Of innocent tumours there are many groups, among them *lipomas*, composed of fatty tissue ; *fibromas*, of fibrous tissue ; *chondromas*, of cartilage ; *osteomas*, of bone ; *myelomas*, of marrow ; *myomas*, of muscle ; *neuromas* and *gliomas*, of nerve tissue ; *angiomas*, of blood-vessels or lymph-vessels (*see* BIRTH-MARKS) ; *adenomas*, of glandular tissue ; and *papillomas*, of epithelium (*see* WARTS). There is scarcely any part of the body in which tumours may not arise, but the organs in which they most frequently occur are the stomach and the womb. All malignant tumours should be thoroughly extirpated at a very early stage, before they have begun to disseminate (*see* CANCER ; SARCOMA). Whether or not the removal of innocent tumours is necessary depends upon their situation and size. If from the one cause or the other they interfere with vital functions, or by pressure on nerves cause great pain, they should obviously, if possible, be excised.

TURKISH BATH (*see* BATHS).

TURPENTINE POISONING.— Oil of turpentine may be taken in mistake for some other medicine, or the liniment prepared from it may be drunk. For treatment, give an emetic (*see* EMETICS), and when this has acted follow it up with half-an-ounce of Epsom salts in half-a-tumblerful of water. Milk, white of egg, and barley water are also useful for their soothing effects on the alimentary canal.

TURPENTINE STUPES (*see* FOMENTATIONS).

TWILIGHT SLEEP.—This is the popular designation of the condition induced in a woman in labour by the injection of scopolamine (also called hyoscine) and morphia. The patient so treated sinks into a condition of semi-consciousness or unconsciousness, and although during the pains she may moan, she has no recollection afterwards of any incident of her ordeal. The treatment has distinct advantages, especially in the case of nervous and highly strung women, and in certain abnormal uterine conditions, but it is not free from danger, and it has other drawbacks, among them its expensiveness, for the doctor must be in closer attendance, and the patient must never be left by the nurse. Whether the treatment is advisable in any given case, it should be left to the doctor to decide.

TYMPANITES (*see* FLATULENCE).

TYPHLITIS (*see* BOWELS, INFLAMMATION OF).

TYPHOID FEVER.—In medical literature this disease is more frequently called enteric fever, from *enteron*, intestine, since it attacks chiefly the intestines—the small intestine, which becomes the seat of ulcers. It is sometimes popularly called *gastric fever*, but this term should be avoided, for in enteric fever the stomach is not specially affected. It may occur at almost any age, but seldom late in life ; the period of greatest frequency is between the ages of fifteen and thirty. Second attacks are infrequent.

Mortality.—As the result of better sanitary conditions, improved methods of treatment and more skilful nursing, the mortality of typhoid fever in this country has gradually diminished. It varies in different epidemics, and is influenced by the age and sex of the patient. The disease is more dangerous in women than in men. In children it is less so, and the mortality is lowest between the ages of five and ten. The patient's previous health is an important factor ; alcoholism, chronic disease of lung and of kidney, obesity and pregnancy are all unfavourable antecedents.

Cause.—The typhoid bacillus, *Bacillus typhosus*, was discovered by Eberth in 1880–1. It is now made use of to distinguish typhoid fever from diseases with which it might in the early stages be confused. This method of diagnosis turns on the discovery made by Widal, a French physician, that when some of the blood serum, i.e. the fluid part of the blood, taken from a patient suffering from this disease, is brought into contact with living typhoid bacilli, they are seen, when examined under the microscope, to become heaped together in masses, and their power of motion is destroyed. This test is known as Widal's reaction.

Infection.—The bacillus is communicated by the intestinal evacuations or the urine ; it is not conveyed by the breath or the perspiration.

Most frequently the infection is water-borne. Thus, the evacuations of a patient suffering from the disease may be thrown, without being disinfected, into a privy or on to the ground and some of the material finds its way into a brook which affords drinking water, or which communicates with a well. Or the water-pipes in a town may be leaky, and at one spot may pass through soil soaked with the sewage from a house where a case of the disease exists. Or linen soiled by the discharges from a case may go to a laundry where the slops leak into a well supplying neighbouring houses. The poison, again, may be sucked up from a water-closet into a cistern which also supplies drinking water.

Milk is another means by which typhoid is disseminated. The infection has been traced to the use of polluted water for diluting the milk or for washing the pans, and sometimes to the milk being contaminated by typhoid " carriers," i.e. persons who, though not themselves suffering from typhoid fever, harbour the germs of the disease. The disease has been contracted by eating oysters infected by the discharge of sewage into the sea in the proximity of oyster-beds. It has also been communicated by the consumption of uncooked vegetables that have been watered during growth, or washed before being brought to the table, with contaminated water. It has been shown, too, that insects, such as the house-fly, may pollute food with infective particles which they carry on their antennæ and legs. It is doubtful whether noxious smells from drains or water-closets are capable of actually causing typhoid, though, by depressing the general health, they may be a contributory factor. In any case, closed and un-ventilated drains are the more harmful. A drain thoroughly open to the air may be offensive but is not dangerous, and a sewage farm, if properly managed, is quite harmless. Evidence has been found that dust may convey the poison in a dry state, and that articles of food and drink may thus be contaminated. This applies more especially to the disease as met with in warm countries.

Incubation period and symptoms.—The incubation period varies from two or three days to three or even four weeks, the average being from ten to fourteen days. The patient feels out of sorts ; he then becomes feverish, the skin hot and dry, and there are pains in the limbs and back, chills, headache, lassitude and drowsiness. He now usually takes to his bed, and is found to have a temperature of 103° or 104° Fahr. ; the pulse is rapid, the tongue swollen, moist and furred. He is thirsty, his abdomen is tender, especially on the right side, and even at this stage there may be some diarrhœa, though constipation is more common. He complains of sleeplessness and of headache, the skin perspires profusely, and the urine is high-coloured. In the second week the fever may reach its height—say 105° Fahr. in the evenings, falling 1° or $1\frac{1}{2}°$ in the mornings. The headache now usually disappears, the pulse is quicker, the skin remains moist, the tongue has a white or yellowish fur but remains red at the edges and the tip, the diarrhœa increases, and the motions have a characteristic " pea-soup " appearance and a very offensive odour. As the second week nears its end the rash may appear. It is present in about 75 per cent. of the cases, and consists of small, separate, round, rose-coloured spots, about the size of a pin's head, which come out on the abdomen, chest and back, occasionally on the arms and legs, in successive crops, generally until about the third week, but sometimes much longer. During the third week the symptoms either gradually subside, as happens in mild cases, or become more severe. Convalescence, in favourable cases, begins in the fourth week. The temperature falls, and natural sleep returns, together with appetite and strength. In some cases, however, the fever does not begin to subside till the end of the fourth week, or even until the fifth or sixth week.

Types of typhoid.—There is great variety in the severity of the symptoms, and some cases are so mild that only with difficulty can they be recognized as typhoid cases; these cases form the *ambulatory* or *walking* types of typhoid. The case may run the same mild course throughout, or very serious symptoms may supervene, with a fatal termination. There is also a *bilious* form of typhoid, in which there is a continuous vomiting of bile. In children, typhoid is sometimes known as *infantile remittent fever*, so called because in the evening the temperature is 2° or 3° higher than in the morning. When the fever comes to an end in the second week it is known as *abortive typhoid* or *fourteen-day fever*.

Relapses.—Typhoid fever is a disease which is peculiarly liable to relapse. This sets in, on an average, about five days after the fever has completely subsided, though it may be deferred for three weeks or longer. It is of shorter duration than the original attack, lasting from nine to twenty-one days; the symptoms are not so severe, and rarely prove fatal. A second, third, or even fourth relapse may occur.

Complications.—The gravest of the complications to be apprehended in typhoid fever is *perforation of the bowel*, due to rupture of an intestinal ulcer; this occurs usually after the second week, more frequently in men than in women, and in about 3 per cent. of the cases. Operation then offers the only chance of recovery. *Hæmorrhage*, another serious complication, which occurs rather more frequently than perforation, is also due to the intestinal ulceration. Even the worst cases, however, may recover. This complication is not usual in children.

Treatment.—All that can be done by the use of drugs is to meet symptoms as they arise. If the temperature rises as high as 102° Fahr. a powder may be taken three times a day in the form of a cachet containing 2 grains of sulphate of quinine, 4 grains of phenacetin and 1 grain of citrate of caffeine. If fever is excessive, the bath and the cold pack must be used (*see* FEVER). If there is sleeplessness, the doctor may order 20 grains of trional, or 10 grains of Dover's powder. Constipation, if severe, should be dealt with, not by purgatives, but by enemas of glycerin, olive oil, or soap and water. During the first week of the illness, however, calomel in 2-grain doses once a day for two or three days in succession is beneficial. Diarrhœa, if excessive, should be treated by injections of 4 ounces of weak starch and water with 20 drops of laudanum, or the latter may be taken by the mouth. Benefit is also obtained from the use of antiseptics to prevent fermentation and flatulence.

In no disease is *good nursing* more important than in typhoid fever. The patient must be kept absolutely at rest in bed from the beginning until convalescence is established.

Diet is of the utmost importance. Typhoid patients used to be restricted to fluids, but statistics show that they do better on a more liberal fare, which better sustains the patient's strength. It was supposed that solid food passing over the ulcers in the intestine might tend to cause hæmorrhage, or perforation; but solid food, if digestible, is reduced to liquid before it reaches the ileum, the part of the intestine where ulceration usually occurs. The patient should have a milk diet for twenty-four or forty-eight hours, the milk being diluted with water or barley-water; if there are curds in the stools the milk may be peptonized (*see* p. 91). Then, if the tongue remains moist and the appetite is good, he may be promoted to such foods as eggs, mashed potatoes and apple sauce, bread and butter, toast and butter, etc., and further additions to the diet may gradually be made as the stools return to normal. He should be encouraged to drink as much cold water or home-made (unaërated) lemonade as possible. Alcohol is sometimes required. If hæmorrhage from the bowel should take place, the patient must be kept absolutely still and flat in bed, the diet should be reduced to the most digestible foods —which must be cold, fluid, and pre-digested, and opium should be given to check all movement of the bowels. Cold must be applied to the abdomen by ice in a bag or by ice-water cloths. Turpentine, in capsules containing 10 drops, may be given every two hours.

The patient must not leave his bed until the temperature has remained normal for a week; he may sit up in an easy chair for a short time, and gradually for longer as convalescence is established. Simple tonics will hasten his recovery.

Various anti-typhoid serums have been tried, but although good results in reducing the mortality of the disease have been reported by some authorities, they have not been confirmed on a large scale. A more favourable account can be given of vaccine treatment, especially if it is begun before the tenth day of the illness. It is contra-indicated if hæmorrhage or perforation threatens, or pneumonia or middle-ear inflammation supervenes.

Prevention.—The best general means of preventing typhoid fever are the provision of a pure supply of water and of milk, the control of the shellfish and ice-cream trades, the proper disposal of sewage, and the destruction of flies and their larvæ. It was mainly, no doubt, because these conditions were secured in the War that our armies were so free from typhoid. But inoculation also counted for something—just how much, it is not easy to say. It is believed that inoculation with a mixed typhoid vaccine, consisting of the bacilli of paratyphoid fever (*see* below) as well as the typhoid germ, confers an immunity that lasts from two to four years, and that in cases in which it fails to avert the disease, the attack is usually mild and uncomplicated.

In some cases symptoms indistinguishable from those of typhoid fever are set up by germs resembling the typhoid bacillus; in such cases the disease is termed *paratyphoid fever*. It is usually milder than typhoid fever, and less protracted; but in other respects it is identical, and prevention and treatment are the same.

TYPHUS FEVER.—Epidemics of typhus fever were frequent, especially in times of war and famine, in the seventeenth and in the early years of the eighteenth century. Since that time the only great epidemic in Europe was that of 1846–7. From the earliest times Ireland has been one of the chief centres of typhus, and Russia another. Formerly England had frequent visitations of the disease, apparently by extension from Ireland; but many years ago it almost disappeared from the southern and midland towns, although it still occurs in the large centres of population in the north and in Scotland, especially those embracing a large Irish population. The predisposing causes are overcrowding, bad ventilation, filth, debility, and privation. As "jail fever," typhus was common in English prisons in the old insanitary days, and as "camp fever" it has often played havoc with armies in the field and beleaguered garrisons. The germ which is the exciting cause of the disease is transmitted by the body louse, and not, as used to be believed, from the patient's breath and other exhalations or from contaminated objects. The mortality of typhus is slightly higher than that of typhoid fever. The eruption, known as the "mulberry rash," appears first on the chest and abdomen, thence spreading to the limbs; it may last from a few days to a fortnight. From the fifteenth to the twenty-first day a crisis takes place, the patient in favourable cases falling into a quiet and deep sleep and awaking calm and refreshed with a normal temperature and a ravenous appetite. The odour emanating from the patient is very offensive, and it is most desirable in the interests both of the patient and of those in attendance that there should be an abundance of fresh air. The disease is indeed eminently suitable for open-air treatment, when the conditions are favourable.

U

ULCER OF STOMACH (*see* STOMACH, ULCER OF).

ULCER, RODENT (*see* RODENT ULCER).

ULCERS.—In ulcers there is a gradual destruction of the tissues of skin or mucous membrane. The *indolent* ulcer is so called because it is slow either to extend or to heal; the *perforating* ulcer eats its way through the tissues of a part, as when a gastric or intestinal ulcer penetrates the walls of the stomach or intestine and allows the contents to escape into the peritoneum; the *phagedænic* ulcer rapidly destroys the tissues it attacks. Gastric (with duodenal) ulcer and rodent ulcer form the subjects of separate articles. The healing of an ordinary ulcer may be promoted by the application of an ointment consisting of boric acid 1 part and vaselin 3 parts, or by dusting it with a powder composed of iodoform and boric acid. In the case of an indolent ulcer, stimulation may be employed in the form of a fly-blister applied to the thickened parts around the edges.

UMBILICAL RUPTURE (*see* RUPTURE).

UNCONSCIOUSNESS.—Consciousness may be lost from many different causes. The symptoms of each variety, and the appropriate treatment, are described in separate articles, but it will be well here to give some general rules for the treatment of unconscious patients.

In the first place, no fluid, whether alcohol, or sal-volatile, or water, must be administered during unconsciousness; it might enter the windpipe instead of the gullet, and cause death by suffocation. If the case is one of fainting, or of shock, a stimulant may be given as soon as consciousness has returned; if the case is one of apoplexy, stimulants must be withheld; they would tend to increase the bleeding on or into the brain.

So much by way of caution. The first thing to do is to lay the patient on his back in a position favourable to easy breathing. If he is wounded, the bleeding, if severe, must at once be arrested. If there is fracture or dislocation, care must be taken that the broken or dislocated limb is not moved. If no injury is present, raise the patient gently on to a bed or couch, if there is one at hand. If the face is pale and the other symptoms make it clear that the case is one of fainting or of collapse, depress the head a little beneath the general level of the body to promote the return of blood to the brain. If this cannot be done, raise the feet. If the face is flushed, as it usually is in apoplexy and in compression of the brain, slightly raise the head, taking care that it does not fall back, or fall forward so that the chin is pressed down : in either case breathing would be obstructed. Loosen all tight clothing from the neck to the waist, unfasten the top buttons of trousers, and unbutton braces in front. See also that the patient has sufficient air. If out of doors and people gather round, try to keep them at a distance ; if indoors, open the doors and windows. It is better not to remove the patient until consciousness has returned, unless this is long delayed ; but if he is out of doors and it is raining, or if he is exposed to the full rays of the sun, he should be protected with a umbrella.

UNDULANT FEVER.—This disease is sometimes spoken of as Malta fever and as Mediterranean fever, but both names are unsuitable, for the fever, though very common in Malta and in other parts of the Mediterranean, has been met with in Western Europe, as far east as China, and as far west as the United States. It is better, therefore, to call it undulant fever, a name which indicates the peculiar behaviour, in many cases, of the patient's temperature, which may ascend and descend at intervals of a few days for several months. Undulant fever is due to infection with one of the varieties of the germ called the *Micrococcus melitensis*, which is believed to be communicated by goats' milk among other media. Treatment is that for fever generally.

URÆMIA.—When the kidneys are diseased or thrown out of working order, they fail to separate from the blood the urea and other waste products formed in the body, and these act as poisons and produce serious effects upon the nervous system, such as delirium, convulsions, violent vomiting and diarrhœa, and drowsiness passing into coma (q.v.). Uræmia may be brought on by pregnancy, as well as by organic disease of the kidney. *Treatment.*— The patient must take to his bed and lie between blankets, and the doctor be called in. He will perhaps give a good dose of Epsom salts, say half-an-ounce, to procure free action of the bowels. Hot poultices and fomentations should be applied to the loins to stimulate the kidneys, while perspiration should be induced by giving hot-water or hot-air baths and injections of pilocarpine nitrate, subject to due precautions. For the nervous symptoms, sedatives and narcotics may have to be employed.

UREA (*see* Urine, Normal and Abnormal).

URETERS (*see* Urinary Organs).

URETHRA, STRICTURE OF.— If the urethra, the canal that conducts the urine from the bladder to the surface of the body, is narrowed, and the walls lose their elasticity, as often happens after gonorrhœa—though this is not the only cause of urethral stricture—a frequent desire is felt to pass water, especially at night, and the act is only accomplished by straining, while after a time it may be attended with pain. The stream may be small and twisted, or forked,

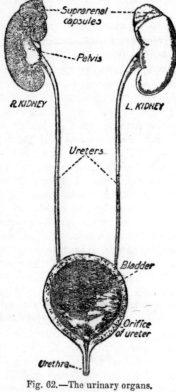

Fig. 62.—The urinary organs.

or sprayed, and may end as a mere dribble. Various complications may also arise, among them inflammation of the prostate, of the bladder, and even of the kidneys. Treatment consists in gradually dilating the passage by passing bougies of larger and larger size. This measure is usually successful, but in some cases it is unsuitable because the stricture is impassable, even to the smallest

bougie. In these and other cases operation is necessary.

URETHRITIS.—Inflammation of the urethra, described under GONORRHŒA.

URIC ACID (*see* URINE, NORMAL AND ABNORMAL ; GOUT).

URINARY CALCULI (*see* STONE IN THE BLADDER ; STONE IN THE KIDNEY).

URINARY ORGANS (Fig. 62).— The urinary organs are the kidneys, the ureters, the bladder and the urethra. The kidneys separate the urine from the blood, the ureters discharge it by little spurts into the bladder, in which it slowly accumulates, and the urethra conducts it from the bladder to the surface of the body. The *kidneys* are situated in the loins, one on each side of the spine and close to it. The ureters are attached to the kidneys above, where they swell out into a funnel-shaped sac, the pelvis ; as they descend to the bladder, they narrow ; their average width is about that of a goose quill, and the length from 14 to 16 in. The *bladder*, when moderately distended, holds about half a pint, but is capable of containing much more. In the walls of the bladder there is a good deal of muscular fibre, and by forcible contraction, aided by other muscles of the body, they can completely empty the bladder into the urethra. At the lowest part of the bladder in men, and surrounding the urethra, is the *prostate gland* (Fig. 48, p. 299), which somewhat resembles a chestnut both in size and shape. It has nothing to do with the urinary functions of the bladder, but forms a secretion which is discharged with the seminal fluid. In the male the *urethra* is about 8 in. long, and into it open ducts connected with the reproductive organs. In the female it is only ¾ inch long, and is embedded in the front wall of the vagina.

URINE, INCONTINENCE OF.— Inability to retain urine in the bladder, so that it dribbles away, even when the bladder is almost empty, is in many cases a symptom of paralysis. In other cases, especially in women, it may be caused by displacement of the surrounding parts, which drag upon the bladder and urethra. It may occur in old age from a weakened sphincter, the muscle which enables the bladder to retain its contents until the time for emptying it has come. The urine may trickle away almost constantly, but most often it only escapes after some slight exertion, as coughing or sneezing, or lifting a weight. Fortunately, incontinence of urine is in most cases amenable to surgical treatment. Another form of incontinence, in which the urine escapes because the bladder is chronically full and runs over, is considered under URINE, RETENTION OF.

For incontinence of urine in children, *see* BED-WETTING.

URINE, NORMAL AND AB-NORMAL.—Urine is secreted from the blood by the kidneys. Normally about 2½ pints (50 ounces) are secreted in the twenty-four hours, but the quantity varies greatly. In hot weather, when much more of the watery portion of the blood escapes through the skin as perspiration, the quantity of urine is diminished ; in cold weather it is increased, as it also is when large quantities of fluid are drunk (*see* POLYURIA). When the quantity is diminished the urine is highly charged with solid constituents and colouring matter. Under ordinary conditions it is a clear, amber-coloured liquid with a saltish flavour and a slight aromatic odour.

But the colour varies much even in health ; the urine may be almost as colourless as water, or dark-brown. As passed, healthy urine is acid, but on standing it becomes alkaline and has an offensive odour. If it is alkaline when freshly passed, the fact points to inflammation of the bladder.

The *specific gravity* of normal urine —i.e. its weight compared with that of pure water—varies from 1015 to 1025, the specific gravity of water being 1000. To test the specific gravity a urinometer is employed, consisting of a glass bulb which is weighted with mercury, and carries at its open end a stem graduated with a scale. If floated in pure water, it sinks until the surface of the water corresponds with the figure 0 of the scale, but if floated in normal urine it comes to rest when the level is somewhere between 15 and 25. That is to say, as urine is denser than water the urinometer does not sink so low in urine as in water. The specific gravity of urine is raised by perspiration and lowered by cold, by mental excitement and by drinking much. Occasional variations in the density of urine may be disregarded, but if the departure from the normal should persist, the urine should be examined by a doctor. Some of the water passed at night and some of that passed in the morning should be preserved for the purpose. A constant high specific gravity may point to diabetes, or to a feverish affection, etc. ; a low specific gravity to hysteria, to gouty kidney, etc.

Deposits in urine.—Of 100 parts of normal urine, 96 are water, and the remaining 4 consist of urea, common salt, phosphates, sulphates and other salts, and colouring matter derived from the blood. *Urea*, which accounts for half the weight of the solids, is a waste material of the body, of which the amount is increased by excessive exercise and in all conditions accompanied by fever. When the water has had time to cool, a sediment of a pale pink or brick-dust colour may be deposited, due to the presence of salts known as *urates* or *lithates*. Though a slight departure from the normal, their occasional presence may be ignored, but if they are frequently observed, the probability is that the diet is too rich, or is indigestible, or that the liver is not doing its work properly, or that some feverish condition is present. In most cases nothing more is necessary than to simplify the diet, drink more fluid, and stimulate the liver with an occasional aperient. If deposit in urine resembles grains of cayenne pepper, it is due to *uric acid*. This again is of little account if it occurs only occasionally and in small quantities, but occurring continually, or in large quantities, it may signify an unhealthy state of the liver or an impending attack of gout. Another urinary deposit sometimes met with is that of *phosphates*, pale-coloured and almost white. They indicate an alkaline state of the urine, and need cause no misgiving unless observed very soon after the urine is passed; in that case they suggest inflammation of the bladder or a state of general debility.

Albumin in urine.—Albumin may be detected in urine after the consumption of too much animal food. Its continuous presence points to Bright's disease (q.v.): some of the fluid part of the blood has escaped through a diseased kidney, and nutritive material which should be retained in the body is therefore lost.

Bile in urine.—When bile does not leave the body by the fæces, it is taken up by the blood, and passes out of the body chiefly in the urine, of which the colour may vary from a saffron yellow to dark brown or even black (*see* JAUNDICE).

Blood in urine. — In large quantities blood in urine is usually recognizable from the colour, but in smaller quantities there may be only a faint pink tint, or merely a thick and smoky appearance. In this case microscopic examination will be necessary; the small red blood-corpuscles can then be detected.

Mucus in urine.—Slight cloudiness, frequently seen in urine as a settlement after it has stood for some time, is caused by the presence of mucus, which comes from the lining membrane of the urinary passages. In slight quantities it has no serious meaning, but if it is passed in dense, stringy masses, so that the urine is very thick and rapidly becomes offensive, it points to inflammation either of the bladder or of the urinary passages.

Pus in urine.—When the bladder or urinary passages are inflamed, not only mucus but pus ("matter") may be present in the urine. In such water, after it has stood for a time, three distinct layers may be observed—clear urine at the top, thickened, cloudy urine containing mucus in the middle, and a yellow or greenish layer—pus—at the bottom.

Sugar in urine.—The consumption of a large amount of sweet or starchy food may explain the presence of sugar, but if it occurs continuously and in large quantities, it is a symptom of diabetes. In this disease the urine is exceptionally clear, has a slight greenish tint, and a peculiar sweetish odour, and enormous quantities may be passed (*see* DIABETES MELLITUS).

URINE, RETENTION OF.—Inability to pass urine, often when the bladder is so full as to cause pain, may be explained by blocking of the urethra, the narrow tube leading from the bladder to the surface, as a result of stricture, the pressure of a tumour, inflammation, enlargement of the prostate gland, etc.; or the trouble may be due to loss of power in the muscles of the bladder owing to actual paralysis or to atony—that is, want of "tone." Atony may result from a habit of disregarding the calls which nature gives for the bladder to be emptied, so that after a time the organ sulks, the calls cease to come, and the bladder becomes so distended that the muscular walls are temporarily paralysed. In some cases, however, retention may be due to nervous causes. A hot bath, or sitting over steam, or the local application of a hot sponge is sometimes sufficient to relieve the disability, at any rate for the time. Another simple remedy consists in taking a rapidly-acting purge, or the doctor may prescribe laudanum. If such measures as these fail, he will draw off the water by passing a catheter.

URINE, SUPPRESSION OF.—This condition is quite different from that just described. Here no urine is secreted, because the kidneys have ceased to act. Suppression of urine is usually a manifestation of acute Bright's disease, but it sometimes follows severe and prolonged operations, or the passing of a catheter. It may, however, be simply hysterical, passing off after a few hours or days, and then being succeeded by a very copious flow.

URINOMETER (*see* URINE, NORMAL AND ABNORMAL).

URTICARIA.—This, the technical name for nettle-rash, is derived from *urtica*, the Latin for "nettle." The disorder manifests itself in eruptions taking the form of wheals very much like those due to the sting of a nettle—slightly-raised patches, firm to the touch, at first red all over but afterwards, as a rule, becoming white in the centre with a bright-red border. As the wheal subsides the centre reddens and the border turns pale. The lesions vary in size from a three-penny piece, or smaller, to a florin, or even much larger.

Causes.—The affection is most common in infancy, owing to the irritability of the skin at that period. Females are more liable than males. Other predisposing causes are indigestion, gout, malaria, jaundice, and the neurotic temperament. The exciting causes may be external, such as the bites or stings of gnats, jelly-fish, wasps, etc., or contact with hairy caterpillars; or they may be internal, these in some cases consisting in the consumption of some article of diet, most often shell-fish, but sometimes a food so generally innocent as oatmeal, mushrooms, strawberries or parsley. In some cases urticaria is caused simply by indigestion quite apart from the consumption of unsuitable food. Often it is very difficult to trace the exciting cause.

Symptoms.—The onset is sudden. As the wheals appear the patient is conscious of an intense itching and burning, and there may be some constitutional disturbance, exhibited in a high temperature, headache, backache, furred tongue, nausea, vomiting and diarrhœa. Ordinarily the wheals last only a few hours at most, and then disappear. In some cases, however, fresh crops continue to appear, so that the attack may last for several days. There are several forms of urticaria. In one of them, *papular urticaria*, or *gum rash* (so called from a theory that it is due to teething), the wheals may be quite small, but may leave behind hard pimples; the eruption may affect all parts of the body, but especially the trunk; there is intense itching; and it may be years before the attacks entirely cease.

Treatment.—If the attack can be traced to unsuitable food, a purgative, such as Epsom salts, should be taken or, if the symptoms are very severe, an emetic. If feverish symptoms are present, the patient should live on milk and milk puddings for two or three days. In these feverish cases the patient should remain in bed, so as to avoid chill and friction of movement, being careful, however, not to get too warm, which would tend to aggravate the itching. This may be allayed by applying lead lotion with a piece of lint, or by dusting on starch powder. Underclothing should be of soft and unirritating material, such as silk or linen mesh. In chronic cases the bowels must be regulated, the food must be light and simple, and alcohol avoided. Sometimes benefit is derived from a holiday. If the attack is of a malarial or gouty or rheumatic character, the antecedent condition must, of course, be dealt with (*see* articles on those subjects).

UTERUS, DISPLACEMENTS OF (*see* WOMB, DISPLACEMENTS OF).

UTERUS, INFLAMMATION OF (*see* WOMB, INFLAMMATION OF).

V

VACCINATION.—The immediate effect of vaccination is to communicate the affection known as cowpox, or vaccinia. The evidence of the utility of vaccination, in diminishing the liability to smallpox and lessening its virulence if contracted, is such as to carry conviction to the great majority of those most competent to judge. Speaking generally, each extension of vaccination, whether in England or abroad, was followed by a reduction in smallpox mortality, and whereas a century ago smallpox was a pestilence of the first magnitude, it is now a comparatively rare disease. That sanitation, with the isolation of infected persons and the surveillance of contacts, has had something to do with the retrogression of smallpox must be conceded. But if the diminution in smallpox were mainly due to these factors, it would be irrespective of age, for all alike are benefited by them. The decline, however, is greater in infants and children, who have more recently been vaccinated, than in adults, though by reason of their age children are more susceptible to infectious disease. It follows, therefore, that the decline is related more to vaccination than to factors which affect children and adults in equal measure.

The Royal Commission on Vaccination (1896) reported strongly in favour of re-vaccination, being of opinion that the protection afforded by vaccination remains at its highest potency for nine or ten years, and then rapidly diminishes, though possibly it never altogether ceases; and that its power of modifying the disease, if contracted, also diminishes, though less rapidly than its protective influence.

The law of vaccination now in force ordains that a child must be vaccinated within six months of birth unless (a) the parent makes a statutory declaration to the vaccination officer that he conscientiously believes vaccination would be prejudicial to its health, or (b) the child is attacked by smallpox, or (c) three or more unsuccessful attempts at vaccination have been made, or (d) the child is in a state of health or is living under conditions that make the little operation undesirable. If no exemption order is obtained, the parent is liable to conviction, but not to re-conviction. If the child's health or environment makes vaccination undesirable a medical certificate of postponement, for not more than two months at a time, is given. A parent may require the public vaccinator to vaccinate the child at its home. Re-vaccination is not compulsory in this country, as it is in Germany; but facilities for gratuitous re-vaccination are provided by the health authorities.

Lymph is now, as a rule, obtained direct from the calf, and is glycerinated to free it from impurities. In an infant the best situation for vaccination is on the shoulder, and for choice the left side, as it is then not liable to pressure against the body of the nurse. If desired, vaccination may be performed on the leg, so that the scars may not show, but it is difficult to keep the leg of an infant always clean, dry, and at rest. Occasionally vaccination is done over birth-marks with the intention of destroying them by the inflammation and subsequent scarring. Apart from keeping the spots clean and protected, no treatment is usually necessary, but if the redness, swelling, and pain are troublesome, they may be relieved by the application of a compress of boric lint soaked in warm water, and covered with oil-silk. A useful lotion to paint over the spots and redness is made by mixing oxide of zinc powder and water to the consistency of cream; this is astringent and sedative. The general symptoms usually require no treatment, but the bowels must be kept regular. If the fever runs at all high, 1-drop doses of tincture of aconite or 10 drops of solution of acetate of ammonia in water are useful. Vaccination is occasionally followed by skin eruptions, but they seldom last more than a few days.

VACCINE AND SERUM TREATMENT.—The reader who is curious to understand the very interesting theory upon which these kinds of treatment are based should refer to the article on IMMUNITY, where he will find it simply expounded. There also he will find explained the essential difference between vaccines and serums. *Vaccines*, usually consisting of dead bacteria or their poisons, are injected into the loose tissue that lies beneath the skin. Preventively, they are beneficial in smallpox (vaccination), typhoid fever, hydrophobia, etc.; remedially, in acne, nasal catarrh, influenza, gonorrhœa, inflammation of the bowels, pyorrhœa alveolaris, boils and carbuncles, erysipelas, abscess, etc. Tuberculin is a vaccine, and is of undoubted benefit in certain cases of consumption, while in other cases it would be harmful. *Serums* are usually injected beneath the skin, like vaccines, but they may be injected into the muscles, while in tetanus and meningitis they are injected into the canal that contains the spinal cord. Preventively, they have been brilliantly successful in tetanus; remedially, in diphtheria. They have also given good results in the form of dysentery which is due to bacilli, and in some cases of cerebro-spinal meningitis ("spotted fever").

VACCINIA (*see* VACCINATION).

VAGINAL INJECTIONS (*see* INJECTIONS).

VALVULAR DISEASE (*see* HEART DISEASE).

VARICELLA (*see* CHICKEN-POX).

VARICOCELE.—In many youths and young men the veins which form part of the spermatic cord are varicose: this is varicocele. For reasons which are not clearly understood, it arises more often on the left side than on the right. In slight cases the patient may be unaware of anything abnormal ; in severe cases a sensation of weight and dragging is experienced, especially in standing or taking exercise, or in hot weather ; there may also be pain of a neuralgic character. A varicocele is easily recognized : the scrotum (the bag containing the testicles) is long and lax, the veins feel to the touch " like a bag of worms," and those on the surface of the scrotum may be enlarged. It tends to disappear spontaneously, and is very rarely met with in old men. In mild cases nothing more is necessary than cold baths and the wearing of a suspensory bandage or an indiarubber ring through which the lower part of the scrotum is drawn. In severer cases, or if the varicocele prevents the patient from being accepted for one of the public services, a slight operation is called for.

VARICOSE VEINS.—When any of the veins of the body become distended and tortuous the condition known technically as *varix* arises. If the veins of the spermatic cord are varicose, the affection is called *varicocele* (q.v.) ; if those of the rectum, *hæmorrhoids* or *piles* (*see* PILES). The veins of the leg are those which most often become varicose, and it is persons whose occupations involve a great deal of standing, or much muscular exertion without walking, who most often suffer from this affection. Men engage in such occupations more than women, and hence it is, no doubt, that varicose veins are met with more frequently in men. Other causes are the use of tight garters, habitual constipation, and congestion of the liver. For the most part varix is an affection of middle life, but it

sometimes occurs in young people, and this suggests that in certain cases there is an inherent weakness in the tissues of the veins which predisposes them to give way under strain.

Symptoms.—Veins may be varicose without causing trouble, but usually pain is felt in the leg, if it is the veins of the leg that are affected, or the patient complains of fatigue on slight exertion. The pain is of an aching character, and is often accompanied by a sense of weight and fullness, and sometimes by numbness and weakness. The feet are always cold, and after walking or a hard day's work the ankles are liable to swell. The dangers to be feared from varicose veins are (1) that, as the result of exertion or a slight accident, a vein may burst, and (2) that a clot of blood may become detached and be swept on by the blood-stream until it blocks a channel too small for it to pass through, thus cutting off the blood supply of the part where its progress is checked.

Treatment. — If the trouble is traced to some definite cause, such as constipation or the wearing of tight garters, this must, of course, be removed. The diet of full-blooded and over-fed persons must be reduced ; if, on the other hand, the patient is ill-nourished, the feeding must be improved and a quinine and iron tonic taken, the bowels being kept open by a mild aperient. Either a perforated rubber bandage (Martin's) should be applied to the leg, or an elastic stocking worn. If a bandage is preferred, it should be put on evenly, beginning at the foot and ankle, and the pressure exerted should be but slight. The bandage should be put on before getting out of bed, while the legs are horizontal. If ulcers are present, a wet " leno " bandage is suitable ; the discharge can be washed away through the meshes. Such measures are sufficient in many cases to produce some amelioration of symptoms and prevent the condition from becoming worse, but nothing short of an operation will rid the patient of the trouble. Operation should be submitted to if ulceration is intractable, or if bloodclots are present or recur time after time, or if pain is considerable, or if the varix debars the patient from entering the public service.

VARIOLA (*see* SMALLPOX).

VEINS (*see* BLOOD, CIRCULATION OF).

VELD SORE.—This is an infectious ulceration of the skin which is met with in South Africa ; it resembles the barkoo rot which occurs in Australia. First there is a hard itching pimple, which presently becomes soft and watery, and then pustular, finally bursting and leaving an ulcer which is covered by a yellow crust. There is very little pain, and the patient complains chiefly of itching. The legs and feet are the parts most often attacked, but sometimes the hands or arms. The crusts should be removed by fomentations, and the surface then rubbed with lint soaked in perchloride of mercury, 1 in 1,000. The perchloride may also be used as a dressing.

VENEREAL DISEASES.—The diseases forming the venereal group are three in number—syphilis, gonorrhœa, and soft sore ; they are considered in separate articles. Medical men have always known how frequent these diseases are, and how seriously the health of the community is affected by two of them, syphilis and gonorrhœa, but it used to be thought indelicate and even improper to make any reference to these subjects in writings intended for the general public, and the result was that of the general public few had any real knowledge of the facts. At last it was felt that this policy was a great mistake, and in 1913 a Royal Commission was appointed to investigate the whole subject, with special reference to its bearing on the public health. In 1916 the Royal Commission reported, advising that in connexion with general hospitals centres should be established for the gratuitous diagnosis and treatment of venereal diseases, and that only one-fourth of the expense should fall upon the rates, the other three-fourths being borne by the State. This recommendation was at once adopted, and now in most parts of the country free diagnosis and treatment centres are at work. The treatment of venereal diseases by quacks or other unqualified persons has also been made illegal, as well as the advertising of so-called venereal remedies. A further recommendation of the Royal Commission that the facts relating to venereal diseases should be brought to the knowledge of the nation by competent speakers and writers has been carried out by voluntary organizations.

VENEREAL WARTS (*see* WARTS).

VENOUS BLOOD (*see* BLOOD, CIRCULATION OF).

VENOUS HÆMORRHAGE (*see* HÆMORRHAGE).

VENTILATION.—The need for ventilation arises partly from the fact that the lungs and other parts of the body give off impurities in the form of carbonic acid gas and animal matter. The carbonic acid is taken up by the blood from the oxidized (burnt) tissues of the body, escapes from the blood into the lungs, and is discharged in the act of expiration.

It is not, however, the accumulation of carbonic acid that gives to the air of a stuffy room its disagreeable smell, but the minute particles of animal matter which come partly from the lungs and partly from the skin of the occupants. Further, close air is rendered more deleterious by the warmth from the breath and the body-heat, by the moisture contained in the breath, and by the presence of harmful bacteria. It must be added that the air of a room will become offensive from mere stagnancy, as anyone may discover by returning to an empty room after it has been shut up for a few hours. One who lives in an ill-ventilated room — and this applies especially to the bedroom—cannot maintain a high standard of health. A warm moist atmosphere tends to produce lassitude, drowsiness, and headache, and the conditions are favourable to the activities of noxious germs, such as those of nasal catarrh and consumption. Sir William Broadbent used to say that the death-rate from consumption would be halved if everyone could be induced to sleep with the windows open, and the success of the open-air treatment of

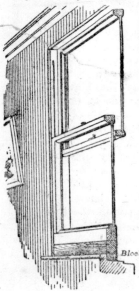

Fig. 63. — The Hinckes - Bird method of ventilation by inserting a block of wood beneath the lower sash, so that air is able to enter between the two sashes.

this disease suggests that there is little exaggeration in the dictum, for if open air can cure the disease it is probably efficacious in preventing it. How deplorably architects have ignored the laws of hygiene in designing buildings, especially buildings in which large numbers of people are to congregate, is matter of common knowledge. Things are not now so bad as they used to be, but too little attention is still paid to ventilation. In a well-ordered community architects who, in designing buildings, gave no proper attention to ventilation would be liable to prosecution.

The amount of space in a room should not be less than one thousand cubic feet for each adult. Even so, the air ought to be changed three times every hour, for one thousand cubic feet are used up in twenty minutes by each grown-up person. Take the case of a bedroom for one person. If it is to conform to the rule just stated, it ought to be ten feet in length, breadth and height, and it should have outlets for the used-up air and inlets for the fresh air. The chimney may be regarded as a "natural" outlet. When an ordinary fire is burning, the chimney extracts from ten to fifteen thousand cubic feet of air per hour, the current flowing at a rate of three to six feet per second. Even without a fire the chimney acts as an extractor; it should never, therefore, be blocked with a register, nor should the free passage of air be obstructed by screens of any kind. For windows, the rule should be to keep them open. This can almost always be done without discomfort by adopting the *Hinckes-Bird* device (Fig. 63). A bar of wood about four inches deep, and extending the whole width of the window, is placed on the sill beneath the lower sash so that this may be raised four inches, and thus a current of air passes between the two sashes. The air-current has, of course, an upward direction; it is carried to the ceiling and then rebounds to the lower part of the room, having been warmed by its passage through the topmost layer of air in the room. Another useful means of ventilation is afforded by *perforated bricks;* the holes are conical in shape, with the narrow ends outside, so that the current of incoming air slackens as it traverses the wall, and enters without causing draughts. *Shering-ham's valve* (Fig. 64) is a small upright flap in the wall near the ceiling, hinged below so as to fall forward towards the room; the current there-fore, as in the Hinckes-Bird flap, can only pass upwards. *Tobin's ventilator* (Fig. 65) is a large upright tube, rising at least 5 ft. from the floor, with an opening at the bottom to admit the air from the outside and another at the top to discharge the air upwards into the room. It is important, of course, to ensure that the air brought in is free from risk of contamination.

VERTIGO (*see* GIDDINESS).

VITAMINS (*see under* FOOD).

VITREOUS CHAMBER (*see* EYE).

VITRIOL, OIL OF (*see* SUL-PHURIC ACID POISONING).

VITILIGO (*see* LEUCODERMIA).

VOICE, LOSS OF.—Aphonia, or voicelessness, may be due to serious organic causes, such as tumour of the brain, or lesions of the nerves governing the muscles of the larynx (voice-box), or it may be due to over-use or misuse of the voice, but in many cases it is simply a functional affection due to hysteria. When, for instance, a soldier in battle loses his

voice as a result of the shock of gun-fire, the case is one of hysteria, but all that is meant by this term is that the condition is of nervous origin, and is not due to any traceable organic damage. In ordinary life aphonia occurs chiefly in young women, though it is sometimes met with in girls as young as 8 years; it also occurs occasionally in boys, and even in strong healthy men. It is pre-disposed to by anæmia, nervous ex-haustion (neurasthenia), indigestion, and intestinal worms, and the "last

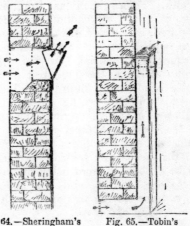

Fig. 64.—Sheringham's valve.   Fig. 65.—Tobin's ventilator.

straw" may be some mental or physical shock, or the strain of pregnancy. When the voice is lost after a fright, an outburst of anger, or the receipt of news which occasions intense joy or grief, the voice is lost suddenly, and the patient may not be able even to whisper. In such cases the power of speech is recovered suddenly, as has so often been re-ported in cases of aphonia due to shell-shock; but if the trouble comes on gradually, the recovery will pro-bably be gradual also.

In some cases the voice is lost, or becomes very hoarse, as a result of excessive use, in preachers and speakers, public singers, school teachers, etc., but generally there is faulty use as well as over-use, as when a singer does not " produce " his notes properly, or sings in a register beyond his capacity.

Treatment.—In the hysterical group of cases a great deal depends upon the personal influence of the medical man. It would serve no good purpose to describe the various methods of treatment in detail; but, whatever special method is adopted, it is important to attend to the general health. Tonics such as iron, nux vomica, and strychnine are often required, and active out-door occupation and plenty of amusement are frequently beneficial. In the other group of cases, thorough rest of the voice is obviously indicated. Treatment should follow the general lines indicated in the article SORE THROAT. A few days of silence will often be sufficient, but if nodules have formed on the larynx the patient may have to be prohibited from using his voice for some months, and the nodules may have to be removed with a special kind of forceps.

VOLVULUS (*see* BOWELS, OB-STRUCTION OF).

VOMITING.—Involuntary emptying of the stomach through the œsophagus (gullet) is usually due to some temporary derangement of the stomach, but it may mark the onset of measles, scarlet fever, or some other infectious fever; it may be a symptom of chronic inflammation of the kidney (Bright's disease), or it may denote some grave affection of the brain, such as cerebral tumour, cerebral abscess, or meningitis.

Treatment.—The chief indication, in cases of ordinary vomiting, is to humour the stomach by putting no food into it for a time. Very hot water may be taken in sips, or small pieces of ice may be sucked, and a mustard plaster applied to the pit of the stomach. When vomiting is the result of such serious diseases as those mentioned, treatment must be directed to the antecedent disease rather than to this symptom, but the doctor may find it necessary to prescribe morphia or some other potent drug. When sickness is due to mere indigestion, 3 to 6 minims of dilute hydrocyanic acid may be given in a dessertspoonful of water. Other remedies are chloretone, in a 5-grain cachet, repeated, if necessary, in two hours; carbonate of bismuth in a 10-grain powder; tincture of nux vomica in 2-drop doses, or spirit of chloroform in 3-drop doses, each with a teaspoonful of water. If the vomiting is due to some irritating or unwholesome food, it should not be checked, but rather encouraged by drinking freely of warm water, until the stomach has been cleared, when one of the remedies mentioned may be taken. The vomiting having ceased, and the stomach having had a complete rest for a few hours, milk and soda-water or milk and lime-water may be begun, first in teaspoonfuls, then in larger quantities, and the patient may return to ordinary diet by way of broths, and light milk foods such as Benger's, arrowroot, and milk-puddings.

A special form of vomiting, known as *morning sickness,* usually comes on as soon as the patient gets out of bed. It is usually due either to alcoholism or to pregnancy. If to the former, the remedy is, of course, to give up alcohol. The morning sickness which is so frequently an accompaniment of pregnancy demands more consideration. It comes in the second month of pregnancy, and usually ceases in six or eight weeks. In some cases, however, especially in first pregnancies, it may continue all day, be accompanied by pain in the pit of the stomach, cause loss of appetite and wasting, and be accompanied by violent retching. Sometimes the sickness can be averted by breakfasting in bed and lying on for half an hour or so, and then dressing in leisurely fashion ; or it may be sufficient to have a cup of strong tea or coffee before getting up to breakfast. In some cases an effervescing drink or milk and soda-water, milk and lime-water or thin barley-water is found to soothe the stomach. So long as any irritability remains, the diet must be limited to such simple and easily digested foods as are nourishing—for example, milk-puddings, broths, meat jellies and, later, fish, chicken and the lightest meats. The bowels must be kept in regular action, for constipation is likely to make the trouble worse. In troublesome cases relief may be found by applying to the pit of the stomach a compress made of half-a dozen folds of lint wrung out of warm water and covered with oil-silk, and wearing it at the time of day when vomiting is likely to occur.

The vomiting of sea-sickness is considered in a separate article (*see* SEA-SICKNESS).

Vomiting in children is most often due to dyspepsia and bad feeding. For infants about a year old the following mixture may in such cases be recommended :

Carbonate of bismuth .... 36 grains
Bicarbonate of soda .... 24 grains
Compound tragacanth powder 10 grains
Spirit of chloroform .... 16 minims
Caraway-water to 1½ ounces.
A teaspoonful every 3 or 4 hours. For a child 1 year old.

In older children vomiting may sometimes be checked by giving a mineral acid, such as dilute hydrochloric acid, after meals, from two to three drops, according to age, in two teaspoonfuls of sweetened water.

VULVAL WARTS.—Warts on the external female genital organs, described under WARTS.

VULVITIS.—Inflammation of the female organs external to the vagina frequently occurs in quite young girls who are debilitated and neglected. It may be set up by dirty diapers, by insufficient washing of the parts, or by threadworms which find their way from the anus to the front passage. In older girls and women, vulvitis is often associated with menstruation, or with confinement ; in other cases it is due to gonorrhœa or syphilis. If the skin is chiefly affected, the inflammation is probably eczematous, or a form of acne, or due to the irritation set up by the sugar in the urine of diabetics.

Treatment.—In young children the parts should be syringed with an antiseptic lotion such as a saturated solution of boric acid (15 grains to an ounce of water), and frequently washed with perchloride of mercury (1 in 2,000 of warm water). They should then be dusted with a powder containing half an ounce each of boric acid and oxide of zinc to an ounce of starch. Small pads of absorbent wool or antiseptic gauze may be inserted between the parts to keep them from contact with each other. The general health must receive attention. Plenty of food must be given, with cod-liver oil and steel wine. In adults also the boric-acid solution may be used, or the parts may be washed with carbolic or sulphur soap, and then bathed with a bicarbonate of potash and rose-water lotion (10 grains to the ounce).

W

WARTS (PAPILLOMATA).—The cause of the *common wart* is not known, but there is a good deal of evidence that blood from one wart may cause another, or others, to appear in the same patient, and this supports the theory that warts are due to the action of some germ as yet undiscovered. Another popular belief, that the wart may be made to disappear by the use of charms—as by rubbing it with a piece of meat and then burying the meat—is obviously a superstition without other foundation than the fact that warts often disappear spontaneously. As we have no knowledge of their cause, it is not surprising that we should be unable to account for their spontaneous disappearance. They occur most frequently on the hands and fingers, either singly or more than one at a time, but they may appear under the nails or on the scalp or, indeed, anywhere. Sometimes they seem to show an hereditary tendency; they are certainly met with most often in childhood. At first the colour is that of the skin, but in the course of time it turns brown, or in uncleanly persons black. If the wart has a distinct stalk, it may be snipped off with a pair of sharp clean scissors, after tying the base with a fine silk ligature. In other cases, after protecting the surrounding skin with oil or vaselin, glacial acetic acid or salicylic acid in collodium may be applied with a brush. If more drastic measures are necessary, the doctor may destroy the warts by carbon dioxide snow, which freezes them, or by cauterization.

Other kinds of warts are (1) the *flat wart*, (2) the *seborrhœic wart*, both of which are more common in old age than in the young, and may give rise to severe itching; and (3) *venereal warts*, which occur about the genitals and sometimes in the armpits and other moist, warm parts in both sexes. Venereal and seborrhœic warts may be treated in the same way as an ordinary wart. Flat warts may be left alone; occasionally they are the starting-point of malignant growths, and it is better not to irritate them.

In women, especially those who are not careful to keep the parts scrupulously clean, warts which are not venereal frequently occur on the external genital organs; they are not infective, and are due simply to irritating discharges. The little growths in their turn cause a discharge which has an offensive odour. If pregnancy comes on, they grow rapidly, but often disappear after labour. If they are small, nothing more is necessary than the free use of soap and water, followed by the application of oxide-of-zinc powder by means of a little bit of cotton-wool, alum water—a teaspoonful of alum to a pint of water—being injected into the vagina to stop the discharge. Larger growths may often be destroyed by painting them with glacial acetic acid, the surrounding parts being protected with a smearing of vaselin, but if very large it may be necessary for the doctor to snip them off with scissors. This little operation must not be attempted by the unskilled on account of the free bleeding which it may cause.

WASP-STINGS (*see* STINGS AND BITES).

WASTING IN CHILDREN.—In infants the commonest cause of *marasmus*, or wasting, is unsuitable food. The food may consist largely of starch, which at this age cannot be digested and may set up vomiting or diarrhœa; or the trouble may be due to premature weaning, underfeeding or over-feeding, or irregular feeding. Wasting may also be produced by digestive disturbance. In children from 1 to 3 years of age, either rickets or tuberculosis of the intestinal glands (tabes mesenterica) may be responsible for the wasting ; the latter condition indeed may cause extreme emaciation. At the age of five or six a chronic form of tuberculosis may produce the same result. Yet another cause of defective nutrition is the presence of worms in the intestine. The only way of checking the wasting is to discover the cause to which it is due and, if possible, remove it. This it may not be easy even for the doctor to do.

WATER FILTRATION (*see* FILTRATION OF WATER).

WATER-BED (*see* NURSING, DOMESTIC).

WATERBRASH.—Waterbrash denotes the rising into the mouth of a quantity of tasteless, watery fluid, following a painful cramp or spasm in the pit of the stomach. The fluid may be small in quantity, or may gush into the mouth in great abundance. The symptom most often occurs in those, especially women, who eat too much and consume food not easy of digestion, such as oatmeal and green vegetables. Such foods, if they have this effect, should be avoided, or reduced to a minimum, and the patient should eat in strict moderation and masticate thoroughly. Limewater is a favourite remedy, or the bismuth and citrate of ammonia prescription on p. 204 may be tried. This condition is sometimes called *pyrosis* (from a Greek word meaning to burn), a term more appropriately applied to those scalding eructations which are described under HEARTBURN.

"WATERY EYE" (*see* EPIPHORA).

WAX IN THE EAR (*see* EAR, WAX IN).

WEANING.—Many mothers who suckle their babies, as every healthy mother ought to do, are tempted to defer weaning too long. In some cases the motive is the mother's reluctance to deny her child what she gladly regards as his right. In other cases nursing is protracted in the mistaken belief that it prevents another pregnancy. As a rule, it should cease between the eighth and tenth months. If it is continued longer, the mother's health is likely to suffer, and the child as a natural consequence will suffer also. Even if the mother's health is not prejudiced, the milk becomes less nutritious with the lapse of time. After the eighth month the effects of nursing on both mother and child should be carefully watched, and as soon as any indication that the one or the other is not flourishing is observed, it should be discontinued. Weaning is, of course, a rather considerable change in the child's mode of life which may cause a little constitutional disturbance ; it should therefore be instituted, if possible, when he is at his best, and not suffering, say, from a cold or from teething trouble. The stage of dentition when the child has cut his eight front teeth is, in ordinary cases, a suitable one for making the change.

Some mothers prepare the way gradually for weaning by giving the child one meal a day from the bottle early in life. This is a very sensible plan, not only because it makes weaning a gradual instead of an abrupt process, but also because, if the mother has to be away from the child at feeding time, or if her flow of milk should become defective, the bottle can at once be brought into use. If necessity arises, there must be no hesitation in weaning the child abruptly. He may show some temper, but the fits of screaming will cease, and hunger will come in to reconcile him to the change of habit. Hints as to the food suitable for the newly-weaned child will be found under INFANTS AND YOUNG CHILDREN, FEEDING OF; directions for the relief of distension of the breasts, under SUCKLING.

WEBBED FINGERS AND TOES. —In these malformations of ante-natal life there is either a partial extension of the web at the point of junction of the digits with the hand or foot, or two or more of the digits may be completely joined together. Webbed toes need not be interfered with, but webbed fingers should be separated by operation.

WEIGHT OF BODY (*see* BODY-WEIGHT).

WEIR-MITCHELL TREATMENT (*see* " REST CURE ").

WET PACK.—A pack may be either cold or hot. The former is used in fevers in which the temperature runs very high (hyperpyrexia); the latter, in such conditions as dropsy and uræmia. To give a *cold pack*, remove the top bedclothes except the sheet, put a mackintosh and blanket under the patient and remove his body linen, wring two sheets out of cold water and place one under and the other over him, then fold the under-blanket over him, and put more blankets above it. The pack may last from twenty minutes to half an hour or, if given by a trained nurse, even longer, but the patient's temperature must be watched, and if it falls to 100° Fahr., the treatment must be discontinued. Stimulants may have to be given to favour reaction if the patient is exhausted, or to promote perspiration.

The method of giving a *hot pack* is as follows : Close the windows so that the patient may not be exposed to draughts, remove the top bedclothes except the blanket covering the patient, place a mackintosh over the bottom sheet, cover with a warm blanket, remove the patient's body linen and put it near the fire, wring a thin blanket or sheet out of water at a temperature of 105° Fahr., quickly roll the patient into it, cover him with a warm mackintosh, fold the under-mackintosh and blanket over him, put on another blanket and tuck it in. The quilt can be replaced. The patient may remain in a hot pack for about an hour, and longer if comfortable. In taking him out, remove the mackintoshes and damp blankets, and leave him rolled in a warm dry blanket for a short time. Then wash him quickly all over with hot water, replace the warmed body linen and make up the bed as usual. All this time the windows should have been kept closed. The wringing of the blanket or sheet out of hot water, as described above, can be done much better by two persons than by one. It is folded lengthwise, the ends are held, and the rest of it is dipped in the water, the ends being then turned in opposite directions until it is wrung out.

WHITE LEG.—What is technically known as *phlegmasia alba dolens* is a serious complication of labour, serious because, if the usual antiseptic precautions are neglected, suppuration may occur, and because, if the affected leg is not kept absolutely at rest until the swelling has disappeared, the clot of blood which is the cause of the trouble may be carried to some vital organ, with a fatal result ; serious also because it is necessary for the patient to keep her bed for many weeks, and even then the limb may remain wasted and feeble for months, and may be the seat of aching, especially after exercise or in damp cold weather. The affection is predisposed to by the tendency of the blood to coagulate after labour and by stagnation of the circulation in the veins as the result of lying in bed. The exciting cause is probably of an infective character. Thus it comes about that a blood clot forms in the large vein of the leg, nearly always the left leg, and usually during the second or third week of the lying-in. The vein becomes inflamed, and in typical cases the lymphatics (the channels for lymph) are blocked so that the leg swells, and becomes hard and brawny and white. The inflammation usually starts in the womb and spreads along the veins to the leg. The onset may be gradual, with a feeling of chilliness and a rise of temperature, or sudden, with a violent shivering fit. Pain is felt in the groin, which is very tender to pressure, the inflamed vein can often be felt, towards the inner side of the thigh, standing out like a cord, and the patient feels thoroughly ill.

Treatment.—The doctor should at once be summoned. A flannel wrung out of poppy fomentations may be rolled round the leg, which should be supported on pillows some 15 inches above the level of the bed, and protected by a cradle. Here it must remain until the swelling has subsided, but even then the doctor will only permit gentle movement. So long as the fever persists, the diet must be limited to slops, and gentle aperients should be given to regulate the bowels. In ordinary cases, under this treatment, the symptoms will begin to abate in a week or ten days. When the pain and swelling have disappeared, a bandage may be applied and

massage instituted. Convalescence may be aided by giving as much light but nutritious food as the patient can take, and a quinine and iron tonic.

WHITLOW (*see* NAILS, DISEASES OF).

WHOOPING-COUGH.— Epidemics of *pertussis*, or whooping-cough, may occur in any climate, but they appear to be less frequent in hot countries. No age is completely exempt, but the vast majority of cases occur in children. Only about five out of every hundred cases end fatally—almost always from some complication of the disease, such as bronchitis, broncho-pneumonia, or convulsions, rather than from the disease itself. But whooping-cough has so high a prevalence that although the percentage of fatal cases is small, the total number of deaths is considerable. Whooping - cough and measles, in fact, are bracketed together as being responsible for more deaths of children than all the other infectious diseases combined. Whooping-cough is probably due to the *Bacillus pertussis*. The disease is highly infectious, and is usually conveyed by actual contact, and sometimes, it may be, by contaminated clothes, toys, books, etc. So far as is known, it is not transmitted by water, milk or other food, nor does bad hygiene, such as overcrowding and exposure to weather, appear to play any part in its propagation, although such conditions increase the danger to life when the disease has been contracted. It is infectious in the early stage, when it cannot be distinguished from a mere cold in the chest ; hence the rapidity with which it spreads. It is not one of the diseases that have been made universally notifiable. One attack almost always confers lifelong immunity. The average incubation period is believed to be about a fortnight, but sometimes is not more than three or four days. Children who have been exposed to infection should be kept in quarantine for three weeks.

Symptoms.—The onset takes the form of a feverish cold in the head and chest with a bad cough, which is worse at night, but is not attended with much expectoration. Dryness and tickling of the throat are felt. This is the first or *catarrhal* stage, which at the end of a week or ten days is succeeded by the second or *paroxysmal* stage, so called because of the paroxysms that characterize the cough. Each paroxysm consists of a number of short coughs, rapidly repeated and ending in the " whoop," a long-drawn, high-pitched, full note which can be heard at a great distance. The paroxysms may occur from a dozen to fifty or sixty times in the twenty-four hours, and the child soon learns to know what is coming and to dread it. He tries to avoid coughing, the face meanwhile assuming an expression of painful apprehension. At last he can restrain himself no longer, and the cough begins, and continues until he may become blue or black in the face, with swollen veins, protruding eyes, dribbling mouth and sweating skin. The paroxysm may be repeated several times in quick succession, and is followed by the bringing-up of thick, stringy phlegm, and with this, probably, the contents of the stomach. The coughing may be brought on by a fit of crying, by the act of swallowing, by lying down in bed or by breathing a dusty atmosphere. Having lasted about a month, the second stage passes into the third, the stage of *decline*, in which the paroxysms become fewer and less severe, and finally cease, although the cough remains for

some time longer and may again become paroxysmal. *Complications* are most prone to occur in delicate and rickety children. They include broncho-pneumonia, convulsions, rupture, bleeding from the nose and throat and elsewhere, diarrhœa, and spasm of the glottis. In this way convalescence may be prolonged for many weeks. The average duration of an attack of whooping-cough, however, may be given as six or seven weeks ; the child probably ceases to be infectious when the coughing and whooping have been absent for a week.

Treatment.—Until the temperature becomes normal the patient must remain in bed and be fed on milk and broth. He should not leave the sick-room until the coughing has ceased to be violent. The room temperature should be kept at 65° Fahr., and sufficient ventilation should be provided, for it is important that the air should be fresh as well as warm. The child must be dressed warmly, and it is a wise precaution against lung complications to cover the chest with a little jacket of gamgee tissue. Washing should not be neglected, but the greatest care must be taken against chill. Until the feverish symptoms have disappeared the diet must be entirely fluid : afterwards it may be of a more nutritious kind, so long as it is quite digestible. Sweets and fruits are better avoided, and starchy foods should be given in moderation. After vomiting the stomach will most easily retain warm milk and water, or Benger's Food. The doctor may order the throat to be sprayed for one minute every three hours with a 2-per-cent. solution of resorcin. Small ulcers on the tongue may be painted two or three times a day with glycerin and carbolic acid. If there is much phlegm, the front and back of the chest may be rubbed until red with compound camphor liniment. The nose should be kept clean, a little boric acid ointment, to which 20 grains of menthol may be added, being introduced into the nostrils twice or thrice daily. If an expectorant is needed, ipecacuanha wine, in 4-minim doses, may be given every four hours. A good sedative to mitigate the paroxysms is powdered belladonna root 1½ grains, sulphate of quinine 8 grains, and white sugar ½ drachm, divided into ten powders, one to be given three times a day. Others are antipyrin, in doses of 1 grain for each year of age in children, and bromide of soda, 5 grains three times a day.

Vaccine treatment has given results which, though not conclusive, suggest that it deserves further trial. It is employed both for prevention and for cure.

Not only must the patient, as soon as the nature of the illness is discovered, be strictly isolated, but every precaution should be taken against spread of the infection. The expectoration and the vomit should be caught in a vessel containing disinfectant, poured into boiling water and buried, or received on sawdust and burnt, and soft paper handkerchiefs that can be burnt should be used for cleansing the nose and mouth. When the patient leaves the sick-room, it and its contents must be thoroughly disinfected (*see* DISINFECTANTS AND DISINFECTION).

WIDAL REACTION (*see* TYHPOID FEVER).

WIND (*see* FLATULENCE).

WOMB, DISPLACEMENTS OF.— The abnormal positions of the uterus which cause trouble are the displacement downwards (prolapse or "falling " of the womb) and the displacement backwards (retroversion, retroflexion).

Prolapse in its milder forms is a not uncommon displacement. In its rarer and severer forms the neck of the womb, or even the whole organ may protrude. It is due to causes which weaken the supports of the womb—the ligaments that support it from above, the muscular wall of the vagina below, and the underlying muscles. Prolapse may occur suddenly, as the result of lifting a heavy weight, violent coughing or vomiting, or the convulsions in an epileptic fit. But more often it comes on as a gradual result of slight downward pressure, acting frequently or continuously. Pregnancy, especially if often repeated, is one of the commonest antecedents of prolapse ; the condition may also be set up by congestion and inflammation of the womb. The most characteristic symptom is a sense of dragging pain felt in the lower part of the abdomen, the back and the thighs, especially the left thigh, and aggravated by standing, by the monthly periods, and by the action of the bowels. Water is passed with difficulty, and the patient can only walk with great discomfort. As soon as she lies down, all the symptoms subside. Treatment in ordinary cases consists in rest in bed, returning the womb to its proper position, and keeping it there by a pessary, which has to be worn continuously, night as well as day. A good astringent injection for tightening up the parts should be used night and morning as hot as it can be borne. Decoction of oak bark, undiluted, may be recommended, or alum, a dessertspoonful to a pint of water. General tonics also are useful to tone up the muscular system. The bowels should be kept regular, and if necessary an aperient should occasionally be taken.

In most cases treatment on these lines will suffice, but in some an operation is necessary.

Backward displacement is called **retroversion** if the womb is simply displaced, and **retroflexion** if bent as well as displaced. The causes are much the same as those which account for prolapse. Many of the cases are a sequel of carelessness during confinements and miscarriages, and of too short a period of rest afterwards. As in prolapse, the womb must be returned to its proper position, and kept there by a pessary. The patient must rest in the recumbent position, but not necessarily in bed, until she is free from pain. Exercise must be gentle, and moderate in amount. Downward pressure of clothes on the abdomen and compression by tight stays and belts must be avoided, but a well-fitting abdominal belt which supports the weight of the intestines may be worn. As in prolapse, it is sometimes necessary to resort to operation.

WOMB, INFLAMMATION OF.

—*Acute* inflammation of the uterus (*metritis*) may be due to a great variety of causes. Many attacks originate in injuries to the womb sustained during confinement, especially if antiseptics are not efficiently applied afterwards. Other cases are traceable to some cause acting upon the womb at the time of menstruation, such as exposure to cold, getting the feet wet, over-exercise from long walks or dancing, or the use of cold or strong astringent injections. Blows, falls and other injuries to the abdomen are yet other causes. The condition may also be due to the wearing of pessaries which are too large or do not fit properly. Another group of cases is due to gonorrhœa.

Symptoms.—The attack is ushered in by a shivering fit, with high fever, nausea, and sickness. Severe pain is felt in the back, the lower part of the abdomen, and the thighs, with a sensation of burning heat internally. The abdomen is distended by gas in the intestines. There is frequent and painful micturition, and the patient's sufferings are aggravated by every movement. The womb becomes large and heavy, is exceedingly tender, and the patient has a sensation of " bearing down." If the attack is associated with menstruation, there is disturbance of this function : the loss may be very profuse, or may be altogether suppressed.

Treatment.—The patient should at once take to her bed and send for the doctor. Fomentations should be applied to the lower part of the abdomen, and warm injections of poppy decoction or of boric acid and water, a tablespoonful to a pint, given. The bowels should be cleared with an enema of warm water and soap, or by giving a mild aperient—castor oil or Apenta water. To subdue the abdominal pain, suppositories of belladonna may be introduced into the bowel, or, if the pain is acute, the doctor may give morphia. When the pain is subdued, warm hip-baths are beneficial, and counter-irritation may be employed by painting tincture of iodine on alternate days over the lower abdomen. The patient should make a point of remaining in bed until all pain and discomfort has disappeared, otherwise, the cure may be imperfect and the inflammation become chronic.

Chronic inflammation of the womb is usually a sequel of an acute attack. In some cases it follows confinement or miscarriage in which the uterus does not return to its normal size and state, either from local injuries and infection with germs, from insufficient rest, or from retention in the womb of some of the products of conception. In other cases it may be due to cold or to excessive exercise during menstruation, or to displacements of the womb. The monthly losses may be increased in the early stages, but after a time may almost cease. A discharge known as " the whites " occurs in many cases, or it may consist of a thick yellowish " mattery " fluid, or, on the other hand, may be pale, watery, and irritating. Usually, for a week before each menstrual period the abdominal pains and other symptoms increase, while during the week following it they diminish or may disappear, only, however, to return. There is great danger of the patient sinking into a state of invalidism. In bad cases she may become sterile, or if pregnancy occurs she may miscarry.

Treatment.—The pain in the back and lower part of the abdomen may be relieved by wearing a pessary. A great deal of rest is necessary, though it is not necessary for the patient to lie up entirely. Change of air to a dry, bracing climate is often helpful.

In *local treatment*, heat will be found of great value in the form of hot salt or bran bags or compresses, applied to the abdomen, or of hot douches, of a temperature of 105° to 115° Fahr., to the womb. The douches may be medicated with tincture of iodine or boric acid, a teaspoonful to a pint of water. Condy's fluid in the same strength will neutralize any unpleasant odour from the discharge. Hot baths of a temperature of 90° to 103° Fahr. are beneficial, especially when followed by cool sponging. Congestion of the uterus may be relieved by tampons : a pledget of cotton-wool about 1½ inches long and 1 inch thick is tied in the middle with a piece of string, one end of which is left 3 or 4 inches long with a loop at its end. Having been soaked in glycerin, it should be passed well into the vagina as far as the finger will reach. One should be used at night and another in the morning, and the patient should lie down for half-an-hour after placing it in position ; or one may be inserted on going to bed and retained all night, being withdrawn in the morning by pulling on the free end of the string, either while lying down or when in a stooping position. Tincture of iodine may with advantage be added to the glycerin. A hot douche should be used when the tampon is withdrawn. For *internal administration*, extract of ergot, 30 minims in a tablespoonful of water, may be taken thrice a day.

A less common form of inflammation of the womb is that in which, instead of the muscular walls of the womb, the mucous membrane which lines its interior is inflamed (**endometritis**). It is due to much the same causes as those already enumerated, but it may be caused also by some congenital deformity of the womb, especially an unusually narrow opening to its neck. The symptoms may appear in childhood, but seldom attract attention until menstruation begins, when irritation and pain are felt. As a rule, pain is not severe, but a sensation of internal heat and bearing down, perhaps with backache, may be experienced. During the first few hours of each period there may be pain, which gradually passes off. As a rule, there is a discharge, which may be white or yellow, or sticky and mixed with pus, or watery and stained with blood ; there may also be bleeding between the monthly periods, or the loss may be excessive.

Treatment.—The patient should take to her bed and remain there until the symptoms have subsided. Night and morning warm sedative and antiseptic douches, such as the boric-acid douche mentioned above, should be given. When the pain subsides, the douche may consist of an astringent, such as chloride of zinc, 5 grains to a pint of water, or alum, a dessertspoonful to a pint. Attention to the general health should follow the lines already described. In most cases such treatment as this will be effectual, but in some cases surgical measures will be necessary.

WOOLSORTER'S DISEASE (*see* ANTHRAX).

WORMS.—The worm which most often infests the human intestine is the *threadworm* (*Oxyuris vermicularis*), which lives chiefly in the large bowel. Threadworms resemble little bits of thread or cotton. In a freshly-passed evacuation they can be seen in active movement, but they soon die, and are then less easily recognized. The eggs of threadworms enter the body on unwashed fruit, raw vegetables, and other foods that have been handled by infected persons, and are hatched in the stomach. In infected children who are uncleanly they are carried on the fingers to the mouth, and so a fresh brood is introduced.

Symptoms.—Heat and irritation are felt about the orifice of the bowel, followed by itching in that region, restlessness and irritability, and later by spasm, St. Vitus's dance, and even convulsions. The child—for it is chiefly children who are affected—complains of stomach-ache, the bowels act irregularly, mucus and blood may appear in the stools, and the appetite becomes capricious or excessive. Other symptoms are cough, hiccough, grinding of the teeth in sleep, and night terrors. In girls the worms may find their way from the anus to the front passage, where they may cause great irritation.

Treatment.—One of the best drugs is santonin in tablet or lozenge, or mixed with castor oil. A 1-grain lozenge may be taken every night for two or three nights, followed by a dose of salts in the morning. A pint or more of warm water, with a tablespoonful of salt to the pint, may also be injected into the bowel every other night for a week. As a tonic, a steel mixture may be given—one-third dose in the case of children:

Tincture of perchloride of iron 80 minims
Spirit of chloroform ...... 2 drachms
Glycerin .... 1½ drachms
Water to 8 ounces.
For an adult two tablespoonfuls three times a day after meals.

Scrupulous cleanliness, with the regular washing of the skin round the anus, must be observed; the finger-nails should be kept short and clean, and drawers should be worn in bed to prevent scratching.

The *roundworm* (*Ascaris lumbricoides*) has a general resemblance to the earthworm; it is from 4 to 14 inches long, or somewhat longer. It dwells for the most part in the small intestine, but may wander to other parts. Treatment is similar to that for threadworms. A child should take a 2-grain lozenge or tablet of santonin twice a day for two days, followed by a dessertspoonful of castor oil. The dose for an adult is 5 grains taken early in the morning for three successive days, with a dose of castor oil to follow.

Tapeworms (*Tæniæ*) are acquired by eating imperfectly cooked beef or pork containing tiny, bladder-shaped bodies which, when they reach the human intestine, develop into flat worms many feet long. Besides causing stomach-ache and diarrhœa, or constipation, they may set up nervous symptoms similar to those mentioned in connexion with threadworms, and the patient may waste and become debilitated. Segments of the worms may be seen in the motions. The favourite remedy is male fern, which should be taken at night in the form of capsules of the liquid extract, one to four according to age, and a tablespoonful of castor oil in the morning. If necessary, the dose of castor oil may precede as well as follow the male fern. The latter kills the worms, and the castor oil expels them from the body. Another favourite remedy is the bark of pomegranate root ; a cachet containing 8 grains of pelletierine, the active principle of the bark, should be taken on rising, and a couple of hours later two tablespoonfuls of castor oil.

WOUNDS.—The simplest form of injury is an *abrasion*, in which only the skin or the mucous membrane is damaged. Injuries affecting deeper tissues may be *contused* wounds, inflicted with a blunt instrument which damages the underlying parts more than the surface ; *incised* wounds, caused by a sharp instrument ; *punctured* wounds, as from a needle, a dagger, a bayonet, etc., or *lacerated* wounds such as those caused by machinery, the edges being irregular and ragged. To these may be added *gunshot* wounds, which, whether inflicted with shot or with bullets, are punctures associated with more or less bruising and laceration.

Treatment of wounds.—The bleeding having been stopped (*see* HÆMORRHAGE) the wound must be carefully cleansed, if possible with an antiseptic, such as boric acid, a dessertspoonful to a pint of water, permanganate of potash, enough to give water a purple colour, Condy's Fluid, or Sanitas (*see* ANTISEPTICS).

If no antiseptic is available, the wound may be washed with clean water and then covered with boric lint or cyanide gauze, either dry or wetted, this in turn being covered with cotton-wool (*see* DRESSINGS AND STRAPPING FOR WOUNDS). *Contused* wounds should be firmly bandaged to check the oozing of blood. The edges of *incised* wounds should be drawn together with narrow strips of plaster, with intervals between the strips, while the lower end of the wound should be left unclosed for the escape of discharge. If the wound is large, it must be stitched up by a doctor after this first-aid treatment. *Punctured* wounds should not be closed up with strapping, and it must be left to the doctor to do whatever is necessary in the way of removing shots, or fragments of clothing, etc., which may have been carried into the wound. *Lacerated* wounds should be dressed with lint and a thick layer of cotton-wool and bandaged firmly, like contused wounds, to prevent oozing of blood.

Any wound in which a breach, slight though it be, is made in the skin or mucous membrane is liable to be poisoned by the introduction of harmful germs ; it then becomes a *septic* wound. Its edges are red and swollen, there is a constant discharge of pus and the patient's temperature is raised. Such wounds require skilled treatment, but it may be said generally that each time the dressing is changed the pus should be carefully removed with swabs wrung out of some antiseptic fluid such as peroxide of hydrogen. Cyanide gauze, wrung out of carbolic lotion (1 in 40) is often used to dress septic wounds (*see* ANTISEPTICS ; DRESSINGS AND STRAPPING FOR WOUNDS).

If a wound is soiled with mud or road-dust, or with fertilized earth, especially if it is a lacerated wound, there is the possibility of lock-jaw to be remembered, and in addition to the cleansing described above, tetanus antitoxin should be injected.

Healing of wounds.—When an injury is inflicted Nature does the best that circumstances permit to repair the injury. The quickest process of repair is that known as *healing by immediate union*, which sometimes occurs when a wound is treated without delay, and is not unknown even in the case of large operation wounds. No inflammation is set up, and the divided parts grow together without the formation of new material. A more frequent method of repair is *healing by first intention*. Here, with some amount of inflammation, there is a slight discharge of sticky fluid which unites the separated surfaces. In *healing by second intention*, the fluid which is exuded by the wound forms a layer of small red masses—granulations, which are gradually changed into fibrous tissue, and as this is done the wound closes up. As a rule, this is the way in which contused and lacerated wounds, and also ulcers, heal.

WRITER'S CRAMP.—This is but one of a large group of what are called occupation neuroses, which include "cramps" that attack the hands of telegraphists, violinists, typists, pianists, cigarette-makers, painters, plasterers, and those who sew and knit. If the leg is used in the occupation, as by sewing-machinists and lathe-workers, that limb may be similarly affected. In most cases the seat of the trouble appears to be the brain rather than the nerves or muscles of the limb. The chief sufferers from writer's cramp are clerks who have to be continually copying long documents in a stiff, copybook hand.

Treatment.—Cramp seldom comes under treatment at an early stage, and unless it does there is little hope of complete recovery. The right hand may still be used for other purposes, but the patient should learn to write with his left hand. Every effort should be made to improve the general health by rest and a nutritious diet into which milk freely enters. If pain or spasm continues, one of the bromides, or phenacetin, or antipyrin may be taken. Massage, galvanism, and appropriate exercises are worth a trial. When the right hand has been rested for, say, six months, and writing can be resumed, it will be well to use a thick cork penholder, and to hold it between the first and second fingers, a freer style of writing should be employed, and the movement should come more from the shoulder and less from the fingers.

WRY-NECK.—Torticollis, as this affection is also called, may be *congenital*, the result of faulty development of the muscles of the neck, or of injury received during birth. More often, however, it is an *acquired* affection. Of this there are two main forms—the paralytic and the spasmodic.

Paralytic wry-neck, known also as stiff-neck, is due to exposure to cold, and mostly affects the young. Although unpleasant, and sometimes distinctly painful, it is usually only a passing trouble. The head is drawn downwards and backwards on one side, the chin pointing towards the shoulder on the other side. If treatment is begun early, the spasm soon disappears. The bowels should be freely opened, as with a blue pill at night and a black draught next morning, and the salicylate-of-soda mixture (*see* p. 312) then started, the patient remaining indoors while the medicine is being taken so as to avoid the risk of chill. Hot fomentations may be applied to the neck, liniment of equal parts of extract of belladonna and glycerin being first smeared over the part to lessen the pain. When the pain has gone the stiffness may be reduced by rubbing in a liniment of belladonna and chloroform (equal parts). Galvanism may be of service.

Spasmodic wry-neck, a distinctly nervous affection, is much more serious. It usually occurs at about middle life, frequently in persons who are apparently quite healthy. The muscles of the neck are constantly contracting and relaxing, the contractions drawing the head to the affected side. In some cases, besides this rotatory movement, the head is drawn backwards and the shoulder dragged up. At first the disease may give little trouble, but afterwards, unless it is checked at an early stage, the spasms may be violent and painful. During sleep, as is the case with some other morbid movements, they cease, and they may be less severe when the patient's mind is preoccupied, while they are often worse when the presence of strangers makes him especially anxious that they should not occur. For treatment, operation upon the nerves or muscles is sometimes necessary. Short of this, electricity and massage are often useful. Nerve sedatives, such as bromide of potash, combined with tonics, may do good.

X

X-RAYS (*see* ELECTRICAL TREATMENT; DIAGNOSIS).

Y

YAWS.—This contagious disease, sometimes called *frambœsia,* has a wide distribution in warm climates. It is caused by inoculation with a microbe of the spirochæte group, the group to which the germ of syphilis belongs. The germ enters through a breach of the skin, chiefly by direct contact, as in kissing and sexual intercourse, but also indirectly as when it is conveyed by flies or by insect bites to an ordinary ulcer. The course and some of the symptoms are not unlike those of syphilis, and salvarsan and its substitutes are as efficacious in the one disease as in the other.

YEAST POULTICES (*see* POULTICES).

YELLOW FEVER.—Of the great infectious fevers, yellow fever, so called from the jaundiced colour of the patient's skin, etc., has the most restricted geographical range. Cases have occasionally occurred in seaport towns in this country and in some Continental ports, but yellow fever has never succeeded in finding a foothold in Europe. Nor is it met with in Asia. The germ is believed to be the *Leptospira icteroides;* it is communicated by the bite of the common mosquito of the West Indies which has been infected by sucking the blood of a patient suffering from the disease. As in other fevers, more depends upon careful nursing and diet than upon drugs.

Z

ZINC POISONING.—Zinc, in the forms (1) of white vitriol and zinc chloride, and (2) zinc chloride with a little iron chloride (Burnett's disinfecting fluid), is used as a disinfectant. If it is drunk in mistake, or suicidally the symptoms are those of an irritant poison. The lips and throat are burned, so that swallowing is difficult, burning pain is felt in the stomach, blood-stained fluid is vomited. An emetic must not be given. Get the patient to drink freely of milk and white of egg, washing soda or carbonate of potash dissolved in water, and strong tea or tannic acid. To relieve the pain, apply hot linseed poultices to the abdomen. The doctor when he arrives may give laudanum.

Made and Printed in Great Britain by
The Greycaine Book Manufacturing Company Limited, Watford

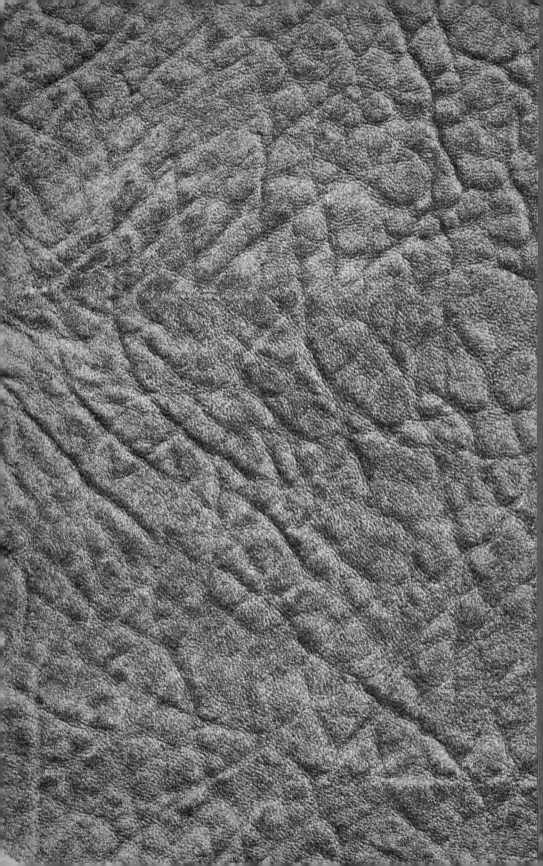